THE PHYSIOLOGY
OF PERIPHERAL
NERVE DISEASE

AUSTIN J. SUMNER, M.Med.Sc., M.B., F.R.A.C.P.

Department of Neurology
University of Pennsylvania
Philadelphia, Pennsylvania

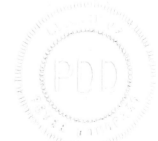

1980

W.B. SAUNDERS COMPANY
Philadelphia London Toronto

W. B. Saunders Company: West Washington Square
                            Philadelphia, PA   19105

                            1 St. Anne's Road
                            Eastbourne, East Sussex BN21, 3UN, England

                            1 Goldthorne Avenue
                            Toronto, Ontario M8Z 5T9, Canada

Library of Congress Cataloging in Publication Data

Main entry under title:

The physiology of peripheral nerve disease.

1. Nerves, Peripheral—Diseases.   2. Neurophysiology.
   I. Sumner, Austin J. [DNLM: 1. Peripheral nerve diseases—
   Physiopathology. WL500 P578]

RC409.P49   616.8'7   79–67796

ISBN 0–7216–8639–7

The Physiology of
Peripheral Nerve Disease   ISBN   0-7216-8639-7

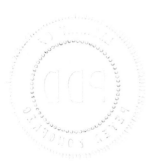
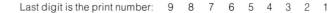

Last digit is the print number: 9   8   7   6   5   4   3   2   1

Contributors

Arthur K. Asbury, M.D.
Professor and Chairman, Department of Neurology, University of Pennsylvania School of Medicine, Philadelphia
THE CLINICAL VIEW OF NEUROMUSCULAR ELECTROPHYSIOLOGY

Robert L. Barchi, M.D., Ph.D.
Associate Professor of Neurology and of Biochemistry and Biophysics, University of Pennsylvania School of Medicine, Philadelphia; Attending Neurologist, University of Pennsylvania and Graduate Hospitals; Consulting Neurologist, Philadelphia Veterans Administration Hospital, Pennsylvania
EXCITATION AND CONDUCTION IN NERVE

R. E. Burke, M.D.
Chief, Laboratory of Neural Control, National Institute of Neurological and Communicative Disorders and Stroke, National Institutes of Health, Bethesda, Maryland
MOTOR UNITS IN MAMMALIAN MUSCLE

Roger W. Gilliatt, D.M., F.R.C.P.
Professor of Clinical Neurology, Institute of Neurology, University of London; Consultant Neurologist, The National Hospital for Nervous Diseases, London; Consultant Neurologist, The Middlesex Hospital, London, England
ACUTE COMPRESSION BLOCK; CHRONIC NERVE COMPRESSION AND ENTRAPMENT

A. J. Harris, Ph.D.
Department of Physiology, University of Otago Medical School, Dunedin, New Zealand
TROPHIC EFFECTS OF NERVE ON MUSCLE

William R. Kennedy, M.D.
Professor of Neurology, University of Minnesota; University of Minnesota Hospitals, Minneapolis
MAMMALIAN MUSCLE SPINDLES

W. I. McDonald, Ph.D., F.R.C.P., F.R.A.C.P.
Professor of Clinical Neurology, Institute of Neurology, London; Honorary Consultant Physician, National Hospitals; Honorary Consultant Neurologist, Moorfield's Eye Hospital, London, England
PHYSIOLOGICAL CONSEQUENCES OF DEMYELINATION

A. K. McIntyre, M.B., B.S., D.Sc., M.D.
Professor of Physiology, Medical School, Monash University, Clayton; Honorary Consultant Physiologist, Alfred and Prince Henry's Hospitals, Melbourne, Victoria, Australia
CUTANEOUS RECEPTORS

iii

CONTRIBUTORS

J. G. McLeod, M.D., D.Phil. (Oxon.)

Professor, Department of Medicine, University of Sydney, Australia

AUTONOMIC NERVOUS SYSTEM

Jackson B. Pickett, M.D.

Assistant Professor of Neurology, University of California, San Francisco; Attending Neurologist, University of California, San Francisco, San Francisco General Hospital, and San Francisco Veterans Administration Hospital, California

NEUROMUSCULAR TRANSMISSION

David Pleasure, M.D.

Professor of Neurology, Pediatrics, and Orthopaedic Surgery, University of Pennsylvania; Attending Neurologist, Hospital of the University of Pennsylvania and Children's Hospital of Philadelphia

AXOPLASMIC TRANSPORT

Richard E. Poppele, Ph.D.

Professor of Physiology, University of Minnesota, Minneapolis

MAMMALIAN MUSCLE SPINDLES

D. C. Quick, Ph.D.

Assistant Professor, Departments of Neurology and Anatomy, University of Minnesota, Minneapolis

MAMMALIAN MUSCLE SPINDLES

Michael E. Selzer, M.D., Ph.D.

Associate Professor of Neurology, University of Pennsylvania School of Medicine; Attending Neurologist, University of Pennsylvania and Graduate Hospitals, Philadelphia

REGENERATION OF PERIPHERAL NERVE

Preface

This volume was written for clinical electromyographers, but it is hoped that it will also prove useful to a more general audience interested in the peripheral nervous system. It contains a comprehensive review of experimental studies that provide a scientific basis for the use and interpretation of electrodiagnostic testing of patients with neuromuscular diseases.

Clinical electrodiagnosis is a relatively recent and expanding subspecialty. As an extension of the neurological examination, it draws upon the skills of clinical neurology. But it is even more dependent on the application of basic neurophysiological techniques and observations, especially those made in studies of experimental animal models of human diseases.

In preparing this book, I have been fortunate to have been able to call upon a group of distinguished contributors, some of whom are former teachers, and all of whom are colleagues and friends. Four contributors have played especially important roles in my professional life—A. K. McIntyre, W. I. McDonald, R. W. Gilliatt, and A. K. Asbury—and I acknowledge my deep indebtedness to them.

During the preparation and editing of this volume, I have had tireless help from Mrs. Karen Tyagi, Mrs. Kamlesh Rai, Ms. Leslie Hansen, and Ms. Grace Karreman. The editorial and publishing staff of the W. B. Saunders Company has provided much support and encouragement.

AUSTIN SUMNER

Contents

vii

CONTENTS

1

Excitation and Conduction in Nerve

Robert L. Barchi

The fundamental property of nerve which distinguishes it from other cells in the body is its ability to produce and conduct the regenerative electrical signals known as action potentials. The generation of an action potential takes place at the neuronal surface membrane as a predictable response to any of a number of external stimuli. Once initiated, the signal may be conducted over relatively long distances at high velocity without distortion or decrement, a feat which would be envied in any modern telecommunication system. Before we can reasonably expect to understand the factors which cause this transmission system to break down when diseased, it is necessary to understand the normal functioning of this complex yet hardy machine.

We should start by outlining some of the unusual properties associated with the mammalian neuron. When a very fine microelectrode is used to probe the electrical field around a nerve cell, an abrupt change in potential between the microelectrode and an indifferent electrode in the extracellular space is noted just as the active electrode penetrates the apparent cell surface. This potential difference across the boundary between the cell and its environment usually ranges between 70 and 90 mV, with the interior of the cell negative with respect to the extracellular space, and remains constant with time. If the potential-measuring electrode is allowed to remain within the cell and small current pulses are injected through a second intracellular microelectrode, asymmetry is found in the membrane response. Small current pulses that cause the membrane potential to deviate in a more negative direction (that is, to hyperpolarize) produce changes in potential whose amplitude can be related to the magnitude of the applied current in a linear fashion. Depolarizing current pulses, however, elicit large nonlinear voltage responses of a stereotyped amplitude and duration; these responses appear to be self-perpetuating and propagate along the cell surface independent of further stimuli.

1

In a typical nerve cell, potassium is the predominant internal cation, although there is little potassium in the extracellular space; conversely, little sodium is present within the cell, although high concentrations are found without. Measurements of apparent ionic mobility using various physical techniques indicate relatively free movement for small monovalent cations within the cell but highly restricted movement for these same ions across the boundary between the cell and its environment.

In this chapter we will examine the physical basis for these experimental observations and integrate them according to modern concepts of excitable membrane function.

PASSIVE PROPERTIES OF THE NEURONAL SURFACE MEMBRANE

The boundary between cell and environment in nerve, as in most eukaryotic cells, is formed by a highly integrated surface membrane composed of lipids, proteins, and small quantities of carbohydrates (Singer, 1974). In the electron microscope this boundary appears as a pair of dark lines separated by a lighter central region. The width of this complex, usually referred to as the unit membrane, averages 75 Å in most cells. The matrix of this membrane is formed by a stable bilayer of phospholipid molecules (Fig. 1–1) organized with their hydrophobic hydrocarbon chain ends gathered together in the membrane interior, and their polar glycerol-phosphate-head group ends oriented towards the aqueous environment on either side of the bilayer. Such an organization represents a stable low energy configuration for these lipid molecules, and can be formed spontaneously in vitro from the component lipids. The hydrocarbon end of a phospholipid molecule cannot interact effectively with water molecules, and the major driving force for the spontaneous organization of phospholipids into a bilayer is the need to remove these hydrocarbon chains from the water environment (Lee, 1975). Under normal conditions this lipid bilayer is in a fluid state, with individual phospholipid molecules able to undergo rapid translational and rotational movement within the plane of the membrane; flip-flop movements of phospholipids between halves of the bilayer, however, occur only at relatively slow rates (Edidin, 1974). The ease with which individual molecules can move within the plane of the membrane is often discussed in terms of apparent membrane "fluidity" or "microviscosity." The fluidity of a phospholipid bilayer depends upon several factors, including ambient temperature and sterol content, and can be extensively modified by altering the chain length or degree of unsaturation of the fatty acid esters comprising the hydrophobic portion of the phospholipid molecules.

Studies of the electrical properties of artificial bilayers composed purely of lipid reveal certain passive characteristics similar to those of the nerve cell membrane.

Membrane Organization

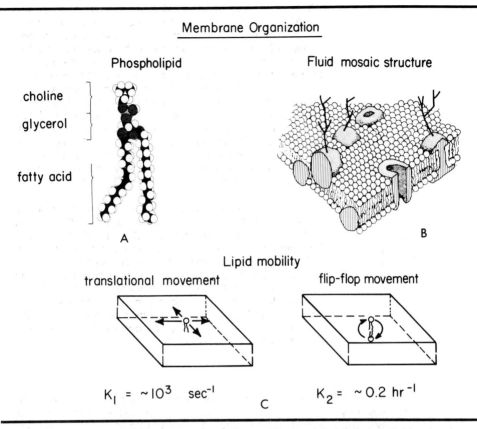

Figure 1–1 *A,* Space-filling model of a phospholipid molecule (phosphatidyl-choline). *B,* The fluid mosaic concept of the cell membrane, demonstrating the continuous lipid bilayer in which integral membrane proteins are anchored by hydrophobic interactions with adjacent phospholipid hydrocarbon chains. *C,* Translational movement of individual phospholipid molecules is usually quite rapid while inside to outside, or "flip-flop," transitions occur only at a much slower rate.

These bilayers exhibit a capacitance of approximately 1 $\mu F/cm^2$ and effectively limit the movement of small and large polar molecules between the two aqueous regions which they separate (Henn and Thompson, 1969). However, their electrical resistance is very high (that is, their conductance to ionic species is very low), much higher than that measured in a native cell membrane.

The addition of small concentrations of certain proteins to an artificial bilayer can selectively increase its conductance to specific ions by several orders of magnitude and thus reduce its resistance by a comparable figure (Mueller and Rudin, 1969). It appears that, in the natural membrane, many complex functions such as ionic conductance, active ion transport, and cell-cell recognition are controlled by specialized proteins which comprise an integral part of the membrane structure. These proteins appear to be positioned within the membrane by virtue of hydrophobic interactions between their surface amino acid residues and the acyl chains of the membrane lipids, and consequently are in a thermodynamically stable state under normal conditions. Some protein molecules span the membrane from surface to surface while others are embedded in one or the other half of the bilayer, thus rendering them accessible only on a single side (Singer, 1974). Like the small lipid molecules, these proteins undergo lateral movement within the plane of the membrane, although their larger size restricts the time scale of these movements (Edidin, 1974).

The nerve cell membrane may be depicted as a random mosaic of protein molecules embedded in a fluid matrix of highly mobile phospholipid molecules (Singer and Nicolson, 1972). This membrane is a dynamic structure; both proteins and phospholipids possess significant freedom of rotational and translational movement. Many generalized membrane properties are determined by the phospholipid matrix, but specialized functions are probably attributable to the intrinsic membrane proteins. A summary of this fluid mosaic model for membrane structure is presented in Figure 1–1.

The Resting Membrane Potential

Let us turn now to the origin of the potential differences observed in the resting state between the cell interior and extracellular space. Microelectrode studies indicate that this potential difference is generated almost entirely across the 75- to 100-Å thickness of the surface membrane. Monovalent ions are distributed asymmetrically across the membrane and, as noted previously, this plane represents a barrier to their free movement.

Concentration gradients of ions in solution can themselves produce electrical gradients. Thus, when two solutions containing respectively high and low concentrations of NaCl are brought into contact, a potential difference is recorded across their interface. This potential arises from the difference in mobility in aqueous solution of the two major charge-carrying species, the negative Cl^- ion and the postive Na^+ ion. Although both species experience the same driving force from their respective chemical gradients, the sodium ion will move slightly faster due to its smaller radius of hydration.*

---

*The radius of hydration is the effective diameter of an ion with its most tightly bound sphere of water molecules in solution.

EXCITATION AND CONDUCTION IN NERVE

A very slight separation of charge develops, with positive charges leading negative as they move down the concentration gradient. This separation creates an electrical gradient at the diffusion boundary such that the less concentrated domain is positive with respect to the more concentrated region. This electrical gradient will tend to retard the movement of the faster Na^+ ion and accelerate the slower Cl^- ion. The net effect is that a balance is achieved between concentration and electrical gradient motive forces, resulting in both ion species moving at an equal rate. The observed electrical potential (referred to as diffusion potential) persists as long as the concentration gradient is present in solution and its magnitude will be related to the size of the gradient and the relative mobilities of the constituent ions by the equation

$$\Delta V = \frac{\mu^+ - \mu^-}{\mu^+ + \mu^-} \frac{RT}{F} \ln \frac{[a_1]}{[a_2]} \qquad (1-1)$$

where μ is the mobility of a given ion in water, [a] is the concentration of salt at either end of the gradient, R is Raoult's gas constant, T is absolute temperature, and F is the Faraday constant relating ion concentration to electrical charge.

Diffusion potentials are, however, intrinsically transient; the ion movements by which they are generated eventually dissipate the initial concentration gradient and the potential falls to zero. It is unlikely that a simple diffusion potential could explain the resting potential in nerve, since movement of all ions across the membrane is extremely limited relative to their movement in solution, since there are essentially equal and opposite gradients formed for sodium and potassium across the membrane, and since the observed potential is constant with time.

Consider a situation in which a membrane separates two solutions having differing compositions, as depicted in Figure 1-2. Assume that this membrane is impermeant to all ions. Under these conditions no ion detects a concentration gradient, there will be no net ionic movement across the membrane, and no potential difference is recorded between the two solutions. If the membrane is suddenly allowed to be permeant selectively to K^+ ions, the situation is dramatically altered. Potassium now experiences a driving force down its concentration gradient from side A to side B. As each K^+ ion moves across the membrane, however, a charge imbalance is created, since Cl^- is not free to accompany it as a counter ion. This charge imbalance, with an excess of positive charge on side B and an excess of negative charge on side A, creates a potential gradient across the membrane such that side B is now positive with respect to side A. This field retards the movement of K^+ ions passing from A to B

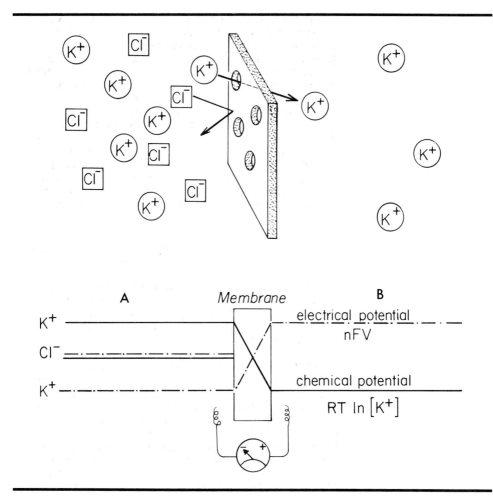

Figure 1–2 A semipermeable membrane which allows passage of only positive ions will result in the generation of a transmembrane potential when it is placed between two salt solutions of differing concentrations. The movement of positive ions down their concentration gradient will result in a separation of charges across the membrane, producing a potential gradient which tends to retard movement of the positive ion. At equilibrium forces due to concentration and potential gradients on the positive ions balance exactly, and no net ion movement occurs.

and accelerates the movement of K^+ ions passing in the reverse direction.

The net result is a situation in which equal numbers of K^+ ions move in either direction across the membrane, thus maintaining a stable electrical potential and concentration gradient. Unlike a simple diffusion potential in solution, this represents a true equilibrium; that is, the gradient and potential will not change with time as long as the permeability characteristics of the membrane are maintained. Stated another way, the change in free energy for a single K^+ ion, which is the sum of the changes in chemical and electrical potentials, is zero, whether moving from A to B or from B to A. The equation which relates the transmembrane potential to the concentration gradient of a permeant species for such a semipermeable membrane is the well-known Nernst relationship

$$V_m = \frac{RT}{nF} \ln \left\{ \frac{[S_B]}{[S_A]} \right\} \qquad (1-2)$$

where $[S_A]$ and $[S_B]$ are the concentrations of S on either side of the membrane, n is the number of charges on each ion, and R, T, and F have their usual meanings.

For a membrane in equilibrium this relationship must hold individually for all ions to which the membrane is permeant, independent of the relative permeabilities of the various ion species. For mammalian nerve, the observed concentration gradients for K^+ and Cl^- are very close to those predicted from the Nernst equation. Variation of external K^+ concentration with constant internal concentrations produces predictable changes in membrane potential which conform fairly well to the Nernst relationship between external K^+ concentrations of 10 and 200 mM (Fig. 1-3). Below 10 mM, however, consistent deviations are seen from predicted values of V_m. In addition, measurements with radioactive ^{22}Na indicate that the membrane is measurably permeant to this ion, and the concentration gradient across the membrane for sodium is indeed very far from equilibrium (Hodgkin and Keynes, 1955). The equilibrium description of the resting excitable membrane and its associated Nernst relationship must be at best an approximation which can be applied only with reservations in particular cases, and is insufficient to describe the true state of the excitable membrane.

A more general description of the relationship between permeability, concentration gradients, and potential can be derived when the membrane is assumed to be permeant to each ion species in varying degrees. For each individual species, the net effect of all the driving forces acting on a given ion within the membrane can be expressed by the general relationship

$$I_s = -\mu_s \left(\frac{RT}{Z} \nabla C_s + \frac{Z}{|Z|} C_s F \Delta\psi \right) \qquad (1-3)$$

where I_s is the net current carried by ion s, ∇C is the concentration gradient of s in three dimensions, $\nabla\Psi$ is the gradient of the potential field in three dimensions, Z is the charge on the ion, and the other terms have their usual meanings. If only ionic movement in the direction perpendicular to the membrane is considered (e.g., flux through the plane of the membrane) for a monovalent cation such as Na, this equation can be reduced to

$$I_s = \mu_s \left(\frac{RT}{dx} \frac{dC_s}{dx} + C_s F \frac{d\psi}{dx} \right) \tag{1-4}$$

The initial solution of this equation for the case of an excitable membrane was proposed by Goldman based upon the simplifying assumption that the potential field through the membrane was constant; that is $\frac{d\psi}{dx} = \frac{V_m}{D}$, where V_m is the measured transmembrane potential and D is the membrane thickness (Goldman, 1943). Using this assumption, the current equation reduces to a simple

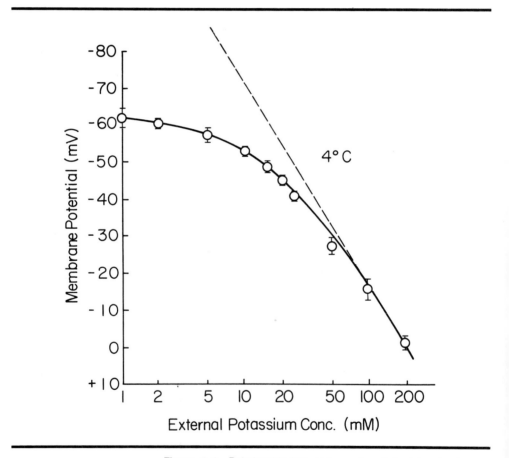

Figure 1–3 Relationship between experimentally determined membrane potential in a molluscan neuron (o) and external K^+ concentrations. The dashed line indicates the slope predicted by the Nernst equation for K^+; the solid line is the solution for the Goldman equation if the ratio of P_{Na}/P_K is assumed to be 0.033. (Modified from Marmor and Gorman, 1970.)

differential which can be integrated across the membrane. When terms are included to relate bulk solution concentrations to intramembrane concentrations of a given ion and mobility of that ion within the membrane, the following general expression is derived:

$$I_s = P_s \frac{F^2 V}{RT} \left(\frac{[S_{out}]e^{-VF/RT} - [S_{in}]}{1 - e^{-VF/RT}} \right) \qquad (1\text{-}5)$$

This is independently applicable to each ion species to which the membrane is permeant. In this equation, P_s represents the apparent membrane permeability to the ion s and is an experimentally measurable parameter which includes experimentally inaccessible factors such as intramembrane mobility and partition coefficient (Hodgkin and Katz, 1949).

Since the membrane potential in nerve remains constant and concentration gradients appear stable as a function of time, the system must either be in equilibrium or represent a steady state. If the former is true then the net ionic movement or current for each ion species will be zero. That is,

$$I_{total} = 0 = I_A = I_B. \ldots \ldots \ldots = I_n$$

When the general equation (1-5) is substituted for each current, set equal to zero, and reduced the result is, as expected, an expression identical to the Nernst equation. We have already seen, however, that this cannot apply to all permeant species and that the equilibrium solution must be rejected.

The alternative hypothesis would be one in which the net current for all ions across the membrane is zero, but currents ascribable to individual ion species may not be zero. Such a stable situation is defined as a steady state and usually implies a net requirement for external work to be done (energy provided) in order to maintain that state. Under these conditions, total membrane current is given as

$$I_{total} = 0 = I_A + I_B + \ldots \ldots \ldots I_n$$

If, once again, individual current terms are substituted and the entire equation reduced, the following relationship is derived:

$$V_m = \frac{RT}{F} \ln \left(\frac{\alpha_a[A^+]_o + \alpha_b[B^+]_o + \alpha_c[C^-]_i \ldots + \alpha_n[N^-]_i}{\alpha_a[A^+]_i + \alpha_b[B^+]_i + \alpha_c[C^-]_o \ldots + \alpha_n[N^-]_o} \right) \qquad (1\text{-}6)$$

This form of flux equation is often referred to as the Goldman-Hodgkin-Katz relationship, after the investigators who first demonstrated its derivation and application (Goldman, 1943; Hodgkin and Katz, 1949). In this expression, transmembrane potential is related collectively to the concentration gradient of each permeant species as modified by the membrane's permeability to that species (α). This equation provides an accurate description of the resting potential and its variation in response to changing ionic conditions over a wide range of concentrations of permeant species (see Fig. 1–3).

The importance of the permeability terms in this equation must be emphasized. If one assumes that the nerve membrane is permeable only to Na^+ and K^+, and that the permeability coefficients for these two ions are equal, then the measured transmembrane potential would be calculated to lie midway between the equilibrium potential for the two ions (about −10 mV). If the membrane is much more permeant to K^+ than to Na^+, the terms $\alpha_{Na}[Na]$ become insignificant and can safely be ignored; under these circumstances, the membrane potential will closely approximate the equilibrium potential for K^+ (about −70 to −80 mV in most nerves). Conversely, if permeability in the same nerve is altered such that permeability to Na^+ greatly exceeds that to K^+, the potential will approximate the sodium equilibrium potential (+30 to +50 mV in most nerves). The membrane potential can thus be controlled by altering permeability without changing concentration gradients. The implications of this concept will soon become evident (Fig. 1–4).

How well does the equation predict the behavior of excitable membranes *in vivo*? Referring back to Figure 1–3, it can be seen that the observed V_m in a neuronal membrane as a function of $[K^+]_{out}$ is fit precisely by the Goldman equation when relative permeability values of $K^+:Na^+$ of 1:0.033 are chosen. Similar results have been found in other tissues and, in general, this mathematical description works quite well for most nerve and muscle surface membranes.

Unidirectional Ion Fluxes

The individual terms of the Goldman equation define an ionic current; that is, the *net* movement of ions across the membrane. Expressions can be derived from these terms to describe unidirectional ionic fluxes in either the inward or outward direction under a given set of conditions; from these expressions the absolute number of ions moving in a given direction per unit time can be predicted. Under appropriate experimental conditions such fluxes can be measured directly. Substitution of these measured values into the equation allows the calculation of an apparent membrane permeability; this may be done in the following manner .

If an axon is equilibrated in a solution containing ^{42}K, the K^+ in the axoplasm will become uniformly labelled with

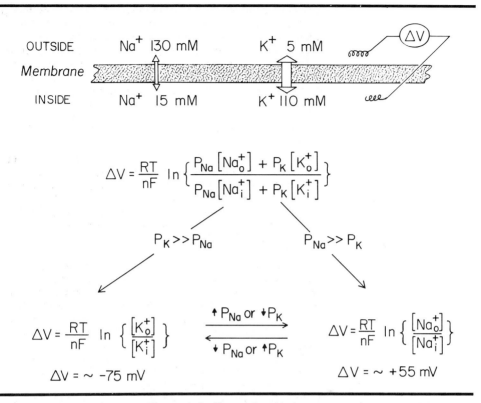

Figure 1-4 The relationship between membrane potential, ion concentration gradients, and membrane ion permeabilities is best expressed by the Goldman-Hodgkin-Katz equation. Given the concentration gradients for Na^+ and K^+ usually found in nerve, it can be seen that membrane potential can vary between -75 mV and $+55$ mV solely on the basis of changing membrane permeabilities, with no change in concentration gradients. Such changes in permeability underlie the generation of an action potential.

this isotope. If the axon is transferred rapidly to a solution containing no isotope, experimental conditions are established in which the external $^{42}K^+$ concentration is zero and the internal $^{42}K^+$ concentration can be determined directly (Hodgkin and Keynes, 1955). Modification of the Goldman equation to reflect this situation and conversion of the current term to a flux term yields

$$J_{K_{outward}} = P_K[K_{in}]\left(\frac{VF}{RT}\ \frac{1}{1 - e^{-VF/RT}}\right) \qquad (1-7)$$

Now J_K outward can be measured by monitoring the appearance of radioactive K^+ in the bathing solution. Using these data a permeability constant P of the membrane for potassium can be calculated.

11

EXCITATION AND CONDUCTION IN NERVE

The reverse situation can also be investigated, beginning with an unlabelled axon and immersing it in a solution containing $^{42}K^+$ at known specific activity. The axon can be removed periodically and monitored to determine the amount of K^+ uptake. Under these conditions $[^{42}K^+_{out}]$ is known and $[^{42}K^+_{in}]$ is initially zero, and a net K^+ influx is measured. The modified flux equation thus becomes

$$J_{inward} = P_K [K_{out}]\left(\frac{VF}{RT} \ \frac{1}{e^{\ VF/RT} - 1}\right) \qquad (1-8)$$

Again, an apparent permeability can be calculated. If the ion being studied is moving through the membrane passively, then the permeability of the membrane will be identical in either direction. If the values do not agree within reasonable experimental limits, this suggests that an active process is in some way contributing to ionic movement asymmetrically.

Experiments of this type have been performed using squid axon (Hodgkin and Keynes, 1955) and muscle (Hodgkin and Horowicz, 1959); typical results for muscle are summarized in Table 1-1. The calculated permeability of the membrane to K^+ is the same whether K^+ influx or efflux is used as the starting point. Sodium permeability calculated from Na^+ influx data yields a value some 100-fold smaller than that for K^+, close to the relative permeability predicted from our comparison of the Goldman equation with membrane behavior *in situ*. Apparent permeability for Na^+ moving in the outward direction is, on the other hand, several orders of magnitude higher than for Na^+ moving inward. Clearly, separate processes must be involved in the vectorial outward movement of this ion.

The high outward Na^+ permeability is remarkably sensitive to temperature and to certain potent cardiac glycosides such as ouabain (Glynn, 1964; Hodgkin and Keynes, 1955). Treatment of the axon with ouabain re-

Table 1-1 Unidirectional Fluxes and Calculated Permeabilities for Na^+ and K^+ Movement Across an Excitable Membrane*

Ion	Direction	Flux	Calculated Permeability
K^+	Inward	5.4×10^{-12} moles/cm²sec	5.8×10^{-7} cm/sec
K^+	Outward	8.8×10^{-12} moles/cm²sec	6.2×10^{-7} cm/sec
Na^+	Inward	3.5×10^{-12} moles/cm²sec	7.9×10^{-9} cm/sec
Na^+	Outward	3.5×10^{-12} moles/cm²sec	3.9×10^{-6} cm/sec

*Data are from isotopic flux measurements made by Hodgkin and Horowicz (1959) on single frog muscle fibers. Similar conclusions can be reached from data obtained with axonal preparations (cf. Hodgkin and Keynes, 1955).

duces apparent permeability to Na^+ moving outward nearly to the level of that moving inward. The correlation between the high outward Na^+ permeability and a membrane ATPase whose activity is stimulated by Na^+ and K^+ has been clearly established. It is now apparent that a portion of Na^+ moving out of the axon under normal conditions does so via an active chemical pump which requires a supply of high energy phosphate in the form of ATP for its action (Skou, 1965).

The overall steady state of the resting excitable membrane can now be described. K^+ exists in a distribution very close to its equilibrium position with respect to membrane potential. Membrane permeability to K^+ is quite high, and K^+ ions move freely in either direction across the membrane. Net current (that is, the algebraic sum of inward and outward fluxes) is, however, close to zero. A similar situation exists for Cl^-, although in nerve its permeability and hence its relative unidirectional fluxes are lower than those of Na^+ or K^+. Sodium is distributed far from its equilibrium position, but membrane permeability to this ion is quite low. Passive sodium influx greatly exceeds passive efflux, resulting in a net inward passive sodium current. There exists in parallel with this passive pathway an active energy-requiring pump mechanism that extrudes sodium at a rate which exactly balances the net passive inward current, thus maintaining the total membrane current at zero and the ionic gradients constant. For completeness a small active inward movement of K^+ must be included, directly linked to Na^+ extrusion via the Na^+ pump. The overall result is a steady state distribution of ions, with the membrane potential reflecting their relative permeabilities and concentration gradients; all of this is maintained at the expense of a constant infusion of metabolic energy in the form of ATP (Fig. 1–5).

What would happen if this source of metabolic energy were removed? Without ATP the active outward transport of Na^+ would no longer be possible. There would therefore be a slow but continuous net inward movement of Na^+ ions. Gradually the Na^+ concentration gradient would decrease and the counterbalancing K^+ gradient would simultaneously begin to dissipate. As predicted by the Goldman equation, membrane potential would progressively fall. Eventually both Na^+ and K^+ would be distributed nearly symmetrically across the membrane, and V_m would fall to zero. This doomsday process does not occur immediately when ATP is withdrawn, however. Since membrane permeability to Na^+ is very low, many minutes or even hours are required for the redistribution of ions to take place, and apparently normal membrane resting potentials will be recorded during the early portion of this event. Many thousands of action potentials can also be generated during this interval.

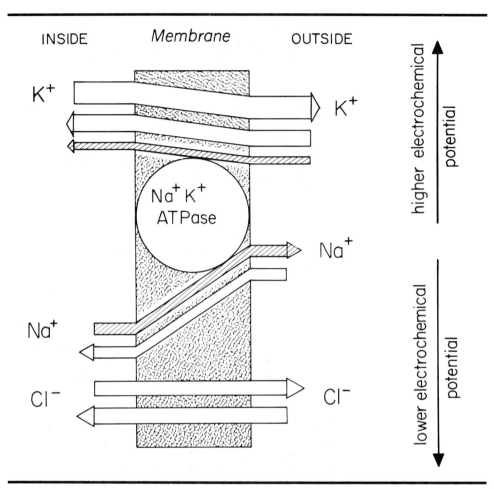

Figure 1–5 Relative electrochemical potential gradients experienced by the major monovalent ions across the nerve cell membrane. K+ is close to equilibrium while Na+ is maintained far from equilibrium by an energy-dependent ATPase. A fraction of inward K+ movement is coupled to the outward movement of Na+ through this pumping system.

The final conception of the resting membrane involves a fluid mosaic of lipid and protein having selective and variable permeability to small charged molecules. Concentration gradients and a transmembrane potential are related by a steady state expression involving a relative permeability term for each ion species, and membrane potential at a given moment depends not only upon the magnitude of the concentration gradients but also upon the relative permeabilities to the ions involved.

Passive Membrane Electrical Properties

Neural membranes respond characteristically to electrical stimulation, as previously discussed. Hyperpolarizing square current pulses injected into an axon result in a time-dependent increase in membrane potential that plateaus at a value proportional to the magnitude of the injected current. On abrupt termination of the applied current, the membrane potential decays exponentially back to its initial resting level. This behavior is characteristic of a circuit containing both a capacitance and a resistance in parallel, and such a model configuration adequately describes the passive hyperpolarizing response of the neuronal membrane. The amplitude of the steady state change in potential at the point of current injection can be related to the membrane resistance. The time, τ, required for membrane potential to achieve $1/e$ of its final value after the onset of a square current pulse is related to membrane capacitance and resistance by the simple expression

$$\tau = RC \qquad (1-9)$$

where R is the membrane resistance and C the membrane capacitance, both expressed per unit area of surface membrane. τ is referred to as the time constant of the membrane, and can be considered as indicative of the time required to alter the charge on the membrane capacitance during an attempted transition in membrane potential.

If simultaneous measurements of membrane potential are made at several points along a hypothetical axon, at increasing distances from the point of stimulation, two observations will be made. First, the steady state amplitude of membrane potential attained with a given current pulse decreases exponentially with distance and, second, the time required to achieve the plateau amplitude increases with distance.

These observations are of considerable importance in conduction of impulses in peripheral nerve, and thus should be discussed more fully. Consider the axon as symmetrical in two dimensions about the point of current injection and extending in either direction towards ground at infinity. Of a given quantity of current injected at point $\times = 0$, half will flow in either direction along the axon. At each point within the axon two potential paths toward ground are available — one continuing down the axonal interior, the second travelling radially across the axonal surface membrane. At each point, therefore, a percentage of the current available will move across the membrane toward ground in the low resistance extracellular fluid, while a constantly decrementing amount will continue down the axon, fractionating further into axial and radial components at each step along the way. The fraction of total current which will flow radially as opposed to axially is determined by the ratio of the effective radial and axial resistances. Radial resistance (R_m) will be due almost entirely to the resistance of the surface membrane; axial resistance (R_i) is determined both by the conductivity of the axoplasm and the cross-sectional area of the axon. The following equation, which can be derived by application of classical cable theory to our axon (Hodgkin and Rushton, 1946), describes the decay of steady state potential as a function of distance, x, from the current sources:

$$V - V_0 e^{-\frac{x}{\lambda}} \quad \text{where } \lambda = \sqrt{R_m/R_i} \quad\quad (1\text{--}10)$$

V_0 is the amplitude of the potential change at $x = 0$, R_m is the membrane resistance, and R_i is the axial resistance. The quantity λ is called the space constant and, in concrete terms, is the distance at which the steady state potential will have decayed to the $1/e$ of its initial value (Fig. 1–6). It can be appreciated that the higher the membrane resistance relative to the internal resistance of the axon, the larger the space constant and hence the further a given steady state signal will spread along the axon before decaying to unmeasurable levels. Conversely, reducing membrane resistance or increasing axial resistance will decrease the effective passive propagation distance for such a signal. It will be seen that optimization of conduction rates in real axons involves selection of optimal values for R_m and R_i.

The increasingly long time required for membrane potential at point x to reach its plateau value after injection of a step current pulse reflects the summated effects of membrane capacitance for all the membrane between that point and the point of current injection which must be charged or discharged before the measured potential can change. Increasing effective membrane capacitance will prolong this delay time, while decreasing effective capacitance will reduce it.

ACTIVE MEMBRANE RESPONSES TO DEPOLARIZATION

Current injection in an axon which results in depolarization of the surface membrane will produce linear responses exactly symmetrical to those seen for hyperpolarizing pulses, as long as the membrane potential does not vary by more than 5 to 10 mV from its resting level. With larger depolarizing pulses, marked nonlinearities develop in the observed membrane response. Following termination of a current pulse the potential may remain depolarized or oscillate slightly about a depolarized level for varying periods before decaying exponentially back to resting levels. With slightly bigger pulses, a larger stereotyped depolarization results which actually continues through zero to a point at which the interior of the axon is positive with respect to the outside. Once initiated, this regenerative spike or action potential will proceed independently, regardless of whether the stimulating current is terminated or continued. The fun-

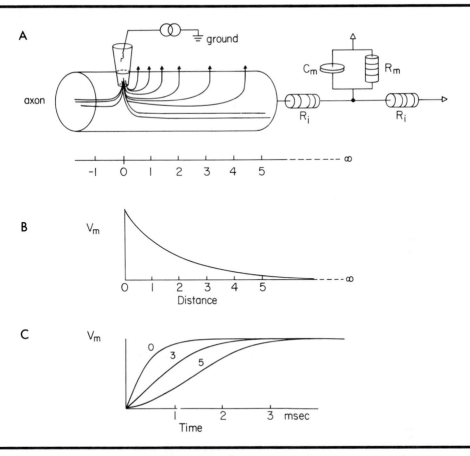

Figure 1–6 *A,* The passive or electrotonic spread of current along an axon or cell process is governed by the relative values of the axial resistance (R_i), mostly due to cytoplasm, and the radial resistance (R_m) and capacitance (C_m), attributable to the surface membrane. *B,* With constant current injection at a single point, the membrane potential produced will decline with distance in an exponential fashion. *C,* In response to an abrupt square current pulse, membrane potential rises to a new steady state in a manner which reflects the time required to change the membrane capacitance. This time-dependent function can be explicitly defined in terms of R_m, C_m, R_i, distance, and time.

damental processes which make excitable membranes unique are those which underlie this nonlinear regenerative response.

The observed nonlinearity in membrane response implies that one of the normally constant membrane properties such as capacitance or resistance is varying in an unexpected manner with voltage or time. Early insight into this process was gained through an incisive experiment performed by Cole in the late 1930's (Cole and Curtis, 1939). Cole arranged a squid axon in a chamber

17

between two plate electrodes in such a manner that the axon could be excited at will. The plates were then connected into a bridge circuit in which the effective impedance (composed of capacitance and resistance contributions) of the axon was just balanced by known resistance and capacitance standards (Fig. 1–7). Changes in axonal impedance would be reflected in resultant imbalance produced in the bridge circuit. Since capacitance changes are dependent upon the frequency used to activate the bridge, while resistance changes are not, these contributing factors can be separated experimentally. This elegantly simple approach clearly revealed that a large change in membrane impedance occurred sychronously with the appearance of an action potential between the bridge electrodes (Fig. 1–7). The change was independent of the activation frequency used in the bridge circuit, indicating that a change in membrane resistance was occurring.

In an axon membrane, a change in membrane resistance implies a change in membrane conductance to one or more ion species. We have seen that information about relative ion permeabilities in the resting membrane may be obtained by observing the effect of variation in exter-

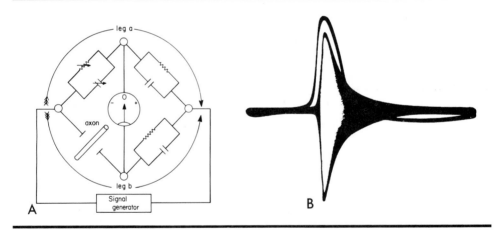

Figure 1–7 *A,* Schematic representation of a bridge circuit incorporating an excitable squid axon in one leg. Initially, the variable resistance and capacitance are adjusted so that the impedance drops along the two legs of the bridge are symmetrical and the potential difference recorded is zero. Subsequent alterations in resistance or capacitance of the axon will unbalance the bridge and produce a signal in the recording device. *B,* A recording of a squid action potential and bridge signal from such an experimental setup. Note that the change in membrane potential is accompanied by a change in membrane impedance. Further studies have shown that this is due to an abrupt alteration in R_m while C_m remains constant. (Modified from Cole and Curtis, 1939.)

nal ion concentration upon membrane potential. Similar experiments can be performed to evaluate the sensitivity of the action potential spike height to ion gradients across the membrane. Variations in K^+ concentration within limits which allow excitation to take place have little effect on the action potential amplitude. Peak height, however, varies markedly when external Na^+ concentration is altered. Lowering external sodium concentration reduces action potential amplitude, and vice versa (Hodgkin and Katz, 1949). A little reflection will indicate that this ion sensitivity is exactly the opposite of that in the resting state. Such a change could be produced (Fig. 1–4) either by a decrease in membrane conductance to K^+ or an increase in conductance to Na^+. Since Cole's experiment demonstrated a decrease in membrane resistance (that is, an increase in conductance or permeability), it can be reasonably anticipated that the latter of these two possibilities holds. Understanding the mechanism whereby the action potential is generated, then, will require defining the manner in which ionic conductances in the membrane change in response to changes in membrane potential.

Voltage Clamp Analysis of Excitable Membrane Currents

Total membrane current in an axon will be composed of at least two terms, one related to ionic currents flowing through the membrane conductance pathways and the other related to currents charging and discharging the membrane capacitance. The total membrane current may be described in its simplest form by

$$I_{total} = I_{ion} + I_{cap.} = (G_{ion} \cdot V_m) + \left(C_m \cdot \frac{dV}{dt}\right) \quad (1-11)$$

where G is the membrane ionic conductance, which is simply the reciprocal of the electrical resistance of the membrane to the flow of ionic current ($G = 1/R$).

Since capacitative currents are proportional to the rate of change of voltage rather than to absolute voltage level, they will be significant whenever potential is changing but will be zero when potential is constant. Ionic currents, on the other hand, depend only upon the magnitude of the potential gradient and upon the membrane conductance to the current-carrying ion. In the unconstrained action potential capacitative and ionic currents are inevitably intermixed, since potential is rapidly changing. Under these conditions analysis of ionic current is very difficult. The single major technological advance which allowed understanding of the excitation process to proceed was the development of a method for separating the capacitative and ionic components of the membrane regenerative response. This method, referred to as voltage clamping, was originally developed by Cole and was successfully applied to the squid axon by Hodgkin et al. (1952).

EXCITATION AND CONDUCTION IN NERVE

The concept behind voltage clamping is quite simple. Because capacitive currents flow only when membrane potential is changing, this technique forces the membrane to maintain a steady potential. This potential is changed rapidly on command to a new level and held there (Fig. 1–8). Since $\frac{dV}{dt}$ is zero before and after this transition, no capacitive current flows during these intervals. All capacitive current is confined to the brief period during which potential is altered from one level to another. The capacitive current will have a larger amplitude but be of shorter duration the more rapidly this transition is made (i.e., the greater $\frac{dV}{dt}$). Modern voltage clamp systems are able to change membrane potential from one level to another so rapidly and effectively that all capacitive current flow is complete within 20 μsec of the transition.

Voltage clamp systems monitor the membrane potential, compare that potential to a control standard, and apply negative feedback current to the membrane so that any tendency of the membrane to deviate from the holding potential is immediately and accurately counterbalanced. Thus, any currents which are flowing across the axonal membrane are balanced immediately by equal and opposite currents from the control amplifier. Monitoring control amplifier output currents yields a direct indication of membrane current at any point in time.

Carrying out these complex monitoring and control functions requires the electrodes to be placed within the interior of the axon. When the technique was developed the giant squid provided the ideal experimental material. This animal contains several giant axons reaching diameters of 800 to 1000 μ or more which can be removed intact. With such large axons it was possible to position the necessary electrodes physically down the center of the axon for distances of 1 to 2 cm or more (Hodgkin et al., 1952).

When the membrane potential of an axon in such a voltage clamp setup is rapidly moved from a resting potential of -90 mV to a more hyperpolarized potential of -140 mV, a brief surge of capacitive current is followed by a continuous, steady ionic current whose amplitude may be predicted from the known change in potential and the resting membrane resistance. Larger hyperpolarizing voltage steps produce larger steady ionic current levels, with their amplitude proportional to the voltage step. That is, current flow in response to hyperpolarizing membrane potential steps behaves in a linear manner — Ohm's law is obeyed and nothing unexpected is observed. A voltage clamp step which rapidly shifts the membrane potential 50 mV in a depolarizing direction (from a resting level of -90 to -40 mV) produces

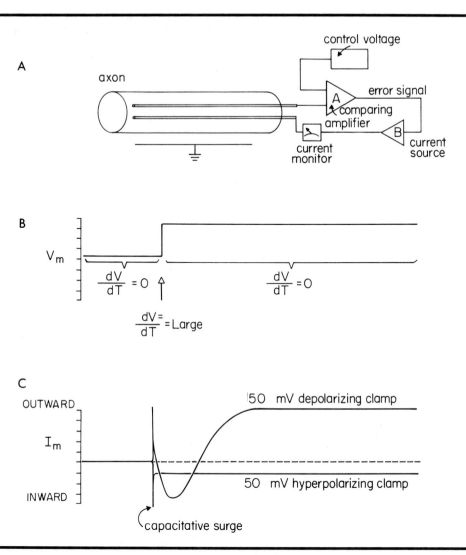

Figure 1-8 *A,* Typical arrangement for electronics required to voltage-clamp a squid axon. An axial electrode senses membrane potential; this potential is compared to a control reference potential by an amplifier, A. Variations from the reference potential generate an error signal which is transformed into a current by a second amplifier, B. This error current is fed back across the membrane by a second axial electrode in such a manner as to force the membrane potential back to the desired control level. Under these conditions in an ideal system, the output of the feedback current source will be equal in magnitude and opposite in sign to any membrane currents which flow as a function of time. *B,* Abrupt step changes in potential are imposed on the axon in order to confine capacitative currents to the brief interval during which voltage is changing. Only ionic currents flow when $\frac{dv}{dt} = 0$. *C,* Membrane currents observed with 50 mV hyperpolarizing and 50 mV depolarizing clamp steps. Large nonlinear currents flow during depolarization.

21

quite different effects. Again, there is the capacitative transient, but now the ionic current component is large and biphasic, changing as a function of time in spite of the constant voltage. Furthermore, the earliest ionic currents seem to be flowing into the cell, in the direction opposite from the linear outward current flow predicted by Ohm's law. With time this early inward current becomes a sustained outward current which is usually maintained until the membrane potential is returned to resting level (Fig. 1–8).

A series of increasingly depolarized steps from the normal resting potential generates a family of current traces which clearly are not proportional in any simple way to the size of the voltage step (Fig. 1–9). The early inward ionic current increases rapidly in maximum amplitude with larger depolarizations between 30 and 60 mV, but then diminishes again and seems to disappear completely when the clamp step approaches 120 mV (that is, membrane potential clamped to +30 mV compared to an initial resting potential of −90 mV). With still larger clamp steps, early current now develops in the outward direction. This voltage point about which early current changes from net inward to zero and then to outward is referred to as the *reversal potential* for this current (Hodgkin and Huxley, 1952a).

Voltage Clamp Sequence

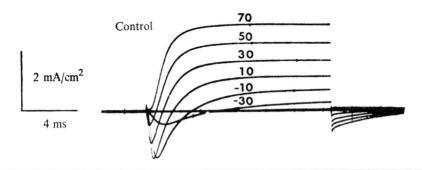

Figure 1–9 A series of current records are shown from a squid axon which has been voltage-clamped to various levels between −30 mV and +10 mV from its resting potential of −70 mV. Note the development and decay of early inward current and the later sustained outward current. With large depolarizing clamp steps, the early inward current disappears. Very large voltage steps which exceed V_{Na} would produce small, early outward currents. (From Rojas and Armstrong, 1971.)

The later current component always appears to develop in an outward direction for depolarizing pulses, but it too is clearly nonlinear. The amplitude of this current is not related in a linear fashion to the size of the step in membrane potential, and the interval after the transition at which this current first develops is a nonlinear function of clamp potential.

Separation of Component Ionic Conductances

Which ions are responsible for carrying these nonlinear currents? Are both early and late components due to the same ion, or are different ions flowing during these periods? Early investigators gained insight into these questions by several simple experiments in which external ionic concentration was modified. They found that when the Ringer's solution being perfused over a voltage-clamped axon was changed to one in which Na^+ ions were totally replaced by those of the impermeant cation choline, the prominent inward current usually seen with a 60-mV depolarizing clamp step disappeared, although the later outward current remained unchanged (Hodgkin and Huxley, 1952a). When perfusion with normal Na^+ Ringer's solution was reinstituted, the early current reappeared exactly as it had been initially.

These observations certainly imply that sodium is the ion responsible for early inward current. Does this explain the apparent reversal of early current which occurs with large depolarizations? One correlation immediately comes to mind. The observed reversal potential in most axons is very close to the calculated equilibrium potential for sodium ions. Could they be directly related? Another experiment was carried out in which several voltage clamp records were obtained at membrane potentials close to the reversal potential for the early current. The external sodium concentration was then changed in several steps and the measurements repeated with each change. A new sodium equilibrium potential could be calculated in each new solution. Analysis of the voltage clamp records showed that the apparent reversal potential had also changed, and that in each solution there was good agreement between the calculated equilibrium potential for Na^+ and the observed reversal potential for the early inward current (Hodgkin and Huxley, 1952a).

These two experiments can be interpreted in the following way. Early current flowing immediately after a depolarizing voltage step is carried by Na^+ ions, and the direction of current flow is dictated not by the degree of depolarization relative to the resting potential but rather by the difference between the clamped membrane potential and the sodium equilibrium potential. Thus, the driving force on the sodium ions is the result of the electrochemical gradient for this ion across the membrane, while the actual magnitude of the current is

23

dependent, in addition, upon the membrane conductance to Na$^+$ at that time

$$I_{Na} = G_{Na}(V_m - V_{Na}) \tag{1-12}$$

where V_{Na} is the sodium equilibrium potential, G_{Na} is the membrane conductance to Na$^+$, and V_m is the membrane potential during the clamp. Sodium conductance increases dramatically with increasing size of depolarizing steps, but the driving force ($V_m - V_{Na}$) progressively decreases. When $V_m = V_{Na}$ this driving force is reduced to zero, and no net sodium current flows in spite of the very large membrane conductance to sodium.

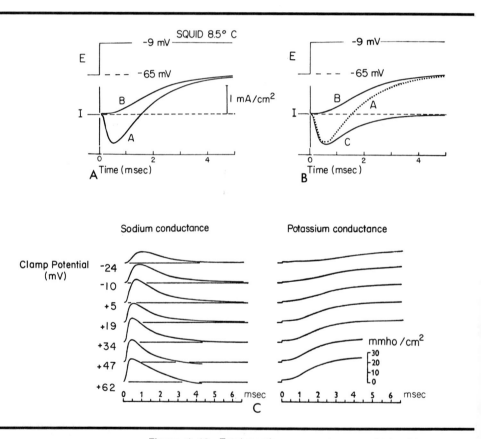

Figure 1–10 Total membrane current curves obtained from voltage clamp experiments must be decomposed into individual ionic currents. *A,* Early inward current is eliminated by replacing normal Ringer's solution with Na$^+$-free Ringer's, leaving only the delayed outward current carried by K$^+$ (B). *B,* Subtraction of delayed K$^+$ current (B) from total ionic current (A) yields true early sodium current (C). *C,* Membrane conductance to Na$^+$ and K$^+$ as a function of time can then be calculated from the ionic currents obtained at each voltage clamp potential. Values shown are for squid axon at 6° C. (Modified from Hodgkin and Huxley, 1952a.)

EXCITATION AND CONDUCTION IN NERVE

So far we have a vague feeling for the voltage dependence of the early current, but any further analysis requires that early and late current components be separated. This can be done quite simply by recording a sequence of voltage clamp steps in the presence and absence of external Na$^+$, and then subtracting the Na$^+$-free records from those recorded in normal Ringer's solution. Such a decomposition yields pure "early" and "late" current records, as shown in Figure 1–10A and B.

At this point the data are in the form of currents. What we would really like to know, however, is the behavior of the membrane conductance to the ion or ions that carry these currents. We can concentrate first on the early currents carried predominantly by Na$^+$. For each current record, V_{Na} can be determined from solution concentrations by using the Nernst equation; V_m is constant and I_m is experimentally obtained. With these values G_{Na} at each point in time can be calculated from Equation 1–12. Similar conversions were carried out for the late currents using the equilibrium potential for potassium (Hodgkin and Huxley, 1952a). The result is the family of curves seen in Figure 1–10C. Membrane conductances for both sodium and potassium increase with increasing depolarization; peak conductances eventually reach a maximum, and are unchanged by further increases in step size. The rate at which peak conductance is reached in each case also increases with increasing depolarization. The most striking difference between the two sets of conductance records lies in their later time-dependent behavior. The delayed potassium conductance increases to a new level after a lag period following a depolarizing step and maintains that new level throughout the duration of the depolarizing step. Early sodium conductance, on the other hand, invariably increases to a maximum and then rapidly reverses back to low predepolarized levels. This inactivation process is of critical importance for excitation.

Inactivation of Sodium Conductance

Inactivation of the sodium conductance system appears to be a voltage-dependent process, and the fraction of the total sodium system available to be turned on by a given depolarization reflects the previous history of the axon membrane potential. An experiment in which the axonal membrane potential was rapidly clamped 50 mV in the depolarizing direction produced the expected early inward sodium current. The amplitude of this current could be compared to currents resulting after identical depolarizing or hyperpolarizing conditioning pulses. Prepulses lasting for 40 msec and ranging between 40 mV in the hyperpolarizing direction and 30 mV in the depolarizing direction were used, and results similar to those shown in Figure 1–11 were obtained (Hodgkin and Huxley, 1952b). It is immediately apparent that the amplitude

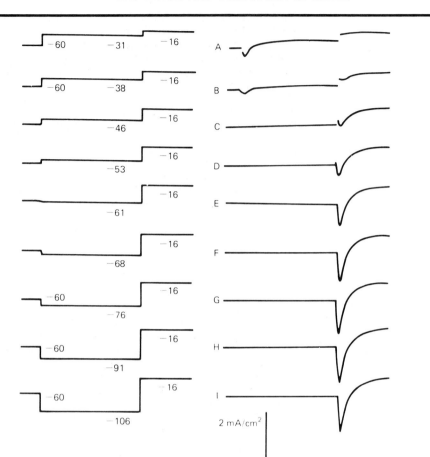

Figure 1–11 The magnitude of the early inward Na⁺ current obtained during a voltage clamp step to a given depolarized potential depends upon the previous membrane potential history of the axon. In these data, a clamp step from −60 mV to −16 mV is separated by a conditioning step to various potentials between −106 mV (a hyperpolarizing step) and −31 mV. Hyperpolarizing preconditioning steps produce larger currents, while depolarizing conditioning pulses reduce the peak sodium currents. (Adapted from Hodgkin and Huxley, 1952b.)

of the peak inward sodium current is dependent not only upon the potential to which the membrane is clamped during the test pulse, but also upon the previous potential history of the membrane. Hyperpolarizing preconditioning pulses tend to increase the amplitude of the resultant sodium current, while depolarizing prepulses reduce its amplitude. When the relative amplitude of the peak inward sodium current is plotted against the membrane potential during the conditioning pulse, a sigmoidal curve is obtained which appears to saturate near holding potentials of -100 to -110 mV and drops to 0 when resting potential is held below -40 or -45 mV prior to a test pulse (Hodgkin and Huxley, 1952*b*). At normal resting membrane potentials, about 75 per cent of the potential peak sodium current is available for use.

In a similar experiment the duration rather than the amplitude of the conditioning pulse can be progressively changed. If either a hyperpolarizing or a depolarizing conditioning pulse is chosen which significantly affects the peak inward current and if the duration of this conditioning pulse is gradually changed from a few milliseconds to 50 or more milliseconds, it is found that the effect of the prepulse is not instantaneous, but requires time to develop. Similarly, if a constant prepulse is separated from the test pulse by varying intervals of time, its effect is reversible with a half-time similar to that noted for its onset in the previous experiment (Hodgkin and Huxley, 1952*b*).

Quantitative Description of Membrane Ionic Currents

The early sodium current which results from membrane depolarization can be considered to be the end product of two sequential processes, both dependent upon time and membrane potential. The first is an activation process whereby the conductance mechanism for sodium in the membrane is "turned on," or opened; the second is a process whereby sodium channels are converted into a nonconducting and inexcitable state, referred to as inactivation. Since activation occurs on a slightly faster time scale than inactivation, depolarization results in the development of an increased membrane conductance to sodium followed by its progressive decline to resting levels. The rapid increase in conductance following a delay period which is observed experimentally is best described as a result of the concerted action of several parallel factors, all of which must be in an activated state for the channel to conduct. This is usually indicated mathematically by relating conductance in the sodium system to the third power of an activation parameter defined as m, where m varies as a function of both time and voltage in some empirically determined manner. The effects of inactivation can be included in a mathematical description by adding another term, h, which can vary between 0 and 1. A zero would represent the state in which all sodium conductance channels are inactive and inexcitable, and a 1 would represent that state in which all channels are potentially activatable. As we have seen, h will also be a function of both voltage and time. Hodgkin and Huxley (1952*c*) developed a general expression for sodium conductance from experimental data using these concepts. This expression, which gives sodium conductance at a single point in time, can be written as

$$G_{Na} = \bar{G}_{Na} m^3 h \qquad (1\text{--}13)$$

27

where $\bar{G}_{Na}$ is the maximal sodium conductance potentially attainable in a given membrane. Since the current carried by sodium ions is related to both the membrane conductance to sodium and the driving force on sodium ions, this expression can be expanded to

$$I_{Na} = \bar{G}_{Na} m^3 h (V_{Na} - V_m) \qquad (1-14)$$

A full description of the sodium current requires additional equations which completely describe the behavior of the variables m and h as a function of membrane potential and time (see Table 1–2). A similar expression can be derived for potassium conductance and, hence, for potassium current. In this case the delayed rise of potassium conductance is best fit by a fourth power dependence upon a voltage- and time-dependent variable, n. A summary of the pertinent equations for m, n, and h are given in Table 1–2. When the individual expressions for Na or K currents are solved at a given membrane potential as a function of time, the experimental voltage clamp current records are reproduced exactly (Hodgkin and Huxley, 1952c).

A complete description of membrane currents as derived by Hodgkin and Huxley includes expressions for sodium and potassium ionic currents, as well as for other currents contributing to the total membrane current.

$$I_{total} = \bar{G}_{Na} m^3 h (V_m - V_{Na}) + \bar{G}_K n^4 (V_m - V_K) +$$

$$G_L (V_m - V_L) + C_m \frac{dV}{dt} \qquad (1-15)$$

This equation includes terms for nonspecific leakage current carried in part by chloride ions and a term for

Table 1–2 Summary of Equations Describing Time and Voltage Dependence of Ionic Currents in the Squid Giant Axon

$$I_m = \bar{G}_{Na} m^3 h (V_m - V_{Na}) + \bar{G}_K n^4 (V_m - V_K) + G_L (V_m - V_L) + C_m \frac{dV}{dt}$$

$$\frac{dn}{dt} = \alpha_n (1 - n) - \beta_n n$$

$$\frac{dm}{dt} = \alpha_m (1 - m) - \beta_m m$$

$$\frac{dh}{dt} = \alpha_h (1 - h) - \beta_h h$$

$$\alpha_n = 0.01 (V + 10) \Big/ \left(\exp\left(\frac{V + 10}{10} \right) - 1 \right) \qquad \beta_n = 0.125 \exp(V/80)$$

$$\alpha_m = 0.1 (V + 25) \Big/ \left(\exp\left(\frac{V + 25}{10} \right) - 1 \right) \qquad \beta_m = 4 \exp(V/18)$$

$$\alpha_h = 0.07 \exp(V/20) \qquad \beta_h = 1 \Big/ \left(\exp\left(\frac{V + 30}{10} \right) + 1 \right)$$

capacitative current. When the entire equation is solved, using simultaneously the appropriate relationships between the variables m, n, and h, and voltage and time, the waveform of the action potential is reproduced (Hodgkin and Huxley, 1952c). This is quite a feat and indicates that, at least in general terms, the quantitative description of ionic conductance events which has been described is valid.

The events which take place during the generation of an action potential may now be summarized (Fig. 1–12.) Sodium conductance begins to increase following depolarization to threshold; the resultant inward sodium current acts to discharge the membrane capacitance and allows the membrane potential to swing towards the

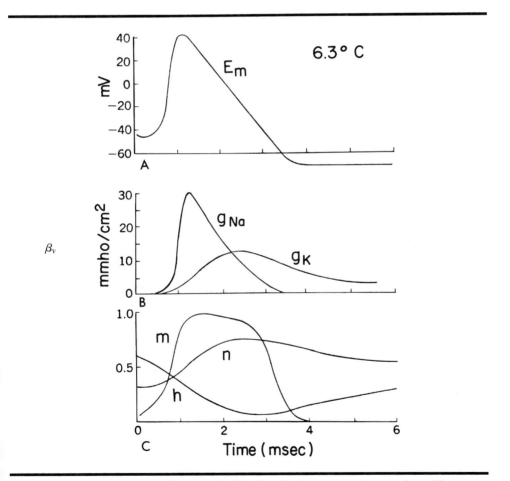

β_v

Figure 1–12 Relationship between membrane voltage (A), sodium and potassium conductance (B), and the variables m, n, and h (C) during a normal action potential. Values shown are for squid axon at 6.3° C. (Adapted from Hodgkin et al., 1952.)

sodium equilibrium potential, as would be anticipated from the Goldman equation. This depolarization produces a further increase in sodium conductance, and a regenerative process is initiated. Several hundred microseconds later, sodium inactivation begins to make its presence felt. Because of progressive inactivation, sodium conductance and, hence, sodium current rises to a maximum and then declines. Maximum sodium current actually occurs slightly before the peak of the action potential. During membrane depolarization, conductance to potassium is increasing towards a maximum at a slower rate. Potassium conductance soon dominates the Goldman expression again and, as expected, membrane potential repolarizes rapidly towards the potassium equilibrium potential. Soon thereafter potassium conductance reaches its maximal value and sodium inactivation reduces sodium conductance to resting levels. At this point the membrane potential will be even closer to V_K than in the resting state, and a hyperpolarizing afterpotential will be seen. The act of repolarization, however, reverses the voltage-dependent potassium conductance and it too returns towards a resting state. Soon G_K and G_{Na} are at their pre-excitation values and membrane potential has returned to the normal resting level. With time, the inactivation process which shut down the sodium system during depolarization will reverse, the sodium system will once again be available for stimulation, and subsequent action potentials can be produced.

During the period immediately following an action potential, when significant sodium inactivation is still present, there will be insufficient sodium conductance available to generate on action potential and the membrane will be inexcitable. This period is referred to as the absolute refractory period of the membrane. As inactivation reverses, there is an interval during which greater than normal depolarization will be required to stimulate an action potential, reflecting the smaller than normal number of channels available for excitation; this corresponds to the classical relative refractory period. In squid axon at 5° C all membrane parameters return to pre-stimulation values within 30 msec. In mammalian nerve at 37° C this interval is considerably shorter.

SEPARATION OF IONIC CURRENTS AND IONIC CHANNELS

A major question for early electrophysiologists studying excitable membranes was whether both sodium and potassium ions moved sequentially through the same pathway in the membrane, or whether separate ion-specific channels existed. Research on a number of naturally occurring toxins which exert their fatal influence by poisoning nerve and muscle membranes has provided a direct answer. The best known of these toxins is tetrodotoxin, a small molecule derived from the Japanse puffer fish, which blocks the generation of action potentials at concentrations as low as 10^{-9} M. Application of tetrodotoxin to a squid axon under voltage clamp conditions completely eliminates the early inward current and leaves a residual current analogous to that seen when external sodium is replaced by choline (Fig. 1–13) (Hille, 1970). The family of voltage clamp patterns observed in the presence of tetrodotoxin can be duplicated exactly by a computer simulation which eliminates the term for sodium current and assumes the presence only of voltage-dependent potassium currents (Hille, 1970). This observation implies that sodium currents can be selectively blocked without interfering with potassium currents and that, therefore, these two current pathways must be independent.

Studies of a complementary toxin, tetraethylammonium ion (TEA), provide further support for this concept. When TEA is applied internally to an axon under similar voltage clamp conditions, the early inward currents are not affected. However, there is a progressive decline and

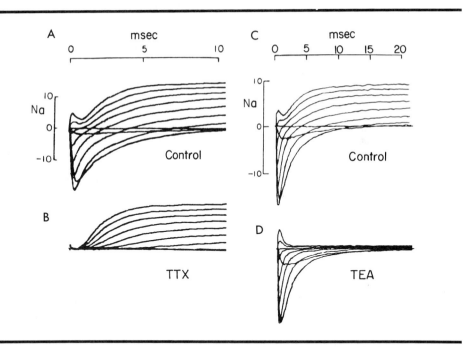

Figure 1–13 Sodium and potassium currents in nerve membrane can be independently blocked by different pharmacological agents. Tetrodotoxin (TTX) selectively eliminates the early currents obtained under voltage clamp conditions *(A, B)* while the late K$^+$ currents are unaffected. Tetraethylammonium (TEA) selectively eliminates the late K$^+$ currents while leaving the magnitude and kinetic characteristics of the early Na$^+$ currents unaltered *(C, D)*. These and similar data strongly support the concept that Na$^+$ and K$^+$ currents flow through the membrane by separate pathways. (Adapted from Hille, 1970.)

eventual loss of all the delayed outward currents normally associated with potassium ions (Hille, 1970). Computer simulations of the voltage clamp patterns obtained after TEA treatment indicate that the membrane has lost its potassium conductance system, although the sodium conductance system appears to be unaffected (Fig. 1–13).

Since both the sodium and potassium conductance systems can be blocked or modified by a number of different agents without affecting their counterpart, most physiologists are convinced that these systems represent separate pathways through the membrane which function independently. Although outside the scope of this discussion at the present time, the preponderance of evidence concerning the number of ions moving through each pathway per unit time, the temperature dependence of this ion movement, and other related factors suggest that the pathways consist of aqueous channels formed by protein molecules extending through the lipid bilayer, rather than carrier molecules which bind and transport ions through the hydrophobic membrane interior.

Activation and inactivation of conductances can be thought of in terms of changes in channel conformation such that ions are either precluded from access or facilitated in their movement through the aqueous interior. One would predict that the "gating" of these channels between on and off states depends upon the movement of charged or polar segments of the molecules comprising the channel according to their voltage-dependent characteristics. Recently, considerable progress has been made in detecting the very small currents associated with the movement of these gating particles (Armstrong, 1975). It appears that channel gating is more complex than originally suggested from simple voltage clamp experiments, but the overall scheme proposed by Hodgkin and Huxley has stood the test of time remarkably well. Nearly 30 years after their initial publication of the ionic conductance theory of action potential propagation, the basic premises remain unchallenged.

THE PROPAGATED ACTION POTENTIAL

With this information the question of propagation of the action potential along an axon can be examined. The simplest form of propagation is found in unmyelinated nerve fibers. Injection of a depolarizing current pulse at a single point along the axon results in a local drop in membrane potential; if threshold is exceeded, an action potential will be produced at this point. Let us assume that the external stimulus is removed immediately after threshold is attained, so that the only current flowing across the membrane will be that associated with the action potential itself. The upstroke of the action potential is accompanied by a significant inward flow of current. This current is dissipated by passive spread along the axon and out across the surface membrane to complete the local circuit (Fig. 1–14). The net result of this local current flow is progressive depolarization of the immediately contiguous areas of membrane until they, too, reach threshold levels and initiate regenerative responses of their own. Thus, a wave of local current

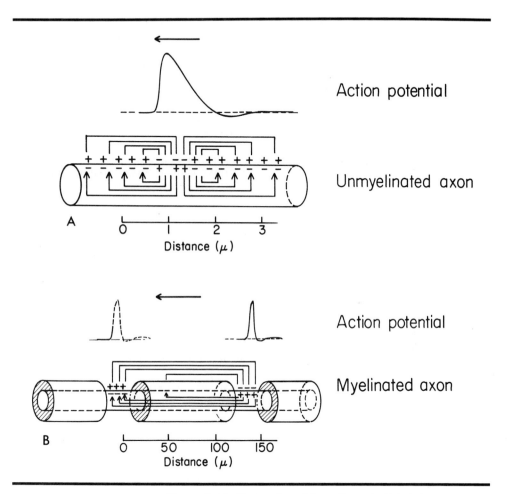

Figure 1–14 Propagation of the action potential. *A,* In unmyelinated nerve fibers local currents flowing as the result of depolarization of a small patch of membrane during an action potential produce depolarization and activation of immediately adjacent membrane. Conduction takes place by sequential activation of adjacent membrane regions in a continuous fashion which involves the entire surface membrane. *B,* In myelinated fibers, action potential generation is confined to the nodal membrane. Local currents spread along the internode due to the excellent passive properties contributed by the myelin, and exit mainly through the low resistance pathway provided by the next nodal region. Here depolarization and activation result in another action potential, although the intervening internodal membrane has not been activated.

moves just ahead of the action potential, continuously invading new areas of unexcited membrane and producing sequential depolarization and excitation. As one point on the membrane approaches the peak of its action potential the area immediately behind it will be in the recovery phase, while the area immediately in front of it will be just initiating its depolarizing upstroke. An instantaneous snapshot of the voltage profile of this propagating wave of depolarization moving along the axon resembles an action potential in reverse, while the time-dependent change in potential recorded at a single point will have the expected waveform of the familiar action potential.

Conduction along unmyelinated fibers is inherently continuous. Each and every point of membrane becomes sequentially activated as the action potential moves along the fiber. What factors determine the speed at which such a signal moves in a given axon? The major determinant will be the time required for current resulting from an action potential at a given point to depolarize an adjacent membrane region to threshold. Conduction will be optimized by factors which minimize the passive decay of the signal with distance along the axon. The passive cable equation (Eq. 1–10) shows that such optimization can be achieved by increasing the ratio R_m/R_i. The passive resistance of a unit area of surface membrane (R_m) is fixed by its biochemical structure and is not readily modifiable *in vivo* if that membrane is to behave in an excitable manner. R_i reflects both the specific resistivity of a unit volume of cytoplasm and the cross-sectional area of a fiber, and can be altered simply by varying axonal diameter. Increasing axonal area will decrease R_i, and vice versa. Since incremental increases in diameter will increase the cross-sectional area of an axon much more than the area of surface membrane associated with a unit length of axon, the ratio R_m/R_i will increase with diameter. One could calculate that the length constant λ should increase with the square of the diameter, and that conduction velocity should follow a similar relationship. Large nonmyelinated axons should conduct faster than small axons and, indeed, this can be experimentally verified (Burrows et al., 1965). However, in order to obtain continued increases in velocity, progressively larger increments in diameter must be made. Thus, the rapid signalling required between ganglia in an invertebrate such as squid containing only unmyelinated fibers requires axons of monumental diameter, an evolutionary quirk of incalculable benefit to modern electrophysiologists.

SALTATORY CONDUCTION

The large fiber diameter required for rapid axonal conduction velocity does not represent a limiting problem in simple invertebrate systems, but introduces severe limitations when the packing density of axons in the mammalian central nervous system is considered. Alternative methods of increasing the velocity of propagation in a more space-conservative manner are required.

In higher organisms a system of axonal conduction has evolved which resembles in its organization the structure of a long distance communications cable. Discrete areas or nodes of excitable membrane capable of generating action potentials are separated by stretches of axon called internodal regions, specially modified to optimize passive propagation of electrical signals. These two regions, respectively, are analogous to the periodic repeater amplifiers in a communications line and the specially shielded cables which interconnect them. The internodal regions must be designed so that the voltage change induced at one node through the production of an action potential is passively propagated to the next node, with small enough losses for the second node to be depolarized past threshold and the process sequentially repeated. Increasing axonal diameter helps to improve passive propagation, but is costly in terms of space. The alternative approach is to increase R_m and decrease C_m in the internode by increasing the thickness of the layer separating the axoplasm from the extracellular space, thus reducing losses due to radial current flow in this region. Such an increase is accomplished *in vivo* by myelination of the axon. Multiple layers of myelin formed from the opposed surface membrane of Schwann cells in the PNS or oligodendroglial cells in the CNS are wrapped around the axon in these internodal regions to form a compact spiral. The thicker the myelin sheath, the greater will be the resistance to radial current flow. In addition, since capacitance depends upon the ability of a material to hold opposite charges very close together while still separated, increasing thickness also reduces membrane capacitance in the internodal region. The net result of these two factors is that less current is required to alter the charge on the residual membrane capacitance, smaller amounts of current flow radially as opposed to axially, and signal degradation as a function of distance is minimized.

In a myelinated fiber, only the nodal membrane appears to be excitable. Current flow along the internode is always in an outward direction, and there is no evidence of active excitation in this region (Huxley and Stämpfli, 1949). The majority of the inward current generated during a nodal action potential passes down the axon and exits across the next nodal region, which represents the lowest resistance pathway to complete the local circuit (Fig. 1–14). Propagation in the internode is passive and serves only to excite the next nodal region in line. The action potential thus jumps from node to node in a discontinuous or "saltatory" fashion. Nonmyelinated fibers which conduct impulses in a continuous fashion may achieve conduction velocities of up to 10 to 15 meters/sec for fibers 10 μ in diameter. An optimally constructed myelinated fiber of the same average diameter can propagate an impulse at speeds in excess of 50 meters/sec.

Optimization of Conduction Velocity in Myelinated Nerve

With a nerve fiber of 10 μ in diameter, how would one best arrange the ratio of myelin thickness to axoplasmic diameter to optimize conduction velocity? Certainly, increasing myelin thickness will increase radial resistance, and that is desired. However, within the confines of a given total diameter, increasing myelin thickness occurs at the expense of decreasing axonal cross-sectional area. This, in turn, is reflected in an increase in axial resistance, R_i, a factor which will retard conduction. A balance must be struck between these two factors. One can carry out theoretical calculations to determine the thickness of myelin which will optimize these two variables, and several authors have reported that peak performance should be expected from a fiber in which 60 per cent of the overall diameter is occupied by the axon cytoplasm and the remaining outer shell by myelin (Deutsch, 1969; Smith and Koles, 1970). If the ratio of axonal diameter to total fiber diameter is measured in myelinated fibers of various sizes in different species one is impressed with the fact that the ratio is very close to 0.6 for virtually all fibers measured (Schnepp and Schnepp, 1971). Natural processes tend, as much as possible, to optimize axon structure for peak conduction efficiency.

A second factor to be considered in optimizing conduction velocity in myelinated axons is the distance between active nodal regions. When the properties of the internodal membrane are such that signals can propagate passively for long distances without decrement, the nodes can be spaced far apart. Conversely, when internodal conditions limit passive propagation, active regions must be placed closer together so that a given node can still be excited by the current flow set up at the penultimate node. It could be anticipated that large myelinated fibers can support long internodal distances, while smaller fibers would require shorter distances between nodes. Experimental measurements confirm an approximately linear relationship between axon diameter and internodal length in myelinated fibers, although there is considerable variability in internodal length among fibers of a given diameter (Rasminsky and Sears, 1972). In most species studied, the internodal length is between 75 and 175 times the fiber diameter (Paintel, 1978).

Consider a fiber 25 μ in diameter and with an internodal length of 2500 μ which nearly optimizes conduction velocity. What would be the effect of subdividing a given internode into two, four, or more shorter internodes with their associated active nodal regions? Propagation through this region would proceed by progressive sequential activation of each node, and the time required to conduct the potential through these short internodes would be longer than that required to traverse the original optimized internode. Thus, it follows that processes which lead to demyelination of an internode and subsequent remyelination with multiple abnormally short internodes will produce conduction slowing (Chapter 8).

Alterations in the properties of the internodal myelin sheath, especially in the immediate vicinity of the nodal region, will have profound effects on conduction velocity in myelinated fibers. Thinning of the myelin either by demyelination or by abnormal initial myelination has two effects: it reduces the effective resistance between axon interior and extracellular fluid, and it increases the capacitance between these two conductors. Both of these actions increase radial flow of current during passive electrotonic spread of an impulse and thereby reduce the current available for excitation at the next node. A longer time must elapse before sufficient current flow occurs at the next node to cause depolarization to threshold, resulting in conduction slowing. If radial current loss is increased sufficiently in the internode, threshold will never be exceeded at the next node, and conduction failure will occur (these phenomena will be discussed in more detail in Chapter 8).

The third factor affecting conduction velocity in myelinated fibers is variation in ambient temperature. The rates at which the sodium and potassium channels undergo their transitions from low to high conductance states is dependent upon temperature in a manner similar to that observed for the temperature dependence of enzymatic reactions (Hodgkin and Huxley, 1952c). These rates increase about threefold for each 10° C increase in temperature. Thus, the time scale over which membrane depolarization and repolarization occur during an action potential at 0° C may occupy 12 msec from onset to return to normal resting potential, while the same process at 30° C requires only 3 msec. Clearly, then, temperature will affect the rate of propagation of the action potential along an axon.

An additional factor must be considered in saltatory conduction along a myelinated axon. Here, passive propagation of electrical transients along the internode is especially important. The length constant of such an internode depends upon the ratio of axial to radial resistances, where axial resistance is attributable to the electrolytic properties of the axoplasm. The resistance of such an electrolyte solution will drop about 1.3-fold for each 10° C increase in temperature. When the temperature dependence of membrane rate parameters and of axoplasmic resistivity are included in computer simulations of saltatory conduction in a myelinated fiber, the effects of changes in temperature on overall conduction velocity can be evaluated. Recently published simulations suggest that the most likely relationship between temperature and conduction velocity in a myelinated fiber over the range between 0° and 40° C will be an exponential function with a Q_{10} (that is, the expected change in value per 10° C change in temperature) of 1.68 (Moore et al., 1978).

Few systematic investigations of the relationship between temperature and conduction velocity in human myelinated fibers have been performed. One recent study found an exponential temperature dependence of conduction velocity for both myelinated sensory and motor fibers in major limb nerves (DeJesus et al., 1973). The Q_{10} for this relationship averaged 1.55, close to that predicted by theoretical simulations. These considerations are of particular importance in the clinical evaluation of nerve conduction velocities. Distal limb temperature can vary considerably as a function of such factors as ambient temperatures, and abnormal distal vasoregulation. These variations in limb temperature, if uncorrected, can be sufficient to reduce the conduction velocity of a

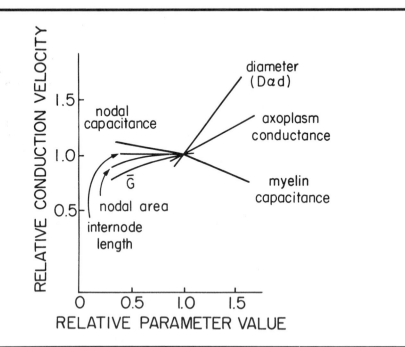

Figure 1–15 A summary of the variation in relative conduction velocity for a theoretical myelinated axon which will result from alteration of various axonal characteristics. (From Moore et al., 1978.)

normal nerve into the abnormal range, resulting in an incorrect diagnosis of neuropathy. This difficulty can be circumvented by routinely monitoring skin temperature and correcting measured conduction velocities using published formulas (DeJesus et al., 1973), or by controlling limb temperature with servoregulated radiant heaters.

Conduction processes in peripheral nerves are optimized for maximal velocity of signal propagation. Pathological processes which alter any of a number of myelin or axonal parameters will result in deterioration or failure of impulse propagation. A summary of the theoretically expected changes in conduction velocity in a typical myelinated fiber for increases or decreases in the various parameters discussed above has been compiled in a single figure by Moore et al. (1978) (Fig. 1–15). Application of the concepts presented here to specific pathophysiological states will be the subject of the following chapters.

References

Armstrong, C. M.: Ionic pores, gates and gating currents. Q. Rev. Biophys., *7*:179–210, 1975.

Burrows, T. M., Campbell, I. A., Howe, E. J., and Young, J. Z.: Conduction velocity and diameter of nerve fibers of cephalopods. J. Physiol., *179*:39P, 1965.

Cole, K. C., and Curtis, H. J.: Electrical impedance of the squid giant axon during activity. J. Gen. Physiol., *22*:649–670, 1939.

DeJesus, P. V., Hausmanowa-Petrusewicz, I., and Barchi, R. L.: The effect of cold on nerve conduction of human fast and slow nerve fibers. Neurology, *23*:1182–1189, 1973.

Deutsch, S.: The maximization of nerve conduction velocity. I.E.E.E. Trans. Sys. Sci. Cybernet., *5*:86–91, 1969.

Edidin, M.: Translational and rotational diffusion in membranes. Annu. Rev. Biophys. Bioeng., *3*:179–201, 1974.

Glynn, I. M.: The action of cardiac glycosides on ion movement. Pharmacol. Rev., *16*:381–407, 1964.

Goldman, D. E.: Potential, impedance and rectification in membranes. J. Gen. Physiol., *27*:37–60, 1943.

Henn, F. A., and Thompson, T. E.: Synthetic lipid bilayer membranes. Annu. Rev. Biochem., *38*:241–262, 1969.

Hille, B.: Ion channels in nerve membranes. Prog. Biophys. Mol. Biol., *21*:1–32, 1970.

Hodgkin, A. L., and Horowicz, P.: Movements of sodium and potassium in single muscle fibers. J. Physiol., *145*:405–432, 1959.

Hodgkin, A. L., and Huxley, A. F.: Currents carried by sodium and potassium ions through the membrane of the giant axon of *Loligo*. J. Physiol., *116*:449–472, 1952a.

Hodgkin, A. L., and Huxley, A. F.: The dual effect of membrane potential on sodium conductance in the giant axon of *Loligo*. J. Physiol., *116*:497–506, 1952b.

Hodgkin, A. L., and Huxley, A. F.: A quantitative description of membrane current and its application to conduction and excitation in nerve. J. Physiol., *117*:500–544, 1952c.

Hodgkin, A. L., Huxley, A. F., and Katz, B.: Measurement of current-voltage relations in the membrane of the giant axon of *Loligo*. J. Physiol., *116*:424–448, 1952.

Hodgkin, A. L., and Katz, B.: The effect of sodium ions on the electrical activity of the giant axon of the squid. J. Physiol., *108*:37–77, 1949.

Hodgkin, A. L., and Keynes, R.: Active transport of cations in giant axons from *Sepia* and *Loligo*. J. Physiol., *128*:28–60, 1955.

Hodgkin, A. L., and Rushton, W. A.: The electrical constants of a crustacean nerve fiber. Proc. R. Soc. Lond. [Biol.], *133*:444–479, 1946.

Huxley, A. F., and Stämpfli, R.: Evidence for saltatory conduction in peripheral myelinated nerve fibers. J. Physiol., *108*:315–339, 1949.

Lee, A. G.: Functional properties of biological membranes: A physical-chemical approach. Prog. Biophys. Mol. Biol., *29*:5–56, 1975.

Marmor, M. F., and Gorman, A. L.: Membrane potential as the sum of ionic and metabolic components, Science, *167*:65–67, 1970.

Moore, J. W., Joyner, R. W., Brill, M. H., Waxman, S. D., and Najar-Joa, M.: Simulations of conduction in uniform myelinated fibers. Biophys. J., *21*:147–160, 1978.

Mueller, P., and Rudin, D. O.: Translocators in lipid bimolecular membranes: Their role in dissipative and conservative bioenergy transductions. *In* Sanadi, D. R. (ed.): Current Topics in Bioenergetics, Vol. 3. New York, Academic Press, 1969, pp. 157–249.

Paintel, A. S.: Conduction properties of normal peripheral mammalian axons. *In* Waxman, S. G., (ed.): Physiology and Pathobiology of Axons. New York, Raven Press, 1978, pp. 131–144.

Rasminsky, M., and Sears, T. A.: Internodal conduction in undissected demyelinated nerve fibers. J. Physiol., *22*:323–350, 1972.

Rojas, E., and Armstrong, C. M.: Sodium conductance activation without inactivation in pronase-perfused axons. Nature [New Biol.], *229*:177–178, 1971.

Schnepp, P., and Schnepp, G.: Faseranalytische Untersuchung an peripherin Nerven bei Tieren verschiedener Grösse. Z. Zellforsch. *119*:99–114, 1971.

Singer, S. J.: The molecular organization of membranes. Annu. Rev. Biochem., *43*:805–835, 1974.

Singer, S. J., and Nicolson, G. L.: The fluid mosaic model of the structure of cell membranes. Science, *175*:720–722, 1972.

Skou, S. J.: Enzymatic basis for active transport of Na^+ and K^+ across cell membranes. Physiol. Rev., *45*:596–617, 1965.

Smith, R. S., and Koles, Z. J.: Myelinated nerve fibers: Computed effect of myelin thickness on conduction velocity. Am. J. Physiol., *219*:1256–1258, 1970.

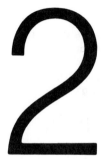

Cutaneous Receptors

A. K. McIntyre

INTRODUCTION

The surface of the skin is found to be a mosaic of tiny sensorial areas . . . . Each, doubtless, coincides with the site of some sensorial "end-organ" or with a tiny cluster of such. Rather, indeed, than to a mosaic may the skin be likened to a sheet of water wherein grow water-plants, some sunken and some floating. An object thrown upon the surface moves the foliage commensurately with the violence of its impact, its dimensions, and with their propinquity to its place of incidence. Where the foliage grows densely, not a pebble striking the surface but will meet some leaf; and beyond that or those directly struck, a number will be indirectly disturbed before equilibrium of the surface is re-established.*

Although written some 80 years ago, these characteristically vivid words of Sherrington can scarcely be bettered as an introduction to the topic of cutaneous sensibility. The skin's rich and complex neural endowment not only provides an effective system for detecting relevant mechanical and thermal events impinging upon it, but also contributes crucially, through reflex and behavioral mechanisms, to the overall protective function subserved by this extensive interface between the organism and its immediate environment. Cutaneous sensory function has been the subject of symposia and reviews in recent years, some of them extensive — for example, Kenshalo (1968), Andres and von Düring (1973), Burgess and Perl (1973), Hensel (1973), Iggo (1974, 1977), Boivie and Perl (1975), Iggo and Ilyinsky (1976), and Zotterman (1976).

These reviews discuss the morphology as well as the functional properties of the array of sensory terminals in the skin and subcutaneous tissues, together with the role of these receptors in signalling the various modalities of sensation, and describe in considerable detail the experimental evidence on which our current understanding of cutaneous sensory function is based. Prominent among the newer findings discussed are matters such as the

*Sherrington, 1900, pp. 920–921.

now incontrovertible demonstration that particular nerve endings show selective sensitivity to particular stimuli, achievement of the technically exacting procedure of recording impulses from single unmyelinated and fine myelinated afferent fibers, substantial progress in disclosure of the fine structure of particular cutaneous receptors and their functional roles, and extension of electrophysiological studies to the primate skin, including that of man. As a result, the ghost of the so-called "pattern theory" of cutaneous sensation (e.g., Sinclair, 1955) — which, at least initially, denied the existence of receptor specificity — has been finally laid to rest, and the Sherringtonian concept of the arrays of cutaneous receptors acting as "peripheral analyzers" has been completely vindicated.

This account, therefore, necessarily draws heavily on reviews such as those cited above, and aims to do no more than provide a reasonably succinct summary of current understanding of cutaneous receptor function.

PATTERNS OF SKIN SENSIBILITY

Since its first disclosure nearly 100 years ago (Blix, 1882), the nonuniformity of the skin's sensitivity has been amply confirmed by psychophysical testing in man; indeed, generations of physiology students have repeated in their laboratory classes at least the essential observations of the early pioneers. Exploration of the skin surface with calibrated bristles (Frey's hairs), fine thermal probes, sharp needles, or with weak discrete electrical stimulation (Bishop, 1946) reveals arrays of separate spot-like regions, each yielding to stimuli not much above threshold one of four recognizably distinct sensations: touch, coldness, warmth, or pain. Maps of the distribution of such spots can be made, both for hairy and glabrous skin. However, with stimulation substantially above threshold for the sensory spots, their specificity is less apparent; for example, strong stimulation of a "touch spot" may be painful. Nor are the skin regions between spots completely insentient. Thus, the sensory spots can better be regarded as foci of maximal sensitivity in areas of responsiveness to a particular type of stimulus, the margins of which may overlap with those of other adjacent sentient zones. Both the density of spot distribution, and the proportions of the different kinds of sensory foci, vary widely from one region of the body surface to another.

REGIONAL DIFFERENCES Tactile spots are more numerous and closely packed in glabrous skin on extremities and face than in hairy skin, and their density is lowest in skin of the proximal limbs and trunk. Spot density increases as more distal regions of the extremities are tested, being greatest in the fingerpads, especially of the index finger. Comparable density of touch spots also occurs in the lips, while they are least densely distributed on the skin of the back. In addition to disclosing its punctate nature, psychophysical testing reveals other aspects of cutaneous sensibility. Apart from recognizing the quality or "modality" of a stimulus, a normal conscious subject of course recognizes, within limits, the site of its application (localization) and also its spatial extent, intensity, and configuration. The latter can be tested by asking a blindfolded subject to recognize patterns (for example, letters or figures) drawn on the skin by a blunt probe. Two point discrimination, or the ability to recognize whether a stimulus is small and confined to a single point or consists of two spatially separated stimuli, is another practical test of the spatial resolution achievable by the skin's sensory mechanisms. This capacity can be shown for any of the four basic modalities, although with differing levels of accuracy; in practice, testing is usually confined to the tactile sense, for which discrimination is best. Striking differences can be demonstrated for different regions of the body surface in accuracy of localization, pattern recognition, and in two point discrimination, doubtless related to the varying density of the array of sensory spots. Regional variations are also apparent in the proportions of foci optimally responsive to different stimulus modalities. For example, tactile spots predominate in glabrous skin of the extremities and head, whereas in hairy skin of the forearm, pain spots are relatively more numerous (Ranson et al., 1935). The relatively sparse tactile spots in hairy skin tend to occur in the vicinity of hairs, especially in the skin regions opposite to the direction taken by the emerging hairs. Temperature-sensitive foci in most regions are the least common, amounting to no more than 3 per cent of the total sensory spots on the volar surface of the forearm. Furthermore, fewer "warm" than "cold" spots can be detected in most regions.

The absolute threshold for perception of a stimulus also differs for different regions of the skin surface. Despite the much greater density of touch spots in glabrous skin, threshold for tactile stimulation of hairy skin may be as low or lower, presumably because of the much thicker epidermis of some glabrous skin areas — for example, the sole of the foot. However, accuracy of localization of a tactile stimulus, and two point discrimination, are much better developed in glabrous than in hairy skin. The minimum distance between the sites of application of a double tactile stimulus (e.g., the blunted points of a pair of dividers) which can be recognized as a double rather than a single stimulus is least at the tip of the tongue, and largest in the skin of the proximal limbs and trunk. For example, the minimal separable distance at the tongue tip is of the order of 1 to 2 mm, for glabrous skin of the finger pads and of the lips, 2 to 5 mm, and for hairy skin in proximal regions of the limbs and the trunk, as much as 50 to 100 mm (Weinstein, 1968).

43

CUTANEOUS RECEPTORS

In view of the punctiform nature of cutaneous sensibility, it is easy to understand the temptation to assign
each of the four distinct qualities of sensation elicited
from these spot-like foci to different, histologically recognizable sensory structures in the skin, and this indeed is what von Frey essayed to do in 1895 (see
Sherrington, 1900; Somjen, 1972). Von Frey suggested
that Meissner corpuscles and endings around hair
shafts subserve tactile sense, Krause end-bulbs and
Ruffini endings cold and warmth, respectively, and
nonspecialized, free branching nerve endings, the
sense of pain. This scheme has held sway in many
editions of standard textbooks until quite recently.
However, histological studies of marked sensory spots
yielding different sensations have not consistently revealed recognizably different organized receptors;
often, only a lacework of free nerve endings can be
seen. Another reason why this relatively rigid association of the different sensory foci with particular types
of end-organ has fallen into disfavor is that repeated
testing of the same skin area in a given subject may
not yield identical maps, the exact location and distribution of the spots apparently changing after an interval of some hours (Dallenbach, 1927). It is nevertheless now widely accepted that, despite being erroneous
in detail, the principle behind von Frey's theoretical
scheme remains valid. This is so despite vigorous attacks on the basic notion that different cutaneous receptors show selective sensitivity to different kinds of
stimulus energy (e.g., Sinclair, 1955), a concept crucial
to the von Frey hypothesis and which, in recent years,
has been proved beyond doubt by electrophysiological
studies of single sensory units.

AFFERENT NERVE FIBERS SUBSERVING CUTANEOUS SENSIBILITY Before discussing the functional properties of the receptor elements responsible for cutaneous sensibility, it is
appropriate to consider the transmission lines along
which nerve signals evoked by skin stimulation travel on
their way to the central nervous system. This is so
because the electrophysiological analysis of sensory
units, on which present understanding of cutaneous
receptor function is largely based, must take into account the size and related properties of the range of
afferent fibers found in cutaneous nerves. Furthermore,
the properties of these cutaneous conducting lines may
be altered by injury or disease, as well as by local
disturbances such as compression, hypoxia, or the action of anesthetic agents. Useful information about the
state of these afferent fibers can be obtained by recording the compound action potential, at least in the more
accessible peripheral nerves.

FIBER COMPOSITION OF CUTANEOUS NERVES The
axons in cutaneous nerves are mostly afferent, with
their cell bodies in ganglia of dorsal spinal roots

or their equivalent in cranial nerves. They originate in the array of sensory terminals in and beneath the epidermis and, for short distances in their initial course, thread their way through two plexuses of nerve fibers, mostly very fine, one superficial and lying just beneath the epidermis and the other a deeper nerve network in the dermis. From the latter spring the peripheral fascicles which combine to form the various cutaneous nerves, or else join mixed sensorimotor nerve trunks. The axons in a purely skin nerve such as the sural or medial cutaneous nerve of the forearm vary widely in size, from fairly large myelinated to small unmyelinated fibers. The latter group includes a substantial number which are not sensory but efferent: postganglionic autonomic axons, with cell bodies in the paravertebral sympathetic ganglia, destined to supply sweat glands and smooth muscle of subcutaneous blood vessels and of hairs. All the myelinated and most of the unmyelinated fibers are afferent and, apart from a few serving joint receptors in some instances, represent the channels of communication between sensory endings in the epidermis and subcutaneous tissues and the spinal cord or brain stem.

The myelinated fibers are easily stained and measured; the unmyelinated component, although detectable by silver staining, demands electron microscopy for reliable counting and measurement. It was first shown by Ranson et al. (1935) that the unmyelinated fibers substantially outnumber those with myelin sheaths in most skin nerves. Even after making allowance for the efferent sympathetic component, sensory unmyelinated fibers constitute some 60 to 70 per cent of the total afferent fiber spectrum of skin nerves supplying the limbs and trunk. However, in cutaneous branches of the trigeminal nerve, the proportion of afferent unmyelinated fibers is substantially lower.

MYELINATED AFFERENT FIBER SPECTRUM The range of diameters of cutaneous afferent fibers extends from a maximum of about 16μm down to less than 0.5 μm for the smallest unmyelinated fibers. For convenience, it is the overall diameter of a myelinated fiber which is usually measured; thus, the figure applies to the axon plus its sheath. The smallest cutaneous myelinated fibers so measured are between 1 and 2 μm in diameter, and the largest from about 10 to 16 μm, depending upon the particular skin nerve. For example, in the study of human nerves by Ranson et al. (1935), the largest fibers in the medial cutaneous of the forearm, lateral cutaneous of the thigh, superficial radial, and dorsal digital nerves were between 15 to 16 μm, 13 to 14 μm, 12 to 13 μm, and 10 to 11 μm, respectively.

The spectra constructed by plotting frequency of occurrence against fiber diameter are essentially bimodal

45

for all mammalian cutaneous nerves, with the smaller fibers grouping about a prominent peak at 2 to 4 μm, and the larger forming a less well defined pile peaking at diameters between 7 and 11 μm, depending upon the species and nerve chosen (e.g., Ranson et al., 1935; Hunt and McIntyre, 1960; Iggo, 1974). The smaller fibers predominate; for example, in the human sural nerve there are approximately twice as many small as large myelinated fibers (Iggo, 1977). With the unmyelinated component also included, the smaller fibers far outnumber the larger in most cutaneous nerves; according to Ranson et al. (1935), the unmyelinated, together with myelinated fibers smaller than 5 μm, constitute 90 per cent of the total number in the medial cutaneous nerve of the human forearm.

CLASSIFICATION OF NERVE FIBERS The terminology of fiber classification is unfortunately confusing, as two systems are in use. The earlier scheme arose from the pioneer work of Gasser and his colleagues (1939) in which fiber groups were designated by letters of the alphabet. Myelinated fibers were subdivided into two groups, labelled A and B; the A fibers included all somatic myelinated fibers, efferent as well as afferent, ranging from the smallest (1 to 2 μm) to the largest, with some 20 to 22 μm in diameter. Several subgroups of the A fibers were labelled with Greek letters — alpha, beta, gamma, and delta — in descending order of size. The B group only occurs in visceral nerves, such as the vagus and white *rami communicantes;* they are small, myelinated preganglionic autonomic axons. Gasser (1960) later showed that the A fibers of cutaneous nerves consist of just two subgroups, A alpha and A delta. Unmyelinated fibers, both somatic afferent and autonomic postganglionic efferent, were designated C fibers.

The other classification was introduced by Lloyd (1943), and applies only to afferent fibers. The largest myelinated fibers (12 to 22 μm) were labelled group I, intermediate-sized (6 to 12 μm) group II, and the smallest (1 to 5 μm) group III; unmyelinated fibers of dorsal root origin constituted group IV. Both systems are used for cutaneous nerves, although the largest (group I) fibers, properly speaking, are only found in muscle or mixed sensorimotor nerves. Thus, the group of largest fibers in skin nerves (those ranging from about 5 to 16 μm) may be designated group II, despite the overlap in diameters between the largest cutaneous and smallest group I muscle afferent fibers (Boyd and Davey, 1968); cutaneous group II fibers thus belong to Gasser's A alpha group. Group III corresponds closely with Gasser's A delta pile which, as already mentioned, peaks at a diameter between 2 to 4 μm.

CONDUCTION VELOCITY The most important factors affecting speed of impulse conduction along a nerve fiber are the axon diameter and the resistance to current flow across its plasma membrane. This is so because impulse propagation depends upon current flow between the zone occupied by an action potential and the region ahead, along the axon's core and across the membrane; the circuit is completed via the extracellular volume conductor. The thinner the fiber, the greater the longitudinal hindrance to current flow along the core, and the larger the transmembrane conductance, the smaller is the effective longitudinal spread of local current. Put differently, the length constant *lambda* (λ) of a fiber is small if its longitudinal core resistance is high, and its transmembrane resistance relatively low, and *vice versa.* Quantitatively, the relationship is expressed as

$$\lambda = \sqrt{\frac{r_m}{r_i}} \tag{2-1}$$

where λ is the length constant,* r_m is the transmembrane resistance, and r_i is the longitudinal core resistance, both per unit fiber length (Katz, 1966). Thus, conduction velocity is directly related to a fiber's length constant; axons of high length constant are of large diameter (low r_i) and have high membrane resistance (r_m) because of the extensive internodal insulation by myelin, and these fibers conduct at high velocity. Conversely, fine unmyelinated fibers have small length constants and their impulses travel slowly.

The range of conduction velocities for mammalian A fibers, at central body temperature, is from 120 m/sec for the largest Aα (group I) fibers down to 3 to 5 m/sec for the smallest Aδ (group III) fibers. Conduction velocity of afferent C fibers (diameters 0.4 to 1.3 μm) ranges from 0.4 to 2 m/sec. As would be expected, *temperature* is a variable which affects conduction velocity in all nerve fibers. Factors related to fiber diameter also determine threshold to external electrical stimulation; for example, the low r_i of large fibers favors flow of stimulating current across the membrane and along the core, so that very weak stimuli can lower membrane potential to trigger level at the cathode. Therefore, when a mixture of afferent axons, as in a dorsal spinal root, is subjected to graded stimulation, only the largest (group I) fibers are activated by weak shocks just above threshold, while those of decreasing diameter are progressively recruited as stimulus intensity is increased. Shocks of 100 or more times threshold intensity may be required to recruit the smallest unmeylinated fibers in a peripheral nerve.

---

*The length constant is the distance from a point 0 at which a steady displacement of membrane potential (V_0) is being imposed by a weak constant current to the point on either side at which the potential displacement has decayed to a value of $1/\epsilon$ of V_0.

THE COMPOUND ACTION POTENTIAL When impulses are set up in all fibers of a nerve trunk by a maximal electrical stimulus, the recorded response represents the summated action of the individual axons. However, the contribution of each is directly related to its diameter, so that potentials of the large A fibers predominate. In this respect the compound action potential is misleading for, as already noted, the great majority of fibers in a cutaneous nerve are small. Impulses in the smaller axons will also, of course, lag behind those travelling in the larger, despite their nearly simultaneous initiation. Recordings by external leads made progressively further away from the stimulating cathode thus present a series of deflections representing increasing temporal dispersion of the individual impulses, and the configuration of this summated response depends upon the distance between the stimulating and recording electrodes. The conditions for studying the compound action potentials in human subjects are far from ideal; stimulation and recording are usually performed percutaneously, and there are the attendant uncertainties concerning precise sites of stimulation and recording in addition to attenuation of signals and other problems. Nevertheless, with the help of modern recording equipment and computer averaging techniques, it is a valuable and widely used procedure for studying normal or disordered peripheral nerve function in man. Recording conditions in animal experiments are naturally much more favorable since the nerves are exposed in situ or maintained as isolated in vitro preparations, making possible monophasic recording, precise location of stimulating and recording leads, and accurate measurement of conduction distance (Fig. 2–1).

Most of our present understanding of the compound action potential is based upon the meticulous pioneer studies of Gasser and his colleagues (1939), in which they succeeded in reconstructing synthetic action potentials from the measured numbers and diameters of fibers in a nerve which matched the actual action potentials recorded remarkably closely, at the chosen conduction distance, from the same nerve before its histological analysis (e.g., Gasser and Grundfest, 1939). The relationship between fiber diameter and conduction velocity agrees with the results of Hursh (1939), obtained by a different method, that conduction velocity in m/sec of a myelinated fiber is approximately six times its (outside) diameter in μm. However, some discrepancies for the small fiber component are apparent. Gasser (personal communication) believed that the Hursh factor was approximately correct for the large but probably too high for the small A fibers. Recent work has confirmed this, a factor of 4.6 for Aδ (group III)

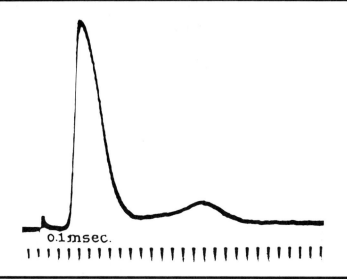

o.1msec.

Figure 2-1 Complete monophasic compound action potential of cat saphenous myelinated fibers, recorded at conduction distance of 3.15 cm, showing large, fast conducting Aα spike, and smaller, slower Aδ deflection. (From Gasser, 1960.)

fibers having been determined by Boyd and Kalu (1979).

One assumption necessary for action potential reconstruction is the duration of the impulse in each fiber. Gasser and Grundfest (1939) assumed, from a small number of recordings made from single axons, that spike duration in all mammalian A fibers is constant and approximately 0.4 m/sec. It is interesting to reflect that, in consequence, the length of fiber occupied at any instant by an action potential must be much greater in the larger fibers. For example, on this basis, an impulse in a myelinated fiber of 10-μm diameter, travelling at 60 m/sec, occupies a stretch of fiber 2.4 cm long. However, the constancy of A spike duration has been questioned by Paintal (1966), who concluded that the time course of action potentials in small myelinated fibers is longer than 0.4 m/sec. This and related matters are discussed in a thoughtful review by Jack (1975).

LOCAL FACTORS INFLUENCING NERVE CONDUCTION One factor already noted is temperature, with conduction velocity, within limits, varying directly with temperature. In a cool environment, temperature of the limbs, particularly their superficial tissues, may be substantially below central body temperature, so that conduction velocity in cutaneous nerves is slower than the

49

value found for the same fibers at 37° C. Taking the latter as 100 per cent, conduction velocity in both myelinated and unmyelinated axons is reduced by approximately 3 per cent for each 1° C of cooling, at least for nerve temperatures above 17° C (Franz and Iggo, 1968). For example, the 10-μm cutaneous nerve fiber conducting at 60 m/sec at 37° C, already referred to in relation to the "wave length" of its action potential, would conduct at 42 m/sec at 27° C. Temperature of the region under investigation must therefore be carefully measured and controlled in studies on human nerve.

Blockage of conduction can be effected by drastic cooling of nerve, and A fibers are more readily blocked than unmyelinated afferent C axons. The mean blocking temperature for a sample of feline saphenous afferent C axons is 2.7° C, whereas conduction in myelinated fibers of the same nerve fails at a mean value of 7.2° C (Franz and Iggo, 1968). Despite some results indicating differential blockade of myelinated fibers according to size, it appears that cooling blocks A fibers in random fashion. However, it must be kept in mind that cooling or other local blocking procedures may be more effective for impulse trains, the more usual physiological situation, than for single electrically evoked action potentials.

Blockade of afferent fibers by other agents, including local pressure, asphyxia, and local anesthetic agents, is also well known, and their actions are to some extent selective for different fiber groups. In general, local pressure or asphyxia blocks the larger members of the myelinated group more readily than the smaller Aδ and C fibers, in this respect having a more differential action than cooling. Local anesthetics, on the other hand, block in the reverse order, with unmyelinated axons being the first to fail, followed by the Aδ and lastly the Aα axons. But none of these procedures has a completely reliable and clearcut differential blocking action. Other more complicated blocking procedures involving, for example, weak constant current pulses, can bring about more reliable differential blockade under special experimental conditions, but these techniques will not be presented here. The effects on nerve conduction of pathological conditions will be discussed only briefly. Obviously, agents which damage myelin sheaths, such as diphtheria toxin and various other neurotoxic agents, must interfere with nerve conduction, either by slowing or complete blockade; this also seems to be the case in the various forms of peripheral neuropathy from other causes — for example, in diabetes. Common to most of these conditions, however, is marked slowing of conduction velocity, especially in the larger myelinated fibers, and greater temporal dispersion of the compound action potential.

**ELECTROPHYSIO-
LOGICAL
ANALYSIS OF
SKIN RECEPTORS**

Real understanding of the way in which sense organs translate the impingement thereon of adequate stimulus energy can be said to have begun with the cracking of the basic sensory code by Adrian and Zotterman (1926), through their successful recording of action potentials from a single sense organ. In the ensuing years, single unit studies have been applied to the examination of almost all known sensory receptors, including those of the skin, with increasing refinement of instrumentation and technical skill. Progress, at first slow, accelerated after World War II and became explosive at about the end of the 1950's, when it became possible to record adequate samples of single unit responses of receptors served by unmyelinated and the smallest myelinated fibers (Iggo, 1959; Iriuchijima and Zotterman, 1960; Hensel et al., 1960). Since then, many other workers have contributed a flood of further and increasingly quantitative information regarding the functional properties of cutaneous and subcutaneous sensory units served by fibers representing all groups present in skin nerves. The bulk of these experiments has been made with animal preparations, ranging from amphibia through reptiles, birds, and mammals, especially the cat and rabbit. However, in recent years, primate skin has been studied increasingly and, with the development of percutaneous microneurography (Vallbo and Hagbarth, 1968), many single unit studies of human cutaneous receptors have been made (e.g., Zotterman, 1976; Gordon, 1978).

The primate experiments have made it clear that there is a basic similarity in the cutaneous receptor mechanisms in all mammals studied so far despite disclosure of some significant differences; consequently, taking all the results together, a fairly clear picture of human cutaneous receptor function has emerged. Furthermore, recent extensive fine structural studies of the neural apparatus in and under the skin in a range of species, often performed in conjunction with electrophysiological analysis, have made possible the morphological identification of some functionally characterized receptors. Such correlations will be discussed subsequently.

Single primary afferent unit recordings can be made either by dissection of fine filaments under a dissecting binocular or by insertion of very fine electrodes into a doral root ganglion or nerve trunk, until an all-or-nothing action potential, derived either intracellularly or extracellularly, appears upon electrical stimulation of the particular skin nerve under study. Conduction velocity of the unit is calculated from the response latency and measured conduction distance between the stimulating cathode and recording site. By using appropriate restricted natural stimulation the axon's receptive field is located, and its extent mapped and measured. Controlled patterns of appropriate stimulation may be applied, such as variable step function or ramp-and-plateau mechanical pulses, or similar patterns of thermal stimulation, to determine the dynamic characteristics of the response. As a result of such studies, three main classes of receptors have been defined, according to the kind of stimulus energy which is effective: (1) *mechanoreceptors,* responding primarily to nondamaging mechanical manipulation of skin or hairs; (2) *thermoreceptors,* with high sensitivity to warming or cooling of their receptive fields; and (3) *nociceptors,* which respond only to strong, potentially or actually damaging mechanical, thermal, or chemical insult.

Within these main groups several subclasses can be defined on the basis of such factors as sensitivity to adequate stimulation, adaptation to a maintained stimulus, presence or absence of background firing, degree of stimulus selectivity, axonal conduction velocity, and size of receptive field. Although still used, the terms slowly and rapidly adapting (SA and RA) are becoming replaced by others which describe response characteristics more accurately. Units which continue responding to a steady stimulus may be designated "displacement receptors," and those purely phasic units which fire only during the dynamic phase of a stimulus are termed "transient receptors." The latter can be subdivided into "velocity" or "acceleration detectors" (Burgess and Perl, 1973). There are considerable regional variations in the proportions of different receptor types, their density, and size of receptive field and of serving axon, but units representative of the three major classes and most of their subdivisions are found throughout, in glabrous as well as in hairy skin (Burgess and Perl, 1973; Iggo, 1974).

Mechanoreceptors　　**MECHANORECEPTORS IN HAIRY SKIN** The most obvious mechanoreceptors in hairy skin are related to the hairs themselves, which extend the range of tactile sensitivity beyond the immediate skin surface. Because deflecting a hair shaft swings it around a subepidermal fulcrum, nerve endings located more deeply on the shaft can be engaged very effectively by this lever action. Hair receptors over the general body surface are all rapidly adapting, transient detectors; however, the complex vibrissal sinus hairs of many mammals — for example, rat or cat whiskers — are equipped with an array of endings which include displacement as well as transient detectors. Even the ordinary hair receptors of the general body surface can be subdivided into several different functional types on the basis of the kind of hair, its degree of dynamic sensitivity, conduction velocity of its afferent fiber, and extent of receptive field (Brown and Iggo, 1967; Burgess and Perl, 1973; Iggo, 1974). In a mammal such as the cat the two principle classes of hair are the thin, closely packed "down" hairs forming the undercoat, which constitute about 90 per cent of the total, and the stouter, much longer "guard" hairs, whose tips project and constitute the glossy outer coat.

Each afferent fiber activated by hair movement supplies, through peripheral branches in the subepidermal plexuses, a variable number of hair follicles in its receptive field, the area of which may be restricted to a few mm² or extend over as much as 600 mm². Furthermore, each of the fiber's terminal receptive ramifications end in similar classes of hair follicles, so that the hair receptor units can be subdivided primarily on this basis. Afferent fibers which discharge in response to movement of *down* hairs are of slow conduction velocity (10 to 30 m/sec), therefore belonging to the $A\delta$ (group III) component of skin nerves. These units (type D hair receptors) are exceedingly sensitive to deflection of groups of down hairs, firing repetitively during the movement and giving an "off" response as the hairs spring back on removal of the stimulus. If deflected by a ramp-and-hold stimulus no discharge takes place during the plateau but, because of hand tremor, irregular firing may occur if the deflection is maintained by a hand-held probe. Type D units may also discharge in response to vascular pulsation, and respond strongly to blowing on the fur.

Fibers responding to *guard* hair deflection belong to the $A\alpha$ (group II) moiety, with conduction velocities ranging from 40 to 90 m/sec. They are not fired by movement of down hairs within their receptive fields. Guard hair units (type G receptors) have been further divided into subgroups on the basis of such properties as critical slope for ramp stimulation and conduction velocity of afferent fiber. Thus, G_1 units respond only when hair movement is rapid (high critical slope), and their axons are among the most rapidly conducting $A\alpha$ fibers. G_2 units have lower critical slopes, give longer trains of impulses during hair deflection at constant velocity, give an "off" discharge, and their axons are more slowly conducting members of the $A\alpha$ group. Like the type D units, type G receptors do not respond to maintained hair deflection. Because in both type D and many type G units discharge frequency, within limits, is proportional to velocity of hair movement, hair receptors in general can be regarded as transient detectors signalling stimulus velocity (Fig. 2–2).

The receptive fields of individual hair receptor units vary considerably in size, as already mentioned. Within each receptive field a single afferent fiber may innervate relatively few hairs or branch extensively to supply a large number of follicles. Because several afferent fibers usually contribute terminals to a given follicle, movement of a single hair may activate several different receptor units. The degree of overlap of hair unit

53

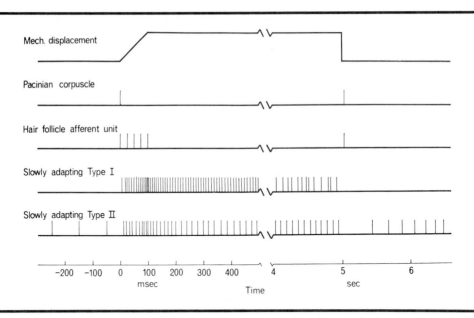

Figure 2–2 Diagram illustrating different discharge patterns of cutaneous transient and displacement mechanoreceptors, in response to "ramp-and-hold" stimulus *(upper tracing.) Abscissa,* time: onset of ramp at zero time (note break and change in time scale). (From Iggo and Gottschaldt 1974.)

receptive fields is quite remarkable; some idea of its extent is conveyed by the field plots in Figure 2–3, showing the fields of 152 hair units with fibers in the cat's sural nerve.

Another type of transient detector in hairy skin has been described, with terminals apparently not associated with hair follicles. These units have relatively large receptive fields and are activated by rapid distortion of the skin surface more readily than by deflection of hairs, although otherwise their properties resemble those of guard hair units. They have been termed *field* receptors (Burgess and Perl, 1973). In addition, receptors exceptionally sensitive to weak rapid transients and to high frequency vibration are found sparsely distributed over hairy skin surfaces; these are termed PC units, being subcutaneously located pacinian corpuscles (Hunt, 1961) which can be classed as acceleration detectors.

Slowly adapting displacement detectors in hairy skin are of three kinds, two with Aα myelinated and one with C unmyelinated afferent fibers. All have small receptive fields, those with myelinated axons being highly localized and spot-like. Of the latter, one variety (the type I or SA I unit) has an extremely discrete field which corresponds with a small dome-like skin elevation; these units respond only when a stimulating probe impinges directly on a dome. Indentations of no more than 1 μm can activate such units. When a suprathreshold step function or ramp-and-hold stimulus is applied, very rapid firing during the dynamic phase of stimulation is followed by continued discharge, adapting to a plateau level with considerable variations in interspike intervals, during maintained indentation. Some units may have an irregular background discharge in the absence of stimulation. The axon of a type I unit may serve only a single tactile dome, or it may branch to supply several (up to five) adjacent domes a few mm apart (Iggo and Muir, 1969).

The second kind of displacement receptor served by Aα myelinated fibers in hairy skin is the type II or SA II unit. These also have discrete receptive fields, but without any specialization of the skin surface. Commonly, they show a very regular background discharge in the absence of stimulation. Their response to controlled skin indentation resembles that of SA I units, but with less pronounced dynamic sensitivity; during steady stimulation, firing declines slowly to a very regular discharge which may be maintained for hours. Frequency

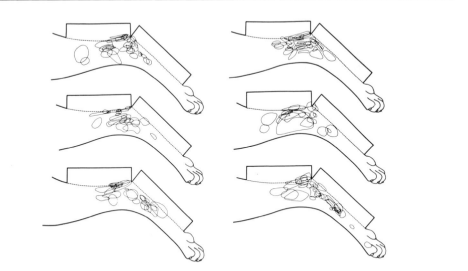

Figure 2-3 Receptive fields of 152 hair receptor units of cat sural nerve plotted, to avoid confusion, on six outlines of the lateral aspect of the leg and foot; skin flaps above allow representation of fields which extend onto medial side. Approximate full extent of overlap in a given animal would be indicated by multiplying the number of plotted fields by 3 or 4, and superimposing all those on one diagram. (From Hunt and McIntyre 1960.)

of the adapted discharge depends upon amplitude of the maintained indentation (Fig. 2–2). Unlike SA I units, which can only be activated from a tactile dome, SA II units respond readily to lateral stretching of nearby skin; this may be directional, stretching one way increasing the discharge, stretching in the opposite direction reducing or silencing it. The axons of both SA I and SA II receptors have conduction velocities characteristic of Aα fibers and these units share another property in that their responses are temperature-dependent. In particular, sudden cooling usually excites, while warming inhibits, a pre-existent discharge, a phenomenon most readily observed with SA II units because of their regular background firing.

The third kind of displacement receptor in hairy skin is one with small receptive fields a few mm^2 in size supplied by unmyelinated C fibers with conduction velocities between 0.5 and 1.0 m/sec. Although of higher threshold than A mechanoreceptors, the units are quite sensitive, responding to probe forces of only about 15 mg. Their discharge shows some dynamic as well as static sensitivity, and a prominent after-discharge follows removal of the stimulus. However, even though slowly adapting, the response declines more rapidly than that of SA I or SA II units, eventually ceasing despite continued indentation. But for periods of about 10 seconds, the firing frequency of these C mechanoreceptors provides direct information about the degree of distortion so that they can act briefly as displacement detectors. One of their most characteristic features is their failure to respond to rapid transients; a stimulus lasting about 0.1 sec is necessary to evoke a response. Related to this property, they are especially responsive to slowly moving stimuli traversing their receptive field, of the kind which could be imposed by a crawling insect parasite (Burgess and Perl, 1973; Iggo and Kornhuber, 1977). It is interesting to note that discharge in C fibers evoked by gentle mechanical stimulation of the skin was reported by Zotterman (1939), who suggested that such receptors could be involved in generating sensations of itch and tickle. Another property of these sensitive C mechanoreceptor units is that, like SA I and SA II receptors, sudden cooling of their receptive fields may evoke firing. The proportion of C fibers serving these sensitive C mechanoreceptors varies in different species. In the cat they account for roughly half the sensory unmyelinated fibers in nerves supplying proximal regions of hairy skin but in primates the proportion appears to be much smaller (Kumazawa and Perl, 1977).

MECHANORECEPTORS OF GLABROUS SKIN Despite the structural differences, especially the absence of appendages, electrophysiological studies have

shown a general similarity between the mechanoreceptor types found in glabrous and hairy skins. However,
there are significant differences, some related to the
density of innervation and, in the extremities, to the
highly folded structural pattern especially characteristic
of primate "fingerprint skin." Like those of hairy skin,
the mechanoreceptors of glabrous skin fall into two
major classes: rapidly adapting (RA) transient detecting
units, and slowly adapting (SA) displacement receptors
which can signal maintained, steady stimulation. These
have been found in hairless skin of the cat's foot pad
(Jänig, et al., 1968), of the monkey's extremities (Lindblom, 1965; Talbot et al., 1968), and of the human hand
(Knibestöl and Vallbo, 1970; Knibestöl, 1973; Johansson, 1978). Results of these and a number of other
investigations (see Burgess and Perl, 1973; Iggo, 1974;
Zotterman, 1976; Gordon, 1978) show a large measure
of agreement, despite species differences.

The *rapidly adapting* (RA) transient detecting units are
of two kinds. One type has a small, sharply demarcated
receptive field ranging from less than 1 mm² to about
10 mm² in area. Upon indentation of the skin, they
respond only during the velocity component of the
stimulus, and in this respect resemble hair receptors.
Thresholds vary from unit to unit, but the most sensitive can be fired by rapid indentations no larger than 3
to 5 μm. Commonly, these units also give a brief "off
response" upon removal of a suprathreshold stimulus.
They are particularly sensitive to brisk, light movement
of a probe across the skin ridges traversing the receptive field. They also respond to vibratory stimulation at
frequencies lower than 100 Hz; optimal response
occurs at about 30 to 40 Hz.

In the human hand the circular or oval fields of these RA
units may cover five to ten papillary ridges, and within
each field are a number of spots of maximal sensitivity.
Obviously, there must be substantial overlap of even these
small and densely packed receptive fields. More distally
located fields tend to be smaller and, correspondingly,
the innervation density becomes greater, particularly of
the fingers. Estimates have been made (Darian-Smith,
personal communication) of receptor density in the volar
surface of the monkey's index finger, which show a
striking increase in density of RA receptors in the terminal
phalanx (225/cm²) as compared with the middle phalanx
(91/cm²); similar gradients are also seen for other types
of glabrous skin mechanoreceptors. Clearly, the richness
of this mosaic of small, closely packed and overlapping
receptive fields relates to the highly discriminatory spatial
resolution of the fingertip's tactile performance.

The other type of quickly adapting transient detector in
glabrous skin has a much broader receptive field, with a
single, centrally located zone of maximal sensitivity where
the threshold to rapid indentation may be no more than

1 to 2 μm. Because these units respond uniquely to high frequency vibratory stimulation (80 to 700 Hz), with optimal responsiveness to a frequency of 200 to 300 Hz, there can be no doubt that they are pacinian corpuscles deeply placed in the dermis. Such units are therefore termed PC units, like those of hairy skin regions. The relatively large receptive fields are a consequence of their great sensitivity to the rapid, wave-like transients spreading through the tissues from the stimulating probe.

The two kinds of slowly adapting mechanoreceptors in glabrous skin behave very similarly to their counterparts in hairy skin; indeed, there is good reason to believe that the same two receptive structures are responsible for the SA responses in both situations, at least for hairless skin of the limbs. SA I receptors of the fingers and hand respond dynamically during onset of an indentation and then adapt to a frequency level which continues to signal the degree of steady displacement; this maintained discharge is somewhat irregular. Their receptive fields, however, have no recognizable surface features and, like RA units, spread over several papillary ridges, have sharply demarcated edges, and have a number of maximally sensitive zones. Their mechanical threshold is some two to four times higher than that of the glabrous RA units (Johansson, 1978). They are also less sensitive than their counterparts in hairy skin.

The SA II displacement detectors have properties similar to those of hairy skin: some dynamic sensitivity, together with the capacity to signal maintained displacement by very regular trains of impulses, at frequencies dependent upon stimulus amplitude. They are also sensitive to lateral stretch of skin and subcutaneous tissues in particular directions, and some respond to manipulation of the nails. Receptive fields of SA II units have a single zone of maximal sensitivity to indentation, and tend to be diffuse, without sharp boundaries (Johansson, 1978). Like those of hairy skin, both types of SA unit in glabrous skin show temperature sensitivity — in particular, excitation by sudden cooling, and reduction or suppression of ongoing discharge upon warming.

The axons supplying the sensitive mechanoreceptors of glabrous skin almost all belong to the myelinated Aα group, with conduction velocities between 40 and 90 m/sec. Fibers of RA units span this whole range of conduction velocities, whereas those of fibers serving PC and both types of SA receptors do not conduct faster than 70 to 80 m/sec. A few mechanoreceptors of the RA or SA type have fibers conducting at velocities between 20 and 40 m/sec and, as in hairy skin, some of the endings served by fibers of intermediate conduction velocity (fast Aδ and slow Aα) may be concerned with signalling stimuli such as firm pressure (Hunt and McIntyre, 1960).

CUTANEOUS RECEPTORS

Unlike hairy skin, especially that of proximal regions of the limbs, no low threshold mechanoreceptors with C afferent fibers have been reported in carnivores or primates (Burgess and Perl, 1973; Iggo, 1974). It would appear that the unmyelinated afferent fibers from glabrous skin are solely concerned with thermoreception, or the signalling of noxious stimulation.

Thermoreceptors

True thermal receptors were first observed by Zotterman (1939), who described units with small myelinated fibers in nerves supplying the cat's tongue which responded selectively to cooling (for references, see Hensel, 1973). Systematic study of adequate samples of skin thermoreceptors could not be undertaken until techniques were developed for recording impulses in the smallest (Aδ and C) fibers in cutaneous nerves reliably. This was achieved by Iggo (1959) and since then by many others. As a result, there is now no doubt that most skin regions are equipped with sensitive thermoreceptors of two kinds, one for signalling cooling and the other for warming. Sensitivity of these specific thermoreceptors is at least ten times greater than that of mechanoreceptors which also have thermal sensitivity, such as the type II slowly adapting receptors of hairy and glabrous skin. Indeed, Iggo (1969) has labelled such mechanoreceptors as "spurious" thermoreceptors. True thermoreceptors, under appropriate conditions, can signal changes in skin temperature of no more than a small fraction of 1 degree Celsius. Criteria for identification of genuine thermoreceptor units include: (1) dynamic response to small thermal changes; (2) background discharge at a frequency dependent upon ambient skin temperature; and (3) insensitivity to mechanical manipulation of the receptive field (Hensel, 1973).

COLD RECEPTORS These units have an ongoing, static discharge at steady skin temperatures between 10° to 15° C and about 34° to 38° C. Discharge frequency is maximal at a temperature below central body temperature, varying for different units from 24° to 32° C (average about 26° to 28° C); as skin temperature is shifted above or below this value, firing frequency declines and ceases at levels below 10° to 15° C or above 34° to 38° C. Plotting discharge frequency against temperature yields a bell-shaped curve. At any temperatures within the unit's static firing range, a small cooling stimulus evokes a dynamic increase in discharge frequency and may provoke firing when no static response is present — for example, at a background temperature of about 40° C. Conversely, a warming pulse reduces or abolishes a cold unit's discharge.

WARM RECEPTORS Warm receptors also have a temperature-dependent static discharge but, unlike cold receptors, the temperature giving maximum firing

59

frequency is above deep body temperature, usually between 41° and 46° C. At skin temperatures below 34° to 36° C or above about 46° C, static firing ceases. Dynamic responses to weak thermal stimuli are the opposite of those seen with cold units; warming evokes firing or increases static discharge, if present, and cooling slows or silences the unit's discharge.

The receptive fields for both warm and cold receptors in glabrous or hairy skin are small and spot-like, rather less than 1 mm² in area and usually single (Iggo, 1969); occasionally, a single afferent fiber may supply two adjacent temperature-sensitive spots. In primates, some cold fibers have been described as supplying a number of spots (up to eight), distributed over a receptive field 1 to 2 cm² in area (Hensel, 1973); these have been observed in transitional regions between hairy and nonhairy skin. Thermoreceptor units either fail to respond to mechanical probing, or only do so feebly when stimulated very strongly.

The afferent axons of thermoreceptors are all of small caliber and slow conduction velocity. In nonprimate mammals, the majority are unmyelinated C fibers with conduction velocities between 0.4 and 1.5 m/sec, both for cold and warm receptors over the general body surface (Iggo, 1969, 1974). However, orofacial skin in carnivores has many cold receptors with small myelinated (Aδ) fibers, with conduction velocity less than 20 m/sec. A few cold units with slowly conducting Aδ fibers have also been reported in glabrous skin of the cat's foot pad. In primates, a major difference is that most cold receptors in all skin regions are served by small myelinated Aδ afferent fibers with conduction velocities between 3 and 20 m/sec. Those supplying hairy skin of the limbs appear to be smaller and more slowly conducting than those supplying glabrous skin. A minority of fibers supplying primate cold receptors have unmyelinated C fibers. Axons of warm units, as in nonprimate mammals, are all unmyelinated; those from the monkey's hand have a mean conduction velocity of 1.25 m/sec. (Darian-Smith and Johnson, 1977).

Although the numbers of thermoreceptive units so far studied in human subjects are limited, there is little doubt that their properties closely resemble those of the monkey's skin. The properties of these thermoreceptors can be compared with the psychophysically determined ability of human subjects to detect and discriminate small changes in skin temperature. Under appropriate testing conditions, and with an indifferent ambient skin temperature of about 24° C, the human hand can discriminate differences of about 0.05° C between successively applied step function thermal stimuli to an area of about 1.0 cm², a discrimination signalled, of course, by a population of units. Individual thermoreceptive units of the monkey's hand have been shown to approach this level of sensitivity. A careful comparison of the ability of a human observer to discriminate small differences in successive thermal stimuli, and the discharge of single thermoreceptive units of monkeys in response to the same stimuli, has shown that the performance of individual units does not fully match the level of human psychophysical discrimination. However, the combined action of a population of 16 to 25 thermoreceptor units could provide the necessary input (Darian-Smith and Johnson, 1977).

Altogether, the properties of cold and warm thermoreceptors in all species so far studied seem to be remarkably constant, there being no indication of different functional types within either of the two classes of thermoreceptors. One special feature has been observed for cold receptors with Aδ axons which is not found in those supplied by C fibers — namely, a strong tendency for their static discharge at temperatures between 20° and 30° to 35° C to be grouped into bursts separated by periods of silence (Iggo, 1969). This occurs particularly in primate cold units, but also in those of the face and tongue of carnivores. The significance of this phenomenon is uncertain, but the pattern of grouping could provide further information about temperatures in this particular range. In the absence of impulse grouping, the bell shape of curves relating static firing frequency to ambient skin temperature means that discharge frequency cannot specify a particular temperature uniquely; the grouping pattern of impulses from cold receptors may be a factor in overcoming this ambiguity in the 20° to 35° C range. But for higher temperatures, within ordinary limits, the inputs from populations of both warm and cold receptors can together specify skin temperature without ambiguity. However, ambiguity can occur for heat stimuli substantially above body temperature — in particular, the phenomenon of paradoxical cold commonly observed on sudden heating of the skin to a temperature of, say 48° to 53° C. Electrophysiological analysis of cold units during heating of the skin to such levels has shown that some, silenced as skin temperature approaches or attains 37° or 38° C, may discharge vigorously when the temperature rises to levels between 46 and 50° C, behavior which could account for the phenomenon of paradoxical cold. At still higher temperatures other receptors classed as heat nociceptive units are recruited, and a sensation of burning pain appears.

Nociceptors These are receptors of high threshold which respond only to stimuli which threaten or cause actual damage to the tissues, and which subserve one of the important protective functions of the skin through the reflex and behavioral consequences of their activation. Despite earlier opposition to the notion (e.g., Sinclair, 1955), there is now no doubt that the skin and subcutaneous tissues are equipped with separate and distinct receptors and afferent fibers which perform this special role. As in the case of thermoreceptors, many studies of receptors with small axons made during the past 10 to 15 years as a result of refinements in electrophysiological technique have settled this matter conclusively. In the words of Boivie and Perl (1975): "High threshold receptors appear to be the sole group of primary afferent fibers from the skin capable of reliably signalling the presence of noxious mechanical and thermal events and differentiating them from innocuous stimuli."

In early experiments (e.g., Zotterman, 1939) multifiber recordings suggested that slowly conducting afferent axons are concerned in signalling strong and noxious stimulation of the skin. Experiments in man as well as in animals also indicated that pain and associated reactions are mediated by way of small myelinated and unmyelinated fibers (e.g., Gasser, 1943; Bishop, 1946). Furthermore, the phenomenon of "double pain" — that is, perception of two successive waves of pain of differing quality after a single, brief painful stimulus — was explained by postulating a dual set of peripheral "pain fibers," one myelinated, the other unmyelinated. Strong support for this view came from the experiments of Collins et al. (1960), who electrically stimulated exposed human sural nerves while monitoring the compound action potential. Only when the stimulus was strong enough to recruit $A\delta$, or $A\delta$ plus C fibers, did their volunteers experience pain. Engagement of C fibers led to "unbearable" pain, even from single shocks. More recent electrophysiological studies of units responding only to noxious mechanical, thermal, or chemical stimulation have fully vindicated these earlier views. They have also made it clear that only some of the slowly conducting $A\delta$ and C fiber populations are concerned with signalling strong and damaging stimuli. Criteria for classing a skin receptor as nociceptive include failure of low intensity mechanical or thermal stimulation to provoke discharge, and a substantial response to stimuli — mechanical, thermal, or chemical — which damage, or threaten injury to, tissue in the receptive field (Zotterman, 1939, 1976; Iggo, 1959, 1974, 1977; Burgess and Perl, 1973). On this basis, the sensitive mechano- or thermoreceptors already described are excluded from any direct role in nociception, apart from a modifying influence upon the central nervous consequences of nociceptive input.

There are two major types of skin receptors responsive to noxious stimulation: *mechanical* nociceptors, which discharge to damaging stimuli, including cutting of the skin or penetration of it by a sharp object such as a needle, or very strong squeezing or crushing maneuvers; and *thermal* nociceptors, of which some respond to strong heating above 45° C, and others to cooling below 10° C (Iggo, 1959). Several varieties of thermal nociceptors have been described, and many respond to mechanical as well as thermal stimulation. The most common of these respond most readily to noxious heat but also to mechanical manipulation or the application of irritant chemicals; they have been labelled *polymodal* nociceptors (Burgess and Perl, 1973).

MECHANICAL NOCICEPTORS These do not respond readily to noxious thermal stimuli, and their axons are either small myelinated or unmyelinated C fibers. Those units with myelinated fibers have oval or circular receptive fields ranging from less than 1 up to 8 cm² in area, containing a variable number of responsive spots separated by unresponsive regions. Strong pressure with a blunt probe is ineffective, but units fire to pressure with a sharp needle, and to forcible pinching with serrated forceps. Increasing skin temperature above 50° C or below 10° C has little or no effect; neither does application of acid to the receptive field. Conduction velocities of their afferent axons are between 5 and 50 m/sec, although most are slower than 25 m/sec and thus belong to the Aδ group. These axons overlap extensively with the many Aδ fibers serving D hair receptors (10 to 30 m/sec), both in monkey and cat; in the latter, fibers of D hairs constitute about 75 per cent of the total Aδ population in cutaneous nerves of hairy skin. Mechanical nociceptors with unmyelinated C fibers have properties similar to those with small myelinated axons; these are relative insensitivity to nondamaging strong punctate probing, vigorous response to penetrating needle prick or forcible pinching, and absence of response to strong thermal stimulation. But they are fewer than those with myelinated fibers, and their receptive fields are smaller, usually consisting of single, discrete regions a few mm² in area. Conduction velocities of the axons are, of course, slower than those of Aδ fibers, ranging from 0.5 to 1.3 m/sec.

THERMAL NOCICEPTORS These are characterized by being most readily activated by noxious heating or cooling; three subgroups have been defined. The first type has been described only in primates, and differs from the others in having fine myelinated axons which are among the slowest of the Aδ group, conducting at velocities between 4 and 10 m/sec. They have small receptive fields a few mm² in area and are most readily fired by noxious heat, but also respond to damaging mechanical manipulation and weakly to noxious cold (0° to 10° C). The other two kinds of thermal nociceptors are found in nonprimate mammals as well as in primates; both are served by unmyelinated C fibers. Units of the first type respond to cooling below 15° C, some continuing to discharge at low frequency with maintained cold. They also respond, although reluctantly, to strong squeezing with forceps or penetrating needle pricks. The second kind of thermal nociceptor with C fibers is the polymodal unit. According to Burgess and Perl (1973) these outnumber other skin receptors served by unmyelinated fibers both in cat and monkey, especially in nerves supplying distal limb regions. They respond vigorously to noxious heating, with thresholds varying from 42° C to about 60° C. They can also be readily activated by strong mechanical stimulation and by the application of irritant chemicals such as strong acid. They give little or no response to severe cooling. Their receptive fields are usually small (1 to 2 mm²) and single. Some nociceptive units of this kind have been found in human subjects using the percutaneous method of microneurography (e.g., Zotterman (1976), p. 480, Fig. 3). A characteristic feature of polymodal units not seen with other nociceptors is the phenomenon of sensitization. After repeated episodes of noxious heating irregular spontaneous firing appears, and the unit's threshold is found on subsequent testing to be lowered to the same or to other noxious stimuli. Furthermore, a given stimulus elicits a more intense response than it did before sensitization. The phenomenon suggests a kinship with inflammatory hyperalgesia, the nerve terminals being sensitized by chemical agents released as a result of tissue damage inflicted by the noxious heating; however, the nature of these remains uncertain.

MORPHOLOGICAL BASIS OF SKIN SENSIBILITY

Despite earlier histological failures to identify recognizable structures matching skin spots giving particular sensations, a great deal of progress has been made in understanding the structural basis of selective receptor sensitivity. Four of the mechanoreceptors of hairy skin can be ascribed with certainty to different, recognizable structures, and three in glabrous skin of the extremities, with a strong probability of identifying a fourth. The endings of afferent axons of the $A\delta$ and C groups present much greater difficulties, and so far only two types of receptor with $A\delta$ fibers have been shown to have structurally recognizable endings: the D hair receptors and the "cold" receptors, at least in one region of the skin surface. The extensive use of meticulous electron as well as light microscopy, together with careful marking of the sites of functionally identified receptors, have been crucial in the successes so far achieved (Andres and von Düring, 1973; Iggo, 1974; Iggo and Ilyinsky, 1976).

In hairy skin the hairs themselves are, of course, a major component of the skin's tactile equipment, as recognized long ago by von Frey and many others. Fine structural studies have revealed details of the arrangement of terminal unmyelinated branches of the several myelinated axons contributing to each hair's sensory equipment, and the close contact which their profusion of longitudinal and encircling branches make, through gaps in their Schwann cell covering, with the epithelial root sheath of the hair. The nerve endings are located just beneath the sebaceous gland openings, where the growing hair shaft has become sufficiently keratinized to be relatively rigid and the epithelial root sheath is thin and attached to the shaft. This placement of the terminal neurites is clearly very favorable for detecting, through lever action, movement or distortion of the deep portion of the shaft in response to hair deflection. So far, however, no structural clues are available to explain the transient (rapidly adapting) nature of their responses.

Both types of slowly adapting tactile endings (the SA I and SA II displacement detectors) have been positively identified in hairy skin. Beneath the dome-like elevations visible on the surface, the type I endings have proved to be a collection of the terminal, expanded (hederiform) endings, first described by Merkel, of the branches of a single myelinated fiber (Fig. 2–4). Each expanded terminal is closely associated with a special, nearly spherical, epithelial cell, the tactile Merkel cell, located at the junction between epidermis and dermis underneath a tactile dome. The expanded nerve plate is invaginated into the deep aspect of the Merkel cell, and makes closely apposed synapse-like contacts with regions of

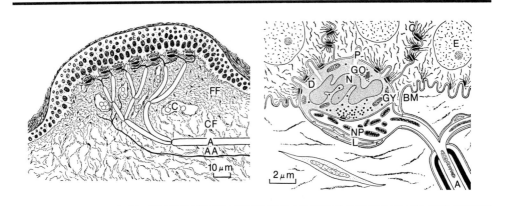

Figure 2–4 Structure of Merkel cell SA I tactile receptor complex. *Left,* Section through tactile dome of hairy skin, with single myelinated parent axon, A, branching to supply expanded tip terminals to seven Merkel cells. *Right,* Diagram showing one expanded nerve terminal (NP) invaginating into a Merkel cell, which contains granules (G) and other inclusions. Merkel cell processes (P) project into basal cells, to which it is anchored by desmosomes (D). E, epithelial cells and nuclei, GO, Golgi apparatus; N, multilobulated nucleus of Merkel cell; GY, glycogen; L, lamellae underlying nerve plate; BM, basement membrane. (From Iggo and Muir 1969.)

65

the cell which contain small spherical granules. It is not known whether these structures are true synapses, but contact with Merkel cells is essential for the characteristic slowly adapting properties of SA I receptors. The irregularity of their firing to maintained indentation is explained by the fact that there are multiple impulse generators among the array of Merkel cell-neurite junctions beneath a single tactile dome (Iggo and Muir, 1969).

The type II displacement detector has also been identified in hairy skin. The receptive fields of type II receptors are small and discrete to vertical probing, and have no detectable surface features. However, histological examination of electrophysiologically identified SA II fields has shown that the receptors are spindle-shaped, encapsulated Ruffini endings in the dermis, each containing the terminal arborization of a single myelinated fiber (Andres and von Düring, 1973). The fine unmyelinated terminal branches of the single afferent fiber ramify among endoneural cells and collagen fibrils of the inner core, which is surrounded by fluid-filled spaces within the capsule. Connections between the collagen fibers emerging from the poles of the spindle and the surrounding dermal connective tissue explain the sensitivity of the type II endings to lateral skin stretching, as well as to vertical probing over their location. The regularity of type II spontaneous firing, or the adapted discharge to maintained displacement, suggests that there is a single impulse-generating zone, in contrast with the multiple endings of type I afferent axons.

The fourth type of mechanoreceptors with fibers in nerves innervating hairy skin to be positively identified are the pacinian corpuscles. Identification is possible because of their unique properties as detectors of rapid transients — that is, as acceleration detectors; this includes their remarkable sensitivity to high frequency vibration. In fact, Hunt (1961) directly identified subcutaneously located pacinian corpuscles under the zone of maximal sensitivity of such units to stimuli applied to the skin surface.

No special structural counterpart has been found for low threshold mechanoreceptors with unmyelinated fibers, nor for nociceptors and the majority of sensitive thermoreceptor endings. These all appear to be served by fine, branching unmyelinated terminals ending in close relationship with basal cell layers of the epidermis, or within the dermal and deeper connective tissue layers. The selective sensitivity of different members of these apparently identical nerve terminals must depend largely upon differences in organization at the molecular level in their membranes.

One kind of thermoreceptor has been histologically identified — namely, the cold receptor in glabrous skin of the cat's nose. As already noted, the axons of these receptors are fine Aδ myelinated fibers. They lose their myelin sheath and branch some distance beneath the epidermis, but each subdivision is accompanied by Schwann cells until it reaches the basal layer of epidermal cells. Each cold receptor axon terminal penetrates for a short distance into a basal epidermal cell, ending within it as a small club-shaped enlargement with special structural features, including small vesicles and a number of mitochondria (Andres and von Düring, 1973; Hensel, 1973; Iggo, 1974).

In *glabrous* skin, the morphological correlation with functional receptor types is less complete. There can be no doubt, however, that the PC rapidly adapting units are indeed deeply placed pacinian corpuscles, because of their highly characteristic properties. The other, very numerous rapidly adapting units of primate glabrous skin, with fields having sharply defined borders, almost certainly consist of the many Meissner corpuscles located just under the dermal-epidermal junction on each side of the down-projecting epidermal "rete pegs" beneath each surface ridge on which the sweat gland ducts open (Fig. 2–5). Each Meissner corpuscle is approximately cylindrical or of oval cross-section, and has a thick lamellated capsule. Internally, flattened lamellar cells are stacked transversely; among and between these interweave the branching, unmyelinated terminals of more than one parent myelinated axon. Also, each Meissner parent fiber gives branches to a number of corpuscles.

The corpuscles lie in niches between the large rete pegs and the smaller limiting ridges beneath the surface grooves of fingerprint skin. The superficial pole of each corpuscle is bound firmly to the epidermis by tonofibrils which pass between cells of the basal layer and enter the corpuscles through fine collagen bundles. The inner poles of these corpuscles are not linked to the surrounding collagenous dermal tissue, so they are mechanically insulated from deformation of the deeper skin layers. This arrangement ensures that the corpuscles are admirably placed to detect small displacements of the skin's surface ridges. It is still not clear why these receptors should be rapidly adapting. An early speculation by Sherrington (1900) is appropriate. In assigning a tactile function to Meissner corpuscles, he said that they "seem to take the place of sensory hairs in hairless parts." In the ridged glabrous skin of the extremities in carnivores, the nonpacinian rapidly adapting receptors are not Meissner corpuscles but are the smaller cylindrical end-bulbs of Krause (Iggo, 1977).

The two types of displacement receptors of glabrous skin appear to be fundamentally the same as those of hairy skin. SA I receptors have essentially the same properties as those in hairy skin and, because Merkel cell-neurite complexes are certainly present in glabrous skin, it can

67

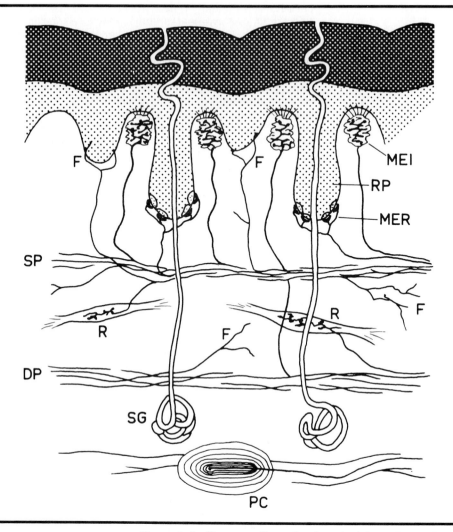

Figure 2–5 Diagrammatic section through glabrous fingerprint skin, indicating afferent innervation and receptor apparatus (not to scale). Horny layer *(dark stippling)*; cellular layers of epidermis *(light stippling)*; RP, rete pegs; SG, sweat glands; SP and DP, superficial and deep plexuses; MEI, Meissner corpuscles; MER, Merkel complexes; R, Ruffini endings; PC, Pacinian corpuscle; F, "free" nerve terminals.

be concluded that the receptor elements are identical. However, the arrangement of the Merkel complexes is different. Instead of being clustered beneath superficial dome-like elevations of the skin surface, the Merkel cells tend to be located more deeply in the epidermis, near the dermal-epidermal junctions at the bottom of the rete pegs (Fig. 2–5). The SA II slowly adapting mechanoreceptors of glabrous skin have identical properties with those of hairy skin, so that the dermal Ruffini spindles are believed to be the structures responsible, but direct correlation of these structures with electrophysiologically identified receptors has not yet been achieved, as it has in hairy skin. Nor has direct identification yet been possible of the nonpacinian RA units of primate glabrous skin. The question of how the many fine, apparently unspecialized, terminal ramifications of small Aδ or C mechanoreceptors and the different kinds of nociceptors are endowed with considerable selective sensitivity remains as obscure as it is in hairy skin. It is, however, quite clear that characteristic structural features of a number of the organized cutaneous and subcutaneous receptors are of crucial importance in determining some of their functional properties, even though they cannot fully explain selective responsiveness to different forms of stimulus energy. It is also very clear that the von Frey hypothesis is inadequate in more than one respect despite the electrophysiological vindication of one of its key tenets, differential sensitivity. Obviously, his choice of Krause end-bulbs and Ruffini endings for detecting cold and warmth, respectively, was very wide of the mark, but a more important defect is the oversimplified notion of "one stimulus, one ending." In fact, the skin has more than one type of receptor which can take part in signalling the impact of a stimulus. For example, even in the very uniform populations of cold and warm receptors, in many instances a small change in skin temperature will be signalled by changes in the firing pattern of groups of both kinds of thermoreceptors. And three different kinds of receptors contribute to the signalling of maintained indentation — the Merkel and Ruffini endings, together with those fine, C fiber terminals sensitive to small mechanical displacements. At the onset of such a mechanical stimulus, at least two transient detectors (pacinian corpuscles, and either Meissner corpuscles or hair receptors), together with the dynamic sensitivity of the Merkel and Ruffini endings, all contribute towards signalling the occurrence of this event and the speed with which the indentation is accomplished. Under most ordinary circumstances, therefore, there can be no doubt that very complex spatial and temporal patterns of impulses in large numbers of cutaneous afferent fibers of different size will be involved in conveying information about most stimuli to the central nervous system. The precise form of this pattern will have been largely determined by the selective sensitivity of the population of receptors involved.

DENERVATION AND REINNERVATION

After a cutaneous nerve is severed there is, of course, a region of total superficial anesthesia, with a marginal zone of altered sensation corresponding to the regions where the fields of neighboring intact nerves overlap with those of their severed fellow. During the months in which sprouting of the cut axons and regrowth into the

69

insentient region take place, sensibility gradually returns to the affected area, however, the threshold to stimulation and quality of sensation evoked are at first grossly different from normal — threshold is high, tactile sensation dull and localization poor. Stimuli which normally are only slightly painful, such as a pinprick, may have a highly unpleasant quality at a certain stage. It seems that this occurs particularly in regions invaded by thin, slowly conducting nerve sprouts following Schwann cell pathways, but still lacking a complement of larger axons and terminals. The situation seems not unlike that which occurs during a more or less differential block of a nerve trunk — for example, by pressure or asphyxia, in which most myelinated fibers from low threshold receptors fail to conduct. Under these circumstances pinprick evokes a peculiarly unpleasant pain, quite different from the normal, mildly painful pricking sensation. Thus, under normal circumstances, noxious mechanical stimulation must elicit a complex discharge pattern from many sense organs of widely varying threshold, and the component of this input in fibers other than those of nociceptors substantially modifies, through central mechanisms, the end results of the nociceptive input itself.

Eventually, when reinnervation is as complete as possible, skin sensibility returns towards normal, but probably never fully regains its previous level of performance. Electrophysiological recording of receptor units in human reinnervated glabrous skin has shown significant increases in threshold (Zotterman, 1976).

The extent to which regenerating sensory axons after nerve severance can reach and make functional connections with appropriate nonneural receptive structures is a matter of great interest. Myelinated fibers regenerating towards denervated Merkel cell cutaneous domes may respond phasically to tactile stimulation of their tips, but do not regain their characteristic high dynamic sensitivity to the onset of stimulation and maintained, slowly adapting irregular discharge, until their branches have established proper connections with the Merkel cells, which themselves require the presence of expanded tip terminals to maintain their structural and functional integrity. A careful study of the regeneration of severed cutaneous afferent fibers supplying the cat's hairy skin has been made by Burgess and Horch (1973). These authors showed that the growing nerve fibers re-establish their peripheral connections with structures such as hair shafts and Merkel cell complexes with a remarkable degree of specificity, although certain abnormalities persist. These include a relative diffuseness of type I receptive fields, which are no longer strictly located in punctate fashion to the Merkel cell domes, and an apparent failure of many type II (Ruffini) slowly adapting receptors to regain their innervation. The possibility of central readjustment of synaptic connections to correct for errors of peripheral reinnervation cannot be excluded, but it seems more likely that the regenerating fibers are able to seek appropriate peripheral targets. The mechanism for this remains obscure.

References   Adrian, E. D., and Zotterman, Y.: the impulses produced by sensory nerve endings. Part 2. The response of a single end-organ. J. Physiol., *61*:151, 1926.

Andres, K. H., and von Düring, M.: Morphology of cutaneous receptors. *In* Iggo, A., (ed.): Handbook of Sensory Physiology, 1st ed., Vol. 2, Berlin, Springer-Verlag, 1973, pp. 3–28.

Bishop, G. H.: Neural mechanisms of cutaneous sense. Physiol. Rev., *26*:77, 1946.

Blix, M.: Experimentela bidrag till lösning af frògan om budnervernas specifika energi. Upsala Läkaref. Förh., *18*:87, 1882. Quoted by Granit, R., *In* Receptors and Sensory Perception, 1st ed., New Haven, Yale University Press, 1955, p. 36.

Boivie, J. J. G., and Perl, E. R.: Neural substrates of somatic sensation. *In* Hunt, C. C. (ed.): International Review of Science, Neurophysiology, Physiology, Series One, 1st ed., Vol. 3. London, Butterworth, 1975, pp. 303–411.

Boyd, I. A., and Davey, M. R.: Composition of Peripheral Nerves, 1st ed. Edinburgh and London, E. & S. Livingstone Ltd., 1968.

Boyd, I. A., and Kalu, K. U.: Scaling factor relating conduction velocity and diameter for myelinated afferent nerve fibres in the cat hind limb. J. Physiol., *289*:277, 1979.

Brown, A. G., and Iggo, A.: A quantitative study of cutaneous receptors and afferent fibres in the cat and rabbit. J. Physiol., *193*:707, 1967.

Burgess, P. R., and Horch, K. W.: Specific regeneration of cutaneous fibers in the cat. J. Neurophysiol., *36*:101, 1973.

Burgess, P. R., and Perl, E. R.: Cutaneous mechanoreceptors and nociceptors. *In* Iggo, A., (ed.): Handbook of Sensory Physiology, 1st ed., Vol. 2. Berlin, Springer-Verlag, 1973, pp. 29–78.

Collins, W. F., Nulsen, F. E., and Randt, C. T.: Relation of peripheral nerve fiber size and sensation in man. Arch. Neurol., *3*:381, 1960.

Dallenbach, K. M.: The temperature spots and end-organs. Am. J. Psychol., *39*:402, 1927.

Darian-Smith, I., and Johnson, K. O.: Temperature sense in the primate. Br. Med. Bull., *33*:143, 1977.

Franz, D. N., and Iggo, A.: Conduction failure in myelinated and non-myelinated axons at low temperatures. J. Physiol., *199*:319, 1968.

Gasser, H. S.: Pain-producing impulses in peripheral nerves. Res. Publ. Assoc. Nerv. Ment. Dis., *23*:44, 1943.

Gasser, H. S.: Effect of the method of leading on the recording of the nerve fiber spectrum. J. Gen. Physiol., *43*:927, 1960.

Gasser, H. S., and Grundfest, H.: Axon diameters in relation to the spike dimensions and the conduction velocity in mammalian A fibers. Am. J. Physiol., *127*:393, 1939.

CUTANEOUS RECEPTORS

Gordon, G. (ed.): Active Touch, 1st ed. Oxford, Pergamon Press, 1978.

Hensel, H.: Cutaneous thermoreceptors. In Iggo, A. (ed.): Handbook of Sensory Physiology, 1st ed., Vol. 2. Berlin, Springer-Verlag, 1973, pp. 79–110.

Hensel, H., Iggo, A., and Witt, I.: A quantitative study of sensitive cutaneous thermoreceptors with C afferent fibres. J. Physiol., *153*:113, 1960.

Hunt, C. C.: On the nature of vibration receptors in the hind limb of the cat. J. Physiol., *155*:175, 1961.

Hunt, C. C., and McIntyre, A. K.: An analysis of fiber diameter and receptor characteristics of myelinated cutaneous afferent fibers in cat. J. Physiol., *153*:99, 1960.

Hursh, J. B.: Conduction velocity and diameter of nerve fibers. Am. J. Physiol., *127*:131, 1939.

Iggo, A.: Cutaneous heat and cold receptors with slowly conducting (C) afferent fibres. Q. J. Exp. Physiol., *44*:362, 1959.

Iggo, A.: Cutaneous thermoreceptors in primates and subprimates. J. Physiol., *200*:403, 1969.

Iggo, A.: Cutaneous receptors. In Hubbard, J. I. (ed.): The Peripheral Nervous System, 1st ed. New York, Plenum Press, 1974, pp. 347–404.

Iggo, A.: Cutaneous and subcutaneous sense organs. Br. Med. Bull., *33*:97, 1977.

Iggo, A., and Gottschaldt, K.-M.: Cutaneous mechanoreceptors in simple and in complex sensory structures. In Schwartzkopff, J. (ed.): Symposium Mechanoreception, 1st ed. Opladen, Westdeutscher Verlag, 1974, pp. 153–176.

Iggo, A., and Ilyinsky, O. B. (eds.): Somatosensory and Visceral Receptor Mechanisms, 1st ed. Amsterdam, Elsevier, 1976.

Iggo, A., and Kornhuber, H. H.: A quantitative study of C-mechanoreceptors in hairy skin of the cat. J. Physiol., *271*:549, 1977.

Iggo, A., and Muir, A. R.: The structure and function of slowly adapting touch corpuscle in hairy skin. J. Physiol., *200*:703, 1969.

Iriuchijima, J., and Zotterman, Y.: The specificity of afferent cutaneous C fibres in mammals. Acta Physiol. Scand., *49*:267, 1960.

Jack, J. J. B.: Physiology of peripheral nerve fibres in relation to their size. Br. J. Anaesthesiol., *47*:173, 1975.

Jänig, W., Schmidt, R. F., and Zimmermann, M.: Single unit responses and the total afferent outflow from the cat's footpad upon mechanical stimulation. Exp. Brain Res. *6*:100, 1968.

Johansson, R. S.: Tactile sensibility in the human hand: Receptive field characteristics of mechanoreceptive units in the glabrous skin area. J. Physiol., *281*:101, 1978.

Katz, B.: Nerve, Muscle and Synapse, 1st ed. New York, McGraw-Hill, 1966.

Kenshalo, D. R. (ed.): The Skin Senses, 1st ed. Springfield, Ill., Charles C Thomas, 1968.

Knibestöl, M.: Stimulus-response functions of rapidly adapting mechanoreceptors in the human glabrous skin area. J. Physiol., *232*:427, 1973.

CUTANEOUS RECEPTORS

Knibestöl, M., and Vallbo, Å. B.: Single unit analysis of mechanoreceptor activity from the human glabrous skin. Acta Physiol. Scand., 80:178, 1970.

Kumazawa, T., and Perl, E. R.: Primate cutaneous sensory units with unmyelinated (C) afferent fibers. J. Neurophysiol., 40:1325, 1977.

Lindblom, U.: Properties of touch receptors in distal glabrous skin of the monkey. J. Neurophysiol., 28:966, 1965.

Lloyd, D. P. C.: Neuron patterns controlling transmission of ipsilateral hind limb reflexes in cat. J. Neurophysiol., 6:293, 1943.

Paintal, A. S.: The influence of diameter of medullated nerve fibres of cats on the rising and falling phases of the spike and its recovery. J. Physiol., 184:791, 1966.

Ranson, S. W., Droegemueller, W. H., Davenport, H. K., and Fisher, C.: Number, size and myelination of the sensory fibers in the cerebrospinal nerves. Res. Publ. Assoc. Res. Nerv Ment. Dis., 15:3, 1935.

Sherrington, C. S.: Cutaneous sensations. In Schäfer's Textbook of Physiology, 1st ed., Vol. 2. Edinburgh and London, Pentland, 1900, pp. 920–1000.

Sinclair, D. C.: Cutaneous sensation and the doctrine of specific nerve energy. Brain, 78:584, 1955.

Somjen, G. S.: Sensory Coding in the Mammalian Nervous System, 1st ed. New York, Meredith Corporation, 1972.

Talbot, W. H., Darian-Smith, I., Kornhuber, H. H., and Mountcastle, V. B.: The sense of flutter-vibration: Comparison of the human capacity with response patterns of mechanoreceptive afferents from the monkey's hand. J. Neurophysiol., 31:301, 1968.

Vallbo, Å. B., and Hagbarth, K. E.: Activity from skin mechanoreceptors recorded percutaneously in awake human subjects. Exp. Neurol., 21:270, 1968.

Weinstein, S.: Intensive and extensive aspects of tactile sensitivity as a function of body part, sex and laterality. In Kenshalo, D. R. (ed.): The Skin Senses, 1st ed. Springfield, Ill., Charles C Thomas, 1968, pp. 195–222.

Zotterman, Y.: Touch, pain and tickling: An electrophysiological investigation on cutaneous sensory nerves. J. Physiol., 95:1, 1939.

Zotterman, Y. (ed.): Sensory Functions of the Skin in Primates. Wenner-Gren Center International Symposium Series, 1st ed., Vol. 27. Oxford, Pergamon Press, 1976.

Mammalian Muscle Spindles*

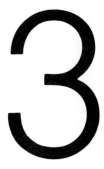

W. R. Kennedy
R. E. Poppele
and D. C. Quick

INTRODUCTION Muscle spindles are among the most widely studied of the peripheral sensory receptors. They have been the subject of over 2000 scientific articles (Eldred et al., 1967, 1977), and several recent reviews (Granit, 1970; Matthews, 1972; Stein, 1974; Barker, 1974; Houk, 1979; Vallbo et al., 1979), in which the accumulated knowledge of their anatomy and physiology has been recounted. In spite of these intense investigations their true significance to the coordination of movement largely remains a mystery. This chapter is an account of our own observations combined with those of other workers. The main morphologic features and physiologic characteristics of spindles are reviewed in an attempt to consolidate these observations into a functional analysis.

Muscle spindles have been the subject of inquiry and controversy since 1851, when these partially encapsulated small diameter muscle fibers were first noticed by Hassall (according to Ruffini, 1898). A more detailed description (Weisman, 1861) and discovery of a nerve supply (Köller, 1862; Kühne, 1863) were soon followed by controversy as to whether spindles were normal components of muscle, centers for development of muscle fibers, or pathological structures. The idea that they were sensory receptors with a sensory and motor nerve supply was espoused by Kerschner (1888*a*, *b*) and Cajal (1888), but

*Preparation of this chapter was supported in part by research grants from the National Institutes of Health, U.S. Public Health Service, No. NS-10969, National Science Foundation, No. B.N.S. 7825168, and the American Diabetes Association (Minnesota chapter).

We are grateful to Professor K.-E. Hagbarth for allowing us to read the reviews of Vallbo et al. (1979) prior to publication.

the first nerve degeneration experiments that supported this view were largely overlooked (Onanoff, 1890). The elaborate degeneration experiments and anatomic description by Sherrington (1894) finally provided convincing proof that the beautifully illustrated primary and secondary nerve endings of Ruffini (1893, 1898) were sensory in nature. Over the next 30 years the motor nature of the plate endings described by Ruffini (1898) were generally accepted but unproven. Finally, Hinsey (1927) and Hines and Tower (1928) firmly established the existence of the motor supply when they demonstrated that end-plate degeneration follows sectioning of the ventral roots. Still, it was not until 1945 that the small motor axons in muscle nerves (Eccles and Sherrington, 1930) were shown to innervate muscle spindles (Leksell, 1945). Further expansion of our knowledge of muscle spindles belongs to more recent times.

It is useful to begin the review with a short overview of spindle structure, size, and location. The shape of the muscle spindle is mainly due to a multilayered capsule that is widest at its central portion and tapers towards both ends (Fig. 3–1). Coursing longitudinally through the capsule there are several slender muscle fibers called intrafusal (IF) muscle fibers to distinguish them from extrafusal (EF) muscle. The larger longer IF fibers extend beyond the spindle to attach to connective tissue or tendon. Sensory innervation is by two types of sensory nerve fibers that place endings approximately midway along the length of the intrafusal muscle fibers inside of the capsule. The main motor innervation is by thinly myelinated gamma efferent axons, also called fusimotor axons. Some spindles also receive beta efferent axons that branch to innervate both EF and IF muscle. Motor endings tend to be located more towards the spindle poles, away from the central or equatorial region occupied by the sensory endings. Excitation of the motor axons results in contractions of intrafusal muscle that greatly influence the sensory outflow. Thus, the spindle has the special property that its sensory input to the central nervous system (CNS) is adjustable by the CNS via the motor outflow to the spindle.

The number of spindles in a muscle is determined in part by muscle function. Muscles responsible for the fine skilled movements of the hand are heavily endowed relative to their size. The first dorsal interosseus and extensor indicis muscles each contain 40 to 45 spindles (Sahinen and Kennedy, 1972; Van Gorp and Kennedy, 1974). Deep muscles of the neck related to head movements contain over 100 spindles and have a density of 30 to 40 spindles per gram (Voss, 1958). Larger muscles, such as triceps brachii and pectoralis major, have about 500 spindles but only 1.5 spindles per gram (Körner, 1960). Within muscle, spindles can be found in the central portion, near the muscle edge, or attached to

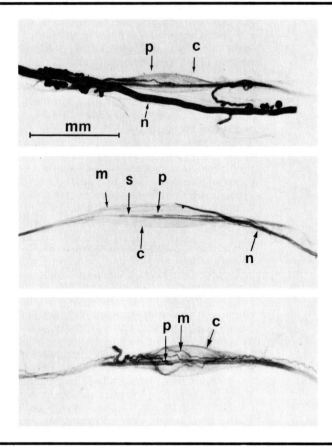

Figure 3–1 Three spindles dissected from glutaraldehyde-fixed third lumbrical muscles of a cat's forepaws. The spindles were postfixed in osmium tetroxide and mounted in Epon. All extrafusal muscle fibers have been removed, leaving only the spindles and parts of adjacent intramuscular nerves (n). Intrafusal muscle fibers run down the centers of the spindle-shaped capsules (c). Primary sensory afferents (p) are identified as thick myelinated fibers terminating at the centers of the spindles. Secondary afferents (s) are thinner and, when present, terminate nearer the spindle poles. Motor efferents (m) are small, thinly myelinated, and terminate in polar regions.

tendon; however, there is usually a concentration of spindles in that part of the muscle where motor endings are found.

Spindle size varies with the species. Spindles from human limbs are from 4 to 10 mm in length and 0.2 to 0.35 mm wide (Kennedy, 1970), and those from the cow are about the same size. Mouse spindles, however, are barely discernible to the naked eye (Chi and Kennedy, in preparation).

MORPHOLOGY

Capsule

The most striking identifying feature of living spindles microdissected from fresh muscle is the long, slender semitransparent fusiform capsule. Under high magnification the thin IF muscle bundle can be observed running longitudinally through the capsule. In the polar region the capsule narrows until only a narrow cleft separates it from the intrafusal muscle (Fig. 3–1). Towards the equator the periaxial space between the IF muscle bundle and the capsule is greatly widened. This space contains a fluid of uncertain composition, probably a thin mucopolysaccharide gel (Brzezinski, 1961). When the capsule of a spindle maintained at body temperature is punctured by a sharp needle the fluid escapes, partly deflating the capsule.

Surrounding the capsule there is a single layer of fibrocytic cells whose thin overlapping processes merge with similar fibrocytes of the interfascicular connective tissue of EF muscle. At the equator the capsule is six or more cell layers thick (Fig. 3–2). The outer capsule cells are flattened, basement membrane-covered, perineurial-like cells with long slender processes that are remarkable for the number of pinocytotic vesicles contained (Fig. 3–2, *inset*). Processes of the same concentric layer abut and form tight junctions. An abundant number of collagen fibers oriented longitudinally and circumferentially are situated between the concentric layers of the capsule (Merrillees, 1960; Landon, 1966).

The innermost capsule layer consists of thin fibrocytic cells and cell processes whose adjoining edges form tight junctions (landon, 1966). Extensions of this layer cross the periaxial space and merge with a similar single cell layer that surrounds the intrafusal muscle fibers individually or in groups. These inner layers are referred to as the inner capsule (Fig. 3–2).

The concentric cell layers of the outer capsule merge imperceptibly with identical-appearing cells that form the perineurium of nerve fibers, entering the spindle through the capsule. In a similar manner the fibrocyte-like cells of the inner capsule merge with the endoneurial cells of entering nerve fibers (Fig. 3–3). The perineurium of nerves is generally viewed as a diffusion barrier between the extracellular and endoneurial spaces (Shantha et al., 1968). Neither ferritin (Waggener et al., 1965) nor horseradish peroxidase (HRP) penetrate perineurium, although the smaller molecule, HRP, does enter between the outer two or three layers (Olsson and Reese, 1971). The barrier is attributed to tight junctions between perineurial cells.

The outer capsule cells of rabbit spindles have been shown to have the same barrier qualities as the perineurium of adjacent intramuscular nerve. HRP injected intra-aortically leaks from EF capillaries and surrounds the spindle. It penetrates the outer two or three layers of the concentric capsule, but never gains entrance to the periaxial space (Kennedy and Yoon, 1979). Direct application of HRP, so as to bathe spindles exposed in vivo, produces the same result (Kennedy and Yoon, 1979). The tight junctions of the capsular cells that are presumably

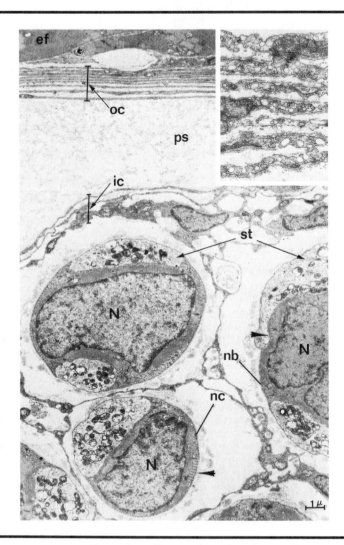

Figure 3–2 Transverse section of a spindle from rabbit tenuissimus muscle showing nuclear bag and chain fibers, inner and outer capsules. Microladders are indicated by arrowheads; N, nucleus; extra fusal muscle, ef; outer capsule, oc; periaxial space, ps; inner capsule, ic; sensory termination, st; nuclear bag muscle fiber, nb; nuclear chain muscle fiber, nc. Glutaraldehyde-OsO$_4$ fixed and Epon embedded; thin section stained with lead citrate and uranyl acetate. *Insert:* Higher magnification of a portion of the capsule from a Chinese hamster spindle.

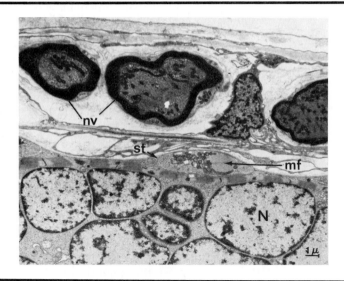

Figure 3-3 Longitudinal section of human muscle spindle from extensor indicis. Three divisions of the Ia sensory nerve, endoneurium, and inner capsule and, above, a nuclear bag fiber. The sensory termination (st) contains a core of microfilaments, mf, and numerous mitochondria. Glutaraldehyde-OsO$_4$ fixed and Epon embedded; this section stained with lead citrate and uranyl acetate. (From Kennedy et al., 1975.)

responsible for the barrier (Kennedy, Quick, and Reese, 1979) are similar in complexity to those of perineurium, as seen in freeze fracture studies (Akert et al., 1976). Penetration of the outer layers of perineurium and spindle capsule of HRP could be explained if the tight junctions of the outer layers were more leaky than tight junctions of inner layers, or if the outer layers were not continuous, or if entering capillaries were more permeable during their course between outer capsule layers than between inner layers.

Vascular Supply The only description of the complete microvascular supply to muscle spindles is for spindles in rabbit tenuissimus muscle (Miyoshi and Kennedy, 1979a). The circulation to rabbit spindles has preferential features and is separate from that to the adjacent muscle and nerve. The arterial pathway is short and direct; the preterminal arteriole arises as a third or fourth order branch from the main muscle artery rather than a sixth to tenth order branch, as do arterioles to EF capillaries. Capillaries in rabbit spindles do not anastomose with capillaries of EF muscle; they do anastomose with each other to form a characteristic vascular loop near the sensory endings. They drain into a venous system that is in close proximity to the main vein.

79

When spindle capillaries are compared to capillaries of EF muscle (Table 3–1) (Miyoshi and Kennedy, 1979b) they are found to be larger in diameter, circumference, and area (Fig. 3–4), principally due to an increase in the number of endothelial cells comprising the vessel walls. Vesicles within the endothelial cells are fewer in number and mitochondrial counts per capillary are greater, but the latter are approximately in proportion to the increased number of endothelial cells. Intercellular junctions are tight, pericyte processes cover a greater proportion of the circumference of IF capillaries, and basement membrane around the endothelial cells of pericytes is thicker and more often multilayered. These features of spindle capillaries are shared by capillaries of the adjacent intramuscular nerve.

HRP injected intra-aortically escapes rapidly from capillaries in EF muscle but does not penetrate the endothelial walls of capillaries in intramuscular nerve or muscle spindles (Kennedy and Yoon, 1979). Olsson and Reese (1971) have shown that capillaries to mouse sciatic nerve are permeable to horseradish peroxidase in their epineurial course but become impermeable as they pass through the perineurium into the endoneurial space.

The similarities between the structure and permeability features of rabbit muscle spindle capillaries and capsule and the capillaries and perineurium of peripheral nerve suggest that the composition of the periaxial fluid that bathes the IF muscle and the sensory nerve endings is closely regulated, and that it differs from extrafusal fluid. The short direct pathway from the central artery of the muscle to the spindle capillaries indicates that it is of some importance to maintain circulation to the spindle under various circumstances. It has been suggested that the microvasculature of the muscle spindle be considered as a miniature model of the blood-nervous system barrier. It was recognized that differences from the barriers to other parts of the nervous system probably exist, but the main mechanisms used to preserve the barrier are likely to be identical (Miyoshi and Kennedy, 1979b).

Capillaries are not present in the periaxial space of spindles in all mammals. In general, the larger mammals are more likely to have capillaries in the periaxial space than are smaller mammals. There are exceptions. For example, capillaries are almost invariably present in rabbit (Banks and James, 1973) but seldom in dog spindles (Banker and Girvin, 1971). The capillaries to smaller spindles often course between layers of the outer capsule but do not enter the periaxial space — e.g., the capillaries to mouse spindles. These are said to be both nonfenestrated and fenestrated in type (Edwards, 1975). Only nonfenestrated capillaries have been observed in spindles from rabbits (Miyoshi and Kennedy, 1979b) and chickens (Ovalle, 1976). In both they lie within the periax-

Table 3–1 Morphometric Analysis of Capillaries

	Intrafusal Cap			Endoneural Cap			Extrafusal Cap			Comparison of Each Parameter: Intrafusal Cap vs. Extrafusal Cap	
	N	Mean	S.D.	N	Mean	S.D.	N	Mean	S.D.	t	p
Luminal diameter (shortest) (μm)	41	4.47	1.45	23	4.00	1.14	41	2.57	0.91	8.65	<0.01
Total capillary diameter (shortest) (μm)	41	5.76	1.58	23	5.03	1.26	41	3.20	1.05	7.07	<0.01
Total capillary circumference (μm)	41	21.49	5.06	23	21.71	6.19	41	12.38	3.67	9.33	<0.01
Luminal area (μm^2)	41	23.92	13.46	23	21.05	8.19	41	8.22	5.53	6.91	<0.01
Endothelial (cytoplasmic) area (μm^2)	41	13.14	6.21	23	11.24	5.20	41	3.98	3.03	8.49	<0.01
Total capillary area (μm^2)	41	37.06	17.73	23	32.29	11.86	41	12.20	7.83	8.21	<0.01
No. of endothelial junctions	40	3.15	0.89	22	3.18	0.85	37	1.95	0.52	7.14	<0.01
Circumference per junction (μm)	40	7.19	2.04	22	7.14	2.35	38	6.69	3.05	0.87	0.3 < p < 0.4
Endothelial area/total capillary area (%)	41	28.78	9.38	23	26.45	6.06	41	26.80	6.17	(−)1.13	0.2 < p < 0.3
Circumference covered by pericytes (%)	41	54.92	19.93	23	57.82	18.45	41	23.61	16.44	7.76	<0.01
Pericyte area (μm^2)	41	5.54	5.64	22	3.58	2.76	40	0.62	0.57	5.49	<0.01
Pericyte area/endothelial area (%)	41	38.48	28.86	22	32.42	15.52	40	16.58	10.31	4.53	<0.01
No. of vesicles per unit area (μm^2) of endothelial cell	32	13.77	6.76	14	16.22	7.24	29	45.98	26.46	(−)6.66	<0.01
No. of mitochondria per capillary	37	6.46	3.07	19	6.00	3.43	35	1.60	1.94	8.12	<0.01
No. of mitochondria per unit area (μm^2) of endothelial cell	37	0.73	0.32	19	0.83	0.57	35	0.53	0.72	1.53	0.1 < p < 0.2

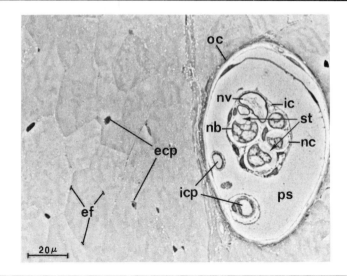

Figure 3–4 Transverse section of rabbit tenuissimus muscle spindle showing most components of a typical mammalian muscle spindle. Extrafusal capillaries, ecp; extrafusal muscle, ef; inner capsule, ic; intrafusal capillaries, icp; nuclear bag muscle fiber, nb; nuclear chain muscle fiber, nc; myelinated nerve, nv; outer capsule, oc; periaxial space, ps; sensory termination, st. Glutaraldehyde-OsO$_4$ fixed and Epon embedded. Phase contrast photograph of 1-μm thick section. (From Kennedy and Yoon, 1979.)

ial space. It seems likely that, as more layers of capsule are placed between the capillary and periaxial space containing the intrafusal muscle and sensory nerve endings, the permeability of the capillary, capsule, or both will be found to be increased.

Intrafusal Muscle Fibers

LIGHT MICROSCOPY Intrafusal muscle fibers are classified as nuclear bag or nuclear chain in type according to the appearance and number of distinctive collections of large vesicular nuclei located in the equatorial region (Figs. 3–2, 3—3, and 3–4). In cat nuclear bag fibers the collection contains 50 to 100 nuclei in a midcapsular segment of muscle that is 200 to 300 μm long (Banks et al., 1972). The nuclear bag segment in human IF fibers is about 1.5 times longer; that in mouse is approximately 0.3 to 0.4 that of the cat (Chi and Kennedy, 1980). Most of the primary sensory terminations of the bag fiber are on this same segment of IF muscle (Figs. 3–2 and 3–3). Transverse sections of the center of a bag fiber show from 2 to 5 nuclei, depending upon the species and the amount of stretch applied at the time of fixation (Fig. 3–4). At each end the collection is not enclosed in a membranous bag. Human nuclear bag fibers are 20 to 30 μm in diameter (Kennedy, 1970). They extend beyond the ends of the capsule to attach to muscle, connective tissue, or tendon. Occasionally a bag fiber enters a second spindle in tandem with the first where it develops a second nucleated equatorial zone.

Nuclear chain fibers in man average 9 to 11 μm in diameter (Kennedy, 1970), with the equatorial zone containing a single chain of nuclei (Figs. 3–2 and 3–4). In cat or rat these number from 20 to 50 nuclei (Banks et al., 1972). Slightly less than half of the chain fibers end inside the capsule, attaching either to it or to adjacent bag fibers. The remainder end within a short distance after penetrating the ends of the capsule except for a "long chain" fiber recently described (Harker et al., 1977).

HISTOCHEMISTRY   The literature describing the histochemical reactions of IF muscle fibers has been collectively plagued by inconsistencies, making it difficult to compare results from different laboratories regarding the several histochemical reactions in IF fibers from various animals. These problems are mainly due to the difficulty in relating an IF fiber stained by histochemical means to the ultrastructure of the same fiber, and to the tendency for the histochemical reactions and the ultrastructural appearance to vary at different sites along the length of the same muscle fiber. Considerable clarification has resulted from the practice of dividing, for reporting purposes, each half-spindle into three parts: segment A — the segment extending from the equator to the end of the periaxial space; segment B — the segment polar to A but still enclosed within the capsule; and segment C — the extracapsular polar segment. Within each segment alternate sections of the intrafusal fibers are processed for various histochemical reactions and for electron microscopy (Banks et al., 1977b).

It has been generally agreed that intrafusal muscle fibers are of three histochemical types (Ogata and Mori, 1964), termed chain, bag 1, and bag 2 (Ovalle and Smith, 1972). The A segment of all three fiber types has the weakest reaction to most histochemical stains. An exception is alkaline ATPase, which shows high activity in chain fibers, medium in bag 2 fibers, and low in bag 1 fibers. This difference in ATPase activity between bag 1 and 2 fibers in segment A continues into segment B, and is the most consistent difference between these two fiber types (Banks et al., 1977b). In all three segments the chain fibers have the highest activity of ATPase, phosphorylase, and glycogen (PAS), bag 2 fibers have moderate amounts of activity, and bag 1 fibers have the least activity; however, with PAS stain bag 1 fibers do stain darker than bag 2 in segments B and C.

In the extracapsular segment C the intensity of the histochemical staining of the three types of fibers is nearly identical.

ULTRASTRUCTURE Much of the fine structure of mammalian IF fibers was described in the initial articles to appear on rat (Merrillees, 1960) and human (Gruner, 1961) spindles. Nuclear chain IF fibers are uniform in structure throughout their length except at the equatorial region, where the chain of nuclei is accommodated by a moderate decrease in the number of myofilaments. Chain fibers resemble fast twitch EF muscle fibers. The myofibrils are packaged in discrete units surrounded by sarcoplasmic reticulum. Sarcoplasm is abundant, and rich in glycogen and large mitochondria. In longitudinal sections numerous diads, triads, and even pentads are observed at the A-I junction or within the A band (Ovalle, 1971). The M line is prominent at all levels. The sarcoplasm between individual chain nuclei at the equator contains ribosomes, Golgi complexes, mitochondria, and occasional lipid bodies. Adjacent nuclear chain fibers may have apparent points of adhesion between their sarcoplasmic membranes, but the membranes are never closer than 15 nm (Corvaja et al., 1969). When seen by light microscopy these areas appear to be unions or branching points between fibers (Barker and Gidumal, 1961). Microladders (leptofibrils), named for their alternating dark and light bands, generally occur near the surface membrane and are often adjacent to nerve terminals (Fig. 3–2). Satellite cells are often found near the spindle poles. These longitudinal cells lie under the muscle basement membrane in shallow depressions of the sarcoplasmic membrane.

Nuclear bag fibers, during their intracapsular course, resemble slower contracting muscle fibers. The myofibrils are large, poorly defined, and merge into one another. The Z lines are often thicker than in chain fibers. Sarcoplasmic reticulum and transverse tubular systems are sparse. There is little sarcoplasm or glycogen. Mitochondria are fewer and smaller than in chain fibers. In the nuclear region there is a striking reduction of myofibrils, and the central nuclei are densely packed (Fig. 3–3). Where space allows, organelles similar to those in chain fibers are inserted between bag nuclei. Microladders and satellite cells are also present. The M line is absent in the equatorial and paraequatorial region. The M line usually appears in bag 2 fibers before they exit from the capsule; bag 1 fibers have an M line only at more polar levels in cat and rabbit and not at all in rat. With appearance of the M line the fine structure of bag fibers becomes indistinguishable from that of chain fibers (see descriptions by Barker, 1974; Banks, et al., 1977b; Banker and Girvin, 1971).

DEVELOPMENT The development of IF muscle fibers has been best studied in the rat (Milburn, 1973; Landon, 1966, 1971, 1972a, b) and man (Cuajunco, 1940). The following account is from Milburn (1973). In rat the first trace of a spindle is seen at 19 days gestation. A thin capsule formed from an extension of the perineurium encloses a single muscle fiber, believed to be a bag 2 fiber. Simple sensory terminals from a large primary afferent are already present. Alongside the bag 2 fiber lie a row of myoblasts that fuse and mature in close association with the bag 2 fiber to form an intermediate fiber (probably bag 1) by birth (21 to 22 days). By postnatal day 4 two chain fibers have formed from the same bag 2 fiber. The fusimotor innervation is seen at birth and matures by the twelfth postnatal day, when myofibrillar ultrastructural differentiation is complete. Development of the sensory innervation is critical for spindle development; denervation in utero prevents normal spindle development. The reinnervated muscle contains a few abnormal receptors, but no normal muscle spindles (Zelená, 1957). If denervation is delayed until the fourteenth postnatal day, the spindles remain to await reinnervation (Zelená and Hník, 1963).

Sensory Innervation

LIGHT MICROSCOPY The light microscopic view of the sensory innervation of cat spindles is almost identical to that illustrated by Ruffini (1898). Each spindle has one primary sensory ending supplied by one Ia afferent nerve fiber. At muscle entry this afferent is 12 to 20 μm in diameter in cats, but decreases to 7 to 11 μm at entry into the spindle capsule, and tapers to 5 to 7 μm before losing the myelin sheath at the distal end (Fig. 3–1, 3–3). The internodal lengths become progressively shorter in the intracapsular parts of the fiber, reaching values of the order of 100 μm for the most distal internodes (Quick et al., 1979a). The primary bifurcation of the nerve usually occurs after penetration of the capsule. Barker (1974) and Banks et al. (1977a) have indicated that one first order branch may innervate the bag 1 fiber exclusively, with the other branch innervating the bag 2 and chain fibers. There are usually three to seven myelinated branches, each giving rise to terminal unmyelinated axons at the last heminode. Here the plasmalemma has a thick granular undercoating that extends for 4 to 5 μm. The unmyelinated segments often branch during their course of 25 to 35 μm before contacting the IF muscle fibers (Kennedy et al., 1975). The granular undercoating and some more recent cytochemical evidence indicates that each myelinated branch may constitute an autonomous sensory unit capable of feeding a spike train into the common afferent fiber (Quick et al., 1979b). This type of circuitry would imply that the independent branches compete with one another for dominance in producing the afferent signals (Eagles and Purple, 1974).

85

The sensory endings wrap around the nucleated portion of the muscle fibers as spirals, incomplete rings, or small sprays, and continue for a short distance onto the striated portions. The spatial configuration of the primary ending is most typically annulospiral in mouse and progressively less so in dogs, cats, and humans. In human and cat spindles the primary ending extends 200 to 400 μm along the IF fibers (Barker, 1974; Kennedy, 1974). Some terminals cross from one chain fiber to another chain fiber or, less often, to a bag fiber (Merrillees, 1960; Adal, 1969; Gruner, 1961; Kennedy et al., 1975).

Secondary sensory units number from zero to four per spindle. The most common arrangement is one secondary unit located adjacent to the primary. The afferent is a group II nerve fiber that is 6 to 12 μm in diameter at muscle entry and 4 to 7 μm inside the capsule. The pattern and degree of branching are more variable than those of primary afferents (Quick et al., 1979a). The arrangement on chain fibers is more spiral, but the flower spray-shaped endings emphasized by Ruffini (1898) are also observed. The sprays predominate on bag fibers. The secondary ending zones are quite variable in length, with an average of about 400 μm (Barker, 1974).

ULTRASTRUCTURE The primary sensory terminals lie in indentations of the muscle membrane. Although Figs. 3–2, 3–3, and 3–5 may leave the misleading impression that these are discrete endings, like motor endings, the true structure more closely resembles interconnected tentacles that wrap about the muscle fiber. The muscle basement membrane covers the sensory terminals and is not found in the nerve-muscle cleft, as is the case with motor endings. The cleft is of irregular width (100 to 200 μm) owing to the corrugated nature of the relaxed sensory membrane (Fig. 3–5). The cleft of spindles fixed during stretch is more uniform. Terminals contain mitochondria, vesicles, glycogen particles, neurotubules, neurofilaments, microfilaments, and cisterns (Figs. 3–2, 3–3, and 3–5) (Kennedy et al., 1975). The mitochondria tend to be clumped together near the central core. Vesicles are fewer than in motor terminals, with a somewhat greater concentration towards the muscle-facing membrane. A few larger vesicles contain dense granules. The matrix contains a microfilamentous network. In man, but not in mouse, rat, cat, rabbit, or baboon, the network takes the form of a dense central core, with microfilaments directed parallel to the course of the encircling terminals (Fig. 3–3). These microfilaments are actin-like in size and form arrowhead complexes in their reaction with heavy meromyosin (Kennedy et al., 1974). Disc-shaped specializations resembling desmosomes are found along the sensory terminal-muscle membrane interface. At

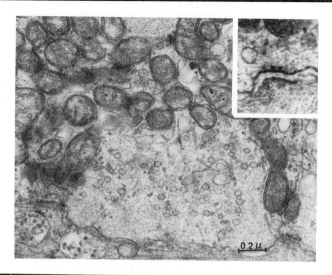

Figure 3–5 Longitudinal section, as in Figure 3–3. There are two junctional complexes between the sensory terminals and intrafusal muscle; both are obliquely sectioned at the I band (not shown) and contain dense bodies shown at higher magnification in the insert (× 83,000). Mitochondria approach the junction. A few tubular structures, cisterns, and vesicles are inside the ending. Two membrane-bound collections of vesicles are in the muscle fiber opposite the junction on the left. (From Kennedy et al., 1975.)

these sites the nerve terminal membrane loses its corrugated nature and becomes straight and thicker, with a few periodic densities (Fig. 3–5). Here the width of the cleft approximates 2.4 nm (Fig. 3–5, *inset*). One or two mitochondria appear to extend from more central clumps of mitochondria, toward the specialization. An occasional cistern is nearby; some appear to open into the extracellular space. These specializations are most often found opposite the I band of the underlying muscle fiber. The muscle membrane is also thickened at these specializations. Cisterns and multivesicular bodies are nearby in the sarcoplasm, and sometimes can be shown to open into the nerve-muscle cleft. The function of these specializations has not been investigated; they may serve as attachment plaques (Kennedy et al., 1975).

The fine structure of the secondary sensory endings is similar to that of the primary. Secondary endings have been described as lying deep within gutters in the muscle to the extent that they present a flat profile with the muscle surface (Hennig, 1969; Corvaja et al., 1969). The prominence of the profile is probably dependent upon the degree of stretch applied at the time of fixation.

CNS PROJECTIONS Projections of spindle primary afferent axons in the central nervous system are highly divergent, with each axon giving rise to hundreds of branches (Mendell and Henneman, 1968). Most of the central branches synapse directly on motor neurons, completing the excitatory stretch reflex loop. In addition to these there are other reflex connections to synergistic and antagonistic muscles, some of which are transsegmental (see review by McIntyre, 1974). Still other branches project to the spinocerebellar pathways (Eccles et al., 1961).

Recently, there has been increased interest in the question of whether spindles project to a cortical afferent pathway. Such projections have been detected physiologically in cats (Landgren and Silfvenius, 1969) and baboons (Phillips et al., 1971). In monkeys it is thought that signals in these pathways are used for control of voluntary movements, but they are not consciously sensed (Polit and Bizzi, 1978; Wolpaw, 1979). On the other hand, humans can be conscious of spindle afferent activation in some circumstances. If spindles are selectively activated by vibration, the alert volunteer will misjudge his limb position (Eklund, 1972; Goodwin et al., 1972 *a, b*). The misjudgment can be so extreme that the subject perceives impossible limb positions (Craske, 1977).

Secondary (group II) spindle afferents are generally thought to have CNS projections similar to those of the primary (group Ia) fibers. At least some of the synapses formed by secondary fibers are monosynaptic on motor neurons, and their effects are excitatory (Kirkwood and Sears, 1975; Stauffer et al., 1976).

The CNS connections of spindles in muscles innervated by the cranial nerves are less well studied and the results are to some extent controversial. Hosokawa (1961) has reviewed this topic rather thoroughly.

Motor Innervation The complexity of the motor control of muscle spindle function makes this organ unique among peripheral receptors. In 1898 Ruffini described small nerve fibers supplying plate endings in spindles. He did not think that enough evidence existed at the time to call them motor endings, and criticized Kerschner (1888 *a, b*) for speculating a motor function without experimental evidence. Later Eccles and Sherrington (1930) described the bimodal distribution of axons in the ventral roots and muscle nerves; the small myelinated axons were erroneously thought to supply small motor units in extrafusal muscle. When Matthews (1933) stimulated the motor nerve with a stimulus intensity beyond that necessary to cause maximal muscle contraction he observed an increase in the excitation of spindle afferents in the dorsal root. He rightly concluded that he had stimulated the small axons of Eccles and Sherrington, and that these were motor to muscle spindles. It was Leksell (1945) who provided the most definitive evidence that these small nerve fibers innervate muscle spindles. He called them gamma efferent fibers because their conduction velocity of about 40 meters/second corresponded to that of Erlanger and Gasser's (1937) gamma group of afferents.

The first indication that gamma axons do not necessarily terminate as typical end-plates was the demonstration by Cöers and Durand (1956) that there was acetylcholinesterase activity over much of the intrafusal muscle fibers, except for the region occupied by the primary ending. The degeneration experiments of Boyd (1962) were particularly important in establishing the presence of a branching gamma network that was responsible for the acetylcholinesterase activity in the paraequatorial zone. The endings of the gamma network are now referred to as the trail axons and endings. Boyd (1962) suggested that the smaller axons, which he called gamma 2, innervated trail endings on the nuclear chain fibers, and that larger axons, called gamma 1, innervated plate endings on the nuclear bag fibers. Adal and Barker (1965) traced the fusimotor axons in cat lumbrical muscles from muscle entry to the spindles but were unable to confirm a consistent sorting out of gamma axons by size. The continuing controversy over the distribution, endings, and action of gamma fibers has stimulated many investigators to attack this problem. The following description is a synthesis of commonly held views (see Boyd, 1962; 1976a; Barker et al., 1970b, 1976a).

There is general agreement that many gamma axons to spindles terminate as "trail" endings. These axons become unmyelinated during their course along the IF muscle fibers, or sometimes before capsule entry (Barker et al., 1970b). Multiple branching results in a diffuse system of endings with different shapes, as seen in silver preparations (Boyd, 1962; Barker, 1967; Kennedy, 1970). In cat, trail endings have been found at all levels between 490 and 2330 μm from the equator of the spindle. Trail endings are found on both bag and chain fibers with about twice the frequency that they are found exclusively on either bag or chain fibers alone (Barker et al., 1973).

There are two recognized types of plate endings on IF fibers; presumably, both were observed but not differentiated by Ruffini (1898). Barker has referred to these as P_2 and P_1 plates (Barker, 1967). Like trail endings, the P_2 plates are also gamma-innervated. They are most often found in the midpolar zone (Barker et al., 1970b, 1976a). The most obvious features of P_2 plates are the knob-like axon terminals and end-plate length, which is about twice that of extrafusal end-plates. Ninety per cent of P_2 plates in cat are on bag fibers and 10 per cent are on chain fibers (Barker et al., 1970b).

89

P_1 plates are the terminations of beta axons, the name given to axons that branch to innervate extrafusal and intrafusal muscle fibers. They are smaller than P_2 plates, and in fact resemble the plates of alpha motor axons on extrafusal muscles in size and conformation. Most are in the midpolar or far polar region in a distribution similar to that of P_2 plates. In cat they are found on both bag (75 per cent) and chain fibers (25 per cent) (Barker et al., 1970*b*).

The activity of the fusimotor axons that supply the various motor endings is discussed below (see the section on functional behavior).

Pathology

Reports by Batten (1897) on natural diseases and Batten (1897) Horsley (1897), and Sherrington (1894) on experimental denervation led to a long-standing belief that neuromuscular spindles are resistant to degeneration. Willard and Grau (1924) reaffirmed that spindle intrafusal (IF) fibers remain essentially unchanged following muscle nerve section. However, Tower (1932) found that, following a nerve section, the IF fibers do eventually atrophy and degenerate, leading to fibrous replacement inside the capsule. It was her opinion (1939) that IF fibers react to denervation to about the same extent as EF fibers, but the changes are less conspicuous. Tower (1932) also did dorsal and ventral root sections and found that the former causes dedifferentiation of the sensory regions of IF fibers, while the latter causes selective atrophy of the spindle poles. Swash and Fox (1974) reported similar observations for wholly or partially denervated human spindles.

Barker et al. (1970*b*) demonstrated that all traces of motor and sensory nerve endings on cat IF muscle fibers disappear 96 hours after muscle nerve section. The endings of the larger diameter nerve fibers degenerate first (see also DeSantis and Norman, 1979). Following denervation of rat muscle, the numbers of intrafusal fibers tend to increase by fiber splitting or by maturation from satellite cells (Schröder, 1974*a*). Reinnervation occurs more readily after nerve crush than after nerve section. Early in regeneration axonal sprouting and unusual associations between muscle, nerve endings, and Schwann cells take place. Later most endings have a normal appearance (Schröder, 1974*b*). Fukami (1972) found that reinnervated snake spindles recover their rapid adaptation to stretch before developing a tonic compoent. Bessou et al. (1965) and Poppele (unpublished data) found that reinnervated cat tenuissimus spindles behaved normally in all respects. Gamma reinnervation may also be specific, for normal function was reported to be reinstated for static and dynamic gamma fibers (Brown and Butler, 1975*a*). Denervation caused by freezing the nerve has different effects. The reinnervated afferents show atypical phasic responses to ramp and hold stretches, and rarely exhibit a regular discharge pause during muscle contraction. Also, there was no evidence of a gamma effect upon the afferent recordings, and no motor fibers with the conduction velocity expected of gamma axons could be detected (Takano, 1976).

The involvement of spindles in human diseases can be characterized by a few generalities:

1. In most disease, pathological changes in spindles are usually nonspecific and do not parallel those in the extrafusal muscle (Lapresle and Milhaud, 1964; Patel et al., 1968). Such changes include thickening of the capsule, generation of collagen inside the capsule, and atrophy of IF fibers (Cazzato and Walton, 1968; Lapresle and Milhaud, 1964; Patel et al., 1968; Swash, and Fox, 1974).

2. The involvement of individual spindles is quite variable; often a single biopsy sample will contain relatively normal-appearing spindles along with markedly abnormal ones (Cazzato and Walton, 1968).

3. In neuropathies, there is often evidence of denervation and reinnervation (Kennedy, 1969, 1971, 1974). This is especially true in severe neurogenic disorders where the intrafusal bag and chain fibers become atrophic. The remarkable degree of collateralization of surviving fusimotor fibers, as seen in amyotrophic lateral sclerosis (Kennedy, 1971), results in reinnervation of intrafusal muscle fibers. This fact and the inherently slow rate of atrophy in even fully denervated IF fibers (Boyd, 1962) are probably the major reasons for the variable degree of IF fiber atrophy found in neurogenic disorders.

A number of studies have focused specifically on muscle spindles in myotonic dystrophy (Daniel and Strich, 1964; Heene, 1973; Maynard et al., 1977; Swash, 1972; Swash and Fox, 1975). In this disease the spindle capsule thickens, the IF fibers split into numerous smaller fibers, the motor endings show extensive sprouting, and the histochemical reactions of the intrafusal muscle fibers are altered.

Except for the experimental denervation studies mentioned above, animal models for spindle pathology have received relatively little attention until recently. Acrylamide (Schaumberg et al., 1974) causes degeneration, first in Pacinian corpuscles and spindle primary sensory endings, later in secondary endings and extrafusal motor terminals, and presumably last in gamma axons (the latter were still normal in the longest time interval studies). A temporal correlation is said to exist between the appearance of symptoms and abnormal spindle function

(Lowndes et al., 1978). Isoniazid (Schröder, 1970), and pyridoxine (Krinke et al., 1978) appear to cause a more specific degeneration of spindle sensory endings. Modified reactions to some chemical reagents may eventually prove useful for physiological experimentation, and perhaps for therapy of human disorders.

Meier (1969) has examined a number of mouse mutants ("Shambling, Ducky, Teetering, Spastic, Lethargic, Disoriented, Rabbit, and Dystrophic") for correlated pathological signs in their muscle spindles, but found none. Another mutant mouse, "Sprawling," has severe deficiency in the number of spindles in the hind limbs (Duchen, 1975). The "Trembler" mouse appears to have relatively normal-looking spindles in the lumbrical muscles of the forelimbs, but a detailed examination has not yet been completed. Abnormalities of sensory innervation are present in the "Wobbler" mouse (Chi and Kennedy, unpublished observations). This mutant was reported as a possible model of anterior horn cell disease of the cervical cord (Duchen and Strich, 1968).

FUNCTIONAL BEHAVIOR

Sensory Behavior

The distinction between primary and secondary endings has not always been as readily apparent to the physiologist as it has been to the anatomist. B.H.C. Matthews (1933) was the first to study the discharge of single afferent fibers from muscle receptors in the cat by recording from dorsal root filaments. He was able to distinguish spindle discharges (type A of Matthews) from Golgi tendon organ discharges (type B of Matthews) by the difference in response to a muscle contraction evoked by stimulation of the muscle nerve. As previously surmised by Fulton and Pi-Suñer (1928) the spindle endings, which are unloaded or shortened by a muscle twitch, cease firing during the twitch and the Golgi tendon organs, which are stretched, are accelerated. Matthews further distinguished two types of spindle responses on the basis of their relative sensitivity to fusimotor activation. As has since been discussed by P.B.C. Matthews (1972), this method did not distinguish between primary and secondary afferent endings. The first reliable physiological identifications of these were made by Hunt (1954) on the basis of the conduction velocities of the afferent nerve fibers (Fig. 3–6). He assigned the classification group I to fibers having velocities greater than 72 m/sec and group II to the fibers of slower afferents, and he suggested that the group I fibers terminated in primary endings and the group II fibers in secondary endings. A significant step in understanding the physiological significance of the dual sensory innervation of the spindle was the recognition that the primary ending exhibits a greater sensitivity to dynamic stretch than does the secondary (Cooper, 1959, 1961); this is illustrated in Figure 3–7.

The difference is particularly evident in the responses of these endings to a ramp-and-hold stretch of the recep-

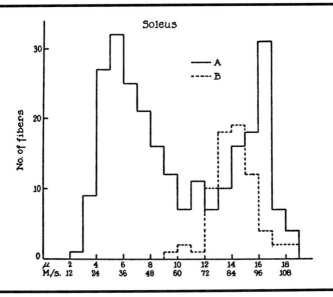

Figure 3–6 Diameter distribution of afferent fibers from muscle spindle *(A)* and tendon organs *(B)*. Note the bimodal distribution of afferent fibers from muscle spindles. (From Hunt, 1954.)

tors. The primary ending exhibits a marked increase in discharge during the ramp phase of the stretch that is much greater than the discharge rate recorded in the hold phase. In contrast, the secondary ending shows a more modest increase in its discharge rate in the ramp phase. The "dynamic index" has been devised to measure these features. It provides a qualitative index of the relative velocity and position sensitivities for a spindle stretched at constant velocity (Crowe and Matthews, 1964). It is defined as the difference between the highest rate of impulse generation (corresponding to the shor-

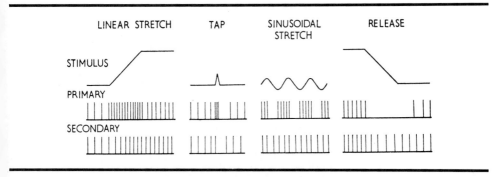

Figure 3–7 Diagrammatical comparison of the responses of "typical" primary and secondary endings to various stimuli. (From Matthews, 1964.)

93

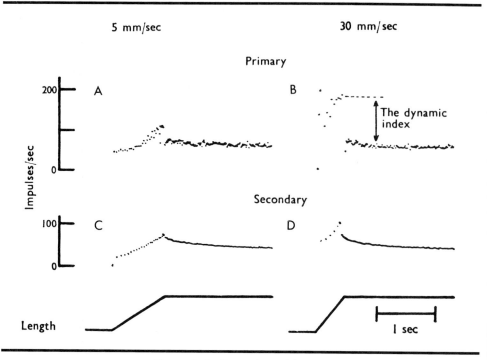

Figure 3–8 Comparison of the response of typical primary and secondary endings to two different velocities of stretch. The dynamic index is defined as shown in *B*. (From Crowe and Matthews, 1964.)

test interspike interval) during a stretch at constant velocity and the rate 0.5 sec after completion of the stretch (Fig. 3–8).

The dynamic index increases with the velocity of applied stretch and is relatively independent of the amount of stretch (Matthews, 1972). It is consistently greater for the primary ending than for the secondary ending by four- to tenfold (Matthews, 1963). The primary and secondary endings are both more sensitive to small amplitude stretches than to large ones in terms of impulses per unit stretch and, for continuous stretching in the range of 2 to 3 per cent of muscle length, primaries are about ten times more sensitive than secondaries (Matthews and Stein, 1969a). The distinction between responsiveness of primary and secondary endings is greatest for small amplitude stretches applied at high velocity, such as may be generated by vibration (Kuffler et al., 1951). Indeed vibration of 100 to 500 Hz applied to a muscle tendon has been shown to activate primary endings selectively to produce a discharge for each vibration cycle (Brown et al., 1967). The spikes occur in a fixed phase relationship with respect to a vibratory sinusoid, and are therefore referred to as phase-locked.

Attempts have been made to provide concise quantitative descriptions of the input-output behavior of the spindle receptors to allow one to predict its response to any arbitrary stretch stimulus and therefore to identify the variables involved in their behavior (Poppele, 1973). The methods of linear analysis that have been used have not been completely successful because of the basic nonlinear nature of the spindle responses. The secondary endings have proved to be better adapted to these methods because their behavior can be closely approximated by a quasilinear model that is given by a transfer function.* Although the transfer function is determined from the responses to small sinusoidal stretches, it describes the way that the receptor operates on any arbitrary stretch to produce a response. For instance, the response to a step change in length, as determined from the transfer function, has a slight overshoot with at least two adaptation time constants — one rapid (around 100 msec), the other slower (about 1 sec). For sinusoidal stretches, the transfer function expresses the fact that the response is nearly proportional to the magnitude of input stretches when they are slow (<1 Hz) and proportional to the velocity of stretch when its angular frequency is greater than 11 rad/sec (1.7 Hz). The output variable given by the transfer function is pulse density, P, which is estimated experimentally from the "instantaneous frequency" (inverse of the interspike intervals). The encoder producing the output pulse train has certain nonlinear properties that become evident when sinusoidal stimuli are used. This behavior is not included in the transfer function under discussion but it is important in explaining the phase-locking behavior that is particularly prominent in the primary ending (Poppele and Chen, 1972).

The primary ending has proved to be more difficult to deal with than the secondary ending in respect to formulating a quantitative description of its behavior. A quasilinear transfer function has been determined for a small range of input stretches; however, this function is

---

*The transfer function is expressed in the frequency domain as (Poppele and Bowman, 1970)

$$H(s) = \frac{P(s)}{X(s)} = K|X| \frac{(s + 0.4)(s + 11)}{(s + 0.8)}$$

or, as determined by a more complete examination of the low frequency behavior (Hasan and Houk, 1975a),

$$H(s) = K|X| \frac{(s + 0.003)(s + 0.16)(s + 11)}{(s + 0.005)(s + 0.34)}$$

In these expressions s is a complex frequency variable ($s = j\omega$) where ω is the angular frequency of the input in rad/sec, P is the response output expressed as impulse density, and X is the applied stretch.

unable to predict responses quantitatively for stretches much greater than 0.1 per cent of rest length.* The transfer function for the primary ending states that the dynamics (or time dependencies) are similar to those of the secondary, with the addition of two components. One is a very slow adaptation (of the order of 20 to 30 sec); the other is an additional rapid adaptation that acts like a response to the acceleration of applied stretch, and which may be seen as an initial burst in the response to a step or ramp stretch.

Within the quasilinear range for which the transfer functions are valid (up to about 0.1 per cent stretch for the primary and 5 per cent or more for the secondary), the dynamics of spindle behavior (i.e., the time constants of adaptation) are independent of input parameters and therefore the response to any kind of stretch (e.g., step, ramp, sinusoid) that is within that range can be predicted from the transfer functions. The scaling of response amplitude is not linear, however, even for a small amplitude stretch. Therefore increases in stretch amplitude do not lead to proportional increases in response amplitude. In general, the sensitivity of the spindle (i.e., the response amplitude per unit stretch) decreases with increasing stretch amplitude (Fig. 3–9). Sensitivity also varies with spindle length, so a small stretch applied to a slack spindle will produce a smaller response than the same stretch applied to a taut receptor (Poppele, 1973) (Fig. 3–10). This behavior has recently been shown to result from the nonlinear length-tension behavior of the intrafusal muscle, which becomes stiffer in the stretched state (Poppele et al., 1979).

In general, the responses to large amplitude stretches cannot be predicted from the transfer functions. If those stretches are combined with relaxations (as in large sinusoidal stretches) then there is a tendency for the receptor to fall silent rather than to produce a negative response, as would be predicted from a linear model. This is an obvious nonlinearity that is introduced by the threshold for action potential production. Even if the stretches are limited to positive stretches (such as ramp-and-hold stretches), the behavior of the receptors can no longer be predicted from the linear analysis when the

---

*The transfer function is given by (Poppele and Bowman, 1970)

$$H(s) = \frac{P(s)}{X(s)} K(x(s)) \frac{s(s + 0.4)(s + 11)(s + 44)}{(s + .04)(s + .8)}$$

and, again, a closer examination of low frequency behavior yields one slightly modified (Hasan and Houk, 1975a)

$$H(s) = K(X(s)) \frac{(s + .004)(s + .12)(s + 11)(s + 44)}{(s + .012)(s + .31)}$$

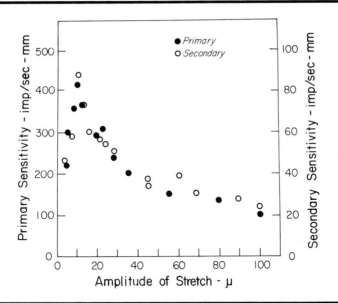

Figure 3–9 Sensitivity of primary and secondary endings from the same tenuissimus spindle as a function of stretch amplitude of a 1-Hz sinusoidal stretch. (From Poppele, 1973.)

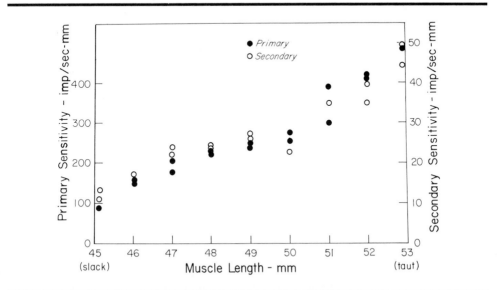

Figure 3–10 Sensitivity of primary and secondary endings from the same tenuissimus spindle as a function of muscle length. The amplitude of sinusoidal stretching at 2 Hz was 12 μm for the primary and 47 μm for the secondary. (From Poppele, 1973.)

stretch exceeds small amplitudes (Hasan and Houk, 1975a; Chen and Poppele, 1978). This problem seems to be different for the primary and secondary endings, although both share certain features.

The most noticeable discrepancy between linear extrapolations and actual responses to large amplitude stretches is the reduction in sensitivity as stretch amplitude is increased. The mechanism of this nonlinearity seems to differ from the nonlinear dependence of response on length because a simple extrapolation of that behavior leads to the prediction that sensitivity should increase with stretch amplitude. Furthermore, the reduction in sensitivity with stimulus amplitude is accompanied by changes in dynamics, at least for the primary ending, so that the time-dependent behavior is no longer predictable from the linear transfer function (Hasan and Houk, 1975a; Chen and Poppele, 1978). Even though it has been shown that the response to large amplitude stretches (triangular, ramp-and-hold in particular) can be described by linear functions (Lennerstrand, 1968a; Windhorst et al., 1976), these functions are different from those describing the linear range (Hasan and Houk, 1975a). Furthermore, there are other effects that have been described, such as discontinuities that do not correspond to linear behavior (Hasan and Houk, 1972; Brown et al., 1969).

A related problem is that most of the studies and observations about nonlinear behavior of spindle receptors have been made using whole muscle preparations. It is not yet clear what aspects of the observed nonlinearities are attributable to intrafusal and extrafusal mechanisms (e.g., Windhorst et al., 1976).

The problems in dealing with spindle nonlinearities are twofold, at least. First, there is no direct or straightforward technique of analysis that can be applied to nonlinear behavior, as there is for linear properties. Some attempts have recently been made to adapt the Weiner-Volterra theory of system identification to this problem (cf. Marmarelis and Marmarelis, 1978; Moore et al., 1976). This involves the use of white noise stimulation, and it does identify spindle nonlinearities satisfactorily. However, unlike linear descriptions, nonlinear descriptions cannot yet be related to functional parameters in a general way. Secondly, there are likely to be several sources of nonlinearity and, indeed, there are several stages in the receptor process in which probable nonlinearities may be identified. There are nonlinearities that involve the neuronal encoder (the possibility that there are multiple encoders serving a single receptor further complicates this) and there are those involving muscle mechanics, those that depend on stimulus amplitude and/or stimulus velocity, as well as those depending upon the previous history of muscle stretch and contraction (Proske, 1975; Eldred et al., 1976). Some attempts have been made to sort out some of these factors.

One hypothesis that has been proposed (Houk et al., 1973; Hasan and Houk, 1975a, b) is that there is a resetting of sensitivity from a high sensitivity to small length changes to a lower sensitivity for large stretches. Both the static and dynamic sensitivities (which are postulated to be different) are said to change, although the linear dynamics are unaffected. The resetting occurs as a sudden transition from a rapid change in firing rate with the initial stretch to a slower change after a certain critical amplitude of stretch is reached. This produces the familiar dynamic response, which appears to be a specific velocity sensitivity. The effect has been attributed to a possible nonlinear friction (called stiction) in the intrafusal muscle (Brown et al., 1969). Models based on that effect can satisfactorily explain many features of the observed nonlinear behavior, particularly for very slow stretches.

Another hypothesis that has been presented (Chen and Poppele, 1978) is that there is a shift in dynamics (a change of time constants) as well as a decrease in sensitivity that accompanies increasing amplitudes of stretch. The evidence that provides the basis for this hypothesis is that the phase of the response to a 0.2-Hz sinusoidal stretch progressively advances as stretch amplitude is increased (Chen and Poppele, 1978; Hulliger et al., 1977). According to this hypothesis, the difference between the dynamics of the small amplitude linear stretch and the large amplitude stretch is due to a shift in the time constant of a velocity response that is sensitive to the amplitude and/or velocity of the stretch. Thus, the response to large amplitude stretches can still be described by linear models, but the time-dependent parameters of those models change with input amplitude. This effect has been attributed to a nonlinear behavior of the intrafusal muscle.

Fusimotor Influence on Sensory Behavior

Since both the sensitivity and dynamics of spindle responses can be altered by intrafusal muscle contractions, it is reasonable to assume that the intrafusal muscle has a major role in the determination of spindle behavior.

With the technique of stimulating single gamma efferent axons in the ventral root developed by Hunt and Kuffler (1951), many details of the nature of the fusimotor innervation have been worked out. A single gamma axon can influence the behavior of several spindles, and each spindle is subject to influences from more than one gamma efferent (Kuffler and Hunt, 1952). Stimulation of fusimotor fibers has two basic effects on sensory endings: it increases their mean level of activity and it changes their sensitivity to stretch. Furthermore, with the work of Matthews (1962), it became evident that there are at least two classes of fusimotor effects, called fusistatic and fusidynamic. Although the dichotomy is not perfect, a recent careful classification of 153 examples of fusimotor action on primary endings confirmed its generality (Emonet-Dénand et al., 1977).

Fusistatic activation influences both primary and secondary endings. It is characterized by an increased static sensitivity to large amplitude stretches with a decrease (or little change) in the dynamic index (Fig. 3–11). Fusistatic action also produces a decrease in the sensitivity to small amplitude cyclic stretches. Fusidynamic action, in contrast, affects only the primary endings, and is characterized by an increase in dynamic index with little effect on static sensitivity. These results are not completely consistent with experimental data obtained with small amplitude sinusoidal stretches, particularly for fusidynamic stimulation. Using that form of stretch there is no significant change in dynamics induced by either fusistatic or fusidynamic stimulation, except for those affected by stretch frequencies greater than 10 to 20 Hz (Goodwin et al., 1975; Chen and Poppele, 1978). Furthermore, the induced changes in sensitivity with fusistatic stimulation are opposite to those seen with ramp stretches. Combined stimulation of fusistatic and fusidynamic fibers leads to a nonlinear interaction of their effects. These interactions have been interpreted as

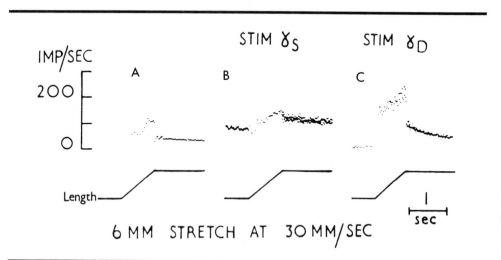

Figure 3–11 Effects of fusistatic (γ_S) and fusidynamic (γ_D) stimulation on the stretch response of the same primary ending. A, No fusimotor stimulation; B, during continuous stimulation of a single static fiber at 70/sec; and C, during continuous stimulation of a single dynamic fiber at 70/sec. (From Brown and Matthews, 1966.)

evidence for the existence of dual pacemakers serving respectively a dynamic and static transducer (Hulliger et al., 1977; Crowe and Matthews, 1964; Lennerstrand, 1968b).

Fusimotor Influence on Intrafusal Muscle

In the past few years efforts have been made to determine the types and locations of the motor endings of the known types of fusimotor axons and the nature of the specific muscle fibers that respond to their stimulation. Different methods have applied to yield important information.

The glycogen depletion method developed by Edstrom and Kugelberg (1968) to plot motor unit territory was first used by Brown and Butler (1973). The method relies upon histochemical (PAS) location of segments of intrafusal muscle fibers that have been glycogen-depleted during rapid repetitive stimulation of the motor axon under ischemic conditions. The segments involved are presumably those contracting during stimulation, and are generally believed to contain the motor ending (but see Banks et al., 1976). Stimulation of static gamma axons resulted in glycogen-depleted segments in chain fibers alone or in chain fibers and the largest bag fiber (Brown and Butler, 1975b). Boyd et al. (1977) suggested that this was the static bag 2 fiber. In similar experiments Barker et al. (1976b) found that chain fibers alone, bag fibers alone, or chain plus bag fibers were depleted by static gamma stimulation. Bag 1 and bag 2 were affected about equally. In activating different spindles a single static gamma could deplete a bag fiber only in one, chain fibers only in another, and bag and chain in a third (Barker et al., 1976b). Both groups of researchers found that the depleted segments were usually intracapsular.

Dynamic gamma stimulation was followed by glycogen depletion that was predominantly in bag fibers (Brown and Butler, 1973), almost always restricted to bag 1 fibers, but rarely in a bag 2 or long chain fiber (Barker et al., 1976b). Depleted segments were rarely on more than one pole and were equally intra- and extracapsular, and therefore generally further from the equator than depleted segments found with static gamma stimulation (Barker et al., 1976b).

Beta fiber stimulation (conduction velocity range, 51 to 77 m/sec) resulted in a dynamic response and glycogen depletion almost exclusively on bag 1 fibers of one spindle pole. Rarely a bag 2 or long chain showed depleted segments (Barker et al., 1977). The branch of dynamic beta axons to extrafusal muscle innervates small motor units of the slow oxidative type (Barker et al., 1977), named according to Ariano et al. (1973). A small number of beta axons have been found to have conduction velocities faster than 85 m/sec. Stimulation of these

101

usually results in depleted zones on long chain fibers, although depletion on bag 1 and bag 2 fibers has been observed (Harker et al., 1977; Jami et al., 1978, 1979). Unlike the slower conducting beta axons, the faster beta axons have a static action and the extrafusal motor units are of the fast glycolytic type (Jami et al., 1979).

The terminals of the different types of fusimotor axons have been studied most directly by nerve degeneration experiments. Following the identification of the action of a single fusimotor axon, all other axons are cut and the animal maintained until degeneration of endings on the intrafusal fibers is complete. The activity of the surviving axons is then reverified, the appropriate muscles are removed, and the surviving endings demonstrated by silver staining (Barker et al., 1970a). By this method all surviving static gamma axons were found to terminate as trial endings distributed to chain and bag fibers. Only rarely did both bag fibers of one pole receive endings. Bag fibers could not be distinguished as bag 1 or bag 2 at the time of the study (Barker et al., 1973; Barker, 1974).

When spindles are deprived of all gamma axon supply by degeneration, leaving the beta axon intact, the motor endings that survive are P_1 plates and these are found on bag 1 fibers (Barker et al., 1971, 1979). The assumption according to several lines of indirect evidence is that dynamic gamma axons end in P_2 plates that are mainly on bag 1 fibers.

IF fiber innervation has also been studied by direct observation of the contraction of individual muscle fibers during stimulation of the fusimotor axons (Bessou and Pagès, 1973, 1975; Boyd et al., 1973, 1977; Boyd and Ward, 1975). It was observed that activation of dynamic gamma axons resulted in contraction of a localized segment of one type of bag fiber, which Boyd et al. (1975a) have called a dynamic nuclear bag fiber. Stimulation of static gamma axons caused contraction of either chain fibers or a second type of bag fiber, called static nuclear bag fiber, or both. Stimulation of a static gamma axon never caused an observable contraction in a dynamic nuclear bag fiber, and vice versa.

Fusistatic stimulation produces contractions that involve discrete segments of the static bag fiber and large intracapsular segments of chain fibers (Bessou and Pagès, 1975; Boyd et al., 1977). These stretch the "in series" sensory endings, thereby increasing the sensory discharge. In fact, the sensory endings respond to individual intrafusal twitches (Bessou et al., 1968). The contraction time for fast bag and chain fibers is relatively short, and the initial velocity is rapid (Boyd, 1976b). Fusidynamic stimulation, on the other hand, produces slow localized contraction in the slow "dynamic" bag fibers (Bessou and Pagès, 1975). A smooth contraction for all bag fibers begins with stimulation at 10 to 20 Hz and is maximal at about 75 Hz (Boyd, 1976b).

Conduction velocity has not proved a useful means of identifying dynamic gamma from static gamma axons, with the exception that fibers conducting below 25 m/sec are almost always static fibers (Brown et al., 1965; Boyd et al., 1977). The conduction velocity of most gamma axons is between 15 and 55 m/sec; this corresponds to a fiber diameter of about 3 to 9 μm (Kuffler et al., 1951). Static gamma axons ending on bag fibers tend to have conduction velocities in the upper part of this range (Barker et al., 1976b; Boyd et al., 1977). Fusimotor axons with conduction velocity of about 50 m/sec are mainly beta axons (Bessou et al., 1965).

Beta axons are now known to comprise from 14 to 30 per cent of the fastest conducting motor axons in cat hind limb (Boyd et al., 1975b; McWilliam, 1974). Beta axons have almost uniformly proven to have a dynamic effect on the primary ending that is indistinguishable from the effect of dynamic gamma axons (Bessou et al. 1965). For 72 of 76 beta axons tested with conduction velocities of 39 to 92 m/sec, the action was found to be dynamic. The remaining four had a static action (Emonet-Dénand et al., 1975). It now appears that the fastest beta axons have a static action (Jami et al., 1978).

In summary, it appears that the dynamic response to gamma axon stimulation is principally effected via P_2 plates on bag 1 fibers, and the dynamic response of beta axons occurs via P_1 plates on the slowly contracting bag 1 fibers. These bag 1 fibers are almost certainly the "dynamic bag" fibers distinguished by Boyd et al. (1975a, 1977). Bag 2 and chain fibers may rarely be involved in the dynamic response in combination with bag 1 fibers. The static response to gamma stimulation is mediated via trail endings which are mainly on the faster contracting chain fibers and bag 2 fibers. The chain and bag 2 fibers are very likely the "static bag" fibers of Boyd and Ward (1975) and Boyd et al. (1977). The fastest beta axons also effect a static response, mainly via long chain fibers (Jami et al., 1979). The type of motor ending is unknown, but may be P_1.

Although this appears to present a clear distinction between the static and dynamic components, as mediated by bag 2, chain, and bag 1, respectively, many trail endings have been observed on bag 1 fibers, thereby leaving open a possible role for bag 1 fibers in the static response (Barker et al., 1973). Furthermore, as noted above, glycogen depletion has been found in bag 1 fibers following stimulation of a gamma fiber shown to elicit a static response (Barker et al., 1976b). Perhaps, though, these findings are not inconsistent with a recent report

Table 3–2

CATEGORY	PHYSIOLOGY			HISTOLOGY		
	Type	Description	%	Glycogen Depletion	Type	%
I	d	Pure dynamic	77	All bag 1	d	81
II	d	Mostly dynamic	23	Bag 1 and bag 2 or bag 1 and chain	d	19
III	?	Unclassified				
IV	s	Static with inc. dynamic index	38	More than half to bag 1	s	33
V	s	Mostly static				
VI	s	Pure static	72	Mostly to bag 2 and chain	s	67

that there are a substantial number of mixed responses elicited by gamma stimulation that are neither pure dynamic nor pure static (Emonet-Dénand et al., 1977). In Table 3–2 that study is summarized and compared with the recent study of Barker et al. (1976b) on the glycogen depletion of identified endings. From Table 3–2 it can be seen that the notion of a static-dynamic dichotomy for bag 2, chain, and bag 1 fibers is supportable, and is still a likely explanation for the present evidence. Intermediate types then simply represent cases in which a particular gamma fiber would activate both bag 1 and bag 2 fibers in some combination (Emonet-Dénand et al., 1977).

FUNCTIONAL MECHANISMS

Despite the fact that the precise anatomy of the mammalian muscle spindle is quite complex, a compartmentalization according to function may be proposed (Fig. 3–12). This hypothetical scheme is presented here to provide a basis for the following discussion of functional mechanisms.

Mechanical Filtering

Most attempts to explain dynamic components of spindle behavior have focused on mechanical filtering, while transduction and encoding have been assumed to be proportional, nonadapting mechanisms. It was Matthews (1933) who first suggested that the viscoelastic properties of the intrafusal muscle might account for the dynamic sensitivity of the spindle receptor. This suggestion, which is still popular today (Matthews, 1972), was reinforced by the finding in another mechanoreceptor, the crayfish stretch receptor (Eyzaguirre and Kuffler, 1955; Terzuolo and Washizu, 1962), that the generator or receptor potential is due to a change in membrane conductance which is proportional to stimulus intensity. If we can assume a similar transducer in the spindle, it is difficult to account for rate sensitivities or adaptations from that process without a series capacitance in the membrane or a changing membrane capacity (Katz,

MAMMALIAN MUSCLE SPINDLE

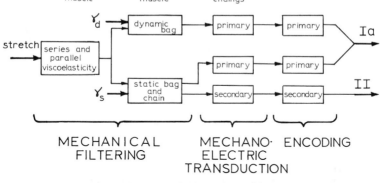

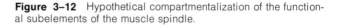

Figure 3–12 Hypothetical compartmentalization of the functional subelements of the muscle spindle.

1950). In addition, the encoder has been considered to provide a direct translation from membrane voltage to impulse rate without adaptation (Terzuolo and Washizu, 1962). These views have now been modified.

Mechanical filtering of applied stretches occurs at at least two levels, the extrafusal muscle lying in parallel and in series with the receptor, and the intrafusal muscle in series with the sensory endings.

As for the extrafusal muscle, evidence has been found to suggest that its contribution to spindle dynamics is negligible for small amplitude stretches. The properties of spindles in such different muscles as the soleus, gastrocnemius, and tenuissimus are nearly identical (e.g., compare Rosenthal et al., 1970 and Poppele and Bowman, 1970). And, the dynamics of the length-tension relationship of the tenuissimus muscle, which reveals the viscoelastic properties of the extrafusal muscle, is like that of a simple spring within the range of frequencies and amplitudes where the receptor exhibits complex dynamics (Poppele and Bowman, 1970). In addition, the behavior of isolated muscle spindles with no extrafusal component is exactly the same as that observed for spindles in the tenuissimus muscle (Kennedy and Poppele, 1972, and unpublished observations).

For larger amplitude stretches the findings are not so clear. By correlating static and dynamic sensitivities with muscle stretch for a number of primary endings, it has been shown that both static and dynamic sensitivities are nonlinearly related to muscle extension, and that this

105

relationship differs for different spindles because of their various locations within the muscle (Windhorst et al., 1976). Thus, passive extrafusal muscle cannot be ruled out as a possible contributor to the determination of spindle response to a given stretch.

The role of intrafusal muscle in determining spindle dynamics has been deduced largely on the basis of morphology. It has been commonly believed, since first suggested by Matthews (1933), that the viscoelastic properties of intrafusal muscle do indeed determine the dynamic behavior of muscle spindle receptors. Furthermore, it has been shown that the input-output characteristics of primary and secondary endings can be fully accounted for if certain *ad hoc* assumptions are made concerning viscoelastic properties of the intrafusal muscle (e.g., Angers, 1965; Houk and Stark, 1962; Gottlieb et al., 1969; Rudjord, 1970). There are, however, only a few quantitative measures of intrafusal viscoelastic properties upon which to base such assumptions. Observations made on isolated muscle spindles from rat (Smith, 1966) and cat (Boyd, 1966; Boyd and Ward, 1969; Beacham et al., 1971) showed a distinct difference in viscoelastic relaxation following a quick stretch for bag and chain fibers. Later studies revealed that only one class of bag fibers, the "dynamic bag" of Boyd (1976a), exhibits a significant mechanical adaptation after a rapid stretch. Other evidence, also derived from direct observation of intrafusal muscle behavior or from measurements of intrafusal muscle tension, suggests that receptor adaptation cannot be fully accounted for by intrafusal muscle properties (Ottoson, 1972; Poppele, 1973; Hunt and Ottoson, 1975). The mechanical adaptation due to intrafusal viscoelasticity will result in a phase lead in the response of the spindle to sinusoidal stretches. This fact provides the opportunity to determine quantitatively whether mechanical adapation is adequate to account for spindle adaptations. Preliminary data have been reported (Poppele et al., 1979) which show that the phase lead of stretch directly across the primary ending in bag fibers is consistently less than the phase lead of the afferent activity from primary endings. Therefore, if mechanical filtering is to account for spindle adaptation, it must be associated with structures within the sensory area and not with the viscoelasticity of the spindle poles.

Transduction The most popular model of mechanoelectric transduction comes from the work done on crayfish stretch receptors, the Pacinian corpuscle, and frog spindles (Edwards et al., 1963; Loewenstein, 1961; Katz, 1950; Ottoson, 1964). The hypothesis is that the mechanical stimulus somehow alters the structure of the membrane so that it becomes ion-permeable. Ions are then relatively free to move along their electrochemical gradient, which is largest for Na^+. This current flow then results in proportional voltage changes. It has been found that a local depolarization is produced by a local mechanical stimulus and the response involves a local change in membrane conductance which depends, at least in part, on the presence of extracellular Na^+ (Edwards et al., 1963). Other hypotheses have been suggested to explain mechanoelectric transduction which are also consistent with this evidence. One is that mechanical deformation leads to the release of a chemical transmitter which acts on the sensory endings. However, the only putative transmitters known to have an excitatory effect on spindles (e.g., succinylcholine) act directly on intrafusal muscle rather than on sensory endings (Henatsch, 1962; Smith, 1966).

Recently it has been shown that the receptor response of the primary ending of the mammalian muscle spindle depends upon the presence of specific ions in a way that is consistent with the basic ionic hypothesis, but with significant differences (Hunt et al., 1978). Specifically, there is an increase in permeability to both Na^+ and Ca^{++} that leads to an inward current, followed by a later outward current that is blocked by tetraethylammonium ions. This and other properties of the outward current suggest that it is carried by K^+ ions. Tetrodotoxin, which is known to selectively block Na^+ channels that lead to the production of action potentials, does not affect the magnitude or time course of the generator (except at higher concentrations of the toxin) (Loewenstein et al., 1966; Hunt and Ottoson, 1975; Hunt et al., 1978). For this reason, and because of their permeability to Ca^{++}, sodium conductance channels involved in the generator response are apparently different chemically from those in the axon where spikes are propagated. Both Na^+ channels appear to recognize Li^+ as well as Na^+ ions, since normal generator responses can be obtained in Li^+ Ringer's solution (Obara and Grundfest, 1968) and, in fact, the generator response of the spindle is enhanced in Li^+ (Hunt et al., 1978). However, there are subtle changes occurring in Li^+ Ringer's solution in some species; these are thought to result from the inability of a Na^+-K^+ pump to recognize that ion (Keynes and Swan, 1959). Apparently Li^+ can enter sensory endings in response to a stimulus, but it is not pumped back out. This causes the cell to become loaded with Li^+, thereby reducing the driving force and depolarizing the cell, at least in the crayfish stretch receptor (Obara and Grundfest, 1968). In the case of the muscle spindle, Li^+ does not appear to have an effect on the resting potential, suggesting therefore that an electrogenic sodium pump does not play a role in its generation.

Although the evidence is incomplete and our understanding of the mechanoelectric transduction is evolving rapidly, it seems clear that this process can indeed account for a significant adaptation in the receptor

107

response. The transduction does not appear to be merely a passive gating of ionic flow, as previously supposed, but rather a combination of inward and delayed outward currents.

Encoding

The intracellular currents induced by the transduction mechanism lead to the production of action potentials at a rate that is related to the magnitude of receptor currents. This is the frequency code that has been well known since the work of Adrian (1928), but the mechanisms responsible for repetitive firing are still basically unknown. Neither the Hodgkin-Huxley model nor any simple modification of that model leads to repetitive firing at rates as low as those observed in receptors like the muscle spindle (i.e., 5 imp/sec or less) (Fitzhugh, 1961).

The properties of repetitive firing in the spindle are similar to those observed in other sensory neurons. The rate of impulse activity in both primary and secondary endings is a linear function of the steady state receptor potential (Hunt and Ottoson, 1975). One difference between the primary and secondary afferent discharge that may be attributable to encoder properties is that interval length tends to be more variable for the primary than for the secondary. This may reflect the greater sensitivity of the primary ending to minute disturbances. However, the variability of the primary is increased in proportion to the increased variability of the secondary in the presence of fusimotor activity; in each case the coefficient of variation (mean interval/standard deviation) is increased about fourfold (Matthews and Stein, 1969b). If a greater sensitivity to disturbances were to account for the differential variability, then it might be expected that the increment of disturbance added by fusimotor contractions would cause a proportionally greater increase in primary variability. An alternate explanation for the variability of primary discharges may be related to the proposed existence of multiple encoders for this nerve (this possibility is discussed below).

Under some conditions, impulse activity from the spindle can be "driven" or "phase-locked" on a one-for-one basis with fusistatic stimulation (Kuffler et al., 1951). This apparently does relate to a receptor response to individual intrafusal muscle twitches, and is therefore related to the phase-locking observed in response to a vibrational stimulus (see above).

Phase-locking to a repetitive stimulus is a general property attributable to many pacemaker mechanisms. Theoretical and model studies have shown that some degree of phase-locking is to be expected from any neuronal encoder in which there is a finite conductance in the interspike interval (Rescigno et al., 1970; Knight, 1972).

The tendency to phase-lock can in fact be related to the magnitude of the conductance: the larger the interspike conductance, the greater the tendency to phase-lock (Knight, 1972; Poppele and Chen, 1972). The encoder of the secondary ending has been studied in some detail, both in comparison to the encoder of the crayfish stretch receptor (Fohlmeister et al., 1974, 1977a, b) and in the context of specific models (Poppele and Chen, 1972; Fohlmeister, 1973). Results of those studies led to the conclusion that the average magnitude of the interspike conductance is inversely proportional to the length of the interval. Therefore, the conductance is not constant in the interval but rather is large early in the interval and small thereafter (Fohlmeister et al., 1974). Since the conductance is determined for a period when sodium conductance is likely to be negligible (the interspike interval), it is probably a potassium conductance that is described.

A similar analysis was attempted for the primary ending but was not as successful (Poppele and Chen, 1972). That encoder behaves as though it has a very low interspike conductance, but it also exhibits an extreme sensitivity to phase-locking. Perhaps the nontypical behavior (in that it is not similar to that of other well studied encoders in the secondary ending, crayfish stretch receptor, and *Limulus* lateral eye receptor (Fohlmeister et al., 1977b; Knight, 1972) may be in part due to the presence of more than one encoder for the primary afferent axon. Indeed, there is now an increasing body of circumstantial evidence supporting this notion.

Several investigators have noted the degree of branching that occurs in the primary afferent fiber after it enters the capsule. Recent studies by Quick et al. (1979a) described up to seven myelinated branches in primary Ia fibers. Furthermore, it has now been shown that each of the nodes and heminodes of these branches react histochemically with a specific stain that has been associated only with membrane that produces action potentials (Quick et al., 1979b; Quick and Waxman, 1977).

Physiological support for the concept of several pacemakers comes from several lines of evidence. If a spindle is cooled or treated with moderate doses of lidocaine, the interval histogram derived from primary afferent activity shows several modes that are attributable to different preferred intervals between spikes (Dawis and Poppele, 1976). This has been interpreted as resulting from occasional failures of one or more encoders to produce a spike (Horak, 1977) and the antidromic resetting of failing pacemakers by those with slower rhythms (Eagles and Purple, 1974) (Fig. 3–13).

Banks et al. (1977a) have also suggested that a branch of the first bifurcation of the primary axon goes only to the

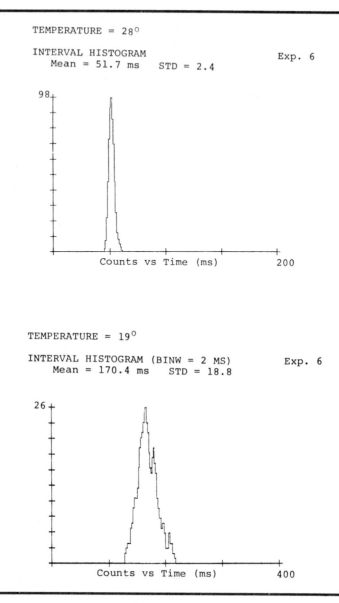

TEMPERATURE = 28°

INTERVAL HISTOGRAM   Exp. 6
    Mean = 51.7 ms   STD = 2.4

98

Counts vs Time (ms)   200

TEMPERATURE = 19°

INTERVAL HISTOGRAM (BINW = 2 MS)   Exp. 6
    Mean = 170.4 ms   STD = 18.8

26

Counts vs Time (ms)   400

Figure 3–13 Interval histograms of the discharge from a primary afferent at 28° C *(upper)* and 19° C *(lower)*. Note the appearance of secondary modes at the lower temperature. (From Horak, 1977.)

bag 1 fiber while the other innervates bag 2 and chain fibers. This would suggest that the primary ending may actually serve two separate receptors, each having its own intrafusal bundle, sensory endings, and encoder (note Fig. 3–12).

Impulse activity in the Ia fiber would then correspond to the activity of the encoder producing the most rapid discharge, since slower encoders would be antidromically reset before they reached threshold by propagated spikes produced at the most rapid rate (Eagles and Purple, 1974). This is indeed a likely explanation for a number of findings involving stretch applied in the presence of fusimotor stimulation. Figure 3–14 shows the effect of gamma static stimulation on the response to a ramp stretch (Crowe and Matthews, 1964). Notice that the dynamic component of the response is completely unaffected. If responses of a dynamic and static transducer are simply summed and encoded at a single pacemaker, the dynamic response will be lifted up and added to the static response. Instead, the pattern observed here is more consistent with a "pacemaker switching" (Crowe and Matthews, 1964) in which the most rapidly firing encoder has absolute control of the output that is propagated along the primary afferent fiber.

More recent data employing static gamma and dynamic gamma stimulation are consistent with this interpretation. By stimulating a spindle with large amplitude sinusoidal stretches and combinations of static gamma and dynamic gamma stimuli, Hulliger et al. (1977) observed that in phases of the cycle for which firing is greater during static than during dynamic stimulation, the static action entirely dominates (Fig. 3–15). Although such behavior might also be attributed to a contraction-induced unloading that is added to stretch-induced unloading during the relaxation phase of the sinusoidal stretch, thereby leaving only chain and static bag fibers stretched in that phase (Hulliger et al. 1977; Schafer, 1974), the alternative explanation of a pacemaker switching cannot be ruled out as a possible mechanism for this

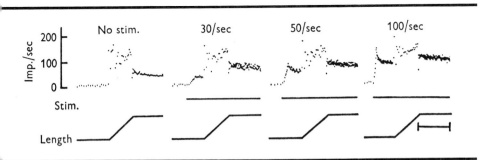

Figure 3–14 Records showing the slight effect of stimulation of a static fusimotor fiber on the frequency of discharge of a primary ending during the dynamic phase of stretching. Frequency of fusimotor stimulation given above each record; stretch was 6 mm at 30 mm/sec; time mark 1 sec. (From Crowe and Matthews, 1964.)

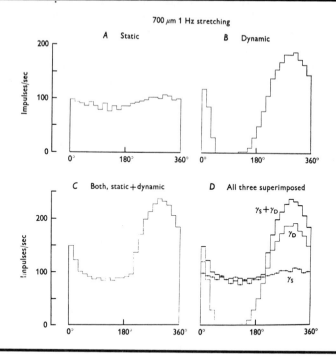

Figure 3–15 Cycle histograms showing the asymmetrical pattern of summation and occlusion of static and dynamic actions during large amplitude stretching. A, Stimulation of static fiber at 56/sec; B, stimulation of dynamic fiber at 100/sec; C, combined; D, superposition of records from A, B, and C. (From Hulliger et al., 1977.)

behavior (cf., Hulliger et al., 1977; Lennerstrand, 1968b).

Returning to the question of spindle adaptation, several attempts have been made to show whether or not some of the receptor adaptation can be accounted for by the encoder. Lippold et al. (1960) used extracellularly applied direct current steps to stimulate the receptor and found no adaptation. A similar experiment by Emonet-Dénand and Houk (1969) gave mixed results and, as they pointed out, one cannot be sure that the currents used are affecting only the encoder. Recent data on this point relate to the finding by Nakajima and Onodera (1969) that there is an electrogenic component of the Na^+-K^+ pump in the crayfish neuron which produces a hyperpolarization after each spike. It was later shown by Sokolove and Cooke (1971) that this mechanism is responsible for the adaptation of repetitive firing activity in response to a step change in depolarizing current. A similar mechanism has now been identified in cat muscle spindles for both the primary and secondary endings, and it would be expected to lead to an adaptation having a time constant of the order of several seconds (Holloway and Poppele, 1978).

FUNCTIONAL STUDIES OF THE HUMAN MUSCLE SPINDLE

Physiological studies using human spindles have been fewer and more limited in scope than those with spindles from experimental animals. Results of in vitro studies of a small number of spindles were reported by Poppele and Kennedy (1974). They recorded from the intramuscular type Ia and type II sensory nerves of spindles that were partially dissected from biopsies of extensor indicis of normal volunteers. The behavior of the human primary and secondary sensory endings conformed precisely to the dynamics reported by Poppele and Bowman (1970) for cat spindles. The dynamics of primary but not of secondary endings were dependent upon temperature, as in the cat. Sensory behavior was also normal in one spindle recorded from a patient with amyotrophic lateral sclerosis in whom the extensor indicis biopsied had only a few functional motor units and severe, neurogenic extrafusal muscle atrophy (Poppele and Kennedy, 1974).

In vivo recording from human nerves has become practical with the technique introduced by Vallbo and Hagbarth (1967) and Vallbo (1970a). By placing a tungsten microelectrode percutaneously into the nerve, they were able to record activity from sympathetic nerve fibers and from a variety of sensory nerve fibers, including types Ia and type II nerves from muscle spindles. Most recordings of nerve fibers from muscle spindles have been made on normal subjects, either at rest, while receiving sensory stimuli, during limited voluntary contractions, or during elicitation of reflex movement. A few studies from patients with movement disorders or neuromuscular disease have been done. The results from this research have contributed greatly to our understanding of spindle function, but the techniques are not yet in use for clinical diagnosis. Much of this work was reviewed recently by Vallbo et al. (1979).

The experiments from the Swedish laboratories have provided convincing evidence that muscle spindles in completely relaxed muscles are not under active fusimotor bias (Vallbo et al., 1979; but see Burg et al., 1973, 1974, 1976 for conflicting views). This conclusion is suggested by several findings. First, the position sensitivity of spindles in resting human muscle is extremely low, in the range of one fifth of that in cat ankle extensors (Vallbo, 1974a), and a majority of the spindle afferents recorded from muscle relaxed at midlength are silent (Hagbarth et al., 1973; Vallbo, 1970a, 1972, 1973a, 1974a). Next, those primary and secondary endings that are discharging do so at rates lower than the discharge rates of de-efferented cat hind limb spindles (Vallbo, 1972, 1973a, 1974a). Their discharge lacks the spontaneous

113

variations in rate expected for spindles with an active fusimotor outflow. That is, the rate is regular, as in de-efferented cat spindles (Matthews and Stein, 1969b) and, related to this, the responses to standard ramp stretches are reproducible (Hagbarth et al., 1975a; Vallbo, 1973a, 1974a). Lastly, virtual elimination of all fusimotor influence by lidocaine block does not significantly change the afferent responses of the spindles to stretch of the muscle or to vibration applied to the tendon (Burke et al., 1976a; Hagbarth et al., 1975b). It is a daily observation of the electromyographer that the skeletal motor system is silent in completely relaxed limb muscles; now it may be concluded that the fusimotor system is also silent.

Human spindles in relaxed muscles without fusimotor bias are found to maintain a high dynamic sensitivity to mechanical stimuli, such as light taps on the skin overlying the muscle belly or tendon percussion. This is analogous to the dynamic sensitivity of the primary sensory endings of cat spindles. Some endings are modulated by the arterial pulse (Burke et al., in press) or by respiratory movements (Hagbarth et al., 1975a). Like unbiased cat spindles (Goodwin et al., 1976; Matthews and Stein, 1969a; Poppele and Bowman, 1970) human primary endings have greater sensitivity (impulses per unit of stretch) to small stretches than to larger length changes (Poppele and Kennedy, 1974; Vallbo, 1973a). The primary sensory endings maintain a high sensitivity to vibratory stimuli that is greatest during application of passive stretch. This is unaffected by lidocaine treatment, which blocks mainly the smaller diameter fusimotor fibers (Burke et al., 1976a).

Using the intraneural recording method, it has been possible to study spindle behavior during voluntary and reflex movement of the receptor-containing muscle. Spindle behavior during isometric contraction has received the most attention, partly because the microelectrode position remains relatively stable, allowing for adequate recording sessions. In their initial studies, Hagbarth and Vallbo (1968) demonstrated that during voluntary isometric contraction sensory activity increases as torque increases and, at the height of the contraction, the activity wavers in proportion to the torque (Vallbo, 1973a). Even minute variations in movement result in corresponding fluctuations of the afferent discharge (Vallbo, 1973a). The first electromyographic (EMG) burst precedes the afferent discharge by several milliseconds (Vallbo, 1971, 1972). This increase in spindle afferent activity during voluntary muscle contraction is best explained by an associated fusimotor outflow that excites the sensory endings. The outflow must be powerful enough to overcome the unloading effect that characterizes sensory behavior of unbiased spindles during muscle contraction (Hagbarth and Vallbo, 1968; Vallbo,

1970*a*, *b*). Blockage of fusimotor axons with lidocaine obliterates the phenomenon. The spindle discharge then decelerates with the isometric contraction (Burke et al., 1976*a*; Hagbarth et al., 1970, 1975*b*).

The above findings are inconsistent with the notion that voluntary movement results from fusimotor-initiated, spindle-mediated, direct reflex excitation of motoneurons; instead, the indication is that descending excitation acting directly upon skeletomotoneurons is responsible for voluntary movement. The time delay observed between the first EMG burst and the later spindle discharge with rapid movement is consistent with the idea that alpha and gamma motoneurons are excited almost simultaneously (Vallbo, 1971) and, as indicated by further experiments, the excitation is parallel in intensity (Vallbo, 1974*b*). The coexcitation of alpha and gamma systems is called alpha-gamma coactivation. It was recently found that during slow isometric contractions the time lag between the initial EMG activity and the afferent burst from individual afferents was different for each afferent recorded; the individual afferents were activated at defined strengths of contraction that were constant for each particular spindle ending (Burke et al., 1978*b*). There was no correlation between externally applied length changes and the ease of activation of individual endings by isometric contraction. It was concluded that the activation threshold of spindle endings is determined by the recruitment order of fusimotor neurons similar to the orderly recruitment of alpha motoneurons during contractions (Burke et al., 1978*b*). This is additional support for the idea that alpha and gamma motoneurons are acted upon in parallel (by descending tracts), and that the descending drives determine the desired muscular force rather than the desired muscular length (Evarts, 1973).

The fusimotor drive during isometric contractions is likely conveyed mostly by gamma rather than beta axons, because spindle discharge continues to increase during attempts at voluntary contraction after the large nerve fibers, alpha and presumably beta included, are blocked by nerve compression (Burke et al., 1979). Conversely, the spindle discharge is abolished by a partial lidocaine block that spares most large fibers, allowing muscle contraction to continue (Hagbarth et al., 1970, 1975*b*).

Alpha-gamma coactivation has been found present for all voluntary movements yet studied. Although shifts in the intensity of outflow of one over the other appear possible and even probable, none have been demonstrated. Two movements, both initiated reflexly at the periphery, do not adhere to the alpha-gamma coactivation principle. Neither the tendon jerk reflex (Burg et al., 1973; Szumski et al., 1974) nor the tonic vibration reflex (TVR) (Burke et al., 1976*b*) are accompanied by demonstrable fusimotor

115

coactivation. Both result in spindle unloading. The TVR is an example of movement due to intense prolonged activity of the spindle afferents. The movement is not strong, and can be voluntarily inhibited.

The Jendrassik maneuver is a means of facilitating a tendon reflex by having the subject contract a remote muscle while the reflex is being tested. The origin of the facilitation is the subject of a controversy that can be traced in part to Sommer's (1940) report that the Jendrassik maneuver did not facilitate the H (Hoffmann) reflex. Because the electric stimulus that elicits the H reflex activates the afferent nerve fibers proximal to the muscle spindle, the spindle itself is bypassed. Sommer inferred that reflex reinforcement by the Jendrassik maneuver was not the result of central potentiation at the common excitatory synapse on the motoneuron. He postulated that excitation of a motor outflow specific to the spindle resulted in increased afferent input onto the anterior horn cells, and produced a state of readiness in the spindle to react to tendon taps. Shortly afterwards the fusimotor system was demonstrated (Leksell, 1945). Sommer's view and logic were challenged by Landau and Clare (1964) and Clare and Landau (1964), whose reflex studies strongly suggested that the reinforcement was not due to increased afferent activity but to centrally originating changes in the excitation of the motoneuron pool. Intraneural recordings from afferent nerves supported the conclusions of Clare and Landau (1964), since evidence of increased fusimotor tone was not found, as judged by frequency of the afferent discharges, during the Jendrassik maneuver (Hagbarth and Vallbo, 1968; Hagbarth et al., 1975a) or during changing levels of mental activity (Vallbo, 1972). There was no decline in afferent discharge after lidocaine block of the muscle nerve (Hagbarth et al., 1975b).

Contradictory findings were reported by Burg et al. (1973, 1974), who did find that spindle afferent activity was increased when their subjects contracted remote muscles or underwent mental drive or acoustic stimulation. The postulated fusimotor drive appeared to have a strong dynamic component because it increased the dynamic sensitivity of the affected spindles (Burg et al., 1974, 1975). These results imply that alpha and gamma outflow are not in parallel in the above circumstances.

Resolution of these conflicting results may require close intramuscular EMG monitoring and high gain measurement of muscle torque, as suggested by Hagbarth et al. (1975a), to detect small contractions that could escape clinical detection and result in afferent volleys during reinforcement. At present most evidence suggests that reinforcement of the tendon jerk by contraction of a remote muscle is due to: (1) altered processing of the afferent volley in the spinal cord (Clare and Landau,

1964); and (2) (in subjects who are not completely relaxed) increased afferent input to the cord from a fusimotor outflow that is synchronous with small unintentional contractions of the receptor-containing muscle (Hagbarth et al., 1975a; Vallbo et al., 1979).

In nonisometric contractions the intensity of sensory discharges from spindles depends upon a combination of factors in addition to the fusimotor outflow. The velocity and amount of muscle shortening or lengthening and the external load assume increasing importance (Vallbo, 1973a; Burke et al., 1978a). Still, the discharge is not as great as in an isometric contraction. With lighter loads and faster contractions the intensity of the sensory discharge lessens, but it is seldom silenced (Burke et al., 1978a).

Vallbo's studies of slow isotonic contractions provide additional insight into spindle function (Vallbo, 1973a, b). At the onset of such a contraction the spindle discharge increases rapidly, then remains approximately steady even though muscle shortening continues to unload the receptor slowly. It also remains steady at the end of the contraction. Presumably the muscle shortening is compensated for by a continuous increase of fusimotor drive that keeps spindle response to a steady level. In addition to the generally increased level of spindle afferent activity there are small bursts and lags of afferent discharge that correspond to minute joint movements. This suggests that during alpha-gamma coactivation the fusimotor system maintains a certain sensitivity level within the receptor to even the smallest superimposed joint movement. The resultant afferent bursts probably affect the anterior horn cells in a manner that tends to eliminate larger irregularities. This functional relationship may smooth variations in the velocity of movement, whether they arise by changes of motoneuron excitation from central sources or peripherally by irregularities of the load, or from joint and tendon friction (Vallbo, 1973a, b).

The general conclusions drawn from the afferent recordings during movement are that the alpha motor outflow is accompanied by a simultaneous proportionate fusimotor outflow. The two are related spatially and in intensity (Vallbo, 1974a, b). The fusimotor outflow drives the spindle afferents so as to provide a background upon which variations in position are presented to the CNS for rapid correction (Granit, 1973; Vallbo et al., 1979). The time relationship between the afferent discharge and the preceding muscle activity recorded by EMG excludes the possibility that the initiation or continuation of voluntary movement depends upon the fusimotor system. Rather, voluntary contractions must be the result of descending impulses from supraspinal structures influencing segmental cellular activity.

117

References

Adal, M. N.: The fine structure of the sensory region of the cat muscle spindles. J. Ultrastruct. Res., *26*:332–354, 1969.

Adal, M. N., and Barker, D.: Intramuscular branching of fusimotor fibres. J. Physiol. (Lond.), *177*:288–299, 1965.

Adrian, E. D.: The Basis of Sensation. The Action of the Sense Organs. London, Christophers, 1928.

Akert, K., Sandri, C., Weibel, E. R., Peper, K., and Moor, H.: The fine structure of the perineural epithelium. Cell Tissue Res., *165*:281–295, 1976.

Angers, D.: Modèle mécanique de fuseau neuromusculaire deeferenté: Terminaisons primaries et secondaires. C. R. Acad. Sci. [D], (Paris), *261*:2255–2258, 1965.

Ariano, M. A., Armstrong, R. B., and Edgerton, V. R.: Hindlimb muscle fiber populations of five mammals. J. Histochem. Cytochem., *21*:51–55, 1973.

Banker, B. Q., and Girvin, J. P.: The ultrastructural features of the mammalian muscle spindle. J. Neuropathol. Exp. Neurol., *30*:155–195, 1971.

Banks, R. W., Barker, D. W., Bessou, P., and Stacey, M. J.: Serial-section analysis of cat muscle spindles following observation of the effects of stimulating dynamic fusimotor axons. J. Physiol. (Lond.), *263*:180–181P, 1976.

Banks, R. W., Barker, D., and Stacey, M. J.: Intrafusal branching and distribution of primary and secondary afferents. J. Physiol. (Lond.), *272*:66–67P, 1977*a*.

Banks, R. W., Harker, D. W., and Stacey, M. J.: A study of mammalian intrafusal muscle fibers using a combined histochemical and ultrastructural technique. J. Anat., *123*:783–796, 1977*b*.

Banks, R. W., and James, N. T.: The blood supply of rat muscle spindles. J. Anat., *114*:7–12, 1973.

Banks, R. W., James, N. T., and Meek, G. A.: Morphometric studies on intrafusal and extrafusal muscle fibers. J. Anat., *111*:489P, 1972.

Barker, D.: The innervation of mammalian skeletal muscle. *In* de Reuck, A. V. S., and Knight, J. (eds.): Ciba Foundation Symposium on Myotatic Kinesthetic and Vestibular Mechanisms. London, Churchill, pp. 3–15, 1967.

Barker, D.: The morphology of muscle receptors. *In* Hunt, C. C. (ed.): Handbook of Sensory Physiology. Berlin, Springer Verlag, Vol. III/2. pp. 1–190, 1974.

Barker, D., Banks, R. W., Harker, D. W., Milburn, A., and Stacey, M. J.: Studies of the histochemistry, ultrastructure, motor innervation, and regeneration of mammalian intrafusal muscle fibers. Prog. Brain Res., *44*:66–88, 107–109, 1976*a*.

Barker, D., Emonet-Dénand, F., Harker, D. W., Jami, L., and LaPorte, Y.: Distribution of fusimotor axons to intrafusal muscle fibres in cat tenuissimus spindles as determined by the glycogen-depletion method. J. Physiol. (Lond.), *261*:49–69, 1976*b*.

Barker, D., Emonet-Dénand, F., Harker, D. W., Jami, L., and LaPorte, Y.: Types of intra- and extrafusal muscle fibre innervated by dynamic skeleto-fusimotor axons in cat peroneus brevis and tenuissimus muscles, as determined by the glycogen-depletion method. J. Physiol. (Lond.), *266*:713–726, 1977.

Barker, D., Emonet-Dénand, F., LaPorte, Y., Proske, U., and Stacey, M.: Identification des terminaisons motrices des fibres fusimotrices statiques chez le chat. C. R. Acad. Sci. [D] (Paris), *271*:1203–1206, 1970*a*.

Barker, D., Emonet-Dénand, F., LaPorte, Y., Proske, U., and Stacey, M. J.: Identification of the endings and function of cat fusimotor fibres. J. Physiol. (Lond.), *216*:51–52P, 1971.

Barker, D., Emonet-Dénand, F., LaPorte, Y., Proske, U., and Stacey, M. J.: Morphological identification and intrafusal distribution of the endings of static fusimotor axons in cat. J. Physiol. (Lond.), *230*:405–427, 1973.

Barker, D., Emonet-Dénand, F., LaPorte, Y., and Stacey, M. J.: Identification of the intrafusal endings of skeleto-fusimotor axons in the cat. Persistence of P_1 plates in cat muscle spindles after degeneration of their supply. J. Physiol., *296*:110P, 1979.

Barker, D., and Gidumal, J. L.: The morphology of intrafusal muscle fibres in the cat. J. Physiol. (Lond.), *157*:513–528, 1961.

Barker, D., Stacey, M. J., and Adal, M. N.: Fusimotor innervation in the cat. Philos. Trans. R. Soc. [Biol.], *258*:315–346, 1970*b*.

Batten, F. E.: The muscle-spindle under pathological conditions. Brain, *20*:138–179, 1897.

Beacham, W. S., Fukami, Y., and Hunt, C. C.: Displacement of elements within mammalian muscle spindles. Proc. Int. Union Physiol. Sci. (XXV International Congress), *9*:46, 1971.

Bessou, P., Emonet-Dénand, F., and LaPorte, Y.: Motor fibres innervating extrafusal and intrafusal muscle fibres in the cat. J. Physiol. (Lond.), *180*:649–672, 1965.

Bessou, P., LaPorte, Y., and Pagès, B.: Observations sur la ré-innervation de fuseaux neuro-musculaires de Chat. C.R. Soc. Biol. (Paris), *160*:408–11, 1966.

Bessou, P., LaPorte, Y., and Pagès, B.: Frequency grams of spindle primary endings elicited by stimulation of static and dynamic fusimotor fibres. J. Physiol. (Lond.), *196*:47–63, 1968.

Bessou, P., and Pagès, B.: Nature des fibres musculaires fusales activées par des axones fusimoteurs uniques statiques et dynamiques chez le chat. C. R. Acad. Sci. [D] (Paris), *277*:89–91, 1973.

Bessou, P., and Pagès, B.: Cinematographic analysis of contractile events produced in intrafusal muscle fibres by stimulation of static and dynamic fusimotor axons. J. Physiol. (Lond.), *252*:397–427, 1975.

Boyd, I. A.: The structure and innervation of the nuclear bag muscle fibre system and the nuclear chain muscle fibre system in mammalian muscle spindles. Philos. Trans. R. Soc. [Biol.], *245*:81–136, 1962.

Boyd, I. A.: The mechanical properties of mammalian intrafusal fibres. J. Physiol. (Lond.), *187*:10–12P, 1966.

Boyd, I. A.: The mechanical properties of dynamic nuclear bag fibres, static nuclear bag fibres and nuclear chain fibres in isolated cat muscle spindles. Prog. Brain Res., *44*:39–49, 1976*a*.

Boyd, I. A.: The response of fast and slow nuclear bag fibres and nuclear chain fibres in isolated cat muscle spindles to fusimotor stimulation, and the effect of intrafusal contraction on sensory endings. Q. J. Exp. Physiol., *61*:203–254, 1976*b*.

Boyd, I. A., Gladden, M. H., and McWilliam, P. N.: 'Static' and 'dynamic' fusimotor action in isolated cat muscle spindles with intact nerve and blood supply. J. Physiol. (Lond.), *230*:29–30P, 1973.

Boyd, I. A., Gladden, M. H., McWilliam, P. N., and Ward, J.: 'Static' and 'dynamic' nuclear bag fibres in isolated cat muscle spindles. J. Physiol. (Lond.), *250*:11–12P, 1975*a*.

Boyd, I. A., Gladden, M. H., McWilliam, P. N., and Ward, J.: Study of β innervation and of β and γ control of isolated muscle spindles in the cat hind limb. J. Anat., *119*:198, 1975*b*.

Boyd, I. A., Gladden, M. H., McWilliam, P. N., and Ward, J.: Control of dynamic and static nuclear bag fibres and nuclear chain fibres by gamma and beta axons in isolated cat muscle spindles. J. Physiol. (Lond.), *265*:133–162, 1977.

Boyd, I. A., and Ward, J.: The response of isolated cat muscle spindles to passive stretch. J. Physiol. (Lond.), *200*:104–105P, 1969.

Boyd, I. A., and Ward, J.: Motor control of nuclear bag and nuclear chain intrafusal fibers in isolated living muscle spindles from the cat. J. Physiol. (Lond.), *244*:83–112, 1975.

Brown, M. C., and Butler, R. G.: Studies on the site of termination of static and dynamic fusimotor fibres within muscle spindles of the tenuissimus muscle of the cat. J. Physiol. (Lond.), *233*:553–573, 1973.

Brown, M. C., and Butler, R. G.: The motor innervation of normal and reinnervated muscle spindles. J. Anat., *119*:199P, 1975*a*.

Brown, M. C., and Butler, R. G.: An investigation into the site of termination of static gamma fibres within muscle spindles of the cat peroneus longus muscle. J. Physiol. (Lond.), *247*:131–143, 1975*b*.

Brown, M. C., Crowe, A., and Matthews, P. B. C.: Observations of the fusimotor fibres of the tibialis posterior muscle of the cat. J. Physiol. (Lond.), *177*:140–159, 1965.

Brown, M. C., Engberg, I., and Matthews, P. B. C.: The relative sensitivity to vibration of muscle receptors of the cat. J. Physiol. (Lond.), *192*:773–800, 1967.

Brown, M. C., Goodwin, G. M., and Matthews, P. B. C.: Aftereffects of fusimotor stimulation on the response of muscle spindle afferent endings. J. Physiol. (Lond.), *205*:677–694, 1969.

Brown, M. C., and Matthews, P. B. C.: On the subdivision of the efferent fibres to muscle spindles into static and dynamic fusimotor fibres. *In* Andrew, B. L. (ed.): Control and Innervation of Skeletal Muscle. Edinburgh-London, Livingston, pp. 18–31, 1966.

Brzezinski, Von D. K.: Untersuchungen zur Histochemie der Muskelspindeln, II. Mitteilung Zur Topochemie und Funktion des Spindelraumes und der Spindelkapsel. Acta Histochem. (Jena), *12*:277–288, 1961.

Burg, D., Szumski, A. J., Struppler, A., and Velho, F.: Afferent and efferent activation of human muscle receptors involved in reflex and voluntary contraction. Exp. Neurol. *41*:754–768, 1973.

Burg, D., Szumski, A. J., Struppler, A., and Velho, F.: Assessment of fusimotor contribution to reflex reinforcement in humans. J. Neurol. Neurosurg. Psychiatry, *37*:1012–1021, 1974.

Burg, D., Szumski, A. J., Struppler, A., and Velho, F.: Observations on muscle receptor sensitivity in the human. Electromyogr. Clin. Neurophysiol., *15*:15–28, 1975.

Burg, D., Szumski, A. J., Struppler, A., and Velho, F.: Influence of a voluntary innervation on human muscle spindle sensitivity. *In* Shahani, M. (ed.): Motor Systems: Neurophysiology and Muscle Mechanisms. Amsterdam, Elsevier, pp. 95–110, 1976.

Burke, D., Hagbarth, K.-E., Löfstedt, L., and Wallin, B. G.,: The responses of human muscle spindle endings to vibration during isometric contraction. J. Physiol. (Lond.), *261*:695–711, 1976*a*.

Burke, D., Hagbarth, K.-E., Löfstedt, L.: Muscle spindle activity in man during shortening and lengthening contractions. J. Physiol. (Lond.), *277*:131–142, 1978*c*.

Burke, D., Hagbarth, K.-E., Löfstedt, L., and Wallin, B. G.: The responses of human muscle spindle endings to vibration of non-contracting muscles. J. Physiol. (Lond.), *261*:673–693, 1976*b*.

Burke, D., Hagbarth, K.-E., and Skuse, N. F.: Recruitment order of human spindle endings in isometric voluntary contractions. J. Physiol. (Lond.), *285*:101–112, 1978*b*.

Burke, D., Hagbarth, K.-E., and Wallin, B. G.: Alpha-gamma linkage and the mechanisms of reflex reinforcement. *In* Desmedt, J. E. (ed.): Progress in Clinical Neurophysiology, Vol. 8, Basel, Karger, in press.

Burke, D., Hagbarth, K.-E., and Skuse, N. F.: Voluntary activation of spindle endings in human muscles temporarily paralyzed by nerve pressure. J. Physiol. (Lond.), *287*:329–336, 1979.

Cajal, S. R.: Terminaciones nerviosas en los husos musculares de la rana. Riv. Trim. Histol. Norm. y Patol., *1*, 1888.

Cazzato, G., and Walton, J. N.: The pathology of the muscle spindle. A study of biopsy material in various muscular and neuromuscular diseases. J. Neurol. Sci., *7*:15–70, 1968.

Chen, W. J., and Poppele, R. E.: Small-signal analysis of response of mammalian muscle spindles with fusimotor stimulation and a comparison with large-signal response. J. Neurophysiol., *41*:15–27, 1978.

Chi, C., and Kennedy, W. R.: Mouse muscle spindles: HVEM of the IA sensory ending. 1979 (in preparation).

Clare, M. H., and Landau, W. M.: Fusimotor function. Part V. Reflex reinforcement under fusimotor block in normal subjects. Arch. Neurol., *10*:123–127, 1964.

Cöers, C., and Durand, J.: Données morphologiques nouvelles sur l'innervation des fuseaux neuromusculaires. Arch. Biol. (Liège), *67*:685–715, 1956.

Cooper, S.: The secondary endings of muscle spindles. J. Physiol. (Lond.), *149*:27–28P, 1959.

Cooper, S.: The responses of the primary and secondary endings of muscle spindles with intact motor innervation during applied stretch. Q. J. Exp. Physiol, *46*:389–398, 1961.

Corvaja, N., Marinozzi, V., and Pompeiano, O.: Muscle spindles in the lumbrical muscle of the cat. Arch. Ital. Biol., *107*:365–543, 1969.

Craske, B.: Perception of impossible limb positions induced by tendon vibration. Science, *196*:71–73, 1977.

Crowe, A., and Matthews, P. B. C.: Further studies of static and dynamic fusimotor fibres. J. Physiol. (Lond.), *174*:132–151, 1964.

Cuajunco, F.: Development of the neuromuscular spindle in human fetuses. Contrib. Embryol. Carnegie Inst., *28*:95–128, 1940.

Daniel, P. M., and Strich, S. J.: Abnormalities in the muscle spindles in dystrophia myotonica. Neurology (Minneap.), *14*:310–316, 1964.

Dawis, S., and Poppele, R. E.: Evidence for multiple encoder sites in primary endings of mammalian muscle spindles. Neurosci. Abstr., *1*:182, 1975.

DeSantis, M., and Norman, W. P.: An ultrastructural study of nerve terminal degeneration in muscle spindles of the tenuissimus muscle of the cat. J. Neurocytol., *8*:67–80, 1979.

Duchen, L. W.: "Sprawling": A new mutant mouse with a failure of myelination of sensory axons and a deficiency of muscle spindles. J. Neuropathol. Appl. Neurobiol., *1*:89–101, 1975.

Duchen, L. W., and Strich, S. J.: An hereditary motor neurone disease with progressive denervation of muscle in the mouse: The mutant Wobbler. J. Neurol. Neurosurg. Psychiatry, *31*:535–542, 1968.

Eagles, J. P., and Purple, R. L.: Afferent fibers with multiple encoding sites. Brain Res., *77*:187–193, 1974.

Eccles, J. C., Oscarsson, O., and Willis, W. D.: Synaptic action of group I and II afferent fibres of muscle on the cells of the dorsal spinocerebellar tract. J. Physiol. (Lond.), *158*:517–543, 1961.

Eccles, J. C., and Sherrington, C. S.: Numbers and contraction-values of individual motor-units examined in some muscles of the limb. Proc. R. Soc. Lond. [Biol.], *106*:326–357, 1930.

Edstrom, L., and Kugelberg, E.: Histochemical composition, distribution of fibres and fatiguability of single motor units. J. Neurol. Neurosurg. Psychiatry, *31*:424–433, 1968.

Edwards, C., Terzuolo, C. A., and Washizu, Y.: The effect of changes of the ionic environment upon an isolated crustacean sensory neuron. J. Neurophysiol., *26*:948–957, 1963.

Edwards, R. P.: An ultrastructural study of neuromuscular spindles in normal mice: With reference to mice and man infected with *Mycobacterium leprae*. J. Anat., *120*:149–168, 1975.

Eklund, G.: Position sense and state of contraction; the effects of vibration. J. Neurol. Neurosurg. Psychiatry, *35*:606–611, 1972.

Eldred, E., Hutton, R. S., and Smith, J. L.: Nature of the persisting changes in afferent discharge from muscle following its contraction. Prog. Brain Res., *44*:157–170, 1976.

Eldred, E., Yellin, H., DeSantis, M., and Smith, C. M.: Supplement to bibliography on muscle receptors: Their morphology, pathology, physiology and pharmacology. Exp. Neurol. *55*: (No. 2):1–118, 1977.

Eldred, E., Yellin, H., Gadbois, L., and Sweeney, S.: Bibliography on muscle receptors: Their morphology, pathology and physiology. Exp. Neurol., Suppl. 3:1–154, 1967.

Emonet-Dénand, F., and Houk, J.: Some effects of polarizing current on discharges from muscle spindle receptors. Am. J. Physiol., 216:404–406, 1969.

Emonet-Dénand, F., Jami, L., and La Porte, Y.: Skeleto-fusimotor axons in hind-limb muscles of the cat. J. Physiol. (Lond.), 249:153–166, 1975.

Emonet-Dénand, F., LaPorte, Y., Matthews, P. B. C., and Petit, J.: On the subdivision of static and dynamic fusimotor actions on the primary ending of the cat muscle spindle. J. Physiol. (Lond.), 268:827–861, 1977.

Erlanger, J., and Gasser, H. S.: Electrical Signs of Nervous Activity. Philadelphia, University of Pennsylvania Press, 1937.

Evarts, E. V.: Motor cortex reflexes associated with learned movement. Science, 179:501–503, 1973.

Eyzaguirre, C., and Kuffler, S. W.: Processes of excitation in the dendrites and in the soma of single isolated sensory nerve cells of the lobster and crayfish. J. Gen. Physiol., 39:87–119, 1955.

Fitzhugh, R.: Impulses and physiological states in models of nerve membrane. Biophys. J., 1:445–466, 1961.

Fohlmeister, J. F.: A model for phasic and tonic repetitively firing neuronal encoders. Kybernetik 13:104–112, 1973.

Fohlmeister, J. F., Poppele, R. E., and Purple, R. L.: Repetitive firing: Dynamic behavior of sensory neurons reconciled with a quantitative model. J. Neurophysiol., 37:1213–1227, 1974.

Fohlmeister, J. F., Poppele, R. E., and Purple, R. L.: Repetitive firing: A quantitative study of feedback in model encoders. J. Gen. Physiol., 69:815–848, 1977a.

Fohlmeister, J. F., Poppele, R. E., and Purple, R. L.: Repetitive firing: Quantitative analysis of encoder behavior of slowly adapting stretch receptor of crayfish and eccentric cell of Limulus. J. Gen. Physiol., 69:849–877, 1977b.

Fukami, Y.: Electrical and mechanical factors in the adaptation of reinnervated muscle spindles in snake. In Banker, B. Q., et al. (eds.): Research in Muscle Development and the Muscle Spindle. Amsterdam, Excerpta Medica, 1972, pp. 379–399.

Fukami, Y., and Hunt, C. C.: Structures in sensory regions of snake spindles and their displacement during stretch. J. Neurophysiol., 40:1121–1131, 1972.

Fulton, J. F., Pi-Suñer, J.: A note concerning the probable function of various afferent end-organs in skeletal muscle. Am. J. Physiol., 83:554–562, 1928.

Goodwin, G. M., Hulliger, M., and Matthews, P. B. C.: The effects of fusimotor stimulation during small amplitude stretching on the frequency-response of the primary ending of the mammalian muscle spindle. J. Physiol. (Lond.), 253:175–206, 1975.

Goodwin, G. M., Hulliger, M., and Matthews, P. B. C.: Studies on muscle spindle primary endings with sinusoidal stretching. Progr. Brain Res., 44:89–98, 1976.

Goodwin, G. M., McCloskey, D. I., and Matthews, P. B. C.: The

123

contribution of muscle afferents to kinaesthesia shown by vibration-induced illusions of movement and by the effects of paralysing joint afferents. Brain, 95:705–748, 1972a.

Goodwin, G. M., McCloskey, D. I., and Matthews, P. B. C.: Proprioceptive illusions induced by muscle vibration: Contribution by muscle spindles to perception? Science, 175:1382–1384, 1972b.

Gottlieb, G., Agarwal, G. C., and Stark, L.: Stretch receptor models I-single-efferent single-afferent innervation. I.E.E.E. Trans., MMS-10:17–27, 1969.

Granit, R.: The Basis of Motor Control. London and New York, Academic Press, 1970.

Granit, R.: Linkage of alpha and gamma motoneurons in voluntary movement. Nature [New Biol.], 243:52–53, 1973.

Gruner, J.-E.: La structure fine du fuseau neuromusculaire humain. Rev. Neurol. (Paris), 104:490–507, 1961.

Hagbarth, K.-E., Hongell, A., and Wallin, B. G.: The effect of gamma fibre block on afferent muscle nerve activity during voluntary contractions. Acta Physiol. Scand., 79:27A–28A, 1970.

Hagbarth, K.-E., and Vallbo, Å. B.: Discharge characteristics of human muscle afferents during muscle stretch and contraction. Exp. Neurol., 22:674–694, 1968.

Hagbarth, K.-E., Wallin, B. G., Burke, D., and Löfstedt, L.: Effects of the Jendrassik manoeuvre on muscle spindle activity in man. J. Neurol. Neurosurg. Psychiatry, 38:1143–1153, 1975a.

Hagbarth, K.-E., Wallin, B. G., and Löfstedt, L.: Muscle spindle activity in man during voluntary fast alternating movements. J. Neurol. Neurosurg. Psychiatry, 38:625–635, 1975b.

Hagbarth, K.-E., Wallin, B. G., and Löfstedt, L.: Muscle spindle responses to stretch in normal and spastic subjects. Scand. J. Rehabil. Med., 5:156–159, 1973.

Harker, D. W., Jami, L., LaPorte, Y., and Petit, J.: Fast conducting skeletofusimotor axons supplying intrafusal chain fibers in the cat peroneus-tertius muscle. J. Neurophysiol., 40:791–799, 1977.

Hasan, Z., and Houk, J. C.: Nonlinear behavior of primary spindle receptors in response to small, slow ramp stretches. Brain Res., 44:680–683, 1972.

Hasan, Z., and Houk, J. C.: Analysis of response properties of deefferented mammalian spindle receptors based on frequency response. J. Neurophysiol., 38:663–672, 1975a.

Hasan, Z., and Houk, J. C.: Transition in sensitivity of spindle receptors that occurs when muscle is stretched more than a fraction of a millimeter. J. Neurophysiol., 38:673–689, 1975b.

Heene, R.: Histological and histochemical findings in muscle spindles in dystrophica myotonica. J. Neurol. Sci., 18:369–372, 1973.

Henatsch, H.-D.: Effects of chemically excited muscle spindles on spinal motoneurones in cats. In Barker, D. (ed.): Symposium on Muscle Receptors. Hong Kong, Hong Kong University Press, 1962, pp. 67–80.

Hennig, G.: Die nervenendigungen der rattenmuskelspindel im elektronen-und phasenkontrastmikroskopischen. Bild. Z. Zellforsch., 96:275–294, 1969.

Hines, M., and Tower, S. S.: Studies on the innervation of skeletal muscles. II. Of muscle spindles in certain muscles of the kitten. Bull. Johns Hopkins Hosp., 42:264–307, 1928.

Hinsey, J. C.: Some observations on the innervation of skeletal muscle of the cat. J. Comp. Neurol., 44:87–195, 1927.

Holloway, S. F., and Poppele, R. E.: Evidence for electrogenic pumping in cat muscle spindle. Brain Res., 154:144–147, 1978.

Horak, F. M. B.: Multiple encoder sites on the primary afferent of the mammalian muscle spindle. M.S. thesis, University of Minnesota, 1977.

Horsley, V.: Short note on sense organs in muscle and on the preservation of muscle spindles in conditions of extreme muscular atrophy, following section of the motor nerve. Brain, 20:375–376, 1897.

Hosokawa, H.: Proprioceptive innervation of striated muscles in the territory of cranial nerves. Tex. Rep. Biol. Med., 19:405–464, 1961.

Houk, J. C.: Regulation of stiffness by skeletomotor reflexes. Ann. Rev. Physiol., 41:99–114, 1979.

Houk, J. C., Harris, D. A., and Hasan, Z.: Non-linear behavior of spindle receptors. In Stein, R. B., Pearson, K. G., Smith, R. S., and Redford, J. B. (eds.): Control of Posture and Locomotion. New York, Plenum Press, 1973, pp. 147–163.

Houk, J. C., Jr., and Stark, L.: An analytical model of a muscle spindle receptor for stimulation of motor coordination. M.I.T. Res. Lab. Electronics, Q. Prog. Rep., 66:384–389, 1962.

Hulliger, M., Matthews, P. B. C., and Noth, J.: Effects of combining static and dynamic fusimotor stimulation on the response of the muscle spindle primary ending to sinusoidal stretching. J. Physiol., 267:839–856, 1977.

Hunt, C. C.: Relation of function to diameter in afferent fibers of muscle nerves. J. Gen. Physiol., 38:117–131, 1954.

Hunt, C. C., and Kuffler, S. W.: Stretch receptor discharges during muscle contraction. J. Physiol. (Lond.), 113:298–315, 1951.

Hunt, C. C., and Ottoson, D.: Impulse activity and receptor potential of primary and secondary endings of isolated mammalian muscle spindles. J. Physiol. (Lond.), 252:259–281, 1975.

Hunt, C. C., Wilkinson, R. S., and Fukami, Y.: Ionic basis of the receptor potential in primary endings of mammalian muscle spindles. J. Gen. Physiol., 71:683–698, 1978.

Jami, L., Lan-Couton, D., Malmgren, K., and Petit, J.: "Fast" and "slow" skeleto-fusimotor innervation in cat tenuissimus spindles; a study with the glycogen-depletion method. Acta Physiol. Scand., 103:284–298, 1978.

Jami, L., Lan-Couton, D., Malmgren, K., and Petit, J.: Histophysiological observations on fast skeleto-fusimotor axons. Brain Res., 164:53–59, 1979.

Katz, B.: Depolarization of sensory terminals and the initiation of impulses in the muscle spindle. J. Physiol. (Lond.), 111:261–282, 1950.

Kennedy, W. R.: Innervation of human muscle spindles in patients with polyneuropathy. Trans. Am. Neurol. Assoc., 94:59–63, 1969.

Kennedy, W. R.: Innervation of normal human muscle spindles. Neurology (Minneap.), 20:463–475, 1970.

Kennedy, W. R.: Innervation of muscle spindles in amyotrophic lateral sclerosis. Mayo Clin. Proc., 46:245–257, 1971.

Kennedy, W. R.: The innervation of muscle spindles in a case of hypertrophic polyneuropathy. Neurology (Minneap.), 24:788–794, 1974.

Kennedy, W. R., Quick, D. C., and Reese, T. R.: Freeze-fracture of muscle spindles. Abstract. Soc. Neurosci., 5:304, 1979.

Kennedy, W. R., and Poppele, R. E.: Sensory activity of human muscle spindles. Electroencephalogr. Clin. Neurophysiol., 34:802–803, 1972.

Kennedy, W. R., Webster, H. DeF., and Yoon, K. S.: Human muscle spindles: Fine structure of the primary sensory ending. J. Neurocytol., 4:675–695, 1975.

Kennedy, W. R., Webster, H. DeF., Yoon, K. S., and Jean, D. H.: Human muscle spindles: Microfilaments in the group Ia sensory nerve endings. Anat. Rec., 180:521–532, 1974.

Kennedy, W. R., and Yoon, K. S.: Permeability of muscle spindle capillaries and capsule. Muscle & Nerve, 2:101–108, 1979.

Kerschner, L.: Bemerkungen über ein besonders Muskelsystem im Willkürlichen Muskel. Anat. Anz., 3:126–132, 1888a.

Kerschner, L.: Beitrage zur Kenntniss der sensiblen Endorgane. Anat. Anz., 3:288–296, 1888b.

Keynes, R. D., and Swan, R. C.: The effect of external sodium concentration on the sodium fluxes in frog skeletal muscle. J. Physiol. (Lond.), 147:591–625, 1959.

Kirkwood, P. A., and Sears, T. A.: Monosynaptic excitation of motoneurones from muscle spindle secondary endings of intercostal and triceps surae muscles in the cat. J. Physiol. (Lond.), 245:64–66P, 1975.

Knight, B. W.: Dynamics of encoding in a population of neurons. J. Gen. Physiol., 59:734–766, 1972.

Kölliker, A.: On the terminations of nerves in muscles, as observed in the frog: and on the disposition of the nerves in the frog's heart. Proc. R. Soc., 12:65–84, 1862.

Körner, G.: Untersuchungen über Zahl, Anordnung und Länge der Muskelspindeln in einegen Schulterden Oberarmmuskeln und im Muskulus sternalis des Menschen. Anat. Anz., 108:99–103, 1960.

Krinke, G., Heid, J., Bittiger, H., and Hess, R.: Sensory denervation of the plantar lumbrical muscle spindles in pyridoxine neuropathy. Acta Neuropathol. (Berl.), 43:213–216, 1978.

Kuffler, S. W., Hunt, C. C.: The mammalian small-nerve fibers: A system for efferent nervous regulation of muscle spindle discharge. Res. Publ. Assoc. Res. Nerv. Ment. Dis., 30:24–47, 1952.

Kuffler, S. W., Hunt, C. C., and Quilliam, J. P.: Function of medullated small-nerve fibers in mammalian ventral roots: Efferent muscles spindle innervation. J. Neurophysiol., 14:29–54, 1951.

Kühne, W.: Über die Endignung der Nerven in den Muskeln. Virchows Arch. [Pathol. Anat. Physiol.], 27:508–523, 1863.

Landau, W. M., and Clare, M. H.: Fusimotor function. Part IV: Reinforcement of the H reflex in normal subjects. Arch. Neurol., *10*:117–122, 1964.

Landgren, S., and Silfvenius, H.: Projections to cerebral cortex of group I muscle afferents from the cat's hind limb. J. Physiol. (Lond.), *200*:353–372, 1969.

Landon, D. N.: Electron microscopy of muscle spindles. *In* Andrew, B. L. (ed.): Control and Innervation of Skeletal Muscle. Edinburgh-London, Livingston, 1966, pp. 96–111.

Landon, D. N.: A quantitative study of some fine structural features of developing myotubes in the rat. J. Anat., *110*:170–171, 1971.

Landon, D. N.: The fine structure of developing muscle spindles in the rat. J. Anat., *111*:512–513, 1972*a*.

Landon, D. N.: The fine structure of the equatorial regions of developing muscle spindles in the rat. J. Neurocytol., *1*:189–210, 1972*b*.

Lapresle, J., and Milhaud, M.: Pathologie du fuseau neuro-musculaire. Rev. Neurol. (Paris), *110*:97–122, 1964.

Leksell, L.: The action potential and excitatory effects of the small ventral root fibres to skeletal muscle. Acta Physiol. Scand. [Suppl.], *10*(31):1–84, 1945.

Lennerstrand, G.: Position and velocity sensitivity of muscle spindles in the cat. I. Primary and secondary endings deprived of fusimotor activation. Acta Physiol. Scand., *73*:281–299, 1968*a*.

Lennerstrand, G.: Position and velocity sensitivity of muscle spindles in the cat. IV. Interaction between two fusimotor fibres converging on the same spindle ending. Acta Physiol. Scand., *74*:257–273, 1968*b*.

Lippold, O. C. J., Nichols, J. G., and Redfearn, J. W. T.: Electrical and mechanical factors in the adaptation of a mammalian muscle spindle. J. Physiol. (Lond.), *153*:209–217, 1960.

Loewenstein, W. R.: Excitation and inactivation in a receptor membrane. Ann. N.Y. Acad. Sci., *94*:510–534, 1961.

Loewenstein, W. R., Terzuolo, C. A., and Washizu, Y.: Separation of transducer and impulse-generating processes in sensory receptors. Science, *142*:1180–1181, 1966.

Lowndes, H. E., Baker, T., Cho, E.-S., and Jortner, B. S.: Position sensitivity of de-efferented muscle spindles in experimental acrylamide neuropathy. J. Pharmacol. Exp. Ther., *205*:40–48, 1978.

Marmarelis, P. Z., and Marmarelis, V. Z.: Analysis of Physiological Systems: The White-Noise Approach. New York, Plenum Press, 1978.

Matthews, B. H. C.: Nerve endings in mammalian muscle. J. Physiol. (Lond.), *78*:1–53, 1933.

Matthews, P. B. C.: The differentiation of two types of fusimotor fibre by their effects on the dynamic response of muscle spindle primary endings. Q. J. Exp. Physiol., *47*:324–333, 1962.

Matthews, P. B. C.: The response of de-efferented muscle spindle receptors to stretching at different velocities. J. Physiol. (Lond.), *168*:600–678, 1963.

Matthews, P. B. C.: Muscle spindles and their motor control. Physiol. Rev., *44*:219–288, 1964.

Matthews, P. B. C.: Mammalian Muscle Receptors and Their Central Actions. London, Arnold, 1972.

Matthews, P. B. C., and Stein, R. B.: The sensitivity of muscle spindle afferents to sinusoidal changes of length. J. Physiol. (Lond.), *200*:723–743, 1969*a*.

Matthews, P. B. C., and Stein, R. B.: The regularity of primary and secondary muscle spindle afferent discharges. J. Physiol. (Lond.), *202*:59–82, 1969*b*.

Maynard, J. A., Cooper, R. R., and Ionaescu, V. V.: An ultrastructure investigation of intrafusal muscle fibers in myotonic dystrophy. Virchows Arch. [Pathol. Anat.], *373*:1–13, 1977.

McIntyre, A. K.: Central actions of impulses in muscle afferent fibres. *In* Hunt, C. C. (ed.): Handbook of Sensory Physiology, Vol. III/2. Berlin, Heidelberg, New York, Springer, Verlag, 1974, pp. 235–288.

McWilliam, P. N.: A quantitative study of β innervation of muscle spindles in small muscles of the hind limb of the cat. J. Physiol. (Lond.), *39*:43–44, 1974.

Meier, H.: The muscle spindle in mice with hereditary neuromuscular diseases. Experientia, *25*:965–968, 1969.

Mendell, L. M., and Henneman, E.: Terminals of single Ia fibers: Distribution within a pool of 300 homonymous motor neurons. Science, *160*:96–98, 1968.

Merrillees, N. C. R.: The fine structure of muscle spindles in the lumbrical muscles of the rat. J. Biophys. Biochem. Cytol., *7*:725–742, 1960.

Milburn, A.: The early development of muscle spindles in the rat. J. Cell Sci., *12*:175–195, 1973.

Miyoshi, T., and Kennedy, W. R.: Microvasculature of rabbit muscle spindles. Arch. Neurol., *36*:471–475, 1979*a*.

Miyoshi, T., and Kennedy, W. R.: Morphometric comparison of capillaries in muscle spindles, nerve, and muscle. Arch. Neurol., *36*:547–552, 1979*b*.

Moore, G. P., Boles, J. A., Reinking, R. M., and Stuart, D. G.: White noise analysis of the dynamic sensitivity of muscle receptor afferents. Soc. Neurosci. Abstr., *2*:945, 1976.

Nakajima, S., and Onodera, K.: Adaptation of the generator potential in the crayfish stretch receptors under constant length and constant tension. J. Physiol. (Lond.), *200*:187–204, 1969.

Obara, S., and Grundfest, H.: Effects of lithium on different membrane components of crayfish stretch receptor neurons. J. Gen. Physiol., *41*:635–654, 1968.

Ogata, T., and Mori, M.: Histochemical study of oxidative enzymes in vertebrate muscles. J. Histochem. Cytochem., *12*:171–182, 1964.

Olsson, Y., and Reese, T. S.: Permeability of vasa nervorum and perineurium in mouse sciatic nerve studied by fluorescence and electron microscopy. J. Neuropathol. Exp. Neurol., *30*:105–119, 1971.

Onanoff, M. I.: Sur la nature des faisceux neuromuscularies. C. R. Seanc. Soc. Biol., *42*:432–433, 1890.

Ottoson, D.: The effect of sodium deficiency on the response of the isolated muscle spindle. J. Physiol. (Lond.), *171*:109, 1964.

Ottoson, D.: Mechanism of spindle adaptation. *In* Banker, B. Q., et al. (eds.): Research in Muscle Development and the Muscle Spindle. Amsterdam, Excerpta Medica, 1972, pp. 341–352.

Ovalle, W. K., Jr.: Fine structure of rat intrafusal muscle fibers: The polar region. J. Cell Biol., *51*:83–103, 1971.

Ovalle, W. K., Jr.: Fine structure of the avian muscle spindle capsule. Cell Tissue Res., *166*:285–298, 1976.

Ovalle, W. K., Jr., and Smith, R. S.: Histochemical identification of three types of intrafusal muscle fibers in cat and monkey based on the myosin ATPase reaction. Can. J. Physiol. Pharmacol., *50*:195–202, 1972.

Patel, A. N., Lalitha, V. S., and Dastur, D. K.: The spindle in normal and pathological muscle. Brain, *91*:737–750, 1968.

Phillips, C. G., Powell, T. P. S., and Wiesendanger, M.: Projection from low-threshold muscle afferents of hand and forearm to area 3a of baboon's cortex. J. Physiol. (Lond.), *217*:419–446, 1971.

Polit, A., and Bizzi, E.: Processes controlling arm movements in monkeys. Science, *201*:1235–1237, 1978.

Poppele, R. E.: Systems approach to the study of muscle spindles. *In* Stein, R. B., Pearson, K. G., Smith, R. S., and Redford, J. B. (eds.): Control of Posture and Locomotion. New York, Plenum Press, 1973, pp. 127–146.

Poppele, R. E., and Bowman, R. J.: Quantitative description of linear behaviour of mammalian muscle spindles. J. Neurophysiol., *33*:59–72, 1970.

Poppele, R. E., and Chen, W. J.: Repetitive firing behavior of mammalian muscle spindle. J. Neurophysiol., *35*:357–364, 1972.

Poppele, R. E., and Kennedy, W. R.: Comparison between behaviour of human and cat muscle spindles recorded *in vitro*. Brain Res., *75*:316–319, 1974.

Poppele, R. E., Kennedy, W. R., and Quick, D. C.: A determination of static mechanical properties of intrafusal muscle in isolated cat muscle spindles. Neuroscience, *4*:410–411, 1979.

Proske, U.: Stretch-evoked potentiation of responses of muscle spindles in the cat. Brain Res., *88*:378–383, 1975.

Quick, D. C., Kennedy, W. R., and Donaldson, L.: Dimensions of myelinated nerve fibers near the motor and sensory terminals in cat tenuissimus muscles. Neuroscience, *4*:1089–1096, 1979*a*.

Quick, D. C., Kennedy, W. R., and Poppele, R. E.: Anatomical evidence for multiple sources of action potentials in the afferent fibers of muscle spindles Neuroscience, *5*:109–115, 1979*b*.

Quick, D. C., and Waxman, S. G.: Ferric ion, ferrocyanide, and inorganic phosphate as cytochemical reactants at peripheral nodes of Ranvier. J. Neurocytol., *6*:555–570, 1977.

Rescigno, A., Stein, R. B., Purple, R. L., and Poppele, R. E.: A neuronal model for the discharge patterns produced by cyclic inputs. Bull. Math. Biophys., *32*:337–353, 1970.

129

Rosenthal, N. P., McKean, T. A., Roberts, W. J., and Terzuolo, C. A.: Frequency analysis of stretch reflex and its main subsystems in triceps surae muscles of the cat. J. Neurophysiol., 33:713–749, 1970.

Rudjord, T.: A second order mechanical model of muscle spindle primary endings. Kybernetik, 6:205–213, 1970.

Ruffini, A.: Sur la terminaison nerveuse dans les faisceaux musculaires et sur leur signification physiologique. Arch. Ital. Biol., 18:106–114, 1893.

Ruffini, A.: On the minute anatomy of the neuromuscular spindles of the cat, and on their physiological significance. J. Physiol. (Lond.), 23:190–208, 1898.

Sahinen, F. M., and Kennedy, W. R.: Distribution of muscle spindles in the human first dorsal interosseus. Anat. Rec., 173:151–155, 1972.

Schafer, S. S.: The discharge frequencies of primary muscle spindle endings during simultaneous stimulation of two fusimotor filaments. Pfluegers Arch., 350:359–372, 1974.

Schaumberg, H. H., Wisniewski, H. M., and Spencer, P. S.: Ultrastructural studies of the dying-back process. 1. Peripheral nerve terminal and axon degeneration in systemic acrylamide intoxication. J. Neuropathol. Exp. Neurol., 33:260–284, 1974.

Schröder, J. M.: Zur Pathogenese der Isoniazid-Neuropathie. II. Phasenkontrast- und elektronen-mikroskopische Untersuchungen am Rückenmark, an Spinalganglien und Muskelspindeln. Acta Neuropathol. (Berlin), 16:324–341, 1970.

Schröder, J. M.: The fine structure of de- and reinnervated muscle spindles. I. The increase, atrophy, and hypertrophy of intrafusal muscle fibers. Acta Neuropathol. (Berlin), 30:109–128, 1974a.

Schröder, J. M.: The fine structure of de- and reinnervated muscle spindles. II. Regenerated sensory and motor nerve terminals. Acta Neuropathol. (Berlin), 30:129–144, 1974b.

Shantha, T. R., Golarz, M. N., and Bourne, G. H.: Histological and histochemical observations on the capsule of the muscle spindle in normal and denervated muscle. Acta Anat. (Basel), 69:632–646, 1968.

Sherrington, C. S.: On the anatomical constitution of nerves of skeletal muscles; with remarks on recurrent fibres in the ventral spinal nerve-root. J. Physiol. (Lond.), 17:211–258, 1894.

Smith, R. S.: Properties of intrafusal muscle fibres. In Granit, R. (ed.): Muscular Afferents and Motor Control. Stockholm, Almquist and Wiksell, 1966, pp. 69–80.

Sokolove, P. G., and Cook, I. M.: Inhibition of impulse activity in a sensory neuron by an electrogenic pump. J. Gen. Physiol., 57:125–163, 1971.

Sommer, J.: Periphere bahnung von muskeleigen reflexen als wesen des Jendrasskschen phanomens. Dtsch. Z. Nervenheilkd., 150:249–262, 1940.

Stauffer, E. K., Watt, D. G. D., Taylor, A., Reinking, R. M., and Stuart, D. G.: Analysis of muscle receptor connections by spike-triggered averaging. 2. Spindle group II afferents. J. Neurophysiol., 39:1393–1402, 1976.

Stein, R. B.: Peripheral control of movement. Physiol. Rev., 54:215–243, 1974.

Swash, M.: The morphology and innervation of the muscle spindle in dystrophica myotonica. Brain, 95:357–368, 1972.

Swash, M., and Fox, K. P.: The pathology of human muscle spindle: Effect of denervation. J. Neurol. Sci., 22:1–24, 1974.

Swash, M., and Fox, K. P.: Abnormal intrafusal muscle fibres in myotonic dystrophy: A study using serial sections. J. Neurol. Neurosurg. Psychiatry, 38:91–99, 1975.

Szumski, A. J., Burg, D., Struppler, A., and Velho, F.: Activity of muscle spindles during muscle twitch and clonus in normal and spastic human subjects. Electroencephalogr. Clin. Neurophysiol., 37:589–597, 1974.

Takano, K.: Absence of the gamma-spindle loop in the reinnervated hind leg muscles of the cat: "Alpha muscle." Exp. Brain Res., 26:343–354, 1976.

Terzuolo, C. A., and Washizu, Y.: Relation between stimulus strength, generator potential and impulse frequency in the stretch receptor of Crustacea. J. Neurophysiol., 25:56–66, 1962.

Tower, S. S.: Atrophy and degeneration in the muscle spindle. Brain, 55:77–90, 1932.

Tower, S. S.: The reaction of muscle to denervation. Physiol. Rev., 19:1–48, 1939.

Vallbo, Å. B.: Slowly adapting muscle receptors in man. Acta Physiol. Scand., 78:315–333, 1970a.

Vallbo, Å. B.: Discharge patterns in human muscle spindle afferents during isometric voluntary contractions. Acta Physiol. Scand., 80:552–566, 1970b.

Vallbo, Å. B.: Muscle spindle response at the onset of isometric voluntary contractions in man. Time difference between fusimotor and skeletomotor effects. J. Physiol. (Lond.), 218:405–431, 1971.

Vallbo, Å. B.: Single unit recording from human peripheral nerves: Muscle receptor discharge in resting muscles and during voluntary contractions. In Somjen, G. G. (ed.): Neurophysiology Studied in Man. Amsterdam, Excerpta Medica, 1972, pp. 283–297.

Vallbo, Å. B.: Muscle spindle afferent discharge from resting and contracting muscles in normal human subjects. In Desmedt, J. E. (ed.): New Developments in Electromyography and Clinical Neurophysiology, Vol. 3. Basel, Karger, 1973a, pp. 251–262.

Vallbo, Å. B.: Impulse activity from human muscle spindles during voluntary contractions. In Gydikou, A. A. (ed.): Motor Control. New York, Plenum Press, 1973b, pp. 33–43.

Vallbo, Å. B.: Afferent discharge from human muscle spindles in non-contracting muscles. Steady state impulse frequency as a function of joint angle. Acta Physiol. Scand., 90:303–318, 1974a.

Vallbo, Å. B.: Human muscle spindle discharge during isometric voluntary contractions. Amplitude relations between spindle frequency and torque. Acta Physiol. Scand., 90:319–336, 1974b.

Vallbo, Å. B., and Hagbarth, K.-E.: Impulses recorded with micro-electrodes in human muscle nerves during stimulation of mechanoreceptors and voluntary contractions. Electroencephalogr. Clin. Neurophysiol., 23:392, 1967.

Vallbo, Å. B., Hagbarth, K.-E., Torebjörk, H. E., and Wallin, B. G.: Somatosensory, proprioceptive and sympathetic activity in human peripheral nerves. Physiol. Rev., 59:919–957.

Van Gorp, P. E., and Kennedy, W. R.: Localization of muscle spindles in the human extensor indicis muscle for biopsy purposes. Anat. Rec., 179:447–452, 1974.

Voss, H.: Zahl und Anordnung der Muskelspindeln in den unteren Zungenbeinmuskeln, dem M. sternocleidomastoideus und den Brauch — und teifen Nackenmuskeln. Anat. Anz., 105:265–275, 1958.

Waggener, J. D., Bunn, S. M., and Beggs, J.: The diffusion of ferritin within the peripheral nerve sheath: An electron microscopy study. J. Neuropathol. Exp. Neurol., 24:430–443, 1965.

Weismann, A.: Über das Wachsen der auergestreiften Muskeln nach Beobachtungen am Frosch. Z. Rat. Med., 10:263–284, 1861.

Willard, W. A., and Grau, E. C.: Some histological changes in striate skeletal muscle following nerve sectioning. Anat. Rec., 27:192, 1924.

Windhorst, U., Schmidt, J., and Meyer-Lohmann, J.: Analysis of the dynamic responses of deefferented primary muscle spindle endings to ramp stretch. Pfluegers Arch., 366:233–240, 1976.

Wolpaw, J. R.: Electromagnetic muscle stretch strongly excites sensorimotor cortex neurons in behaving primates. Science, 203:465–467, 1979.

Zelená, J.: The morphogenetic influence of innervation on the ontogenetic development of muscle-spindles. J. Embryol. Exp. Morphol., 5:283–292, 1957.

Zelená, J., and Hńik, P.: Motor and receptor units in the soleus muscle after nerve regenerration in very young rats. Physiol. Bohemoslov., 12:277–290, 1963.

4

Motor Units in Mammalian Muscle

R. E. Burke

INTRODUCTION

Over 50 years ago, Sherrington (1929) introduced the term "motor unit" to refer to the combination of a motoneuron plus the set of muscle fibers innervated by it. The latter can, for convenience, be called the "muscle unit" portion of the motor unit (Burke, 1967). Sherrington recognized that the motoneuron and muscle unit toether form a functional entity, indivisible in normal motor action, which corresponds to "... a so-to-say quantum reaction, which forms the basis, by combinations temporal and numerical, of all grading of the muscle as effector organ..." (Eccles and Sherrington, 1930).

Because motor units are the quantum elements underlying all muscular action, the motor unit concept is fundamental to present models of motor system organization and the neural control of movement. It is also a critical concept in the interpretation of clinical observations in patients with neuromuscular and peripheral nerve diseases. The clinical manifestations of peripheral nerve diseases include alterations in motor unit structure and function, inferred from electromyographic studies and/or from changes in the strength, structure, or histochemistry of muscles. Thus, it seems appropriate in a text on disorders of peripheral nerve to review some of the evidence currently available concerning the structure and function of normal motor units. Most of this material has been gathered from studies on experimental animals, which continue to serve as essential models for interpretation of data gathered from human subjects using much less direct methods.

DEFINITIONS

In the light of current evidence, some further discussion of the precise meaning of the term "motor unit" is required. Sherrington (1929) originally conceived of the motor unit as including "...an individual nerve-fibre with the bunch of muscle-fibres it activates." It does no

133

violence to history to include the entire motoneuron, dendrites, and cell body, as well as its axon, in the modern definition. However, there are currently three recognized categories of motoneurons and two basic categories of striated muscle fibers; their interrelations are shown in Table 4–1.

The skeletomotor, or alpha, motoneurons are relatively large cells with fast conducting axons that innervate exclusively the large skeletal muscle fibers which make up the bulk of the anatomical muscles. The latter are also called "extrafusal" to differentiate them from the much smaller, specialized "intrafusal" muscle fibers that are present only within the muscle spindle stretch receptors. The motoneurons that innervate only the intrafusal muscle fibers are relatively small cells with slowly conducting myelinated axons; these are usually called "fusimotor" or gamma motoneurons. To these well established and easily differentiated categories must be added a third group, referred to as "skeletofusimotor" or beta motoneurons; these innervate both extra- and intrafusal muscle fibers. The development of these motoneuron categories has been lucidly explained by Matthews (1972; cf. esp. pp. 42–44 and 69–77). The present account will use the designations "alpha," "beta," and "gamma" for motoneurons, and "skeletal" versus "intrafusal" for describing muscle fibers. Unless otherwise noted, the term "motor unit" will refer only to the combination of an alpha motoneuron and its skeletal muscle unit. Consideration of beta motoneurons and their muscle units will be specifically discussed later. The organization of gamma motoneurons and muscle spindles will not be presented in this chapter; the reader is referred to Matthews' (1972) excellent monograph.

The word "motor unit" is frequently used in both the research and clinical literature when discussing only the muscle unit portion. However, the motoneuron is functionally inseparable from the muscle unit it innervates, and this review includes some consideration of the structure and function of motoneurons per se.

Table 4–1 Interrelation Between Categories of
Motoneurons and of Muscle Fibers

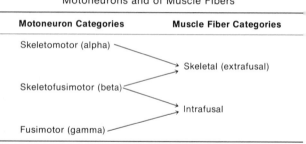

Motoneuron Categories	Muscle Fiber Categories
Skeletomotor (alpha)	Skeletal (extrafusal)
Skeletofusimotor (beta)	Intrafusal
Fusimotor (gamma)	

ANATOMICAL CONSIDERATIONS

Motor Nuclei

There is no question that most of the large neurons found in the ventrolateral horn of the spinal gray matter (lamina IX of Rexed's cytoarchitectonic map of the spinal cord; Rexed, 1952) are in fact alpha motoneurons. These cells, among the largest neurons in the mammalian central nervous system, have remarkably extensive dendritic trees (up to 1 mm or more in length; Aitken and Bridger, 1954; Testa, 1964). Recently developed methods for marking functionally identified motoneurons by intracellular injection of radioactive tracers (Lux et al., 1970) or fluorescent dyes (Barrett and Crill, 1974) have permitted detailed study of the relations between cell anatomy and those functional properties dependent upon it. Alpha motoneurons exhibit a twofold range in average soma diameter (Fig. 4–1; see Burke et al., 1977) and up to a fivefold range in cell body volume (Sato et al., 1977) and total area of the surface membrane (Barrett and Crill, 1974). Gamma motoneurons are significantly smaller, making a second peak in the motoneuron size distribution (Fig. 4–1), and they exhibit histochemical characteristics (rich in oxidative enzymes and poor in phosphorylase) rather different from those of the cells in the alpha size range (poor in oxidative enzymes and rich in phosphorylase; Campa and Engel, 1971). Sato and coworkers (1977) have recently shown that the alpha-gamma size distinction is present in newborn kittens but the differential growth of large and small alpha motoneurons occurs later in postnatal development (third to seventh postnatal week).

With the exception of the axon hillock that gives rise to the motor axon, the entire surface of alpha motoneurons is covered with synaptic contacts, or boutons, and a variety of synaptic types can be recognized in the electron microscope (Conradi, 1969; McLaughlin, 1972). Alpha motoneuron axons usually give off one or more fine axon collaterals before they exit from the spinal cord (Prestige, 1966). Recent evidence indicates that at least some of these collaterals terminate not only on Renshaw interneurons, which produce the well-known recurrent inhibition of motoneurons (Eccles et al., 1954), but also enter the motor nuclei to end directly on alpha motoneurons (Cullheim et al., 1977).

The motoneurons that innervate muscle units within a given anatomical muscle are grouped into longitudinal columns, the motor nuclei (Fig. 4–2), that lie in the ventrolateral gray matter of the cord (Rexed, 1952). The position of the nuclear column for a particular muscle is predictable, and the number of motoneurons in the nucleus is also roughly the same from one individual to another in a given species. As would be expected, most of the available information about the anatomy of motor nuclei comes from animal studies, but the general features of these results are similar in human spinal cords (Elliott, 1942, 1943; Sharrard, 1955).

135

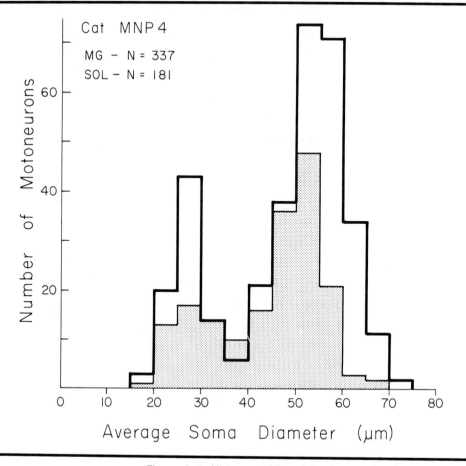

Figure 4–1 Histogram of the relative frequencies of average soma diameters of cat medial gastrocnemius (MG; *heavy lines, open bars*) and soleus (SOL; *lighter lines, stippled bars*) motoneurons, identified by retrograde transport of the exogenous protein tracer, horseradish peroxidase. Note the bimodal character of both distributions, with about 25 per cent of the cells in both MG and SOL nuclei included in the smaller size peak (<38.5 μm average diameter). The smaller motoneurons are assumed to be mostly, if not exclusively, gamma motoneurons and the larger ones, alpha motoneurons. The MG nucleus contains a wider size range of alpha cells than the SOL, with larger mean diameter. (From Burke et al., 1977.)

Identification of the motoneurons belonging to individual muscles has been accomplished experimentally by cutting the muscle nerve to produce recognizable chromatolysis in the motoneuron cell bodies (Romanes, 1951; Van Buren and Frank, 1965), or, more recently, by inducing uptake by motor terminals of tracer substances such as the exogenous protein horseradish peroxidase (HRP), which is carried to the cell bodies by the normal process of retrograde axonal transport (Kristensson et al., 1971;

Burke et al., 1977). In a remarkable study, Sharrard (1955) was able to deduce the functional identities of individual motor nuclei in the human lumbosacral spinal cord by studying material from patients affected in different muscle groups with poliomyelitis. In general, the nuclei that innervate muscles of the neck and trunk are located ventromedially throughout the length of the spinal cord, while those supplying the limb musculature are located in the more lateral portions of the cervical and lumbar enlargements (Brodal, 1969). Within the limb enlargements, the position of particular nuclei and their anatomical relations with surrounding nuclei belonging to other muscles are predictable and related both to the function of the muscle (i.e., whether a flexor or extensor) and to the particular joint moved (Romanes, 1951).

Alpha and gamma motoneurons innervating a given muscle are mixed more or less randomly within its motor

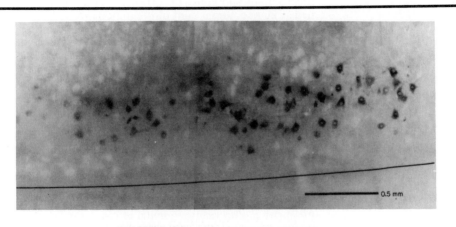

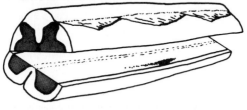

Figure 4–2 Anatomy of the MG motor nucleus in cat spinal cord, determined by motoneuron labelling with horseradish peroxidase. *Upper panel:* Dorsal view of a thick (about 200 μm) section of spinal cord showing the ventral horn gray matter, with gray-white interface indicated by the heavy black line. MG motoneurons show as dark-staining cells arranged in a rostrocaudal cell column amid unstained *(lighter outlines)* motoneurons belonging to other motor nuclei. *Lower panel:* Diagram of three lumbosacral segments (L6, L7, and S1) showing the horizontal section level and approximate position of the MG motor nucleus *(dots).* (From unpublished material of R. E. Burke, P. L. Strick, and M. W. Brightman; see Burke et al., 1977 for methods.)

137

nucleus (Burke et al., 1977). Their numbers, and therefore the number of motor units in the muscle, have been estimated by counting the myelinated axons of different sizes in muscle nerves after degeneration of the afferent fiber component (Eccles and Sherrington, 1930; Boyd and Davey, 1968). The counts found in motoneuron-marking experiments, using either chromatolysis or HRP transport, have been somewhat lower (Romanes, 1951; Burke et al., 1977), possibly because some cells are not detectably labelled. However, at least part of this discrepancy can also be accounted for by the fact that motor axons branch in the peripheral nerves (see review by Sunderland and Lavarck, 1953), a process that increases as the nerve approaches the target muscle (Eccles and Sherrington, 1930; Boyd and Davey, 1969; Wray, 1969). Thus, axon counts in peripheral nerves tend to overestimate the actual numbers of motoneurons present, although the amount of branching that occurs apparently varies from one muscle nerve to another (Peyronnard and Lamarre, 1977). On the average, between 25 and 40 per cent of the motoneurons in a given motor nucleus are likely to be gamma motoneurons (Fig. 4–1). As a numerical example, the medial gastrocnemius nucleus in the cat contains some 250 to 280 alpha motoneurons and between 80 and 170 gamma cells (see Boyd and Davey, 1968; Burke et al., 1977).

Estimates of the numbers of motor units in a variety of human muscles have been made from axon counts in muscle nerves, subtracting an assumed percentage (40 per cent) of afferent fibers (reviewed by Buchthal, 1961). Not surprisingly, large muscles generally tend to possess more motor units than small muscles, but the range of variation is less than might be expected simply on the basis of relative muscle size. For example, the nerve to the bulky medial gastrocnemius of man appears to contain about 580 motor axons and the much smaller first dorsal interosseous nerve has some 119 axons (Feinstein et al., 1955; see also Buchthal, 1961, for other estimates). The latter number seems larger than expected on the basis of relative muscle volumes alone. The nerve to the tiny external rectus oculi may contain over 1700 motor axons (Buchthal, 1961). Thus, function as well as muscle volume apparently condition the numbers of motoneurons present in motor nuclei (Feinstein et al., 1955).

Recently, McComas and coworkers (1971) described an electrophysiological method for estimating the number of motor units in the human extensor digitorum brevis muscle (EDB), and have suggested that this model system can be used to detect alterations in motor unit numbers in neuromuscular disorders (e.g., McComas et al., 1973). The method is limited to the EDB because of technical considerations, and several potentially troublesome sources of error have been identified (McComas et al., 1971; Brown and Milner-Brown, 1976; Peyronnard and Lamarre, 1977). Nevertheless, when tested in the rhesus monkey, fairly good agreement has been found between electrophysiological estimates of EDB motor unit number and counts of alpha motor axons in deaf-ferented EDB nerves (Peyronnard and Lamarre, 1977). The normal human EDB contains, on the average, about 180 motor units (McComas et al., 1971) and that of the rhesus monkey, about 150 units (Peyronnard and Lamarre, 1977).

There is evidence suggesting that a rough somatotopic relationship may exist between the rostrocaudal position of a motoneuron within its nuclear column and the location of its muscle unit within the muscle. For example, motoneurons in the more rostral portions of the medial gastrocnemius nucleus of the cat tend to innervate muscle units in the more proximal and superficial parts of the muscle. Stimulation of cells located progressively more caudal in the nucleus tends to produce contraction of muscle units located progressively more deeply (Swett et al., 1970; see also Burke et al., 1977). The developmental and functional significance of this motor unit somatotopy remains to be elucidated.

Muscle Unit Anatomy

From both anatomical and functional viewpoints, most muscles as defined by the anatomist can be considered to be collections of muscle units, usually (but not always) arranged in parallel to generate force vectors between more or less localized skeletal points (i.e., origin and insertion). It should perhaps be noted, however, that muscles can have very complex internal architecture, including some with complicated multipinnate arrangements (e.g., see Gans and Bock, 1965). The origin and insertion regions can be quite extensive, such that different parts of the same anatomical muscle can have quite different functional effects about a given joint. Some muscles span two joints and can act as flexors in one limb position and as extensors in another. These complications are undoubtedly important to a full understanding (not yet at hand) of functioning motor unit populations and the reasons for the differences between them in various muscles.

In general, a given motor axon innervates muscle fibers within a single anatomically defined muscle — i.e., a muscle unit is limited to one muscle. An exception to this has been demonstrated in the lumbrical slips of the cat hind limb, where one axon may branch peripherally to innervate fibers in adjacent slips (Emonet-Dénand et al., 1971). Motor axons branch repeatedly to provide individual neuromuscular junctions for each innervated muscle fiber. While most of this profuse branching appears to take place within the muscle (see Feindel et al., 1952), axon branching does occur in the peripheral nerve with

139

increasing frequency as the nerve nears the muscle (Eccles and Sherrington, 1930).

Detailed experiments in animals have shown that, in the normal adult, each muscle fiber is innervated by one and only one motoneuron, with little or no polyneuronal innervation (Feindel et al., 1952; Brown and Matthews, 1960, Bagust et al., 1973; Van Harreveld and Tachibana, 1961). Even when two end-plates can be visualized on a single muscle fiber, as sometimes happens, they can usually be traced back to the same parent motor axon (Feindel et al., 1952). In newborn rats and kittens, however, there is considerable polyneuronal innervation which then disappears in the first 6 weeks of postnatal life as motor units mature into their adult patterns (Bagust et al., 1973; Brown et al., 1976). Interestingly, Christensen (1959) found no evidence for polyneuronal innervation in the muscles of stillborn human fetuses of unspecified gestational age, using anatomical methods involving counting muscle fibers and cholinesterase-stained end-plates.

Until relatively recently, it was thought that muscle fibers belonging to a single muscle unit were arranged in localized collections, or "subunits," of eight to ten fibers, and that these subunits were in turn scattered throughout a more extensive motor unit territory (Buchthal, 1961). This view was based in part on histological studies of muscle units remaining in cases of motoneuron disease (Wohlfart, 1949) and on interpretation of electromyographic recordings in human subjects (Buchthal, 1961), although the results of animal experiments were not consistent with the existence of motor subunits (Krnjevic and Miledi, 1958; Norris and Irwin, 1961).

More recently, the muscle fibers belonging to individual muscle units have been identified directly by depletion of intrafiber glycogen following prolonged activation of only that motor unit in both rat (Edström and Kugelberg, 1968; Doyle and Mayer, 1969; Brandstater and Lambert, 1973) and cat muscles (Figs. 4–3 and 4–4; see Burke et al., 1973, 1974; Burke and Tsairis, 1973). All of these studies indicate that the fibers of an individual muscle unit are actually distributed relatively uniformly throughout an extensive territorial volume (Fig. 4–3), with only occasional contiguous fibers (Fig. 4–4). The absence of "subunits" in normal human muscle is also strongly suggested by the results of single fiber electromyography (Ekstedt, 1964; Stålberg and Ekstedt, 1973; Stålberg et al., 1976) and by histochemical studies from a patient with myokymia (see Dubowitz and Brooke, 1973, their Fig. 3.42). Thus, it is now generally agreed that, in normal animals and probably in man, the fibers of a given muscle unit are scattered randomly throughout its unit territory, without local subunits (see Buchthal and Rosenfalck, 1973).

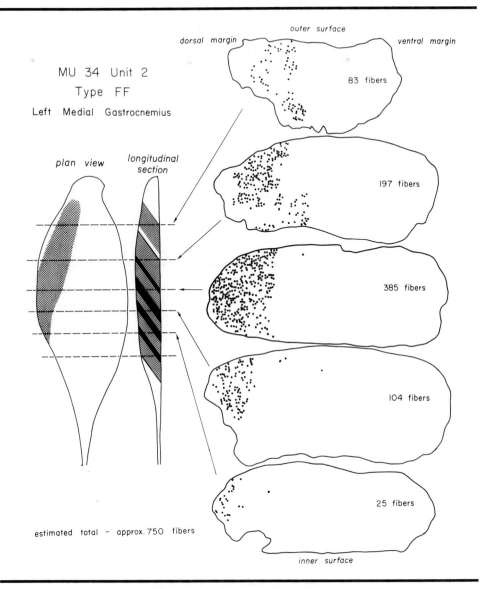

MU 34 Unit 2
Type FF
Left Medial Gastrocnemius

plan view   longitudinal section

outer surface
dorsal margin   ventral margin
83 fibers
197 fibers
385 fibers
104 fibers
25 fibers
inner surface

estimated total – approx. 750 fibers

Figure 4–3 Reconstruction of the muscle unit territory of a type FF motor unit in cat MG muscle. *Left side:* Outline diagrams showing the whole MG muscle in plan and longitudinal section views. Projected extent of the FF muscle unit indicated by shading, with fiber angulation in this unipennate muscle indicated by parallel lines on the longitudinal section view. *Right side:* Outline drawings of five cross sections of the muscle, with positions of glycogen-depleted unit fibers denoted by dots. Fiber counts at each level are given, and the approximate level of each cross section is indicated by arrows and dotted lines referred to the whole muscle diagrams. Estimated total innervation ratio for this unit was 750 fibers. (From Burke and Tsairis, 1973.)

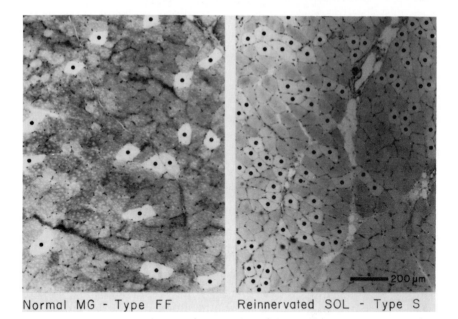

Normal MG - Type FF   Reinnervated SOL - Type S

Figure 4–4 Photomicrographs of frozen sections of medial gastrocnemius (MG; *left panel*) and soleus (SOL; *right panel*), stained for glycogen by the PAS method. Both sections show some muscle fibers completely depleted of glycogen (indicated by dots) after prolonged stimulation of the innervating motoneurons. The MG unit was obtained in a normal muscle and shows the random scattering, with few contiguous fibers, characteristic of normal muscle units (same unit as shown in Fig. 4–3). The SOL unit was obtained in an animal in which the SOL nerve had been cut and rejoined to itself 9 months previously (self-reinnervation). Note here the large number of contiguous depleted fibers within a relatively small area. Same magnification for both photomicrographs (note scale on right). (From unpublished material of Burke and Tsairis.)

The territory of a single muscle unit is usually pictured as a two-dimensional mosaic but it is in fact a three-dimensional volume. Figure 4–3 illustrates a reconstruction of the territory of a fast contracting, fatigue-sensitive muscle unit (type FF, see below) in a medial gastrocnemius muscle in the cat. Observations on this and other similarly studied units indicate that, in this muscle, the average density of fibers belonging to a given muscle unit is between two and five fibers per 100 at any point within the unit territory. Thus, any part of the territorial volume occupied by the fibers of one unit must be shared by at least 20 to 50 other muscle units (Burke and Tsairis, 1973). Electromyographic studies of large human muscles (e.g., biceps brachii) have produced estimates of unit fiber densities and territorial sharing of the same order of magnitude (Buchthal and Rosenfalck, 1973). The density of fibers belonging to individual muscle units appears to increase with age in man, implying possible death of some motoneurons and consequent reorganization of muscle unit architecture (Stålberg and Thiele, 1975).

The boundaries of a normal muscle unit's territory are usually irregular (e.g., Fig. 4–3) and do not appear to conform to fascicular subdivisions within the whole muscle. However, one glycogen depletion study has shown that motor axons travelling together in natural intramuscular branchlets tend to innervate muscle units filling the same region of the muscle, sometimes with sharp boundaries that are, in fact, related to connective tissue fascicles (Letbetter, 1974). Further, the same study has suggested that such local sets of muscle units tend to be innervated by motoneurons clustered together within the motor nucleus, as would be consistent with the somatotopic organization discussed above.

The fraction of total muscle volume occupied by a single muscle unit territory is difficult to estimate with precision, but it can be quite substantial. For example, in the cat medial gastrocnemius, territorial volumes may occupy as much as 15 to 20 per cent of the total muscle volume (e.g., Fig. 4–3), a figure compatible with territorial sharing by 50 different muscle units in a muscle containing some 250 to 300 motor units. The territorial volume of units in the cat soleus muscle may be even more extensive, perhaps as large as 25 to 30 per cent of total muscle volume (see e.g., Fig. 3 in Burke et al., 1974). Territorial volumes of human muscle units are unknown, but electromyographic studies by Buchthal and coworkers suggested that unit territories in limb muscles may be as much as 11 mm in cross-sectional diameter (Buchthal and Rosenfalck, 1973; Buchthal et al., 1959; see also Kato and Tanji, 1972; Stålberg et al., 1976). There is remarkably little difference in the EMG estimates of territorial diameter for muscle units in different human muscles, irrespective of overall muscle size, but within a given muscle there may be a three- to fivefold range in diameter from one unit to another (Buchthal et al., 1959).

The average number of muscle fibers innervated by a single motoneuron, or the "innervation ratio," has been estimated simply by dividing the total number of muscle fibers by the number of large motor axons in the muscle nerve. With this method, Clark (1931) estimated that the average muscle unit in the cat soleus muscle contained 140 to 200 fibers (see also Burke et al., 1974), and Burke and Tsairis (1973) suggested that the average innervation ratios in the three major motor unit types present in cat medial gastrocnemius vary from 440 to 750 fibers per unit. For comparison, Wray (1969) estimated that the average innervation ratio for motor units in the monkey medial gastrocnemius is about 790 fibers/units, while in man it may be up to 2000 fibers/unit (Feinstein et al., 1955). For technical reasons, it is difficult to provide reliable estimates of innervation ratios from study of individual glycogen-depleted muscle units (Fig. 4–3; see Burke and Tsairis, 1973). Nevertheless, comparison of muscle unit force outputs with the fiber counts and average fiber areas in glycogen-depleted soleus muscle (Burke et al., 174, their Table 1) suggests that there is at least a fivefold range of innervation ratios (from about 50 fibers/unit at minimum to over 400 fibers/unit at maximum) among different units in this otherwise homogeneous population.

Estimates of average innervation ratios for a variety of human muscles have been summarized by Buchthal (1961). These suggest that large limb muscles such as gastrocnemius and biceps brachii tend to have large ratios (600 to 1700 fibers per unit), while the ratios in intrinsic hand muscles (e.g., first lumbrical and dorsal interosseous) are somewhat smaller (100 to 340 fibers per unit; Feinstein et al., 1955). Muscle units in extraocular muscles probably have very small ratios (13 to 20 fibers per unit). When looking at different motor unit pools there is evidently no simple relation between the size of a motoneuron or its motor axon diameter and the number of muscle fibers innervated by it. Even within a single muscle there is little evidence for a strong correlation between these features (e.g., Burke and Tsairis, 1973). Rather, average innervation ratios appear to depend mainly upon whole muscle bulk and on the number of alpha motoneurons, reflecting in turn the functional demand for precise grading of force output.

The developmental aspects of muscle unit organization and the control of innervation ratios remain largely unclear. However, as noted above, polyneuronal innervation is widespread in muscles of newborn mammals and disappears over the first few weeks of life (Bagust et al., 1973; Brown et al., 1976), as motor units mature into their adult organization (Hammarberg and Kellerth, 1975). Furthermore, early stages of spinal cord development probably involve the death of a significant proportion of cells in the motor nuclei (see review by Hamburger, 1977). We do not understand the mechanisms controlling such processes of removal of existing connections and cells, but they clearly must affect the final pattern of motor unit structural organization in important ways.

Subsequent to the above processes of connectivity modification, which occur within a few weeks after birth, there may be continued remodelling of motor unit organization. Kugelberg (1976) has found that units in the rat soleus change during the period from 5 to 34 weeks of postnatal age such that many fast twitch motor units appear to "transform" into slow twitch, both physiologically and histochemically. This kind of late developmental change may well reflect patterns of motor unit usage rather than of genetic specification (Kugelberg, 1976).

Muscle Units After Denervation and Reinnervation

The anatomy of muscle units found after motoneuron or motor axon injury and subsequent reinnervation is quite different from the normal situation. Glycogen depletion marking of individual muscle units in reinnervated animal muscle shows marked rearrangement of the normal fiber scattering (Fig. 4–4), with local collections of contiguous fibers (Kugelberg et al., 1970; Kugelberg, 1973; Brandstater and Lambert, 1973). Single fiber electromyography in human muscles indicates a similar reorganization after denervation and reinnervation (Schwartz et al., 1976). This reorganization of the normal muscle unit architecture is also reflected in the occurrence of local groups of histochemically similar fibers (known as "type grouping"; Karpati and Engel, 1968) in reinnervated muscle, which is clearly distinctive when compared to the normal histochemical mosaic in mixed muscles (Fig. 4–5). Presumably, the clustering of fibers innervated by one motor axon is due mainly to intramuscular sprouting of regenerating motor axon collaterals taking over denervated muscle fibers that previously belonged to different muscle units. Edds (1950) has shown that this sprouting process is highly localized and occurs near the terminal regions of the remaining motor axons. Sprouts are evidently "guided" to denervated end-plate regions by the Schwann cell sheaths remaining after degeneration of the cut axis cylinders (see also Warszawski et al., 1975, esp. their Fig. 6). It is clear, however, that reinnervated muscle units are histochemically uniform (Kugelberg et al., 1970), implying apparently complete histochemical and morphological conversions of fibers from one type to another after reinnervation. This process of conversion occurs, however, only after some delay (about 2 weeks) following establishment of functional neuromuscular connections by regenerating axons (Warszawski et al., 1975). The range of physiological properties for individual units after reinnervation is also approximately normal (Bagust and Lewis, 1974). Both observations are important evidence that motoneurons indeed exert powerful "trophic" control over the characteristics of their muscle fibers.

Kugelberg and coworkers (1970) have found that motor unit territories are smaller than normal in total area after experimental reinnervation in the rat. They also suggested that unit territories appear to be determined to some extent by intramuscular connective tissue boundaries, unlike units in normal muscle. Bagust and Lewis (1974) observed that, after self-reinnervation in the cat, individu-

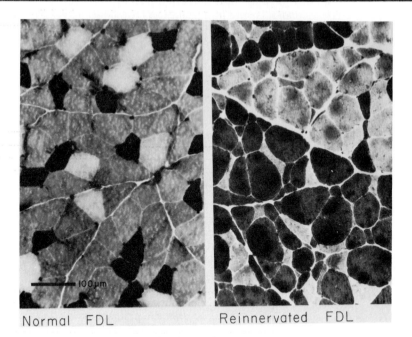

Normal FDL   Reinnervated   FDL

Figure 4–5 Photomicrographs of normal *(left panel)* and self-reinnervated *(right panel)* flexor digitorum longus muscles in cat, showing alteration in the normal histochemical mosaic after reinnervation. Both preparations stained for ATPase activity after acidic preincubation at pH 4.65 (Ac-ATPase; see Table 4–2). Note local aggregates of fibers with similar staining ("type grouping") in reinnervated muscle. From unpublished material of Burke and Tsairis.)

al muscle units exhibited a wider range of tetanic tension than normal, suggesting that innervation ratios may vary over a correspondingly wider range after reinnervation. This is perhaps due to temporal dispersion of arrival of regenerating axons in the target muscle, with the first axons taking over a larger share of denervated fibers than the late-comers.

Following nerve injury and reinnervation, apparently permanent polyneuronal connections can be established with individual muscle fibers when the reinnervating axons contact points on a muscle fiber that are relatively distant from one another. Polyneuronal connections established in close proximity after reinnervation tend to disappear when the different end-plates are located close together, implying the existence of some mechanism of spatial competition between motor axon terminals (Kuffler et al., 1977).

Thompson and Jansen (1977) have recently shown that motor axons in developing rat soleus exhibit the normal process of terminal retraction from some muscle fibers even in partially denervated muscles, leaving large numbers of permanently denervated fibers. Thus, the disappearance of polyneuronal innervation during development cannot wholly be explained by peripheral competition. Remarkably, adult motoneurons appear to be able to sprout about twice as profusely in response to partial denervation as they do in newborn animals. Nevertheless, Thompson and Jansen (1977) have clearly shown that alpha motoneurons cannot expand their field of peripheral innervation indefinitely, even though denervated fibers may remain in the target muscle. In rat soleus, motoneurons appear able to support about four times their normal number of terminal end-plates (and muscle fibers) after partial denervation of adult muscles, but no more than that.

PHYSIOLOGICAL PROPERTIES OF MOTOR UNITS

General Considerations

If all of the motor units in a given population (i.e., those belonging to one anatomical muscle) were similar, consideration of their physiological, structural, and biochemical properties would be simple and rather uninteresting. However, the available evidence indicates that most mammalian muscles are made up of very heterogeneous groups of motor units that exhibit widely varying attributes. Homogeneous populations of basically similar motor units are not unknown (the unit population in the cat soleus is an example; McPhedran et al., 1965; Burke et al., 1974), but these are exceptional. Accordingly, much of the recent active interest in motor units has centered on examination of the range of properties within particular unit populations and on questions of the probable functional significance of motor unit heterogeneity.

For over a century, since Ranvier's classic (1874) work on the correlation between muscle color and contraction speed, physiologists have been interested in the difference between "red, slow twitch" and "pale, fast twitch" muscles. These designations, derived as they are from the overall characteristics of whole muscles, have sometimes been used in a way that implies that the motor unit populations in those muscles are similarly homogeneous — either all "slow" or all "fast" twitch. However, histologists have been aware for many years of the existence of structural heterogeneity among the muscle fibers in most muscles (see Padykula and Gauthier, 1967, for a concise review). The relatively recent development of muscle fiber histochemistry and the identification of muscle fiber "types" (reviewed by Dubowitz and Brooke, 1973; their Chapter 3) have provided a strong impetus for physiologists to examine motor unit populations systematically to determine whether or not there may exist matching categories of motor unit "types," based on

147

physiological criteria. An important early study of this point was done in toad muscle by Lännergren and Smith (1966).

The presence of relatively "slow twitch" muscle units within nominally "fast twitch" mammalian muscles has been known for some time (Gordon and Holbourne, 1949; Gordon and Phillips, 1953). However, systematic study of the full range of properties exhibited by individual motor units in heterogeneous populations really began in the early 1960's, with work on the cat lumbrical muscles by Laporte's group (Bessou et al., 1963) and on the medial gastrocnemius in the cat by Henneman and coworkers (Wuerker et al., 1965; Henneman and Olson, 1965). Since that time there have been a rather large number of studies on motor unit populations in a great variety of muscles, mainly in the cat and rat, that have provided ample evidence for motor unit heterogeneity and have revealed the existence of correlations between a number of motor unit properties that, in all probability, have functional significance. In order to provide a frame of reference for discussion of this data, it seems useful to consider one motor unit population in some detail, both because the available information is extensive and because the pattern of unit organization is reasonably representative of that found in other muscles and species, with some exceptions to be discussed specifically.

Motor Units in the Cat Medial Gastrocnemius

In their 1965 paper on motor units of the cat medial gastrocnemius (MG) population, Wuerker and colleagues (1965) described wide ranges in muscle unit force outputs and twitch contraction times, and suggested that this physiological heterogeneity was related to the histochemical heterogeneity of MG muscle fibers (Henneman and Olson, 1965). Burke (1967) later suggested that MG units might usefully be classified as either "fast twitch" (type F) or "slow twitch" (type S) on the basis of muscle unit contraction times. He confirmed the findings of Wuerker et al. (1965) that the slowly contracting muscle units tended to produce rather small forces and were innervated by slowly conducting motor axons, while the "fast twitch" units could produce either large or small forces but all tended to be innervated by fast conducting motor axons.

In 1971, Olson and Swett (1971; see also 1966) and Burke and coworkers (1971) re-examined large samples of MG motor units in the normal cat and proposed different ways of classifying MG units into three categories, based on the properties of their muscle units. In the latter study, Burke et al. (1971; 1973a) also used the method of glycogen depletion introduced by Edström and Kugelberg (1968) to "mark" the fibers of physiologically characterized muscle units for detailed histochemical analysis.

The three-dimensional diagram in Figure 4–6 illustrates the distribution of four physiological properties in a sample of MG muscle units (Burke et al., 1973). Clearly, the data points (*circles*) cluster in different regions of the data space, and it is this differential clustering that can be used to identify motor unit "types." Note that the units

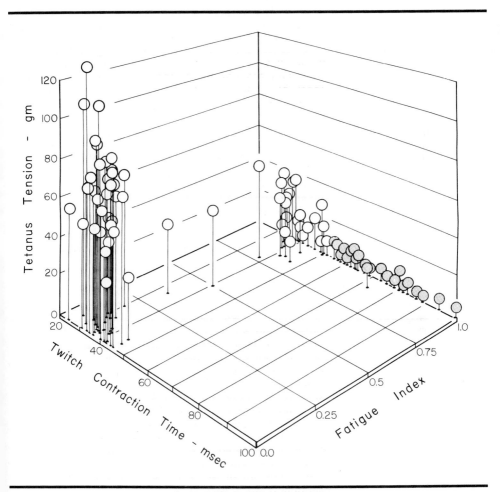

Figure 4–6 Three-dimensional diagram showing the distribution of four physiological properties of cat MG muscle units. Each circle represents a different muscle unit, with open circles denoting the presence of a characteristic shape ("sag" property) in unfused tetanic responses, and stippled circles denoting absence of "sag." The "fatigue index" represents a measure of fatiguability during a standardized stimulation sequence, with increasing values indicating increasing resistance to fatigue. When the distribution of all four properties are taken into account, the units clearly tend to cluster in different regions of the data space, suggesting the existence of definable motor unit types (see text). (From Burke et al., 1973a.)

149

denoted by stippled circles all tend to produce quite small tetanic forces (*vertical axis*) and are all resistant to fatigue (fatigue index >0.75). All of these tend to have relatively long twitch contraction times and, even though their contraction times vary over a twofold range, have therefore been designated simply as "slow twitch," or type S, motor units. The more rapidly contracting units (the "fast twitch" or type F; see Burke, 1967) exhibit two major clusters, one made up of units with little resistance to fatigue (fatigue index <0.25) and generally large force outputs, and the other with greater resistance to fatigue (fatigue index >0.75) but generally smaller tetanic force outputs. The former are referred to as "type FF" (fast contracting, fatigable) and the latter as "type FR" (fast contracting, fatigue-resistant). Two motor units are intermediate between the FF and FR groups in the diagram, and these are now called simply "fast twitch, intermediate," or type F(int) (Burke et al., 1976*b*). The patterns of correlations between muscle unit properties evident in Figure 4–6 are entirely compatible with results from other studies of MG motor units, allowing for differences in methods and experimental objectives (Olson and Swett, 1971; Proske and Waite, 1974; Reinking et al., 1975; Hammarberg and Kellerth, 1976).

The multidimensional diagram in Figure 4–6 clearly demonstrates the existence of cluster groupings resulting from the interrelatedness of muscle unit mechanical properties. It is virtually impossible to communicate such results without applying names to the data clusters ("FF," "FR," etc.) and appending verbal generalizations such as in the preceding paragraph. However, the diagram also shows that each cluster group, or unit "type," contains individual units that exhibit a range of properties. Identification of a "type" involves recognition of a "center of gravity" in the data cluster, which tends to obscure both the variability within the type group and the existence of overlap between groups in certain attributes (e.g., tetanic tension; see Fig. 4–6). Any system of classification tends to blur such realities and should thus be used with a certain degree of caution— that is, with a healthy skepticism.

A data classification scheme is useful when it can predict attributes of the system under study which are not included as classification parameters. This is the case with the FF-FR-S system for cat MG, since these physiological groups are made up of muscle units with distinctive histochemical profiles. Figure 4–7 illustrates glycogen-depleted muscle fibers (PAS stain, *leftmost column, arrows*) from representative FF, FR, and S units, and shows their distinctive histochemical differences in the other enzymatic reactions (Burke et al., 1971, 1973). All of the physiological type FF units showed the same histochemical profile as the unit illustrated in the top row

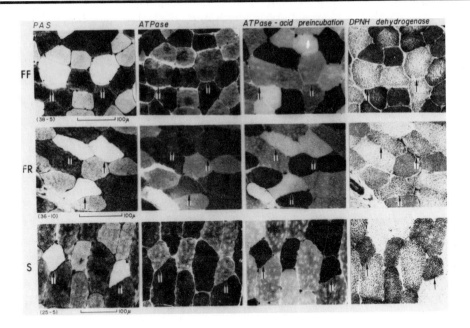

Figure 4–7 Photomicrographs of serial frozen sections *(rows)* from three different cat MG muscles, showing the histochemical profiles characteristic of typical type FF *(top row)*, type FR *(middle row)* and type S muscle units *(bottom row)*. Fibers belonging to physiologically-studied units identified by glycogen depletion (PAS stain, first column, *arrows*). The same fibers can be identified in serial sections stained for myofibrillar ATPase at pH 9.4 (ATPase, second column, *arrows*), for ATPase activity after preincubation in acidic buffer at pH 4.65 (third column), and for the oxidative enzyme DPNH (or NADH) dehydrogenase (fourth column). Each physiological unit type has a characteristic histochemical profile (see Table 4–2). All photomicrographs at the same magnification; note calibration bars. (From Burke et al., 1971. Copyright 1971 by the American Association for the Advancement of Science.)

of Figure 4–7, and the FR and S units similarly examined also had the quite different profiles shown for typical examples of these respective types. Further, all of the fibers belonging to a given unit exhibit the same histochemical profile — that is, muscle units are histochemically homogeneous (see also Edström and Kugelberg, 1968; Kugelberg, 1973, 1976; Doyle and Mayer, 1969). Table 4–2 shows the histochemical profiles that are characteristic of muscle fibers in heterogeneous, or mixed, human and some animal muscles. Also included are two systems of nomenclature based on fiber histochemistry and their concordance with the profiles found for the physiological motor unit types in cat MG.

151

Table 4–2 Concordance Between Systems of Nomenclature for Muscle Fiber and Motor Unit Types and the Histochemical Profiles of Human and Some Animal Muscles

Reference	Muscle Fiber Types			
Dubowitz and Brooke, 1973 (human)	2B	—	2A	1
Peter et al., 1972 (guinea pig, rabbit)	FG	—	FOG	SO
	Motor Unit Types			
Burke et al., 1973 (cat)	FF	F(int)	FR	S
	Histochemical Profiles			
Myofibrillar ATPase (pH 9.4)	High	High	High	Low
Ac-ATPase (pH 4.65)	Medium	Medium	Low	High
Ac-ATPase (pH 4.3)	Low	Low	Low	High
Oxidative enzymes	Low	Medium	Medium-high	High
Glycogen, phosphorylase	High	High	High	Low

The three-dimensional diagram in Figure 4–8 represents a summary of interrelations between a variety of physiological properties of cat MG motor units (including muscle unit, motoneuron, and synaptic organization attributes) and the histochemical profiles of their muscle units. The diagram is based directly on the one illustrated in Figure 4–6 but the type S group is offset on the "resistance to fatigue" axis to emphasize the observation that type S units are, in fact, much more resistant to fatigue than type FR units (Burke et al., 1973a; Burke and Tsairis, 1974). All of the fast twitch group (FF, F(int) and FR units together) have muscle units that stain intensely for myofibrillar ATPase activity at alkaline pH and are therefore histochemically "type 2" according to one widely used system of nomenclature (Table 4–2; see Dubowitz and Brooke, 1973). They also show relatively heavy histochemical staining for enzymes involved in anaerobic metabolism (e.g., phosphorylase), and fibers of these types have a high glycogen content. Conversely, type S muscle units exhibit relatively less intense activity in both of these histochemical categories.

As discussed in some detail elsewhere (Burke and Tsairis, 1974), the difference between fast and slow twitch muscle units in myofibrillar ATPase staining (which reflects fiber biochemistry with some accuracy; see Peter et al., 1972) conforms with the idea that differences in ATPase breakdown rates are important to the control of fiber shortening velocity (Barany, 1964). However, there is nevertheless a range of unit contraction times within both F and S unit groups in the cat, and the "fastest" type S units have almost the same contraction times as the "slowest" type F units (see Figs. 4–6 and 4–8). Thus, myofibrillar ATPase activity as reflected histochemically cannot be the only factor that controls the speed of isometric twitch contraction in these muscle units, at least as measurable at the tendon. In contrast, Kugelberg (1973, 1976) has found that the

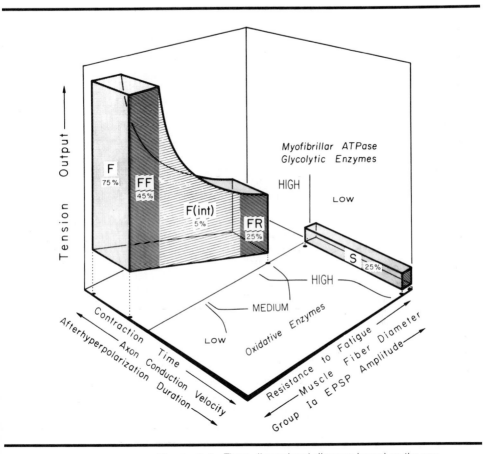

Figure 4–8 Three-dimensional diagram based on the one shown in Fig. 4–6, intended to summarize some of the interrelations found in the motor unit population of cat MG muscle between muscle unit physiological and histochemical profiles, and some characteristics of the innervating motoneurons (axonal conduction velocity and spike after hyperpolarization duration), as well as with the spectrum of amplitudes of the monosynaptic potential produced in these cells by stimulation of the group Ia (primary) muscle spindle afferents (group Ia EPSP). Arrows indicate the direction of increasing magnitude for the features listed. The box-like outlines indicate the positions within the data space of the clusters of points for actual motor units (see Fig. 4–6), with shading and labels indicating the different motor unit types. (Based on data in Burke, 1967; Burke et al., 1973a; Burke and Tsairis, 1973; Burke et al., 1976 a.)

contraction times of muscle units in rat soleus correlate more closely with the relative staining intensities in myofibrillar ATPase preparations. The difference may perhaps be partially explained by mechanical differences between rat and cat muscle preparations.

Differences in patterns of metabolic enzymes are clearly related to physiological motor unit type, especially as determined by relative resistance to fatigue (Fig. 4–8). The intensity of oxidative enzyme staining is closely related to fatigue resistance among the fast twitch unit groups. Such staining is also high in fibers of identified type S units (Burke et al., 173a) but the reaction product is also distributed in a different pattern, perhaps reflecting differences in the density and distribution of mitochondria and other intracellular organelles (e.g., Gauthier, 1969; Dubowitz and Brooke, 1973; Eisenberg and Kuda, 1977). Although caution must be used in interpreting histochemical staining intensities in terms of muscle fiber biochemistry (see Dubowitz and Brooke, 1973), there is evidence that the staining patterns do indeed reflect the relative predominance of aerobic versus anaerobic metabolic pathways (Peter et al., 1972). The physiological-histochemical correlation between high oxidative capacity and high resistance to fatigue (Fig. 4–8; see also Edström and Kugelberg, 1968; Kugelberg, 1973) implies a causal relationship. The fibers of type S and FR units are liberally supplied with capillaries (see also Romanul, 1965), as would be expected if they indeed depend heavily upon oxidative metabolism. In contrast, the fibers of type FF units are much less well supplied with capillaries, and are furthermore considerably larger in diameter than S or FR unit fibers (Fig. 4–9). The latter factor is consistent with the interpretation that, since FF unit fibers appear to depend almost entirely upon self-contained glycogen stores rather than upon bloodborne oxygen and metabolites, there is little need for maintaining the favorable surface-to-volume ratio given by small overall fiber diameter. Presumably, the very rapid fatigue exhibited by type FF muscle units (Burke et al., 1973) reflects exhaustion of intrafiber glycogen stores in fibers poorly adapted for oxidative metabolism.

Stability of Motor Unit Types

The evidence available thus far indicates that the motor unit types found in the adult cat MG are stable under conditions of altered functional demand within the physiological range (see Burke and Edgerton, 1975). Neither compensatory hypertrophy (Walsh et al., 1978), produced by disabling all Mg synergists, nor the atrophy produced by chronic immobilization by joint pinning (Mayer et al., 1976) results in any significant reorganization of the MG unit population. The motor unit types can be recognized by the same criteria as in normal muscles, and their relative frequencies in the MG pool are unaltered. Histo-

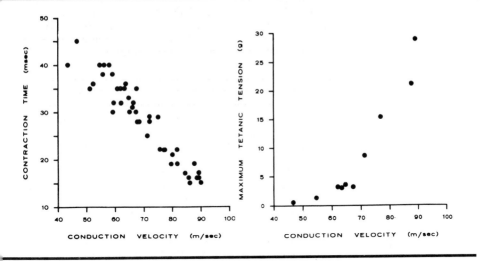

Figure 4–9 Some physiological features of motor units in a small distal foot muscle (superficial lumbrical) in the cat. Note the negative linear correlation between muscle unit contraction time and axonal conduction velocity of the innervating motoneuron *(left)*. The similarly close, although nonlinear, relation between conduction velocity of innervating axons and maximum isometric tension output from individual muscle units is shown in the right-hand graph. Both correlations are similar in general pattern but different in detail from those found in the larger MG muscle (Fig. 4–6). (From Appelberg and Emonet-Dénand, 1967.)

chemical fiber profiles are also apparently unchanged. There are large changes evident in tetanic tension output from individual units in all categories (increases in hypertrophy and decreases in immobilization atrophy) but no apparent alteration of normal twitch contraction times or fatigue resistance.

From studies of muscles after chronic endurance exercise in a variety of animals (e.g., Barnard et al., 1970a; Edgerton et al., 1972; Faulkner et al., 1972), it is clear that muscle fibers can change in oxidative metabolic capacity. This increase is evident in whole muscle histochemistry and biochemistry, and is further reflected in increased resistance of whole muscles to fatigue (Barnard et al., 1970b). There are, however, no changes in myofibrillar ATPase staining with endurance training, suggesting that this physiological overload does not cause interconversion of fast and slow twitch muscle units. The same type of oxidative capacity change is inferred to occur in human muscles after endurance training (e.g., Gollnick et al., 1972). To date, there are no studies available of individual motor units after endurance training. However, Reinking and coworkers (1975) found a greater proportion of fatigue-resistant fast twitch muscle units in the MG of active uncaged cats than was found in that muscle by Burke et al. (1973a; see Fig. 4–6) in animals that had been more confined before examination. The changes in oxidative capacity and fatigue resistance appear to be greatest among the fast twitch muscle units, suggesting that there may be interconversion possible between the FF and FR unit types, depending upon current exercise levels. The type F(int) units might then represent units in transition (see Burke and Edgerton, 1975, and Prince et al., 1976, for discussion of this question).

The apparent stability of motor unit types discussed above holds only for the "physiological" range of functional demand. There is considerable evidence that nerve cross-union (e.g., Buller et al., 1960; Romanul and Van Der Meulen, 1965; Close, 1969; Weeds et al., 1974) can dramatically alter the physiological, histochemical, and biochemical profiles of muscle fibers. The restructuring of muscle units that occurs after reinnervation (see above) has the same implication. Further, chronic stimulation of muscles with various pulse patterns also produces profound changes in muscle fiber biochemistry (e.g., Salmons and Sreter, 1976). The implications of such changes in relation to questions of "trophic" relations between motoneurons and muscles are discussed in Chapter 5.

Motoneuron Characteristics

Included in Figure 4–8 (*left horizontal axis*) are two characteristics of the innervating motoneurons. As noted above, type S muscle units tend to be innervated by relatively slowly conducting motor axons and their motoneurons tend to present greater electrical resistance ("input resistance") to currents passed into them through a micropipet electrode (see Burke, 1967) than is the case with motoneurons of fast twitch units. Both of these physiological characteristics are related to the anatomical size of the motoneurons, the correlation being direct in the case of conduction velocity and inverse in the case of input resistance (Barrett and Crill, 1974; Burke and Rudomin, 1977). Thus, type S motoneurons are inferred to be smaller on the average than type F cells (see also Fig. 4–1). There is, however, no systematic difference between the axonal conduction velocities of FF and FR motor unit groups (Burke et al., 1976b), suggesting that both of these unit types have relatively large motoneurons. It is of interest that there is rather little difference in innervation ratios between the F and S motor unit groups in cat MG (Burke and Tsairis, 1973), suggesting that, if motoneuron volume limits the maximum number of terminal endings possible, this limit is not reached in the normal MG motor unit pool.

The physiological mechanisms underlying the motoneuron action potential and other membrane properties are beyond the scope of this review (for details, see Burke and Rudomin, 1977). However, it is relevant to the present discussion to note that the action potential is followed by a prolonged afterhyperpolarization (AHP) that is a key factor in the control of maximum cell firing rates. The longer the AHP, the slower motoneurons tend to fire, other factors being equal (Kernell, 1965). Figure 4–8 indicates that motoneurons of type S units tend to have AHPs of longer duration than are observed in type F cells (Burke, 1967; see also Eccles et al., 1958; Kuno, 1959), but there is no systematic difference between FF and FR cells in this regard (Hammarberg and Kellerth, 1975). It is well known that slow twitch whole muscles require lower stimulation rates to reach maximum force output than is the case with "fast twitch" muscles (e.g., Cooper and Eccles, 1930), and the same relation exists in individual muscle units (Burke et al., 1976a). Thus, the relatively long AHP durations in type S motoneurons can be viewed as an appropriate functional specialization, limiting maximum firing rates to ranges that efficiently utilize the properties of slow twitch muscle units.

Intrinsic motoneuron properties such as specific membrane resistance, voltage threshold for action potential production, and dendritic electrotonic length are important for a complete picture of the control of motoneuron response to synaptic input, or relative "excitability" (see Table 4–4). Information about the distribution of such properties in the various motor unit groups of cat MG is discussed elsewhere (Burke, 1973; Burke and Rudomin, 1977). Only two points merit specific mention here. The first is that there is a systematic difference between S and F motoneurons in their accommodation to persistent depolarization, such that type S cells tend to fire repetitively to sustained input while the response of many type F cells tends to decrease ("accommodate") with time (Burke and Nelson, 1971). Furthermore, Schwindt and Crill (1977) have shown, with voltage clamp methods, that cat motoneurons with high input resistance (presumably innervating type S muscle units) tend to have a form of intrinsic membrane response that can produce repetitive cell firing irrespective of sustained depolarizing input. These findings again suggest functional specialization by which motoneuron and muscle unit properties are precisely matched.

It would be erroneous to conclude from the preceding discussion that alpha motoneurons can be classified into clearly separable groups, such as the "tonic" and "phasic" categories suggested some years ago (Granit et al., 1956). The existence of such qualitatively separate groups is questionable (see, e.g., Henatsch et al., 1959; Henneman et al., 1965a; Burke, 1967; Burke and Rudomin, 1977) and systematic surveys of motneuron electrophysiological properties have disclosed no set of attributes that provide a basis for the type of cluster

157

analysis classification that can be done with muscle units. Rather, the distribution of alpha motoneuron properities appears to be a spectrum. The motoneurons that innervate type S muscle units are at one end and the cells of type F units are at the other, but between the extremes is a continuum with sufficient overlap between F and S motoneurons so as to negate the possibility of identifying motor unit type through motoneuron properties alone (Burke, 1967, 1973).

Motor Units in Other Limb Muscles: Animal Studies

Although the detailed results of motor unit surveys vary with the muscle, species, and methods employed, the overall pattern of interrelations found in cat MG between motor axon conduction velocity and muscle unit twitch contraction time, force output, and resistance to fatigue are evident in other heterogeneous limb muscles of the cat (e.g., Olson and Swett, 1966; Goslow et al., 1972; Mosher et al., 1972; Bagust et al., 1973). The same can be said for motor units in rat limb and tail muscles (Steg, 1964; Close, 1967; Edström and Kugelberg, 1968; Kugelberg, 1973, 1976). It is, however, difficult to reconcile some aspects of rat and cat muscle unit histochemistry and physiology, presumably because of fundamental species differences. A quite interesting species variation is illustrated by recent data from the skunk (Van de Graff et al., 1977). The mixed gastrocnemius in this animal contains no muscle fibers with the FG or type 2B histochemical profile (see Table 4–2) and no muscle units with the type FF physiological profile. This finding seems to be related to the very different movement pattern of the skunk, which ordinarily neither runs nor jumps as compared to a predator such as the cat, which does both.

The proportion of motor units equivalent to the categories found in the cat appear to vary widely, depending upon the muscle and species in question. For example, over 80 per cent of the fibers in the guinea pig "white vastus" are histochemically type FG, while a similar proportion of fibers in the "red vastus" have the FOG histochemical profile (Peter et al., 1972), implying corresponding variation in the predominance of FF or FR muscle units, respectively. By and large, however, almost all nominally "fast twitch" whole muscles contain some proportion of fibers with the type SO histochemical profile, implying the existence of an equivalent proportion of slow twitch motor units in a variety of animal species (e.g., Ariano et al., 1973) and in man (Buchthal and Schmalbruch, 1970; Edström and Nyström, 1969; Johnson et al., 1973; Edgerton et al., 1975).

A classic example of an exception to the above rule is the soleus muscles of the cat and guinea pig, which are histochemically virtually homogeneous and are made up of type SO muscle fibers (see also Collatos et al., 1977). The motor units of the cat soleus exhibit a relatively restricted range of properties (e.g., McPhedran et al., 1965) as compared to the heterogeneous gastrocnemius, and all so far studied can be classified as type S (Burke et al., 1974). It may be noted, however, that the units in cat soleus are in several respects rather different from the type S units in the heterogeneous MG (Burke et al., 1974). While the details of this distinction are not important here, its existence shows that the characteristics of a motor unit group (in this case, the type S) cannot necessarily be extrapolated accurately from data on a whole muscle, even when it is "homogeneous." It is also useful to point out that the soleus muscle of some species, including the rat (Kugelberg, 1973; 1976), is heterogeneous, as it is histochemically in man (Edström and Nyström, 1969; Edgerton et al., 1975).

It seems pertinent to consider in some detail results from studies of motor units in small distal limb muscles. The organization of units in such muscles is somewhat at variance with that in the larger, more proximal muscles, and this is important to the interpretation of recent studies of human motor units which have concentrated on small distal muscles for technical reasons. The lumbrical slips in the cat each consist of a small number of motor units (three to eight; see Kernell et al., 1975) that nevertheless exhibit a wide range in contraction times and force outputs (Fig. 4–9). Further, both of these muscle unit properties are very closely correlated with the conduction velocity of the motor axon (Fig. 4–9; Bessou et al., 1963; Appelberg and Emonet-Dénand, 1967). The remarkably linear relation between conduction velocity and twitch contraction time demonstrated in these studies (Fig. 4–9) is quite different from that found for these features in cat MG, where there is no clear relation among the large population of fast twitch units (Burke, 1967; Stephens and Stuart, 1975). In addition, lumbrical motor units do not fall exactly into the FF-FR-S classification system (Kernell et al., 1975), providing an example of the caution that must be exercised when trying to formulate comprehensive generalizations about different populations of motor units.

The motor unit populations in muscles innervated by cranial nerves are, as far as most of them have been studied, not very different in basic organization from those in limb muscles (e.g., see Taylor et al., 1973, for a discussion of jaw musculature). Even the tiny muscles of the middle ear have identifiable fast and slow twitch units with appropriate attributes, both physiological and histochemical (Teig, 1972; Teig and Dahl, 1972). The morphology, histochemistry, and physiology of the extraocular muscles are apparently considerably more complex and specialized but, here too, the general patterns evident in limb motor units can be recognized (for details and references see Bach-y-Rita and Ito, 1966; Lennerstrand, 1974; Goldberg et al., 1976; and Barmack, 1977).

159

Mechanical Properties of Human Motor Units

There is an extensive literature on electromyographic (EMG) studies of human motor units, but attention in this review will be focused instead on the relatively small amount of data now available concerning the mechanical properties of units in human muscle and how these relate to results from animal studies.

Fast and slow twitch fiber bundles have been found in in vitro studies of muscle biopsies from a wide variety of human muscles (Eberstein and Goodgold, 1968). While Denny-Brown and Pennybacker (1938) showed that it was possible to correlate unit force records with single unit EMG discharges in some cases of motoneuron disease, systematic attempts to obtain mechanical recordings from individual human motor units comparable to those from animals began only relatively recently. Two types of approaches have been used, one in which motor axons are stimulated electrically, and the other in which force contributions of single motor units are isolated during voluntary contractions.

Buchthal and Schmalbruch (1970) used intramuscular stimulation of motor axons to activate "small bundles" of muscle fibers, and recorded the resulting forces with a transducer system impaled in the tendon of insertion. Mechanical forces were averaged for many responses in order to enhance the signal to noise ratio. While these authors did not claim to have recorded responses to individual motor units, they did demonstrate a wider range of twitch contraction times in some muscles (e.g., biceps brachii) than in others (e.g., triceps brachii, platysma). They noted the prevalence of slower contracting "bundles" in muscles that had relatively high proportions of mitochondria-rich muscle fibers, some proportion of which were assumed to be of the slow twitch type, and they further noted the disappearance of the slower responses after local circulatory arrest, implying dependence upon aerobic metabolism. Intramuscular electrical stimulation has also been used in a study by Taylor and Stephens (1976), who contend that, under certain conditions, the method can indeed activate individual muscle units.

Sica and McComas (1971) used surface electrical stimulation of extramuscular peripheral nerves, combined with mechanical recording of deflections of the great toe, to record all-or-none twitch responses from the extensor hallucis brevis, which were interpreted as reflecting single motor unit action. They observed a wide range of "unit" contraction times (35 to 98 msec) but, surprisingly, found no correlation between these and twitch forces.

A different method of unit recording was exploited by Milner-Brown et al. (1974a), who recorded single unit EMG spikes from the human first dorsal interosseous muscle, and used this signal to trigger an averaged record of the isometric force exerted by the index finger. The mechanical records thus educed from the whole muscle force can be ascribed to the action of an individual motor unit with considerable certainty, as long as EMG identification is secure and there is no statistical synchronization between firings in different motor units (Milner-Brown et al., 1973a). However, this method has the serious disadvantage that the mechanical records in fact represent component responses in unfused tetani rather than true isolated twitches. The resemblance between such components and isolated twitches appears to be reasonably close under some conditions (Milner-Brown et al., 1973a), but it depends significantly upon the rate of unit firing during mechanical averaging — the faster the rate, the less the resemblance (see e.g., Büdingen and Freund, 1976). The mechanical response averaged from the appendage of muscle insertion may also be distorted by the mechanical compliance of the tissues (tendon, skin, et al.) when records are obtained at different force levels (Monster and Chan, 1977).

Milner-Brown and colleagues (1973b) found wide ranges in contraction times (30 to 90 msec) and force outputs (<0.2 gram to >12 grams) in the "twitch" responses of units in the first dorsal interosseous (see also Desmedt and Godaux, 1977a). The latter distribution is quite skewed, however, and the muscle appears to consist largely of quite small force units (true also of many animal muscles, see above) with only a weak correlation between contraction times and force outputs (see Fig. 4–14), unlike the close relation found in the cat lumbrical (see Fig. 4–9; Appelberg and Emonet-Dénand, 1967). In another study of the first dorsal interosseous, using methods similar to those of Milner-Brown et al., Stephens and Usherwood (1977) found a somewhat closer force-contraction time correlation. Moreover, they estimated the relative resistance of individual units to fatigue and found, as in cat MG (Fig. 4–6), that the slower twitch units were not only smaller but also more fatigue-resistant as compared to many fast twitch units. There was a much wider range of force outputs among the faster twitch units than among the slow, and the smaller force fast units tended to be more resistant to fatigue than the larger (see their Fig. 3). Thus, the general pattern of muscle unit organization in the human first dorsal interosseous seems to echo that found in animal studies (Figs. 4–6 and 4–8).

A rather different pattern was obtained by Monster and Chan (1977) in a study of muscle units in the human extensor digitorum communis. Again using EMG-triggered averaging of voluntary contractions, they found a rather narrow (<two-fold) range in unit contraction times and concluded that even this range is an artifact of measurement, due to variable compliance of the measur-

ing system. There was, however, a tenfold range in "twitch" forces. If all of the muscle units in the human extensor digitorum communis are, in fact, fast twitch, with a narrow range of contraction times as has been found in a large sample of units from the same muscle in the baboon (Eccles et al., 1968), then this muscle may be an exception to the rule that histochemical heterogeneity implies the presence of fast and slow twitch muscle units. The histochemical composition of most human arm and hand muscles contains an appreciable proportion (>30 per cent) of type 1 fibers, suggesting that at least some units should be relatively slow twitch (Johnson et al., 1973). A similar lack of a strong contraction time-force correlation was found among units recorded in the human masseter, in which some muscle units are remarkably forceful (up to 200 grams "twitch" force; Goldberg and Derfler, 1977; see also Yemm, 1977).

Skeletofusimotor Units

As shown in Table 4–1, certain motoneurons innervate both extrafusal skeletal muscle fibers and intrafusal fibers within muscle spindles. This skeletofusimotor, or beta, pattern of innervation is the rule in amphibian and reptilian muscle but its existence in mammals was first suggested by physiological results of Bessou et al. (1965). Since contractions of skeletal muscle fibers and of intrafusal fibers both affect muscle spindle afferents (see Matthews, 1972), physiological demonstration of the beta pattern of innervation requires special conditions and precautions. Ordinarily, extrafusal contractions unload and silence muscle spindle afferents which subsequently signal extrafusal relaxation and lengthening by a burst of spikes (Fig. 4–10, records 1 and 2). However, when extrafusal neuromuscular junctions are blocked by curariform agents at doses insufficient to block the more resistant intrafusal junctions, an underlying activation of spindle afferents can be seen (Fig. 4–10, record 3) when beta innervation is present (Bessou et al., 1965; Emonet-Dénand et al., 1970). Using such methods, beta innervation has now been demonstrated in a variety of limb muscles in cat and rabbit (Emonet-Dénand et al., 1970, 1975).

Recently a more direct demonstration of beta innervation was accomplished by Barker, Laporte and their colleagues (1977). They stimulated individual motor axons to the small peroneus brevis or tenuissimus muscles of the cat and found cases in which fiber glycogen was depleted in both intra- and extrafusal muscle fibers. One beta motor unit has also been similarly demonstrated in the soleus muscle in the cat (Burke and Tsairis, 1977).

Because of the technical difficulty in identifying beta motoneurons, there is little information about their specific properties. However, there is clearly a class of beta motoneurons that have relatively slow axonal conduction

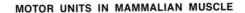

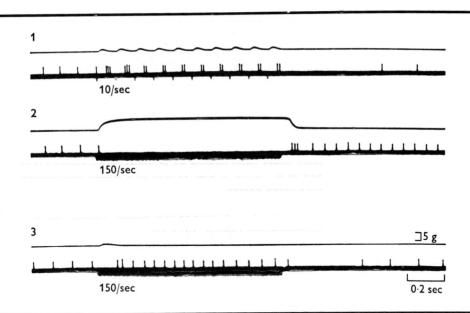

Figure 4–10 Physiological identification of beta innervation. Stimulation of an isolated motor axon at a low rate (10/sec; *record 1*) produces twitch responses of its extrafusal muscle unit (*upper trace;* force recorded at the tendon) and consequent brief discharge of a primary (group Ia) afferent axon *(lower trace)* on the falling phase of each twitch. Higher frequency tetanization (150/sec) of the motor axon silences the spindle afferent during the mechanical tetanus *(record 2),* as expected for ordinary muscle unit-spindle interaction. However, partial curarization of the preparation *(record 3),* with a dose sufficient to block extrafusal but not intrafusal neuromuscular transmission, leads to failure of extrafusal mechanical response and increased firing of the spindle afferent. Such results indicate that the spindle afferent arose in a muscle spindle to which the motor axon contributed functional innervation — i.e., the beta pattern of innervation. (From Emonet-Dénand et al., 1970.)

velocities, in the slower portion of the alpha motoneuron range (40 to 90 m/sec in the cat; Emonet-Dénand et al., 1975). Intracellular records are available for only one documented beta motoneuron (in cat soleus), which had no unusual properties and which clearly received monosynaptic excitation from soleus group Ia muscle spindle afferents (Burke and Tsairis, 1977), a synaptic connection entirely absent in gamma motoneurons (Eccles et al., 1960; Grillner et al., 1969).

With few exceptions, the slow conduction velocity beta motoneurons innervate one of the two types of nuclear bag fibers (bag 1 in the cat spindle; Barker et al., 1977), and their extrafusal muscle units are histochemically type SO (Table 4–2). The one beta extrafusal muscle unit that has been studied thus far physiologically (Burke and

163

Tsairis, 1977) was not unusual when compared to other soleus muscle units. It is interesting to note that the morphology and histochemical profile of bag 1 intrafusal fibers are very different from those of extrafusal (type SO fibers, even though they are sometimes innervated by the same (beta) motoneuron. The slow beta motoneurons usually exert a "dynamic" physiological action on spindle afferent responses (Emonet-Dénand et al., 1970, 1975).

Until recently, the beta innervation pattern was regarded as something of a curiosity, demonstrable only in small distal muscles and of questionable functional importance. However, with continued study in Laporte's laboratory, beta motor units have now been found in larger limb muscles such as soleus, tibialis anterior, and flexor hallucis longus (Emonet-Dénand et al., 1975). Furthermore, the proportion of beta axons in systematic surveys is not small. McWilliam (1975) found that 30 to 40 per cent of spindles in the small tenuissimus and abductor digiti quinti muscles of the cat had beta innervation. In the cat peroneus brevis, 18 per cent of axons supplying extrafusal muscle fibers also innervated intrafusal muscle (Emonet-Dénand and Laporte, 1975). The cat peroneus brevis muscle contains about 20 per cent type SO fibers (Ariano et al., 1973) so that, given the evidence that slow beta axons innervate type S muscle units, a significant fraction of the type S motor units in this muscle may in fact be beta motor units. There is good evidence that type S motor units receive the strongest excitatory projection from group Ia muscle spindle afferent fibers (Burke, 1968; Burke et al., 1976b). The dynamic sensitivity of group Ia afferents is increased by beta activity, so that the beta pattern represents a powerful positive feedback loop, sensitive to muscle length and velocity of stretch. This organization is very different from the gamma motoneuron-spindle-alpha motoneuron loop, which is essentially open insofar as gamma motoneurons receive no direct excitation from spindle afferents. The functional role of the beta organization is still undefined but potentially important.

The story of beta innervation has recently become even more complicated with the demonstration that fast conducting motor axons, innervating type 2 (presumably fast twitch) muscle units, may also innervate intrafusal nuclear chain fibers (cat peroneus tertius muscle; Harker et al., 1977). Very recently, Jami and coworkers (1978) have obtained evidence suggesting that the "fast" beta axons have a static action on spindle afferents, that they may innervate either bag or chain intrafusal fibers, and that their extrafusal muscle units have the 2A histochemical profile characteristic of type FR units. The type FR units generally also receive quite powerful excitatory feedback from group Ia spindle afferents (Burke et al., 1976b)

**FUNCTIONAL
CONSIDERATIONS:
CONTROL OF
MUSCLE FORCE**

Attention in this section will be limited to consideration of two issues: 1) the factors involved in the control of muscle force; and 2) how these factors correlate with motor unit characteristics and the probable functional roles played by units of different types.

The production of force by whole muscles is usually thought of in terms of the numbers of motor units active and the frequency at which they fire. Numbers of active motor units can be discussed under the rubric of "recruitment," another key concept introduced to physiology by Sherrington (see Granit, 1966, p. 71). The role of motoneuron firing frequency has a similarly distinguished history, having been first emphasized by Adrian and Bronk (1929). However, current information makes it clear that these factors are not the whole story.

Table 4–3 shows one way of identifying the factors that control force output from whole muscle. Clearly, the notion of "recruitment" involves not only the numbers of active motor units but also their identities, in terms of their muscle unit characteristics (e.g., isometric contractions times, force outputs, unit types). Perhaps less obvious is the fact that information about the instantaneous firing frequency of an active motoneuron is in itself insufficient to predict the force output from its muscle unit, even if that unit's isometric properties are known. The force produced by a muscle unit can vary with the pattern of interspike intervals in a motoneuron discharge (Fig. 4–12), as well as with frequency (Fig. 4–11). Furthermore, this output also depends on the long-term history (measured in minutes) of previous motoneuron firings, in that force production can be either enhanced by postactivation (or posttetanic) potentiation (PTP), or it may be diminished by the effects of fatigue.

**Firing Rate, Firing
Pattern, and Other
Factors**

An example of the nonlinear effects of frequency and PTP on muscle unit force is shown in the graph in Figure 4–11. The curves labeled $P_T(1)$ and $P_T(2)$ show the plateau force (*right ordinate,* grams) produced during trains of motoneuron pulses at different interspike intervals

Table 4–3 Factors that Influence Whole
Muscle Force Output

---

1. Recruitment of motor units:
   a. Number of active units.
   b. Identity of active units, in terms of their muscle unit characteristics.

2. Activation history for each unit:
   a. Average motoneuron firing frequency.
   b. Pattern of motoneuron interspike intervals.
   c. Postactivation potentiation of force output.
   d. Fatigue.
   e. Effects of active lengthening or active shortening.

165

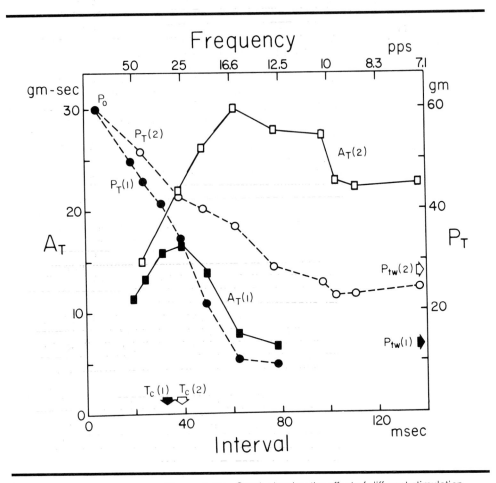

Figure 4–11 Graph showing the effect of different stimulation frequencies *(upper abscissa)* or equivalent interpulse intervals *(lower abscissa)* on the isometric mechanical responses of a fast twitch (probably type FR) muscle unit in cat MG. The curves indicated by circles refer to the right ordinate and denote the plateau force (P_T, grams) measured during the fourteenth response in mechanical tetani at the indicated frequencies (or intervals). The solid symbols are curves obtained from the unit in its initial state [$P_T(1)$] and the open circles [$P_T(2)$] are from responses obtained after the muscle unit had been subjected to repeated high frequency tetanization to induce posttetanic potentiation (PTP) of its mechanical output. The force produced by a single twitch after PTP ($P_{tw}(2)$; open arrow on right ordinate) is about double that of the twitch before potentiation [$P_{tw}(1)$], but the contraction times are not very different ($T_c(1)$ and $T_c(2)$; msec scale on lower abscissa). The force-time integral (A_T, left ordinate, gram-seconds) for 14 stimuli in the same series of isometric tetani before and after PTP are shown by the square symbols and solid lines [$A_T(1)$ and $A_T(2)$]. Note the marked difference in the curves produced by PTP. (From Burke et al., 1976 *b*.)

(lower abscissa) or equivalent frequencies (upper abscissa), before (filled circles; $P_T(1)$) and after force enhancement by PTP (open circles; $P_T(2)$). Both curves have steep slopes but converge to the same force (P_0) when the activation frequency is very high (200 Hz) and the tetanus response is fused. Clearly, force output is modulated over a wide range with input frequencies between 12 and 50 Hz, and PTP significantly affects this modulation. Note that the force produced by the highest frequency of stimulation (P_0) is the same before and after PTP but that, at lower frequencies, the forces are uniformly larger after PTP. The square symbols (curves labelled A_T denote the integral of force and time (left ordinate, gram-sec) measured for tetani, each produced by 14 stimuli recurring at the various input frequencies indicated. There is a considerable difference in the curves produced before (filled squares; $A_T(1)$) and after PTP (open squares; $A_T(2)$). The force-time integral under isometric conditions is equivalent to mechanical momentum, which should in turn reflect the potential work available were the muscle allowed to shorten. It is of interest that both force-time integral curves have well-defined peaks at relatively low input frequencies (16 to 25 Hz), suggesting that the potential work output from this muscle unit is optimized at low frequencies of motoneuron firing, even though it is a fast twitch unit. Similar results have been found in slow twitch units, the only difference being that the frequency and interval curves are shifted to lower values (Burke et al., 1976a).

There is no systematic data on the ranges of motoneuron firing frequencies during movements in intact animals, but hind limb motoneurons can fire at instantaneous rates up to 90 Hz during the alternating bursts of activity produced in "fictive" locomotion in the decerebrate cat (Severin et al., 1967; Zajac and Young, 1976). Sustained firing rates during decerebrate stretch reflexes are generally lower (8 to 25 Hz; Burke, 1968; Grillner and Udo, 1971a) among slow twitch units than among fast, which can fire at up to 50 Hz (Burke, 1968). Much more extensive data is available from human subjects, examined during voluntary contractions. These results all indicate that human motor units usually exhibit rather similar minimum rates of steady firing (6 to 8 Hz). Maximum firing rates during steady isometric contractions of both small distal muscles and larger limb muscles vary from about 15 to 50 Hz, seeming to depend more upon the methods used than upon the identity of the muscle (Bigland and Lippold, 1954; Norris and Gasteiger, 1955; Clamann, 1970; Person and Kudina, 1972; Tanji and Kato, 1973a; Milner-Brown et al., 1973c; Freund et al., 1975; Monster and Chan, 1977). In all cases, however, the steady firing rates are well below what would be required to produce maximum (i.e., fused) tetanic forces.

The situation in rapid or ballistic contractions is rather different. In both isometric contractions and those in

167

which movement is permitted, some high threshold motor units can emit bursts of firing with instantaneous frequencies up to 140 Hz, and sustained firing above 75 Hz is apparently not unusual (Desmedt and Godaux, 1977b; Grimby and Hannerz, 1977). Recent work by Borg and coworkers (1978) indicate that units in the short toe extensor muscle of man that tend to fire in high frequency bursts also tend to have relatively fast axonal conduction velocities, as compared to the lower threshold, continuously firing units. This would, of course, fit the notion that some fast twitch units are specialized for high frequency firing during large force or rapid movements.

The role of firing rate modulation in the control of whole muscle forces has been somewhat controversial. Motor units in red, slow muscles such as the cat soleus show very narrow ranges of firing frequencies, at least in decerebrate stretch reflexes (Grillner and Udo, 1971a), and it has been argued that the control of total output force in such muscles must therefore reside largely in the mechanism of recruitment of new units and in the inherent stiffness exhibited by active muscle fibers (Grillner and Udo, 1971b). Motor units in the human SOL display the same narrow (6 to 10 Hz) range of firing frequency during stance (Mori, 1973). However, in most heterogeneous motor unit populations that have been studied, individual units show three- to fivefold ranges in firing rates during the production of gradually increasing forces, often without systematic differences in firing rates when low threshold units are compared to high. In fact, low threshold units often exhibit wider ranges of firing modulation during ramp contractions, apparently because they are active over a wider range of force outputs (Bigland and Lippold, 1954; Clamann, 1970; Person and Kudina, 1972; Tanji and Kato, 1973a; Monster and Chan, 1977; but cf. Hannerz, 1974). This seemingly paradoxical observation may be due in part to the fact that many studies are done only with slowly varying output forces. High frequency bursting is clearly present in more rapid or ballistic contractions (Grimby and Hannerz, 1977; Borg et al., 1978). Marsden et al. (1971) have in fact seen firing rates as high as 150 Hz for brief periods of maximal voluntary contraction in the human adductor pollicis.

Some studies have suggested that the process of recruitment of new units is prominent only at relatively low output levels (<50 per cent maximum voluntary force), and that modulation of firing rate is the major factor in force modulation at high force levels (e.g., Milner-Brown et al., 1973c). Other results, however, indicate that recruitment is important over the entire range of voluntary force (e.g., Tanji and Kato, 1973b). In general, both mechanisms must be considered relevant to control of the entire range of muscle force, both in steady or slowly increasing forces and in the production of varying levels of very rapid, ballistic forces (Desmedt and Godaux, 1977a, b).

The pattern of motoneuron firing may be as important to unit force modulation as the average firing frequency. Figure 4–12 illustrates an example of the influence of a short interspike interval in the firing pattern on muscle unit force output, in this case from a slow twitch unit. The average firing frequency in each stimulus train was virtually identical and the trains differ in only one or two interspike intervals (*arrows*). A single short (approxi-

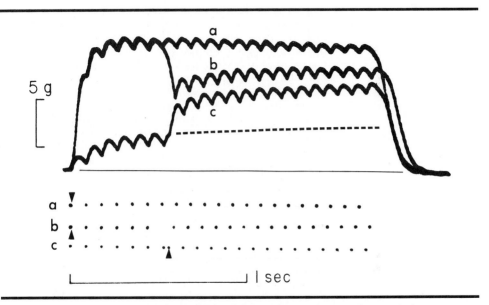

Figure 4–12 "Catch-like" enhancement of isometric force output from an individual type S muscle unit (cat MG muscle), produced by altering only one or two interpulse intervals in an otherwise low frequency stimulus train. The lowermost force trace, continued by the dashed line, shows the isometric response found for a perfectly regular train of stimuli at a frequency of about 12.6 Hz. The addition of a single extra pulse at an interval of 10 msec following the first stimulus (*arrows*, dot sequence "a") produced a very marked and sustained force increase (trace *a*) lasting as long as the basic train. Widening one interval in the basic train, after the initial doublet, produced the fall in force shown in trace *b* (stimulus sequence "b") which was "caught" at a new level as soon as the 12.6 Hz train resumed. Insertion of an interpulse interval only moderately shorter than that of the basic train (sequence "c", record c) produced less marked force enhancement than the short doublet, but nevertheless force output enhancement was similarly sustained. The average stimulus frequencies in each train were almost the same (within 5 per cent of one another) but the resultant force output was clearly very different, demonstrating the dependence of muscle unit force upon the pattern of input as well as upon the average frequency. (From Burke et al., 1970. Copyright 1970 by the American Association for the Advancement of Science.)

169

mately 10 msec) interval (or double discharge) can produce remarkable enhancement of force output (compare records a and c) without changing average frequency significantly. This "catch-like" enhancement of muscle unit force (Burke et al. 1970, 1976b) may well be important in normal activities, since the presence of short interval motoneuron spikes is not unusual in human (Denslow, 1948; Denny-Brown, 1949) and animal muscle (Denny-Brown, 1929; Gordon and Holbourne, 1949; Zajac and Young, 1976), especially during rapid voluntary movements (Gurfinkel et al., 1972). Norris and Gasteiger (1955) in fact found double discharges most commonly among human motor units recruited at low and moderate levels of voluntary force. "Catch-like" enhancement is present in both fast and slow twitch muscle units but is particularly prominent in the latter. It varies greatly, depending upon the state of PTP, and is most marked with relatively low basic input rates in the range at which motor units normally fire under physiological conditions.

The mechanical properties of individual muscle units have been investigated under isometric conditions, largely for experimental convenience. However, it is known that muscle output can be significantly influenced when muscle length changes. The mechanical properties of shortening muscle are rather well known (see e.g., Carlson and Wilkie, 1974, for a succinct review) and many actions certainly involve active shortening. However, it is becoming increasingly clear that stretching of active muscle occurs in many movements, including locomotion (Goslow et al., 1973). The force output of an active muscle during stretch is enhanced because of its stiffness (see e.g., Grillner, 1972). Furthermore, even stretching passive muscle produces a persistent enhancement of force during subsequent activity, above what would be expected without such prior stretch (Cavagna et al., 1971; Cavagna and Citterio, 1974). Thus, the history of length changes prior to the moment of interest must also be taken into account in order to relate motor unit activity to actual force production. It seems fair to say that the dynamic characteristics of moving muscles are not well understood at present. Much needs to be learned before we can go beyond simple qualitative assertions about the relation of motor unit numbers, identities, and firing rates to muscle force outputs.

Recruitment Some 50 years ago, Denny-Brown (1929) demonstrated in decerebrate cats that motor units in the slow, red soleus muscle tended to be recruited more readily by stretch and crossed-extension reflexes than the units in the faster, paler synergistic gastrocnemius. He formulated this result in terms of a hierarchy of functional thresholds, such that

... units of lowest threshold grade are present in the red slow extensors. . . . The units of higher threshold grades, according to their grade, require more subsidiary excitation before responding to proprioceptive excitation by discharge. These units are arranged evenly through the different heads of the compound extensors so that the units of highest threshold are confined almost exclusively to the pale muscles.[*]

This grading of functional threshold was viewed as due to a corresponding scaling of the quantitative organization of central excitatory and inhibitory influences, which clearly implies that the ordering of threshold grades is a stable property, correlated with muscle unit characteristics. These implications have been amply confirmed in a great deal of subsequent work.

Investigations of motor unit recruitment patterns require some means of labelling different units so that they can be compared. The first identifying parameter used was simply the amplitude of the electrical signal from muscle unit or motor axon. Early EMG studies in human subjects revealed that, for a given action, recruitment patterns are relatively stereotyped (Denny-Brown and Pennybacker, 1938; Seyffarth, 1941; Denny-Brown, 1949), and that the muscle units of lowest functional threshold (i.e., those first activated) in voluntary contractions tend to have smaller spike signals than higher threshold units (e.g., Smith, 1934; Denny-Brown and Pennybacker, 1938; see also Norris and Gasteiger, 1955; Tanji and Kato 1973b; Goldberg and Derfler, 1977). This is true also in reflex activation of animal muscle (Olson et al., 1968). The amplitude and shape of the EMG signal produced by an individual muscle unit depends on a complex interplay of technical factors (e.g., electrode configuration, placement) together with factors intrinsic to the muscle unit itself (e.g., innervation ratio, spatial density of unit fibers, average fiber diameter). It seems difficult to draw a general conclusion as to which of these is most important and it may thus be unwise to conclude that, because units with low threshold usually have small EMG spikes, they must therefore have small innervation ratios.

Early studies of motoneuron recruitment patterns in experimental animals showed that the amplitude of motor axon spikes in nerve filament recordings are generally smaller for low threshold motoneurons than for cells of higher threshold (Granit et al., 1956). Henneman and coworkers (1965a, b; Somjen et al., 1965), in an influential series of papers, showed that the order of functional motoneuron thresholds in a variety of reflex responses was closely correlated with the relative amplitude of the extracellular axon spike, and that this ordering was essentially invariant with input source. They inferred, as did Granit et al. (1956), that the size of the

---

[*]Denny-Brown, 1929, p. 295.

axon spike reflects axon diameter and conduction velocity (confirmed in recent work by Clamann and Henneman, 1976) and, further, that axon spike amplitude also indicates relative motoneuron size. Electrophysiological evidence is generally consistent with the latter notion (Eccles et al., 1958; Kuno, 1959; Burke, 1967) but direct anatomical and physiological measurements in the same motoneurons indicate that the correlation between axon and cell sizes is not very precise (Barrett and Crill, 1974). Henneman and colleagues (1965a) proposed that the gradation of functional thresholds in a motor unit population is related quite strictly to a corresponding grading of anatomical cell size, and this hypothesis has come to be known as the "size principle." Later studies from the same laboratory (Clamann et al., 1974) have re-enforced the view that alpha motoneurons in a given pool are ordered in functional threshold into an invariant hierarchy, such that information about the number of motoneurons active at any moment exactly specifies their individual identities (a "law of combination"; Henneman et al., 1974). This conceptual model has great intuitive appeal but it would require that all of the factors that influence functional threshold be graded or scaled equally in each motoneuron in the motor pool, a point not consistent with other evidence (see below).

The ordering of motor unit recruitment has been examined systematically in a number of studies in animals and in man. Many of the results from human subjects are consistent with the idea of relative invariance of recruitment order (and hence, of functional threshold grading) in a variety of muscles and in contractions of different speeds (e.g., Denny-Brown and Pennybacker, 1938; Seyffarth, 1941; Milner-Brown et al., 1973b; Freund et al., 1975; Yemm, 1977; Monster and Chan, 1977; Desmedt and Godaux, 1977a, b; Goldberg and Derfler, 1977). Departures from a rigidly fixed recruitment (threshold) hierarchy in these studies are usually found only among motor units with similar functional thresholds (Tanji and Kato, 1973b; see also Henneman et al., 1965a, 1974).

Recent studies in human subjects have attempted to label active units in terms of relative axonal conduction velocity (Freund et al., 1975; Borg et al., 1978) or the mechanical characteristics of muscle unit "twitch" responses educed by spike-triggered averaging (Milner-Brown et al., 1973a, b; Desmedt and Godaux, 1977b; Monster and Chan, 1977; Goldberg and Derfler, 1977; Yemm, 1977). Figure 4–13 shows an example (Freund et al., 1975) in which the voluntary force needed for unit recruitment (*ordinate*, a measure of functional threshold grade) is clearly related to the relative conduction velocity of the unit motor axon (*abscissa*, scaled such that larger values represent slower conduction velocities), although there is significant scatter about the central trend, consistent with some degree of variability in the

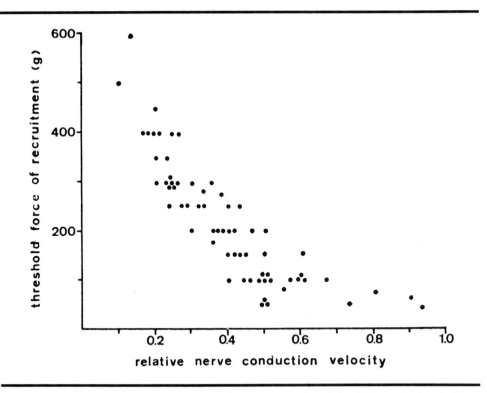

Figure 4–13 Graph showing the relation between the threshold force at which motor units were recruited to steady firing in voluntary contractions *(ordinate)* and the relative conduction velocities of the axons of those units *(abscissa).* The conduction velocity scale is inversely related to actual conduction velocity, such that slower axons tend to have higher abscissa values. Data from 65 different motor units in the human first dorsal interosseous muscle. (From Freund et al., 1975.)

relation of conduction velocity to functional threshold. As noted above, Borg and coworkers (1978) have also found that the low threshold motor units in the human short toe extensor tend to have more slowly conducting axons than the higher threshold units.

An example of the correlation between voluntary recruitment threshold and muscle unit properties is shown in Figure 4–14 (Milner-Brown et al., 1973*b*) in the human first dorsal interosseous. These authors found a very clear relation between the total force output needed for stable unit recruitment ("threshold force"; *abscissae*) and the measured "twitch" force for that unit (*left graph*). There was a less marked trend suggesting that lower threshold units have slower contraction times as well (*right graph*). Qualitatively similar results have been obtained in human masseter (Goldberg and Derfler, 1977;

173

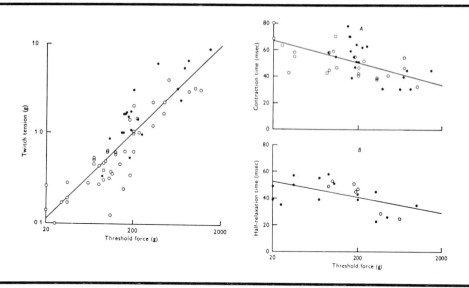

Figure 4–14 Characteristics of the mechanical "twitch" responses of individual muscle units in the human first dorsal interosseous muscle, determined by spike-triggered averaging of muscle force output. The left-hand graph shows the monotonic relation between the voluntary threshold force at which a given unit is recruited and the "twitch" force generated by that unit. The relation is linear when plotted on double logarithmic axes. The graphs on the right show that the recruitment threshold is inversely related (albeit weakly) to the contraction time (A, ordinate) and half-relaxation time (B) of the unit "twitch" responses. Low threshold motor units thus tend to be smaller and slower in twitch responses than higher threshold units. (From Milner-Brown et al., 1973 a.)

Yemm, 1977) and extensor digitorum communis muscles (Monster and Chan, 1977).

Stephens and Usherwood (1977) have recently reexamined recruitment patterns in the first dorsal interosseous, using methods similar to those of Milner-Brown et al. (1973a, b). Their results were basically the same but they added observations on unit fatigue resistance, showing that the lowest threshold units tended to be resistant to fatigue as well as slowly contracting. In contrast, motor units recruited at output forces greater than 25 per cent of maximum voluntary force tended to exhibit large "twitch" forces, fast contraction times, and little resistance to fatigue. Between these extremes were units with moderate force, fast contraction, and relatively high fatigue resistance. If, for convenience, these results are expressed in the motor unit terminology applicable to cat muscle, the recruitment sequence begins with a group of units analogous to type S units, progresses to include type FR, and ends with units analogous to type

FF, which are active only at relatively high force output levels.

This recruitment sequence makes intuitive sense (see, e.g., Henneman and Olson, 1965; Burke and Edgerton, 1975), and it is consistent with observations of Warmolts and Engel (1972) on the contrasting recruitment thresholds and firing patterns for muscle units in regions of human quadriceps, with a predominance of fibers with either high (type 2) or low (type 1) staining for myofibrillar ATPase. The S-FR-FF sequence also fits very well with the ordering of the strength of synaptic input from group Ia (primary) muscle spindle afferents (Burke et al., 1973b, 1976b; see also Fig. 4–8). The relative strength of group Ia input is closely related to the responsiveness of fast and slow twitch motor units in cat MG during stretch reflexes in decerebrate preparations (Burke, 1968). Direct measurements of force output from the MG in intact, freely moving cats show that quiet standing requires only about 5 per cent of the MG maximum force capacity (<500 grams on average), which can be produced by the subpopulation of type S units in this muscle acting alone (Walmsley et al., 1978). Walking and running movements demand up to 20 to 25 per cent of maximum MG force capacity. This magnitude of force can be attributed to the combined action of type S and FR motor units — i.e., the fatigue-resistant units that produce small to moderate forces and which make up about 50 per cent of the medial gastrocnemius pool (see Fig. 4–8). Gallop and vertical jumps, which are actions emitted only in short bursts, require forces between 25 and 100 per cent of maximum MG force capacity (up to 9 kg in jumping), and must involve recruitment of most or all of the MG unit pool, including the type FF units (Walmsley et al., 1978).

While the available evidence is consistent with the notion that the grading of functional thresholds in motoneuron pools is more or less fixed under most circumstances, there is some question as to the precision and rigidity of threshold gradation. Lloyd and McIntyre (1955) showed that the relative excitability of individual motoneurons responding in homonymous and heteronymous monosynaptic reflexes can be quite different. Rall and Hunt (1956) then demonstrated that the probability of reflex firing of a given motoneuron can vary over a sizable range in a manner independent of fluctuations in overall output of the motor pool to which it belongs. Rudomin and Madrid (1972) later showed that the magnitude of such independent fluctuations in motoneuron excitability is, at least in part, due to variations in presynaptic inhibition, which is in turn modulated by sensory input and dependent upon experimental conditions. It is thus not surprising to find some degree of variability in threshold grading, even when conditions appear to be constant

175

and the same input systems can be assumed to activate the motor unit pool (e.g., Wyman et al., 1974).

There is some debate in the literature about the mechanisms that control motoneuron recruitment, so it seems useful to present a brief review of the factors that control the hierarchy of functional thresholds in motor unit populations. Table 4–4 gives a somewhat abridged listing of the major factors involved, which devolve into two basic areas: (1) properties intrinsic to the motoneuron membrane (e.g., true voltage threshold, passive membrane electrical properties); and (2) factors that affect the efficacy of synaptic transmission (measured as synaptic potential amplitude or charge injection to the spike-generating region of the motoneuron). Those factors in the second group all represent an interplay between the characteristics of synaptic terminals and those of the postsynaptic motoneurons. In view of the frequent use of the term "size principle" to describe the hierarchy of functional thresholds (a concept quite distinct from that of the true voltage threshold of the motoneuron), it is important to note that motoneuron size, measured as total membrane area, is relevant only as a determinant of synaptic density. The control of functional threshold clearly involves properties of synaptic elements as well as of motoneurons, so that the hierarchy is not something irrevocably "built into" motoneurons themselves. Rather, it is an emergent property of the interaction

Table 4–4   The Main Factors that Control Motoneuron Response to Synaptic Input

---

Synaptic Potential Amplitude, which depends upon:

---

1. Synaptic density, which depends upon:
   a. The number of synaptic terminals from each functional input system.
   b. The total cell membrane area.
2. The average conductance per terminal, which depends upon:
   a. The average amount of transmitter liberated per terminal.
   b. The average sensitivity of the synaptic receptors.
   c. The driving potential for the synaptic process.
3. Electrotonic attenuation of synaptic potentials, which depends upon:
   a. The spatial distribution of active synaptic terminals.
   b. The geometry of the motoneuron dendritic trees.
   c. The specific membrane resistivity and capacitance.
   d. The electrical resistivity of motoneuron cytoplasm.

Intrinsic Motoneuron Membrane Properties, including:

---

1. The absolute threshold voltage for spike generation.
2. The absolute true resting membrane potential.
3. Nonlinear membrane responses to changes in transmembrane voltage (e.g., anomalous rectification).
4. Membrane responses related to refractoriness (e.g., spike afterhyperpolarization, accommodation, etc.).

The Relative Efficacy, or Synaptic Strength, of all the Input Systems Active at the Moment of Interest

---

between presynaptic and postsynaptic elements. More detailed discussion of this viewpoint and the evidence underlying it is available elsewhere (Burke, 1973; Zucker, 1973; Burke and Rudomin, 1977; Traub, 1977).

When motoneurons in a particular pool respond to a given synaptic input, the observed gradient in functional thresholds is equivalent to a measure of the strength, or efficacy, of that input system. This is in turn dependent upon the quantitative organization of that input system (Table 4–4), and thus one may expect to find some variation in threshold gradients when the pool is activated by different input systems that may not have exactly matching organizations. This sort of variability has been observed by Kernell and Sjöholm (1975) in studies of recruitment of cat lumbrical motor units by afferent versus cortical stimulation. This system has the advantage that the units are few in number and can be identified as individuals with great assurance. A fundamentally similar state-dependent variability of recruitment patterns has been described by Grimby and Hannerz (1970, 1976) in human subjects.

Dislocations in the recruitment process have been sought in human motor pools by comparing output patterns during slow tracking versus rapid tracking movements (Büdingen and Freund, 1976) or ballistic contractions (i.e., moving as fast as possible; Desmedt and Godaux, 1977a, b), and these studies have shown no significant differences between the two processes. Grimby and Hannerz (1977), however, have described a small population (less than 10 per cent of the sample) of motor units in the short toe extensor of normal subjects which are functionally high threshold during ramp contractions and tend to fire only in relatively rapid bursts, but which also tend to be readily activated, and may even act exclusively, in some rapid alternating or ballistic contractions. The existence of a degree of type grouping in this muscle in otherwise normal subjects seems to make it particularly suitable for EMG studies of high threshold muscle units.

Another point of some contention is whether or not human subjects can voluntarily produce isolated activity in individual motor units irrespective of their functional threshold under other conditions. Early experiments of this kind (Harrison and Mortensen, 1962; Basmajian, 1963; Wagman et al., 1965) suggested that up to four to five different motor units can be activated independently under voluntary control. Kato and Tanji (1972) later showed that voluntary isolation was indeed quite easy, but only when the units involved had relatively similar force output thresholds (less than 20 per cent of maximum). Units with higher force thresholds could not be activated in isolation under any conditions.

177

More recent work has tended to find less and less ability to produce voluntarily isolated activity of motor units with even modest differences in functional threshold (Henneman et al., 1975; Thomas et al., 1978). Some of the differences between experimental results probably depend upon technical factors, particularly the difficulty of assured identification of individual units in EMG records, and perhaps partly to the fact that muscle units in some multifunctional muscles may be recordable on a single electrode and yet have disparate functional actions, making voluntary isolation possible but distorting the interpretation of the results (Thomas et al., 1978; cf. Wagman et al., 1965). Person (1974) has shown that there is greater variability in recruitment and derecruitment patterns among units in the human rectus femoris when movements are unconstrained in contrast to much more stereotypy in movements that are themselves rigidly stereotyped (see also Denny-Brown, 1949).

Such interpretive problems are not apparent, however, in a recent study by Stephens and coworkers (1978). They have demonstrated that the recruitment sequence of pairs of motor units in the human first dorsal interosseous muscle can be altered rather markedly during continuous stimulation of the skin of the index finger. During such stimulation, the initially higher threshold unit can be made to fire alone under voluntary control and the force thresholds for motor unit recruitment for the pair are reversed from the usual order.

It is possible to summarize the results of studies of recruitment patterns and threshold gradation, as well as to reconcile some of the apparently discordant observations, by assuming that the critical factor controlling threshold gradients is the quantitative distribution of synaptic inputs to the target set of motoneurons (Table 4–4). There is evidence from animal studies that, of the factors outlined in Table 4–4, the major source of variation between motoneurons is in synaptic organization and not in intrinsic motoneuron characteristics (Burke, 1973; Burke and Rudomin, 1977). In particular, as discussed above, motoneuron cell size does not appear to be a critical factor in determining threshold gradations. Thus, in the diagram in Figure 4–15, the four motoneurons (*circles*) are indicated as equal diameter circles but the arrows denoting synaptic projections vary in width to suggest corresponding variations in efficacy, or input strength. If all of the synaptic systems projecting to a motor unit population, both excitatory (E) and inhibitory (I), were scaled exactly in parallel (*stippled arrows,* representing different input systems with the same scaling), then the ordering of resultant functional thresholds would be the same irrespective of input source. Increasing synaptic drive through any E system would produce a recruitment sequence such as the one shown in the upper set of spike sequences, and reduction of E, or

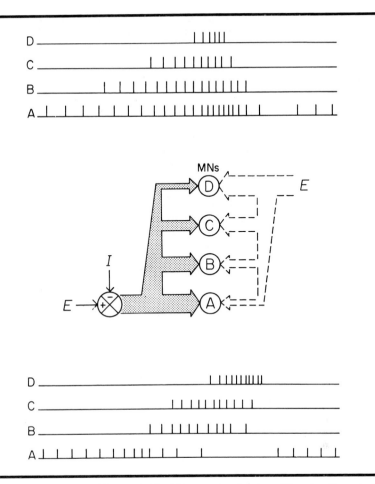

Figure 4–15 Diagram showing two different patterns for the organization of synaptic input to four symbolic motoneurons (MNs, *A* through *D*). The strength, or efficacy, of input in each neuron is indicated by the width of the input arrows. One pattern includes both excitatory (E) and inhibitory (I) input systems, and is organized so that the synaptic effect is scaled $A > B > C > D$. Varying input drive with this pattern of efficacy should produce recruitment patterns similar to those shown in the upper set of spike sequences. The addition of excitation with a reversed pattern of distribution *(dashed arrows)* can produce other patterns of recruitment, as in the lower set of spike sequences. Such unusual patterns have been observed experimentally and there is evidence that the "reversed" pattern of input distribution actually exists, at least in the cat spinal cord. (From Kanda et al., 1977.)

increase in I, would produce derecruitment in a reverse pattern (see Henneman et al., 1965b, 1974). The weight of the available evidence suggests that such parallel scaling is probably characteristic of many synaptic systems. The existence of some statistical uncertainty in individual threshold levels (e.g., Rall and Hunt, 1955; Wyman et al.,

1974), which can be visualized on the diagram as fluctuations in the width of the arrows projecting to individual motoneurons (e.g., Rudomin and Madrid, 1972), does not negate the validity of this general pattern, with its obvious functional advantages.

A complete picture of motor unit recruitments must, however, also account for what appear to be major departures from the "size principle" expectation, even though such departures may require special conditions for their demonstration. Firing patterns such as those shown in the lower set of spike sequences have been observed in cat MG motor units (Kanda et al., 1977) and cannot be accounted for by parallel input scaling. An excitatory synaptic system is present in the cat spinal cord with the distribution pattern equivalent to that indicated by the dashed arrows — i.e., in a pattern roughly reversed from that for muscle spindle input (Burke et al., 1970, 1973b). Such an organization can account for the lower spike sequences (Kanda et al., 1977), but whether a similar synaptic pattern exists in the human cord to account for the occasional occurrence of preferential activation of high threshold motor units (e.g., Grimby and Hannerz, 1977), or recruitment reversals (Stephens et al., 1978), remains to be determined. The functional utility of alternative patterns of synaptic organization is unclear but the evidence for the existence of such patterns seems obvious. Note that, by activating excitatory input systems with both the usual and the "reversed" patterns (Fig. 4–15), synchronous and powerful activation of the entire motor unit pool can be accomplished efficiently. The patterns of motor unit firing in ballistic movements in human subjects are quite compatible with this sort of dual mode activation (Desmedt and Godaux, 1977a; Grimby and Hannerz, 1977).

SUMMARY A motor unit consists of an alpha (or beta) motoneuron together with the set of muscle fibers (muscle unit) innervated by it. The motoneurons that innervate muscle units in a particular anatomical muscle (i.e., a motor unit population) are predictable in number, and are grouped together in longitudinally oriented cell columns located in predictable regions of the spinal gray matter. In normal adult animals there is no significant polyneuronal innervation of muscle fibers. Muscle unit fibers are normally scattered more or less randomly throughout an extensive territorial volume, without local subgroups. The average density of muscle unit fibers in the territory is such that any region of a muscle contains muscle fibers belonging to 20 to 50 different motor units. The anatomy of muscle units changes markedly after reinnervation, apparently due to local axonal sprouting during the reinnervation process.

A few muscles contain relatively homogeneous populations of motor units, but most limb and trunk muscles of mammals are composed of very heterogeneous mixtures of units in which at least three basic types can be recognized. These are: (1) slowly contracting, small force, very fatigue-resistant units, called "type S" in the cat; (2) moderate force, fast contracting, fatigue-resistant units, called "type FR" in the cat; and (3) large force, fast contracting, fatigue-sensitive units, called "type FF" in the cat. There is considerable indirect, and some direct, evidence that human motor units may be organized in a generally similar pattern.

Certain properties intrinsic to motoneurons are matched to the characteristics of the muscle units innervated. Motoneurons of type S units tend to be smaller than the cells of either FR or FF units. The type S units have longer duration afterhyperpolarizations than FR or FF units, and correspondingly lower maximum firing rates under synaptic drive.

Total muscle force output in any motor act is controlled by a number of factors, including the numbers and individual mechanical properties of units active (both included under the rubric of "recruitment"), and by the time history of individual unit firings, of which firing frequency is only one component. The overall weight of available evidence indicates that both recruitment and firing frequency modulations are important over the full range of total force output control in both slow tracking and ballistic movements. The process of recruitment occurs under most conditions according to a more or less fixed sequence of functional thresholds, beginning with units equivalent to type S, progressing to include units equivalent to type FR and ending, at relatively high levels of force output, with units equivalent to type FF. The recruitment sequence is controlled mainly by the efficacy of the relevant synaptic input systems in motor pool elements, which is in turn controlled by a complex interplay of multiple factors. The scaling of synaptic efficacy is apparently similar for many synaptic input systems, accounting for the relative invariance of recruitment ordering. However, large departures from the expected sequence do occur under some conditions, and these can be explained by the existence of alternative patterns of input distribution for a few input systems.

References

Adrian, E. D., and Bronk, D. W.: The discharge of impulses in motor nerve fibres, Part II. The frequency of discharge in reflex and voluntary contractions. J. Physiol. (Lond.), 67:119–151, 1929.

Aitken, J. T., and Bridger, J. E.: Neuron size and neuron population density in the lumbosacral region of the cat's spinal cord. J. Anat., 95:38–53, 1962.

181

Appelberg, B., and Emonet-Dénand, F.: Motor units of the first superficial lumbrical muscle of the cat. J. Neurophysiol., 30:154–160, 1967.

Ariano, M. A., Armstrong, R. B., and Edgerton, V. R.: Hindlimb muscle fiber populations of five mammals. J. Histochem. Cytochem., 21:51–55, 1973.

Bach-y-Rita, P., and Ito, F.: In vivo studies of fast and slow muscle fibers in cat extraocular muscles. J. Gen. Physiol., 49:1177–1198, 1966.

Bagust, J., Knott, S., Lewis, D. M., Luck, J. C., and Westerman, R. A.: Isometric contractions of motor units in a fast twitch muscle of the cat. J. Physiol (Lond.), 231:87–104, 1973.

Bagust, J., and Lewis, D. M.: Isometric contractions of motor units in self-reinnervated fast and slow twitch muscles of the cat. J. Physiol. (Lond.), 237:91–102, 1974.

Bagust, J., Lewis, D. M., and Westerman, R. A.: Polyneuronal innervation of kitten skeletal muscle. J. Physiol. (Lond.), 229:241–255, 1973.

Barany, M.: ATPase activity of myosin correlated with speed of muscle shortening. J. Gen. Physiol., 50:197–216, 1967.

Barker, D., Emonet-Dénand, F., Harker, D. W., Jami, L., and Laporte, Y.: Types of intra- and extrafusal muscle fibre innervated by dynamic skeletofusimotor axons in cat peroneus brevis and tenuissimus muscles as determined by the glycogen depletion method. J. Physiol. (Lond.), 266:713–726, 1977.

Barmack, N. H.: Recruitment and suprathreshold frequency modulation of single extraocular muscle fibers in the rabbit. J. Neurophysiol., 40:779–790, 1977.

Barnard, R. J., Edgerton, V. R., and Peter, J. B.: Effect of exercise on skeletal muscle. I. Biochemical and histochemical properties. J. Appl. Physiol., 28:762–766, 1970a.

Barnard, R. J., Edgerton, V. R., and Peter, J. B.: Effect of exercise on skeletal muscle. II. Contractile properties. J. Appl. Physiol., 28:767–770, 1970b.

Barrett, J. N., and Crill, W. E.: Specific membrane properties of cat motoneurones. J. Physiol., 239:301–324, 1974.

Basmajian, J. V.: Control and training of individual motor units. Science, 141:440–441, 1963.

Bessou, P, Emonet-Dénand, F., and Laporte, Y.: Relation entre la vitesse de conduction des fibres nerveuses motrices et le tempe de contraction de leurs unites motrices. C. R. Acad. Sci.[D] (Paris), 256:5625–5627, 1963.

Bessou, P., Emonet-Dénand, F., and Laporte, Y.: Motor fibres innervating extrafusal and intrafusal muscle fibres in the cat. J. Physiol. (Lond.), 180:649–672, 1965.

Bigland, B., and Lippold, O.: Motor unit activity in the voluntary contraction of human muscle. J. Physiol. (Lond.), 125:322–335, 1954.

Borg, J., Grimby, L., and Hannerz, J.: Axonal conduction velocity and voluntary discharge properties of individual short toe extensor motor units in man. J. Physiol. (Lond.), 277:143–152, 1978.

Boyd, I. A., and Davey, M. R.: Composition of Peripheral Nerves. Livingstone, Edinburgh, 1968.

Brandstater, M. E., and Lambert, E. H.: Motor unit anatomy: Type and spatial arrangement of muscle fibers. *In* Desmedt, J. E. (ed.): New Developments in Electromyography and Clinical Neurophysiology, Vol. 1. Basel, Karger, 1973, pp. 14–22.

Brodal, A.: Neurological Anatomy in Relation to Clinical Medicine. New York, Oxford University Press, 1969.

Brown, M. C., Jansen, J. K. S., and Van Essen, D.: Polyneuronal innervation of skeletal muscle in new-born rats and its elimination during maturation. J. Physiol. (Lond.), *261*:387–422, 1976.

Brown, M. C., and Matthews, P. B. C.: An investigation into the possible existence of polyneuronal innervation of individual skeletal muscle fibres in certain hind-limb muscles of the cat. J. Physiol. (Lond.), *151*:436–457, 1960.

Brown, W. F., and Milner-Brown, H. S.: Some electrical properties of motor units and their effects on the methods of estimating motor unit numbers. J. Neurol. Neurosurg. Psychiatry, *39*:249–257, 1976.

Buchthal, F.: The general concept of the motor unit. Neuromusc. Disord. (*In* Res. Publ. Assoc. Res. Nerv. Ment. Dis.), *38*:3–30, 1961.

Buchthal, F., Erminio, F., and Rosenfalck, P.: Motor unit territory in different human muscles. Acta Physiol. Scand., *45*:72–87, 1959.

Buchthal, F., and Rosenfalck, P.: On the structure of motor units. *In* Desmedt, J. E. (ed.): New Developments in Electromyography and Clinical Neurophysiology, Vol. 1. Basel, Karger, 1973, pp. 71–85.

Buchthal, F., and Schmalbruch, H.: Contraction times and fibre types in intact human muscle. Acta Physiol. Scand., *79*:435–452, 1970.

Büdingen, H. J., and Freund, H. J.: The relationship between the rate of rise of isometric tension and motor unit recruitment in a human forearm muscle. Pfluegers Arch., *362*:61–67, 1976.

Buller, A. J., Eccles, J. C., and Eccles, R. M.: Interactions between motoneurons and muscles in respect of the characteristic speeds of their responses. J. Physiol. (Lond.), *150*:417–439, 1960.

Burke, R. E.: Motor unit types of cat triceps surae muscle. J. Physiol. (Lond.), *193*:141–160, 1967.

Burke, R. E.: Firing patterns of gastrocnemius motor units in the decerebrate cat. J. Physiol. (Lond.), *196*:631–654, 1968.

Burke, R. E.: On the central nervous system control of fast and slow twitch motor units. *In* Desmedt, J. E. (ed.): New Developments in Electromyography and Clinical Neurophysiology, Vol. 1. Basel, Karger, 1973, pp. 69–94.

Burke, R. E., and Edgerton, V. R.: Motor unit properties and selective involvement in movement. *In* Wilmore, J. H., and Klogh, J. F. (eds.): Exercise and Sport Sciences Reviews, Vol. 3. New York, Academic Press, 1975, pp. 31–81.

Burke, R. E., Levine, D. N., Salcman, M., and Tsairis, P.: Motor units in cat soleus muscle: Physiological, histochemical and morphological characteristics. J. Physiol. (Lond.), *238*:503–514, 1974.

Burke, R. E., Levine, D. N., Tsairis, P., and Zajac, F. E.: Physiological types and histochemical profiles in motor units of the cat gastrocnemius. J. Physiol. (Lond.), *234*:723–748, 1973*a*.

Burke, R. E., Levine, D. N., Zajac, F. E., Tsairis, P., and Engel, W. K.: Mammalian motor units: Physiological-histochemical correlation in three types in cat gastrocnemius. Science, *174*:709–712, 1971.

Burke, R. E., and Nelson, P. G.: Accommodation to current ramps in motoneurons of fast and slow twitch motor units. Int. J. Neurosci., *1*:347–356, 1971.

Burke, R. E., and Rudomin, P.: Spinal neurons and synapses. *In* Kandel, E. R. (ed.): Handbook of Physiology, Sect. 1. Vol. I. The Nervous System: The Cellular Biology of Neurons. Washington, D. C., American Physiological Society, 1977, pp. 877–944.

Burke, R. E., Rudomin, P., and Zajac, F. E.: Catch property in single mammalian motor units. Science, *168*:122–124, 1970.

Burke, R. E., Rudomin, P., and Zajac, F. E.: The effect of activation history on tension production by individual muscle units. Brain Res., *109*:515–529, 1976*a*.

Burke, R. E., Rymer, W. Z., and Walsh, J. V., Jr.: Functional specialization in the motor unit population of cat medial gastrocnemius muscle. *In* Control of Posture and Locomotion. Stein, R. B., Pearson, K. B., Smith, R. S., and Redford, J. B. (eds.): New York, Plenum Press, 1973*b*, pp. 29–44.

Burke, R. E., Rymer, W. Z., and Walsh, J. V., Jr.: Relative strength of synaptic input from short-latency pathways to motor units of defined type in cat medial gastrocnemius. J. Neurophysiol., *39*:447–458, 1976*b*.

Burke, R. E., Strick, P. L., Kanda, K., Kim, C. C., and Walmsley, B.: Anatomy of medial gastrocnemius and soleus motor nuclei in cat spinal cord. J. Neurophysiol., *40*:667–680, 1977.

Burke, R. E., and Tsairis, P.: Anatomy and innervation ratios in motor units of cat gastrocnemius. J. Physiol. (Lond.), *234*:749–765, 1973.

Burke, R. E., and Tsairis, P.: The correlation of physiological properties with histochemical characteristics in single muscle units. Ann. N. Y. Acad. Sci., *228*:145–159, 1974.

Burke, R. E., and Tsairis, P.: Histochemical and physiological profile of a skeletofusimotor (β) unit in cat soleus muscle. Brain Res., *129*:341–345, 1977.

Campa, J. F., and Engel, W. K.: Histochemical and functional correlations in anterior horn neurons of the cat spinal cord. Science, *171*:198–199, 1971.

Carlson, F. D., and Wilkie, D. R.: Muscle Physiology. Englewood Cliffs, N. J., Prentice-Hall, 1974.

Cavagna, G. A., and Citterio, G.: Effect of stretching on the elastic characteristics and the contractile component of frog striated muscle. J. Physiol. (Lond.), *239*:1–14, 1974.

Cavagna, G. A., Komarek, L., Citterio, G., and Margaria, R.: Power output of the previously stretched muscle. Med Sport, *6*:159–167, 1971.

Christensen, E.: Topography of terminal motor innervation in striated muscles from stillborn infants. Am. J. Phys. Med. *38*:65–78, 1959.

Clamann, H. P.: Activity of single motor units during isometric tension. Neurology, 20:256–260, 1970.

Clamann, H. P., Gillies, J. D., and Henneman, E.: Effects of inhibitory inputs on critical firing level and rank order of motoneurons. J. Neurophysiol., 34:1350–1360, 1974.

Clamann, H. P., and Henneman, E.: Electrical measurement of axon diameter and its use in relating motoneuron size to critical firing level. J. Neurophysiol., 39:844–851, 1976.

Clark, D. A.: Muscle counts of motor units: A study in innervation ratios. Am. J. Physiol., 96:296–304, 1931.

Close, R.: Properties of motor units in fast and slow skeletal muscles of the rat. J. Physiol. (Lond.), 193:45–55, 1967.

Close, R.: Dynamic properties of fast and slow skeletal muscles of the rat after nerve cross-union. J. Physiol. (Lond.), 204:331–346, 1969.

Collatos, T. C., Edgerton, V. R., Smith, J. L., and Botterman, B. R.: Contractile properties and fiber type compositions of flexors and extensors of elbow joint in cat: Implications for motor control. J. Neurophysiol., 40:1292–1300, 1977.

Conradi, S.: On motoneuron synaptology in adult cats. Acta Physiol. Scand. [Suppl.], 332:1–115, 1969.

Cooper, S., and Eccles, J. C.: The isometric responses of mammalian muscles. J. Physiol. (Lond.), 69:377–385, 1930.

Cullheim, S., Kellerth, J., and Conradi, S.: Evidence for direct synaptic interconnections between cat spinal α-motoneurons via the recurrent axon collaterals: A morphological study using intracellular injection of horseradish peroxidase. Brain Res., 132:1–10, 1977.

Denny-Brown, D.: On the nature of postural reflexes. Proc. R. Soc. Lond. [Biol.], 104:252–301, 1929.

Denny-Brown, D.: Interpretation of the electromyogram. Arch. Neurol. Psychiatry, 61:99–128, 1949.

Denny-Brown, D., and Pennybacker, J. B.: Fibrillation and fasciculation in voluntary muscle. Brain, 61:311–344, 1938.

Denslow, J. S.: Double discharges in human motor units. J. Neurophysiol., 11:209–215, 1948.

Desmedt, J. E., and Godaux, E.: Fast motor units are not preferentially activated in rapid voluntary contractions in man. Nature, 267:717–719, 1977a.

Desmedt, J. E., and Godaux, E.: Ballistic contractions in man: Characteristic recruitment pattern of single motor units of the tibialis anterior muscle. J. Physiol. (Lond.), 264:673–694, 1977b.

Doyle, A. M., and Mayer, R. F.: Studies of the motor unit in the cat. Bull. Sch. Med. Maryland, 54:11–17, 1969.

Dubowitz, V., and Brooke, M. H.: Muscle Biopsy—A Modern Approach. London, W. B. Saunders, 1973.

Eberstein, A., and Goodgold, J.: Slow and fast twitch fibers in human skeletal muscle. Am. J. Physiol., 215:535–541, 1968.

Eccles, J. C., Eccles, R. M., Iggo, A., and Lundberg, A.: Electrophysiological studies on gamma motoneurons. Acta Physiol. Scand., 50:32–40, 1960.

Eccles, J. C., Eccles, R. M., and Lundberg, A.: The action potentials of the alpha motoneurones supplying fast and slow muscles. J. Physiol. (Lond.), *142*:275–291, 1958.

Eccles, J. C., Fatt, P., and Koketsu, K.: Cholinergic and inhibitory synapses in a pathway from motor-axon collaterals to motoneurones. J. Physiol., *126*:524–562, 1954.

Eccles, J. C., and Sherrington, C. S.: Numbers and contraction values of individual motor units examined in some muscles of the limb. Proc. R. Soc. Lond. [Biol.], *106*:326–357, 1930.

Eccles, R. M., Phillips, C. G., and Wu, C. P.: Motor innervation, motor unit organization and afferent innervation of m. extensor digitorum communis of the baboon's forearm. J. Physiol. (Lond.), *198*:179–192, 1968.

Edds, M. V.: Collateral regeneration of residual motor axons in partially denervated muscles. J. Exp. Zool., *113*:507–552, 1950.

Edgerton, V. R., Barnard, R. J., Peter, J. B., Gillespie, C. A., and Simpson, D. R.: Overloaded skeletal muscles of a nonhuman primate (*Galago senegalensis*). Exp. Neurol., *37*:322–339, 1972.

Edgerton, V. R., Smith, J. L., and Simpson, D. R.: Muscle fiber type populations in human leg muscles. Histochem. J., *7*:259–266, 1975.

Edström, L., and Kugelberg, E.: Histochemical composition, distribution of fibres and fatiguability of single motor units. Anterior tibial muscle of the rat. J. Neurol. Neurosurg. Psychiatry, *31*:424–433, 1968.

Edström, L. and Nyström, B. Histochemical types and sizes of fibres in normal human muscles. A biopsy study. Acta Neurol. Scand., *45*:257–269, 1969.

Eisenberg, B. R., and Kuda, A. M.: Retrieval of cryostat sections for comparison of histochemistry and quantitative electron microscopy in a muscle fiber. J. Histochem. Cytochem., *25*:1169–1177, 1977.

Edkstedt, J.: Human single muscle fiber action potentials. Acta Physiol. Scand., *61*(Suppl. 226):1–96, 1964.

Elliott, H. C.: Studies on the motor cells of the spinal cord. I. Distribution in the normal human cord. Am. J. Anat., *70*:95–117, 1942.

Elliott, H. C.: Studies on the motor cells of the spinal cord. II. Distribution in the normal human foetal cord. Am. J. Anat., *72*:29–38, 1943.

Emonet-Dénand, F., Jami, L., and Laporte, Y.: Skeletosfusimotor axons in hind-limb muscles of the cat. J. Physiol. (Lond.), *249*:153–166, 1975.

Emonet-Dénand, F., Jankowska, E., and Laporte Y.: Skeletofusimotor fibres in the rabbit. J. Physiol. (Lond.), *210*:669–680, 1970.

Emonet-Dénand, F., and Laporte, Y.: Proportion of muscle spindles supplies by skeletofusimotor axons (β-axons) in peroneus brevis muscle of the cat. J. Neurophysiol., *38*:1390–1394, 1975.

Emonet-Dénand, F., Laporte, Y., and Proske, U.: Contraction of muscle fibers in two adjacent muscles innervated by branches of the same motor axon. J. Neurophysiol., *34*:132–138, 1971.

Faulkner, J. A., Maxwell, L. C., and Lieberman, D. A.: Histo-chemical characteristics of muscle fibers from trained and de-trained guinea pigs. Am. J. Physiol., 222:836–840, 1972.

Feindel, W., Hinshaw, J. R., and Wendell, G.: The pattern of motor innervation in mammalian striated muscle. J. Anat., 86:35–48, 1952.

Feinstein, B., Lindegard, B., Nyman, E., and Wohlfart, G.: Mor-phological studies of motor units in normal human muscles. Acta Anat. (Basel), 23:127–142, 1955.

Freund, H.-J., Büdingen, H.-J., and Dietz, V.: Activity of single motor units from human forearm muscles during voluntary isometric contractions. J. Neurophysiol., 38:933–946, 1975.

Gans, C., and Bock, W. J.: The functional significance of mus-cle architecture—a theoretical analysis. Ergeb. Anat. Entwick., 38:116–141, 1965.

Gauthier, G. F.: On the relationship of ultrastructural and cyto-chemical features to color in mammalian skeletal muscle. Z. Zellforsch. Mikrosk. Anat., 95:462–482, 1969.

Goldberg, L. J., and Derfler, B.: Relationship among recruit-ment order, spike amplitude, and twitch tension of single motor units in human masseter muscle. J. Neurophysiol., 40:870–890, 1977.

Goldberg, S. J., Lennerstrand, G., and Hull, C. D.: Motor unit responses in the lateral rectus muscle of the cat: Intracellular current injection of abducens nucleus neurons. Acta Physiol. Scand., 96:58–63, 1976.

Gollnick, P., Armstrong, R. B., Saubert, C. W., Piehl, K., and Saltin, B.: Enzyme activity and fiber composition in skeletal muscle of untrained and trained men. J. Appl. Physiol., 33:312–319, 1972.

Gordon, G., and Holbourne, A.: The mechanical activity of sin-gle motor units in reflex contraction of skeletal muscles. J. Physiol. (Lond.), 110:26–35, 1949.

Gordon, G., and Phillips, C. G.: Slow and rapid components in a flexor muscle. Q. J. Exp. Physiol., 38:35–45, 1953.

Goslow, G. E., Reinking, R. M., and Stuart, D. G.: The cat step cycle: Hind limb joint angles and muscle lengths during unre-strained locomotion. J. Morphol., 141:1–42, 1973.

Goslow, G. E., Stauffer, E. K., Nemeth, W. C., and Stuart, D. G.: Digit flexor muscles in the cat: Their action and motor units. J. Morphol., 137:335–352, 1972.

Granit, R.: Charles Scott Sherrington: An Appraisal. London, Nelson, 1966.

Granit, R., Henatsch, H.-D., and Steg, G.: Tonic and phasic ventral horn cells differentiated by post-tetanic potentiation in cat extensors. Acta Physiol. Scand., 37:114–126, 1956.

Grillner, S.: The role of muscle stiffness in meeting the chang-ing postural and locomotor requirements for force develop-ment by the ankle extensors. Acta Physiol. Scand., 86:92–108, 1972.

Grillner, S., Hongo, T., and Lund, S.: Descending monosynap-tic and reflex control of γ-motoneurones. Acta Physiol. Scand., 75:592–613, 1969.

Grillner, S., and Udo, M.: Motor unit acitivity and stiffness of

187

the contracting muscle fibers in the tonic stretch reflex. Acta Physiol. Scand., *81*:422–424, 1971a.

Grillner, S., and Udo. M.: Recruitment in the tonic stretch reflex. Acta Physiol. Scand., *81*:571–573, 1971b.

Grimby, L., and Hannerz, J.: Differences in recruitment order of motor units in phasic and tonic flexion reflex in "spinal man." J. Neurol. Neurosurg. Psychiatry, *33*:562–570, 1970.

Grimby, L., and Hannerz, J.: Disturbances in voluntary recruitment order of low and high frequency motor units on blockade of proprioceptive afferent activity. Acta Physiol. Scand., *96*:207–216, 1976.

Grimby, L., and Hannerz, J.: Firing rate and recruitment order of toe extensor motor units in different modes of voluntary contraction. J. Physiol. (Lond.), *264*:865–879, 1977.

Gurfinkel V. S., Mirskii, M. L., Tarko, A. M., and Surguladze, T. D.: Function of human motor units on initiation of muscle tension. Biofizika, *17*:(No. 2):303–310, 1972.

Hamburger, V.: The developmental history of the motor neuron. Neurosci. Res.. Program Bull., *15*(Suppl.): 1–37, 1977.

Hammarberg, C., and Kellerth, J.-O.: The postnatal development of some twitch and fatigue properties of single motor units in the ankle muscles of the kitten. Acta Physiol. Scand., *95*:243–257, 1975.

Hannerz, J. Discharge properties of motor units in relation to recruitment order in voluntary contraction. Acta Physiol. Scand., *91*:374–384, 1974.

Harker, D. W., Jami, L., Laporte, Y., and Petit, J.: Fast-conducting skeletofusimotor axons supplying intrafusal chain fibers in the cat peroneus tertius muscle. J. Neurophysiol., *40*:791–799, 1977.

Harrison, V. F., and Mortensen, O. A.: Identification and voluntary control of single motor unit activity in the tibialis anterior muscle. Anat. Rec., *144*:109–116, 1962.

Henatsch, H.-D., Schulte, F. J., and Busch, G.: Wandelbarkeit des tonisch-phäsichen reaktionstype einzelner extensor-motoneurone bei variation ihrer antriebe. Pfluegers Arch., *270*:161–173, 1959.

Henneman, E., Clamann, H. P., Gillies, J. D., and Skinner, R. D.: Rank order of motoneurons within a pool: Law of combination. J. Neurophysiol., *34*:1338–1349, 1974.

Henneman, E., and Olson, C. B.: Relations between structure and function in the design of skeletal muscles. J. Neurophysiol., *28*:581–598, 1965.

Henneman, E., Shahani, B. T., and Young, R. R.: Voluntary control of human motor units. Neurology, *25*:368. 1975.

Henneman, E., Somjen, G., and Carpenter, D. O.: Functional significance of cell size in spinal motoneurons. J. Neurophysiol., *28*:560–580, 1965a.

Henneman, E., Somjen, G., and Carpenter, D. O.: Excitability and inhibitibility of motoneurons of different sizes. J. Neurophysiol., *28*:599–620, 1965b.

Jami, L., Lan-Couton, D., Malmgren, K., and Petit, J.: Histophysiological observations on fast skeleto-fusimotor axons. Brain Res., *164*:53–59, 1979.

Johnson, M. A., Polgar, J., Weightman, D., and Appleton, D.: Data on the distribution of fibre types in thirty-six human muscles. An autopsy study. J. Neurol. Sci., 18:111–129, 1973.

Kanda, K., Burke, R. E., and Walmsley, B.: Differential control of fast and slow twitch motor units in the decerebrate cat. Exp. Brain Res., 29:57–74, 1977.

Karpati, G., and Engel, W. K.: "Type grouping" in skeletal muscles after experimental reinnervation. Neurology, 18:447–455, 1968.

Kato, M., and Tanji, J.: Volitionally controlled single motor units in human finger muscles. Brain Res., 40:345–357, 1972.

Kernell, D.: The limits of firing frequency in cat lumbosacral motoneurones possessing different time course of afterhyperpolarization. Acta Physiol. Scand., 65:87–100, 1965.

Kernell, D., Ducati, A., and Sjöholm, H.: Properties of motor units in the first deep lumbrical muscle of the cat's foot. Brain Res., 98:37–55, 1975.

Kernell, D., and Sjöholm, H.: Recruitment and firing rate modulation of motor unit tension in a small muscle of the cat's foot. Brain Res., 98:57–72, 1975.

Kristensson, K., Olsson, Y., and Sjöstrand, J.: Axonal uptake and retrograde transport of exogenous protein in the hypoglossal nerve. Brain Res., 32:399–406, 1971.

Krnjevic, K., and Miledi, R.: Motor units in the rat diaphragm. J. Physiol. (Lond.), 140:427–439, 1958.

Kuffler, D., Thompson, W., and Jansen, J. K. S.: The elimination of synapses in multiply-innervated skeletal muscle fibres of the rat: Dependence on distance between end-plates. Brain Res., 138:353–358, 1977.

Kugelberg, E.: Histochemical composition, contraction speed and fatiguability of rat soleus motor units. J. Neurol. Sci., 20:177–198, 1973.

Kugelberg, E.: Adaptive transformation of rat soleus motor units during growth. Histochemistry and contraction speed. J. Neurol. Sci., 27:269–289, 1976.

Kugelberg, E., Edström, L., and Abbruzzese, M.: Mapping of motor units in experimentally innervated rat muscle. J. Neurol. Neurosurg. Psychiatry, 33:319–329, 1970.

Kuno, M.: Excitability following antidromic activation in spinal motoneurones supplying red muscles. J. Physiol. (Lond.), 149:374–393, 1959.

Lännergren, J., and Smith, R. S.: Types of muscle fibres in toad skeletal muscle. Acta Physiol. Scand., 68:263–274, 1966.

Lennerstrand, G.: Mechanical studies on the retractor bulbi muscle and its motor units in the cat. J. Physiol. (Lond.), 236:43–55, 1974.

Letbetter, W. D.: Influence of intramuscular nerve branching on motor unit organization in medial gastrocnemius muscle. Anat. Rec., 178:402, 1974.

Lloyd, D. P. C., and McIntyre, A. K.: Transmitter potentiality of homonymous and heteronymous monosynaptic reflex connections of individual motoneurons. J. Gen. Physiol., 38:789–799, 1955.

Lux, H. D., Schubert, P., and Kreutzberg, G. W.: Direct matching of morphological and electrophysiological data in cat spinal motoneurones. In Andersen, P. and Jansen, J. K. S., (eds.): Excitatory Synaptic Mechanisms. Oslo, Universitetsforlaget, 1970, pp. 189–198.

Marsden, C. D., Meadows, J. C., and Merton, P. A. Isolated single motor units in human muscle and their rate of discharge during maximum voluntary effort. J. Physiol. (Lond.), 217:12–13p, 1971.

Matthews, P. B.: Mammalian Muscle Receptors and Their Central Actions. Baltimore, Williams and Wilkins, 1972.

Mayer, R. F., Burke, R. E., and Kanda, K.: Immobilization and muscle atrophy. Trans. Am. Neurol. Assoc., 101:1–3, 1976.

McComas, A. J., Fawcett, P. R. W., Campbell, M. J., and Sica, R. E. P.: Electrophysiological estimation of the numbers of motor units within a human muscle. J. Neurol. Neurosurg. Psychiatry, 34:121–131, 1971.

McComas, A. J., Sica, R. E. P., and Campbell, M. J.: Numbers and sizes of human motor units in health and disease. In Desmedt, J. E. (ed.): New Developments in Electromyography and Clinical Neurophysiology, Vol. 1. Basel, Karger, 1973, pp. 55–63.

McLaughlin, B. J.: The fine structure of neurons and synapses in the motor nuclei of the cat spinal cord. J. Comp. Neurol., 144:429–460, 1972.

McPhedran, A. M., Wuerker, R. B., and Henneman, E.: Properties of motor units in a homogeneous red muscle (soleus) of the cat. J. Neurophysiol., 28:71–84, 1965.

McWilliam, P. N.: The incidence and properties of β axons to muscle spindles in the cat hind limb. Q. J. Exp. Physiol., 60:25–36, 1975.

Milner-Brown, H. S., Stein, R. B., and Yemm, R.: The contractile properties of human motor units during voluntary isometric contractions. J. Physiol. (Lond.), 228:285–306, 1973a.

Milner-Brown, H. S., Stein, R. B., and Yemm, R.: The orderly recruitment of human motor units during voluntary isometric contractions. J. Physiol. (Lond.), 230:359–370, 1973b.

Milner-Brown, H. S., Stein, R. B., and Yemm, R.: Changes in firing rate of human motor units during linearly changing voluntary contractions. J. Physiol. (Lond.), 230:371–390, 1973c.

Monster, A. W., and Chan, H.: Isometric force production by motor units of extensor digitorum communis muscle in man. J. Neurophysiol., 40:1432–1443, 1977.

Mori, S.: Discharge patterns of soleus motor units with associated changes in force exerted by foot during quiet stance in man. J. Neurophysiol., 36:458–471, 1973.

Mosher, C. G., Gerlach, R. L., and Stuart, D. G.: Soleus and anterior tibial motor units of the cat. Brain Res., 44:1–11, 1972.

Norris, R. H., and Gasteiger, E. L.: Action potentials of single motor units in normal muscle. Electroencephalogr. Clin. Neurophysiol., 7:115–126, 1955.

Norris, F. H., and Irwin, R. L.: Motor unit area in rat muscle. Am. J. Physiol., 200:944–946, 1961.

Olson, C. B., Carpenter, D. O., and Henneman, E.: Orderly recruitment of muscle action potentials. Arch. Neurol., 19:591–597, 1968.

Olson, C. B., and Swett, C. P.: A functional and histochemical characterization of motor units in a heterogeneous muscle (flexor digitorum longus) of the cat. J. Comp. Neurol., 128:475–498, 1966.

Olson, C. B., and Swett, C. P.: Effect of prior activity on properties of different types of motor units. J. Neurophysiol., 34:1–16, 1971.

Padykula, H. A., and Gauthier, G. F.: Morphological and cytochemical characteristics of fiber types in normal mammalian skeletal muscle. In Milhorat, A. T. (ed.): Exploratory Concepts in Muscular Dystrophy and Related Disorders. Amsterdam, Excerpta Medica, 1967, pp. 117–128.

Person, R. S.: Rhythmic acitivty of a group of human motoneurones during voluntary contraction of a muscle. Electroencephalogr. Clin. Neurophysiol., 36:585–595, 1974.

Person, R. S., and Kudina, L. P.: Discharge frequency and discharge pattern of human motor units during voluntary contraction of muscle. Electroencephalogr. Clin. Neurophysiol., 32:471–483, 1972.

Peter, J. B., Barnard, R. J., Edgerton, V. R., Gillespie, C. A., and Stempel, K. E.: Metabolic profiles of three fiber types of skeletal muscle in guinea pigs and rabbits. Biochemistry, 11:2627–2633, 1972.

Peyronnard, J.-M., and Lamarre, Y.: Electrophysiological and anatomical estimation of the number of motor units in the monkey extensor digitorum brevis muscle. J. Neurol. Neurosurg. Psychiatry, 40:756–764, 1977.

Prestige, M. C.: Initial collaterals of motor axons within the spinal cord of the cat. J. Comp. Neurol., 126:123–136, 1966.

Prince, F. P., Hikida, R., and Hagerman, F. C.: Human fiber types in power lifters, distance runners and untrained subjects. Pfluegers Arch., 363:19–26, 1976.

Proske, U., and Waite, P. M. E.: Properties of types of motor units in the medial gastrocnemius muscle of the cat. Brain Res., 67:89–102, 1974.

Rall, W., and Hunt, C. C.: Analysis of reflex variability in terms of partially correlated excitability fluctuations in a population of motoneurons. J. Gen. Physiol., 39:397–422, 1956.

Ranvier, L.: De quelques faits relatifs à l'histologie et à la physiologie des muscles striés. Arch. Physiol. Norm. Pathol., 1:5–18, 1874.

Reinking, R. M., Stephens, J. A., and Stuart, D. G.: The motor units of cat medial gastrocnemius: Problems of their categorisation on the basis of mechanical properties. Exp. Brain Res., 23:301–313, 1975.

Rexed, B.: The cytoarchitectonic organization of the spinal cord in the cat. J. Comp. Neurol., 96:415–496, 1952.

Romanes, G. J.: The motor cell columns of the lumbo-sacral spinal cord of the cat. J. Comp. Neurol., 94:313–363, 1951.

Romanul, F. C. A.: Capillary supply and metabolism of muscle fibers. Arch. Neurol., 12:497–509, 1965.

Romanul, F. C. A., and Van Der Meulen, J. P.: Slow and fast muscles after cross innervation. Arch. Neurol., 17:387–402, 1967.

Rudomin, P., and Madrid, J.: Changes in correlation between monosynaptic responses of single motoneurons and in information transmission produced by conditioning volleys to cutaneous nerves. J. Neurophysiol., 35:44–64, 1972.

Salmons, S., and Sreter, F. A.: Significance of impulse activity in the transformation of skeletal muscle type. Nature 263:30–34, 1976.

Sato, M., Mizuno, N., and Konishi, A.: Postnatal differentiation of cell body volumes of spinal motoneurons innervating slow-twitch and post-twitch muscles. J. Comp. Neurol., 175:27–36, 1977.

Schwartz, M. S., Stålberg, E., Schiller, H. H., and Thiele, B.: The reinnervated motor unit in man. A single fibre EMG multielectrode investigation. J. Neurol. Sci., 27:303–312, 1976.

Schwindt, P., and Crill, W. E.: A persistent negative resistance in cat lumbar motoneurons. Brain Res., 120:173–178, 1977.

Severin, F. V., Shik, M. L., and Orlovskii, G. N.: Work of muscles and single motor units during controlled locomotion. Biophysics, 12:762–772, 1967.

Seyffarth, H.: Behavior of motor units in healthy and paretic muscles in man. Acta Psychiatr. Scand., 16:79–109, 1941.

Sharrard, W. J. W.: The distribution of the permanent paralysis in the lower limb in poliomyelitis. J. Bone Joint Surg., 37B: 540–558, 1955.

Sherrington, C. S.: Ferrier Lecture—some functional problems attaching to convergence. Proc. R. Soc. Lond. [Biol.], 105:332–362, 1929.

Sica, R. E. P., and McComas, A. J.: Fast and slow twitch units in a human muscle. J. Neurol. Neurosurg. Psychiatry, 34:113–120, 1971.

Smith, O. C.: Action potentials from single motor units in voluntary contraction. Am. J. Physiol., 108:629–638, 1934.

Somjen, G., Carpenter, D. O., and Henneman, E.: Responses of motoneurones of different sizes to graded stimulation of supraspinal centers of the brain. J. Neurophysiol., 28:958–965, 1965.

Stålberg, E., and Ekstedt, J.: Single fibre EMG and microphysiology of the motor unit in normal and diseased human muscle. In Desmedt, J. G. (ed.): New Developments in Electromyography and Clinical Neurophysiology, Vol. 1. Basel, Karger, 1973, pp. 113–129.

Stålberg, E., Schwartz, M. S., Thiele, B., and Schiller, H. H.: The normal motor unit in man—a single fibre EMG multielectrode investigation. J. Neurol. Sci., 27:291–301, 1976.

Stalberg, E., and Thiele, B.: Motor unit fibre density in the extensor digitorum communis muscle. J. Neurol. Neurosurg. Psychiatry, 38:874–880, 1975.

Steg, G.: Efferent muscle innervation and rigidity. Acta Physiol. Scand., 61(Suppl. 225):1–53, 1964.

Stephens, J. A., Garnett, R., and Buller, N. P.: Reversal of recruitment order of single motor units produced by cutaneous stimulation during voluntary muscle contraction in man. Nature, *272*:362–364, 1978.

Stephens, J. A., and Stuart, D. G.: The motor units of cat medial gastrocnemius: Speed-size relations and their significance for the recruitment order of motor units. Brain Res., *91*:177–195, 1975.

Stephens, J. A., and Usherwood, T. P.: The mechanical properties of human motor units with special reference to their fatiguability and recruitment threshold. Brain Res., *125*:91–97, 1977.

Sunderland, S., and Lavarack, J. O.: The branching of nerve fibres. Acta Anat., *17*:46–61, 1953.

Swett, J., Eldred, E., and Buchwald, J. S.: Somatotopic cord-to-muscle relations in efferent innervation of cat gastrocnemius. Am. J. Physiol., *219*:762–766, 1970.

Tanji, J., and Kato, M.: Firing rate of individual motor units in voluntary contraction of abductor digiti minimi muscle in man. Exp. Neurol., *40*:771–783, 1973*a*.

Tanji, J., and Kato, M.: Recruitment of motor units in voluntary contraction of a finger muscle in man. Exp. Neurol., *40*:759–770, 1973*b*.

Taylor, A., Cody, F. W. J., and Bosley, M. A.: Histochemical and mechanical properties of the jaw muscles of the cat. Exp. Neurol., *38*:99–109, 1973.

Taylor, A., and Stephens, J. A.: Study of human motor unit contractions by controlled intramuscular microstimulation. Brain Res., *117*:331–335, 1976.

Teig, E.: Tension and contraction time of motor units of the middle ear muscles in the cat. Acta Physiol. Scand., *84*:11–21, 1972.

Teig, E., and Dahl, H. A.: Actomyosin ATPase activity of middle ear muscles in the cat. Histochemie, *29*:1–7, 1972.

Testa, C.: Functional implications of the morphology of spinal ventral horn neurons of the cat. J. Comp. Neurol., *123*:425–443, 1964.

Thomas, J. S., Schmidt, E. M., and Hambrecht, F. T.: Facility of motor unit control during tasks defined directly in terms of unit behaviors. Exp. Neurol., *59*:384–395, 1978.

Thompson, W., and Jansen, J. K. S.: The extent of sprouting of remaining motor units in partly denervated immature and adult rat soleus muscle. Neuroscience, *2*:523–535, 1977.

Traub, R. D.: A model of a human neuromuscular system for small isometric tensions. Biol. Cybernet., *26*:159–167, 1977.

Van Buren, J. M., and Frank, K.: Correlation between the morphology and potential field of a spinal motor nucleus in the cat. Electroencephalogr. Clin. Neurophysiol., *19*:112–126, 1965.

Van de Graff, K. M., Frederick, E. C., Williamson, R. G., and Goslow, G. E., Jr.: Motor units and fiber types of primary ankle extensors of the skunk (*Mephitis mephitis*). J. Neurophysiol., *40*:1424–1431, 1977.

Van Harreveld, A. and Tachibana, S.: Innervation and reinnervation of cricothyroid muscle in the rabbit. Am. J. Physiol., *201*:1199–1202, 1961.

193

Wagman, I. H., Pierce, D. S., and Burger, R. E.: Proprioceptive influences in volitional control of individual motor units. Nature, *207*:957–958, 1965.

Walmsley, B., Hodgson, J. A., and Burke, R. E.: The forces produced by medial gastrocnemius and soleus muscles during locomotion in freely moving cats. J. Neurophysiol., *41*:1203–1216, 1978.

Walsh, J. V., Burke, R. E., Rymer, W. A., and Tsairis, P.: Effect of compensatory hypertrophy studied in individual motor units in medial gastrocnemius of the cat. J. Neurophysiol., *41*:496–508, 1978.

Warmolts, J. R., and Engel, W. K.: Open biopsy electromyography. I. Correlation of motor unit behavior with histochemical muscle fiber type in human limb muscle. Arch. Neurol. Psychiatry (Chicago), *27*:512–517, 1972.

Warszawski, M., Telerman-Toppet, N., Durdu, J., Graff, G. L. A., and Coërs, C.: The early stages of neuromuscular regeneration after crushing the sciatic nerve in the rat—electrophysiological and histochemical study. J. Neurol. Sci., *24*:21–32, 1975.

Weeds, A. G., Trentham, D. R., Kean, C. J. C., and Buller, A. J.: Myosin from cross-reinnervated cat muscles. Nature, *247*:135–139, 1974.

Wohlfart, G.: Muscular atrophy in diseases of the lower motor neurones. Contribution to the anatomy of motor units. Arch. Neurol. Psychiatry, *61*:599–620, 1949.

Wray, S. H.: Innervation ratios for large and small limb muscles in the baboon. J. Comp. Neurol., *137*:227–250, 1969.

Wuerker, R. B., McPhedran, A. M., and Henneman, E.: Properties of motor units in a heterogeneous pale muscle (m. gastrocnemius) of the cat. J. Neurophysiol., *28*:85–99, 1965.

Wyman, R. J., Waldron, I. and Wachtel, G. M.: Lack of fixed order of recruitment in cat motoneuron pools. Exp. Brain Res., *20*:101–114, 1974.

Yemm, R.: The orderly recruitment of motor units of the masseter and temporal muscles during voluntary isometric contraction in man. J. Physiol. (Lond.), *265*:163–174, 1977.

Zajac, F. E., and Young, J. L.: Discharge patterns of motor units during cat locomotion and their relation to muscle performance. *In* Herman, R. M., Grillner, S., Stein, P. S. G., and Stuart, D. G. (eds.): Neural Control of Locomotion. New York, Plenum Press, 1976, pp. 789–793.

Zucker, R. S.: Theoretical implications of the size principle of motoneurone recruitment. J. Theor. Biol., *38*:587–596, 1973.

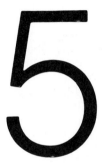

Trophic Effects of Nerve on Muscle*

A. J. Harris

INTRODUCTION Denervation of muscles produces profound changes in both their structure and function, changes which are said to demonstrate the existence of a "neurotrophic" influence of nerve on muscle. The effects of denervation have been studied and described extensively; much less is known about how this neurotrophic influence is actually exerted.

Wasting of muscles has long been a useful clinical sign of denervation and, as muscles also atrophy when disused, and become enlarged and more effective as a result of exercise, many authorities have argued that the effects of denervation are simply those of extreme disuse. On the other hand, clinical and experimental situations exist in which muscles may remain paralyzed in the presence of an otherwise intact innervation, and not show the usual signs of denervation. These observations have been explained by postulating some "specific agency in the motor innervation of skeletal muscle" which "may involve substantial transfer from the nerve to the muscle" and "is not activity as such" (Tower, 1939).

This debate, as to whether or not there exists "an influence of nerve not mediated by impulses" (Miledi, 1963), is not merely of historical interest but still continues, particularly in regard to the normal state of mature skeletal muscles. Lømo & Westgaard (1975) have shown that appropriate patterns of direct electrical stimulation can completely reverse the effects of denervating rat soleus muscles, and proposed that a separate trophic mechanism need not be supposed to exist in any other situation. This extreme view is countered by many observations which are difficult to explain in terms other than a nonelectrical influence of nerve. Mechanisms by which

*Work in the author's laboratory is supported by the New Zealand Medical Research Council.

195

such an influence might be exerted have not been described in other than the broadest detail, so that the relative importance of electrical and nonelectrical forms of communication between nerves and muscles in maintaining muscle in its normal state is yet to be determined.

The Role of Innervation in Muscle Development

Skeletal muscle fibers are long multinucleate cells which begin to form during the late stages of embryogenesis by fusion of mononucleate myoblasts. Nerve fibers are present in developing muscle masses from the earliest stages (Kelly and Zacks, 1969; Landmesser and Morris, 1975), before fusion has begun. The initial induction of mesodermal tissue to form myogenic tissue may depend on its proximity to primitive neural tissue (Holtzer and Detwiler, 1953). However, both in vitro and in vivo, considerable further development of muscle can occur in the absence of nerves, although innervation is essential for the final maturation of muscle in neonates (Engel and Karpati, 1968).

Myoblasts from disaggregated embryonic muscle (Konigsberg, 1963) or from permanent cell lines (Yaffe, 1968) will multiply in tissue culture and eventually fuse into multinucleate myotubes which can develop further into striated muscle fibers. All this occurs in the total absence of nerve although the full cycle of multiplication, fusion, and maturation occurs more readily if embryo extract or some form of fetal or placental serum is present in the culture medium.

Removal of a length of spinal cord from chick embryos at stages 16 through 22 (Hamburger and Hamilton, 1951), before motoneurons have extended processes to presumptive muscle tissue, does not prevent muscles from developing to the myotube stage although they are atrophic and infiltrated with fat (Pockett, 1977). Similar results are seen following destruction of motoneurons by β-bungarotoxin injection (Abe et al., 1976) into 5-day-old chick embryos (Pockett, 1977) or by injection of 3-acetylpyridine into stage 25 embryos (Shellswell, 1977).

It has similarly proved possible to destroy rat embryo motoneurons in vivo, with the result that mammalian skeletal muscles can be seen to develop without innervation. Also, rat embryos can be chronically paralyzed by inserting slow release capillaries containing tetrodotoxin, so that their nerves and muscles develop without action potentials (Braithwaite and Harris, 1979a, b). Aneural and paralyzed rat embryo muscles examined at the time embryos would normally be born are relatively atrophic, but in a better state than aneural chick muscles: this may not reflect any important species difference in mechanism, but simply the relatively advanced state of development in newly hatched chicks as compared to neonatal rats.

Although development to the myotube state may be possible in the absence of innervation, further maturation does require the presence of the nerve. Denervation of chick embryo muscle or treatment with neurotoxic drugs prevents later survival of myotubes, so that by the time of hatching muscle tissue is virtually absent (Eastlick, 1943; Drachman, 1967). Muscles denervated in newborn rats (Engel and Karpati, 1968; Stewart, 1968) continue to grow but at a rate slower than normal, with many fibers remaining in the myotube stage instead of developing further. Muscles denervated in neonates may atrophy completely if not reinnervated within a few weeks, and even those that do become reinnervated suffer some permanent reduction in fiber number and fiber size (McArdle and Sansone, 1977).

Muscle fibers are slow contracting at birth (some differentiation into slow or fast has already begun in newborn rats (Close, 1969)). In cats, all muscle fibers become faster contracting during the first 6 postnatal weeks and then fibers destined to be slow contracting in the adult progressively get slower, while fibers destined to be fast contracting continue to get faster (Buller et al., 1960a). Both denervation and disuse have little effect on changes up until 5 weeks after birth, after which time all muscles remain in a similar relatively fast contracting state. Denervation of adult muscles, in contrast, leads to all fiber types, both slow and fast, becoming slower (Eccles et al., 1962).

Effects of Denervating Adult Muscles

Many of the changes which result from denervation are due to an altered expression of the muscle cell genome, an actual change in expression of the differentiated state of skeletal muscle cells, not simply a running down of normal metabolism. Much detailed information about the effects of denervation is available (Gutmann, 1962, 1976; Gutmann and Hnik, 1963; Guth, 1968; Harris, 1974).

In addition to gross muscle atrophy, denervation produces at least five changes in muscle membrane properties. Earliest is a reduction in muscle resting potential; this is followed by the appearance of a tetrodotoxin (TTX)-resistant action potential mechanism, an increase of acetylcholine (ACh) sensitivity in extra-junctional regions, spontaneous fibrillary action potentials arising from the end-plate region and, finally, an increase in specific membrane resistance. Blocking RNA or protein synthesis prevents the development of TTX-resistant action potentials and the development of extrajunctional ACh sensitivity (Grampp et al., 1972), but not the fall in resting potential (Bray et al., 1976).

197

RESTING POTENTIAL DECREASE The fall in resting potential which follows denervation is first seen close to the end-plate region, and only later in more distal regions of the muscle (Albuquerque et al., 1971; Bray et al., 1976). The time course of the decrease has been variously described by different investigators, but there is qualitative agreement as to its occurrence. The most interesting point of conflict concerns the question of whether onset of the fall may precede degeneration of nerve terminals (Albuquerque et al., 1971; Bray et al., 1976; Deshpande et al., 1976), or whether it can be seen only after nerve terminal degeneration has begun (Card, 1977). The reduction in potential appears to be the result of loss of an electrogenic component which accounts for about 20 mV of normal resting potential (Locke and Solomon, 1967; Bray et al., 1976). Agents such as epinephrine, which increases activity of the electrogenic pump in normal muscle (Clausen and Flatman, 1977), restore the resting potential of denervated muscle. Conversely, ouabain induces a rapid fall in resting potential of normal muscle to the denervated level, but induces only a slow rate of decrease of potential in denervated muscle (Bray et al., 1976). Robbins (1977) has used an indirect method of estimate Na^+ permeability and suggested that this permeability is increased following denervation, and accounts for the fall in potential. The electrogenic pump has been well characterized by Clausen and Flatman (1977), and certainly is significant in maintaining normal potentials. The assumptions inherent in Robbins' technique of measuring permeability, and the variations in his control data, make it difficult to assess whether his suggested increase in Na^+ permeability actually exists; no change in membrane impedance has been seen to accompany it (Albuquerque et al., 1971). It still is difficult to understand how, in a steady state, resting potential can remain much in excess of K^+ equilibrium potential without passive movement of K^+ bringing E_{K+} close to resting potential, and thus removing the presumed basis for the rapid component of ouabain-induced depolarization.

ACTION POTENTIALS Within 2 days of denervation TTX fails to block action potentials initiated near old end-plates and, within a week of denervation, action potentials can be evoked at any part of a muscle fiber in the presence of this drug (Redfern and Thesleff, 1971). TTX does reduce the rate of increase of action potentials in denervated muscles, and action potentials still require the presence of Na^+ in the external medium, showing no sensitivity to Ca^{++} levels.

INCREASED SENSITIVITY TO ACh Denervated muscles become hypersensitive to ACh (Frank et al., 1922; Brown, 1937) principally because of the appearance of ACh receptors outside the synaptic region (Axelsson and Thesleff, 1959; Miledi, 1960*a*). Extrajunctional ACh sensitivity is not detectable outside the end-plate regions of fast skeletal muscle fibers (Kuffler and Yoshikami, 1975) but slow muscles, in particular rat soleus, are measurably sensitive to ACh in extrajunctional regions, with a response about four orders of magnitude less than that at the end-plate (Miledi and Zelena, 1966). Extrajunctional sensitivity increases in a fairly uniform way after denervation of both fast and slow muscles, showing that the increase in sensitive area is not due simply to a spread of receptors away from the end plate (Albuquerque and McIsaac, 1970). The use of snake venoms which bind strongly and specifically to the ACh receptor molecule (Lee et al., 1967; Miledi and Potter, 1971) has made it possible to isolate ACh receptor molecules and to provide a sophisticated analysis of their synthesis, incorporation into cell membranes, and degradation (Devreotes and Fambrough, 1975; Brockes at al., 1975; Fambrough and Devreotes, 1978). Receptors are synthesized on polyribosomes and are immediately incorporated into membranes which form vesicles of the Golgi apparatus. These vesicles migrate to and fuse with the external cell membrane, exposing ACh receptors on its outer surface. Degradation involves their internalization from the cell membrane and proteolysis, presumably in lyosomes. Extrajunctional and embryonic receptors (Burden, 1977) have a turnover time of the order of 1 or 2 days, but junctional receptors are extremely stable even in denervated muscles, and only a lower estimate of their lifetime, of at least a week, can be given. In rat muscles extrajunctional ACh receptors begin to increase in number about 48 hours after denervation and reach maximum density after about 2 weeks (Hartzell and Fambrough, 1972; Berg et al., 1972).

FIBRILLATION A spontaneous and usually unsynchronized twitching of single muscle fibers (for exceptions see Harvey and Kuffler, 1944*b*; Purves and Sakmann, 1974*b*) is first seen about 2 days after denervation of rat muscles (Salafsky et al., 1968) and increases in intensity during the first week or so after denervation. Fibrillary potentials usually arise near old end-plates (Hayes and Woolsey, 1942; Belmar and Eyzaguirre, 1966; Purves and Sakmann, 1974*a, b*; Smith and Thesleff, 1976) and propagate from there along the whole length of muscle fibers (Eccles, 1941). Subthreshold fibrillary origin potentials (FOPs) may be recorded near points of origin (Purves and Sakmann, 1974*b*; Smith and Thesleff, 1976), and these are suggested to be spontaneous events in the t-tubule system. Fibrillary action potentials may occur at a fixed regular frequency in the range 0.1 to 30 Hz (most commonly 5 to 10 Hz in both animal and human muscle) or as bursts, and studies of single fibers in cultured rat diaphragm muscles showed that individual fibers fibrillated for about

20 hours and then were quiescent for the next 40 to 60 hours (Purves and Sakmann, 1974*b*). Only a proportion of fibers in muscles denervated in vivo are fibrillating at any one time (Thesleff and Ward, 1975; Cangiano et al., 1977), indicating that a cyclical pattern of activity is present, as in organ culture.

MUSCLE ATROPHY   The most striking effect of muscle denervation is the rapid and extensive muscle atrophy. Rates of atrophy in different muscles and different species vary considerably. For example, rat limb muscles are reduced to half their original weight within 2 weeks of denervation (Solandt and Magladery, 1940), whereas rat diaphragm may undergo a transient hypertrophy before it finally atrophies (Stewart et al., 1972). A rapid increase in the whole muscle content of DNA following denervation is principally due to mitosis in interstitial cells, but labelled DNA precursor molecules also appear in satellite cells (Zak et al., 1969), and mononucleate myoblasts are seen in interstitial spaces (Lee, 1965). At longer times after denervation some muscles disappear altogether, becoming replaced by connective tissue and fat. Others survive indefinitely; Weddell et al. (1944) recorded fibrillatory potentials from leg muscles in a man whose limb was paralyzed 18 years previously by an attack of poliomyelitis. The general effect of denervation is to decrease the rate of synthesis of muscle proteins, and to increase their rate of degradation. This contrasts with the effect of work-induced hypertrophy, in which the rate of protein synthesis is increased and the rate of degradation decreased (Goldberg, 1969*a, b*). Goldberg (1969) found the loss of myofibrillar proteins to be greater than the loss of sarcoplasmic proteins.

Reinnervation of Adult Muscle

Reinnervation of denervated muscle partly or wholly reverses the changes induced by denervation. Resting potentials are restored, ACh sensitivity becomes restricted to the end-plate region, fibrillation stops, TTX sensitivity of the action potential is restored, and there is substantial, although not necessarily complete, recovery of muscle size and weight. Incomplete restoration of muscle size is most obvious after denervation of muscles in young animals; it is due to a permanent reduction in muscle fiber diameter (McArdle and Sansone, 1977) as well as to the reduction in the number of muscle fibers that is common to muscles denervated at all ages (although more marked in newborn animals, perhaps due to motoneuron cell death (Romanes, 1946)). Fibers may be smaller as a consequence of reduced muscle use resulting from the permanent deficit in muscle sensory innervation that follows denervation in neonates (Zelena and Hnik, 1960).

Reversal of the denervated state is sometimes seen to be initiated before the ingrowing nerve can evoke activity in the muscle. Miledi (1960b) and Bennett et al. (1973) found that extrajunctional ACh sensitivity was reduced in frog sartorius and chick anterior latissimus dorsi muscles, respectively, after nerve-released miniature endplate potentials had returned but before nerve stimulation could evoke an end-plate potential. This is not true of denervated rat skeletal muscles (McArdle and Albuquerque, 1973), but is seen during the prolonged course of recovery from botulin poisoning in rat diaphragm muscle (Bray and Harris, 1975). It is also seen in an analogous situation in which supersensitivity is lost from denervated sympathetic ganglion cells in the frog heart in the early stages of reinnervation, before synaptic transmission is restored (Dennis and Sargent, 1978). There is a 2- or 3-week stage in the development of salamander muscles during which they cannot give action potentials but are caused to contract by the large end-plate potentials evoked at their multiple points of synaptic contact. They remain supersensitive throughout this period, until they gain the ability to give action potentials (Dennis and Ort, 1977). Frog slow muscle fibers do not possess an action potential mechanism even when mature but gain this capacity and become supersensitive if they are denervated. Upon reinnervation both supersensitivity and the action potential mechanism are lost, in direct contrast to the events in developing salamander muscle (Miledi et al., 1971).

Cross-Reinnervation Muscle fibers can be divided into the two general categories of slow and fast contracting or, using histochemical criteria, type I and type II (Engel, 1974). The physiological response to stimulation of individual motor nerve fibers indicates that motor units are homogeneous in their properties. For example, Anderson and Sears (1964) detected fast and slow motor units in cat intercostal muscles when they stimulated individual ventral root fibers. More recently it has become possible to demonstrate the homogeneity of muscle fibers within a single motor unit with respect both to contraction speed and histochemical profile (Edstrom and Kugelberg, 1968; Burke et al., 1971). Because muscle fibers of more than one type can coexist within a muscle, it is appealing to assume that the properties of the fibers in each unit are conferred upon them by their nerve. This idea is strongly supported by the finding that cross-reinnervation of slow and fast contracting muscles causes a considerable transformation in muscle properties, from slow to fast and fast to slow (Buller et al., 1960b; Close, 1969).

Muscle Regeneration Muscles can regenerate even after severe damage — for example, being literally minced up and then replaced in the animal (Studitsky et al., 1963; Carlson and Gutmann, 1976). The initial stages of regeneration are similar whether or not regenerating nerves are present, but later stages of regeneration are impeded in the absence of nerve. Regeneration in denervated limbs proceeds as far as the myotube stage, with some fibers developing striations and peripherally placed nuclei. However, this is followed by prolonged atrophy and eventual disappearance of the tissue (Jirmanova and Thesleff, 1972; Carlson and Gutmann, 1976), in contrast to the complete restoration of muscle that can occur in innervated limbs (Carlson, 1976).

EXPERIMENTAL ANALYSIS OF NERVE TROPHIC MECHANISMS

The phenomena described above make it clear that an intact and functional innervation is of vital importance for maintaining muscle in a normal healthy state. The question remains as to whether this influence is fully accounted for by activation of the electrical and mechanical events associated with muscle contraction, or whether some other influence of the nerve must be proposed.

Two major periods of interest in this problem coincided with the two world wars, as physiologists and clinicians sought research projects relevant to the war effort. During the first war the famous English physiologist J. N. Langley, together with visiting Japanese researchers Kato, Itayaki, and Hashimoto, considered the possibilities of whether denervation atrophy was due to loss of muscle activity, loss of some nutritive influence of nerve, or some other factor. They were unable to show any marked effect of direct stimulation in maintaining denervated muscle weight (Langley, 1916). Langley's extensive researches into functions of the autonomic nervous system (Langley, 1900) left him with no sympathy for the idea of the existence of special motor nerve impulses affecting nutrition, but he was struck by the presence of fibrillatory activity in denervated muscles (Langley and Kato, 1915). Fibrillation was first seen by Schiff (1851) who noticed spontaneous surface twitchings on the surface of dogs' tongues over a period 3 days to 6 months after cutting both hypoglossal nerves. Langley proposed that denervation atrophy was not the result of disuse but of overuse — of fatigue due to the continuous fibrillation.

This view was still popular at the beginning of World War II (Tower, 1939) although Tower, as a result of experiments with innervated but disused muscles in puppies, proposed that fibrillation in turn resulted from the loss of an influence of nerve independent of activity. During the war experiments with drugs that suppressed fibrillation without affecting muscle atrophy (Solandt and Magladery, 1940) caused a loss of interest in Langley's proposal. Also, improvements in techniques for direct muscle stimulation enabled several workers to retard or even prevent denervation atrophy (Solandt et al., 1943; Eccles, 1944). Evidence for an influence of nerve independent of impulses still appeared strong (Tower et al., 1941; Weddell et al., 1944), and this was strengthened by Miledi's (1960a) observation that if one of the end-plates of a multiply innervated muscle was denervated a local supersensitivity of ACh appeared, despite maintained use of the muscle fiber via its other end-plates.

A dramatic change in view arose in the early 1970's. Lømo and Rosenthal (1972) found that anesthetic block of a motor nerve evoked muscle changes similar to those of denervation, while direct stimulation of a denervated muscle reversed those changes. Extension of this work, in the form of the careful quantitative analysis of Lømo and Westgaard (1975), led to the proposal that the effects of denervating muscles were purely those of disuse. On the other hand Albuquerque et al. (1972) blocked axonal transport in the same preparation (rat sciatic nerve) used by Lømo and Rosenthal, and found that muscles which continued to be activated by nerves in which transport was blocked reacted as if denervated.

Direct Stimulation of Denervated Muscles

Direct electrical stimulation of denervated rat soleus muscles resulted in reversal of all effects of denervation that were examined — ACh hypersensitivity, resting potential, etc., but not atrophy, TTX sensitivity, or end-plate AChE levels; results of these experiments were summarized by Lømo and Westgaard (1975). Two important points can be made based upon this work: first, that electrical activation of rat soleus muscle can effectively substitute for the presence of the nerve; and second, that the temporal pattern of activation is at least as important as the total amount of stimulation delivered. For example, a mean frequency of stimulation at 1 Hz was much more effective when delivered in the form of 100-Hz trains every 100 seconds, instead of continuously. Nothing is known about which aspect of the muscle response to stimulation is involved, nor have such well executed experiments been performed on other muscles or in other species. Lømo and Westgaard's results effectively eliminate all current arguments against muscle activity being capable of acting as an important regulatory factor on normal muscle. Muscle activity has not been shown to be involved in regulation of end-plate structure and function.

Effects of Muscle Disuse

If muscle structure and function are regulated solely by activation, then a sufficient reduction in muscle use should give rise to symptoms of denervation. Alternatively, if nerves provide a trophic influence on muscle independently of muscle activation then even total disuse of an innervated muscle should not provoke a response quantitatively similar to that of denervation.

203

TROPHIC EFFECTS OF NERVE ON MUSCLE

Disuse of muscle due to bed rest, limb immobilization (Solandt et al., 1943; Fischbach and Robbins, 1969), isolation of motoneurons by combined spinal cord section and dorsal root section (Tower, 1939; Eccles, 1941; Solandt and Magladery, 1942; Johns and Thesleff, 1961), hibernation (Moravec et al., 1973), or in cases of hysterical paralysis (Harvey and Kuffler, 1944a) may give rise to some degree of muscle atrophy (which varies in some histological details from denervation atrophy (Tower, 1939)), but does not otherwise reproduce the effects of denervation. In none of these cases is it possible to state unequivocally that no very brief high frequency bursts of muscle action potentials could not have occurred two or three times a day, even when attempts to record such activity were unsuccessful. While the results of such experiments may give rise to doubts regarding the adequacy of Lømo and Westgaard's hypothesis, they do not invalidate it.

Disuse of muscle can also be effected by blocking the propagation of action potentials in an otherwise intact muscle nerve. To give meaning to the results of such experiments it is essential to ensure that the procedure used does not affect axonal transport; otherwise the effects on muscle could be due to lack of delivery of a trophic factor, in addition to inactivity. Very few experiments presently satisfy this criterion.

Robert and Oester (1970a, b) developed the technique of placing an anesthetic-impregnated silicone rubber cuff around a nerve in order to produce a prolonged block of conduction. They used lidocaine-impregnated cuffs, and reported that up to 14 days of paralysis of rabbit leg muscles did not produce fibrillation or hypersensitivity to ACh. Their technique was later applied to rat leg muscles (Lømo and Rosenthal, 1972) where it produced the opposite result: denervation was mimicked. Lømo and Rosenthal also blocked impulses and mimicked the effect of denervation with a demyelinating block induced by diphtheria toxin. The discrepancies between these results, and between those of others using the same technique, as well as reflecting possible species differences, may be accounted for by several technical factors. Tightly fitting cuffs, with or without anesthetic impregnation, will by themselves block both axonal transport and nerve impulses, presumably as a result of local anoxia of the nerve. Ochs (1974) has shown that anoxia blocks both impulses and transport with the same threshold. Cangiano et al. (1977) have shown a good example of misapplication of this technique. Even when loosely fitting cuffs are used, local anesthetics can block axonal transport as well as impulses (Byers et al., 1973; Bisby, 1975). Diphtheria toxin also has this action, totally blocking fast axonal transport while leaving the demyelinated axons physically intact (Kidman et al., 1978). All these difficulties make the use both of nerve cuffs and of local anesthetics of limited utility; only if each individual case is checked for the integrity of fast axonal transport through the region of the cuff can a useful interpretation of results be given.

A recent improvement in technique has been to use tetrodotoxin to block conduction (Lavoie et al., 1976, 1977; Pestronk et al., 1976; Bray et al., 1979). This drug does not have any direct effect on axonal transport, but does block nerve impulses effectively. The technique of application is critical: local injection under the nerve sheath gives rise to blocks of short duration; cuffs provide blocks of longer duration, but with the attendant difficulties listed above. The best technique so far devised is that of Bray and Mills (1979), in which a short length of fine glass capillary, closed at one end and open with a small pore at the other, is filled with a concentrated solution of TTX and slipped under the nerve sheath. The capillary sits in place without compressing nerve fibers or affecting blood flow or axonal transport. Diffusion of TTX from the small pore maintains a local nerve block of a week or more in duration, and the capillary is easily replaced to give nerve blocks of several weeks duration. The initial effect of the block is to give rise to a denervation-like increase in muscle ACh receptors (Lavoie et al., 1976, 1977; Pestronk et al., 1976; Bray et al., 1979), with the difference that the magnitude of the response is much less than that of denervation. ACh receptor levels reach a peak of about 50 per cent of the denervated level after 10 days and then slowly decline, for example, by 15 days being lowered to about 20 per cent of denervated levels in rat soleus muscles (Bray et al., 1979). Muscle fiber resting potentials fall much more slowly than after denervation, and stabilize with about 50 per cent of the decrease that occurs in denervated muscles (Bray et al., 1979). Inactive muscle fibers in rats fibrillate in much the same manner as denervated fibers, and fibrillation is maintained when ACh receptor levels are declining. Fibrillation was not seen in an analogous experiment in baboons (Fowler et al., 1972; Gilliatt et al., 1977, discussed below) nor is it thought to occur in clinical cases of conduction block in man (Harvey and Kuffler, 1944a; Weddell et al., 1944), indicating that there may be species differences in this response.

Another technique for inducing a long-lasting conduction block in peripheral nerve is to apply pressure to a nerve locally for a period of 30 to 60 minutes (Fowler et al., 1972). This produces a condition similar to pressure palsy in man (Weddell et al., 1944), in which action potentials will not pass the block but the nerve remains intact and electrically excitable below the point of block. The block appears to be due to local deformation of the axon giving rise to damage to nodes of Ranvier and to local demyelination (Ochoa et al., 1972); it is not due to ischemia. The effects of such a block when applied to the

205

limb of a baboon are similar to those of TTX application to rat limb nerve in that ACh sensitivity develops, but only to an extent less than 20 per cent of that resulting from denervation (Gilliatt et al., 1977). Fibrillation is of low degree and perhaps attributable solely to a small number of nerve fibers caused to degenerate by the block. Muscle atrophy is also much less marked than following denervation.

These studies of disused muscles show that the effects of denervation do not result solely from inactivity. Lømo and Westgaard (1975) pointed out that they do not, however, immediately demonstrate the existence of a trophic action of nerve on muscle. The products of nerve terminal degeneration may have a direct action on muscle, exacerbating or accelerating the effects of inactivity. The effects of denervation are seen later if a nerve is sectioned far from rather than close to a muscle (Deshpande et al., 1976); there is a corresponding delay before the isolated nerve terminal degenerates (Miledi and Slater, 1970). Direct stimulation of denervated muscle does not fully substitute for the nerve within the first few days of denervation, when products of nerve terminal degeneration are present, although it is effective at later times (Lømo and Westgaard, 1975). Small pieces of degenerating nerve, when laid on the surface of a normal muscle, cause a temporary and localized hypersensitivity to ACh (Jones and Vyskocil, 1975), but as this response is quite nonspecific and occurs in reaction to virtually any foreign body the significance of such experiments is not clear. Although it may seem a strange inversion to argue that while normal nerve terminals do not release any material that has a trophic action on muscle, degenerating terminals do release a highly potent substance that rapidly and irreversibly has an effect that is additive to the effects of inactivity, there is at present no evidence that completely refutes this hypothesis (see Cangiano and Lutzemberger, 1977, and Tiedt et al., 1977a, for conflicting opinions on this point).

Effects of Blocking Axonal Transport

If the normal neurotrophic regulation of muscle properties depends both upon activation and delivery to the muscle of some substance transported down the nerve and released from its terminals, then blocking axonal transport while leaving the muscle normally activated should produce some denervation-like effects. Many experiments of this kind have been done, using various techniques to apply colchicine or vinblastine to nerves. These drugs are said to interfere with fast axonal transport without affecting action potentials (Albuquerque et al., 1972; Hoffman and Thesleff, 1972; Fernandez and Ramirez, 1974; Kauffman et al., 1974; Tiedt et al., 1977b). These experiments can all be criticized on the basis that colchicine and vinblastine, when applied directly to an innervated muscle, produce some changes similar to those of denervation even when axonal transport has not been blocked (Lømo, 1974; Cangiano and Fried, 1977). The mechanism of this direct action is not known.

Investigators have become aware of the problem of direct action of these drugs, and some careful experiments have been done in which the use of Silastic cuffs was avoided (Fernandez, 1973; Fernandez and Ramirez, 1974; Tiedt et al., 1977b), together with controls that might account for any direct action. These experiments gave results indicating that application of colchicine or vinblastine to a nerve partially mimicked the effect of denervation, despite continued use of the muscles. A number of technical difficulties, such as fragility of the treated nerves, are associated with the use of these agents (Warnick et al., 1977) and the results of the experiments are still difficult to interpret unambiguously.

Embryonic Development of Muscles

A possible explanation for the coexistence of both trophic and activity-related mechanisms for maintaining adult skeletal muscles could be the advantage, in the course of evolution, of having the size, strength, and endurance of muscles reflect the extent to which they have been needed and used. It could then be argued that trophic actions independent of activity are of greater importance during embryonic development, before there is opportunity for interaction with the external world.

Certainly muscles in newborn animals are particularly sensitive to the effects of denervation (McArdle and Sansone, 1977; Robbins et al., 1977). However, comparison of the development of aneural and paralyzed muscles in rat embryos (Braithwaite and Harris, 1979a, b) shows that inactivity alone could account for many of the effects of deprivation of muscle innervation during development. Aneural and paralyzed muscles are both relatively atrophic, being thinner and shorter than controls. They contain areas of unfused myoblasts, which makes it difficult to estimate the relative effects of these treatments on muscle fiber numbers. Junctional ACh receptor clusters, and junctional deposits of AChE, appear at the appropriate time and place even in aneural muscles, showing that the position of nerve-muscle junctions is determined by factors intrinsic to the muscle (perhaps encoded in basement membrane; Sanes et al., 1978; Sanes and Hall, 1979; Burden et al., 1979). At later times extrajunctional clusters of ACh receptors also appear. In the case of paralyzed muscles this appearance is transitory and they are removed with a half-life of 2 or 3 days; this removal is hastened by allowing muscles to recover from paralysis. Junctional clusters progressively increase in size in paralyzed innervated muscles, but retain only their initial dimensions in aneural muscles.

207

Thus the embryonic nerve, by a trophic action, regulates the number and position of ACh receptor molecules on muscle fibers, but activity is an absolute necessity for normal physical growth of embryonic muscles. The embryonic nerve, independently of nerve impulses, promotes the normal growth of junctional receptor clusters and inhibits the formation of extrajunctional clusters. Dispersed extrajunctional receptors in paralyzed muscles are present at a greater density than in controls, but at half the density found in aneural muscles. These trophic actions require the continuous presence of the nerve. If embryo muscles are allowed to become innervated and then denervated, junctional receptor clusters stop growing within 2 days and extrajunctional clusters appear within 1 day. The trophic signal regulating AChE has longer lasting effects. Muscles from rat embryos whose motoneurons have been destroyed at day 12 gestation, before muscle development can be recognized, develop extremely faint deposits of AChE. Each muscle fiber has only a single deposit, near its midpoint. In contrast, muscles denervated at day 15 gestation, after nerve-muscle transmission has developed but before any junctional AChE can be recognized, not only develop junctional AChE deposits with roughly normal histological staining properties but also develop many extrajunctional deposits of the enzyme (Harris, unpublished).

The results of these experiments indicate that the relative contributions of nerve trophic actions and of activity to the development of embryonic muscles are not strikingly different from those in the maintenance of mature muscles.

Muscles in Organ Culture In the hope that a greater degree of experimental control might give rise to a clearer understanding of the effects of denervation, muscles have been maintained in organ culture (Miledi and Trowell, 1962; Harris and Miledi, 1972; Fambrough, 1970; Berg and Hall, 1975; Purves and Sakmann, 1974a, b; Bray et al., 1976; Ziskind and Harris, 1978) and subjected to various manipulations, including direct electrical stimulation (Purves and Sakmann, 1974a; Ziskind and Harris, 1978) or reinnervation (Ziskind and Harris, 1978). Purves and Sakmann (1974a, b) in an elegant quantitative study, showed that fibrillatory activity in denervated rat diaphragm muscles is self-regulating. Individual fibers fibrillate for about 20 hours and then stop fibrillating for about 60 hours before beginning again. Direct stimulation of muscles for a similar period stops fibrillation in all muscle fibers. Prevention of fibrillation, with TTX paralysis, produces fibrillation in nearly all fibers once the paralysis is relieved. ACh sensitivity of the cultured fibers is similarly affected, and the study as a whole demonstrated why it is that fibrillation in denervated muscles does not relieve the gross symptoms of denervation: as soon as fibrillation does begin to have an affect it inhibits itself and the muscle fiber relaxes. As the authors pointed out, the study does not, of course, provide information about how much activity an innervated muscle requires to maintain itself in a healthy state.

Ziskind and Harris (1978) maintained denervated adult mouse diaphragm muscle strips in organ culture and caused them to become reinnervated by nerve fibers growing out from small explants of fetal mouse spinal cord. In order to support growth of the nerve fibers a culture medium enriched with fetal and placental serum and embryo extract is used, and muscle strips cultured alone in these circumstances do not fibrillate. Once reinnervation has occurred discrete bundles of muscle fibres begin to fasciculate, presumably because of spontaneous discharges in the spinal cord neurons. Muscle fibers that have become reinnervated lose the resistance to TTX blockage of the action potential that is present in all denervated fibers in the cultures. This restoration to normal of the action potential mechanism also occurs in cultures which have become reinnervated in the continual presence of curare, which blocks all muscle contraction, showing that in these circumstances the nerves can exert a trophic influence that is independent of electrical or contractile activity in the muscles. The authors pointed out that exertion of this action by developing or regenerating nerves does not constitute evidence that similar mechanisms are of quantitative importance at normal nerve-muscle junctions.

Summary of Experimental Techniques

Experimental evidence has been presented to show that the pattern of electrical activation of muscle fibers can affect many of the changes that result from denervation. A small amount of viable evidence and much that is suggestive but inconclusive exists to show that muscles that are innervated but disused show the symptoms of denervation in an attenuated form, and in a pattern that varies between different muscles and species. In a literature in which vehemence has recently come to be substituted for evidence (Warnick et al., 1977; Cangiano et al., 1977), no clear-cut evidence has emerged to settle the question of the extent to which fast axonal transport is involved in trophic regulation of muscles when normally innervated and functioning. Knowledge of control pathways whereby expression of the muscle cell genome is affected by activity and by other factors is so rudimentary as to preclude any attempt to estimate the relative importance of nerve activity and nerve trophic mechanisms in normal unmanipulated muscles. The presence of transient responses to disuse (Bray et al., 1979), of nerve actions independent of activity during regeneration (Miledi, 1960b; Ziskind and Harris, 1978; Dennis and Sargent, 1979), of species differences in muscle response to nerve paralysis (Robert and Oester, 1970b; Lømo and Rosenthal, 1972; Gilliatt et al., 1978), and of large alterations of metabolic patterns in nerve cells in response to changes in the peripheral environment of their terminals (Watson, 1974) make it impossible to extrapolate from experimental circumstances back to the normal state.

MUSCLE DISEASE Earlier studies of the effects of nerves on muscles, particularly those performed during times of war, were inspired by concurrent clinical interest in caring for patients who had suffered trauma to nerve and muscle. Much present day concern is based upon interest in problems of congenital muscle disease. Understanding what it is that nerves do, and how they do it, may make it possible to devise replacement therapies, either electrical or chemical, that will at least alleviate symptoms of disorders such as hereditary muscle dystrophy. In this regard it is important to determine whether particular human dystrophies are partly or wholly neurogenic. Given the lack of consensus as to the mechanism of neurotrophic actions in animals, it is no surprise to find even less agreement as to the possible role of neurogenic deficits in inducing or exacerbating human dystrophies. Interesting work has been done, however, with some hereditary mouse dystrophies.

The *med* (motor end-plate) dystrophy has an obviously neurogenic component (Duchen and Stefani, 1971) in that nerve-muscle transmission fails. The 119 ReJ and C57Bl/6J strains of dystrophic mice have a disorder which is said to resemble human Duchenne dystrophy in some respects. Although there is debate, it seems likely that nerve-muscle transmission is still intact in younger animals at a stage when other signs of dystrophy have already become apparent (Parry, 1977; Harris and Ribchester, 1978). Nevertheless, muscles in these animals show signs of denervation, such as TTX-resistant action potentials and extrajunctional ACh receptors (Harris and Montgomery, 1975; Howe et al., 1977). That some aspects of innervation may be instrumental in allowing these changes is indicated by the finding that dystrophic muscles transplanted into normal hosts develop a better functional state than after autotransplantation (Neerunjun et al., 1976). There are difficulties of interpretation in these experiments, and even greater difficulties in assessing their relevance to human disorders, but they still are of interest in directing attention to the question of whether treatments of an electrical or biochemical nature may ever be applicable to human disease.

EFFECTS OF MUSCLE ON NERVE The chromatolytic reaction of motoneurons to axotomy is associated with the synthesis of new RNA and an enhanced capacity for protein synthesis in the cell body (Watson, 1965, 1968), together with the breakdown of some pre-existing RNA (Mathews and Raisman, 1972). Watson has shown that this reaction can also occur without the axon being physically damaged, but in response to paralysis of nerve terminals with botulin toxin, or at the time a regenerating nerve begins to form synapses in denervated muscle (Watson, 1969, 1970). In other words, a mature motoneuron can change its pattern of metabolism and the amount and kind of protein it exports to its periphery in response to changes in its functional relation to the muscles it innervates. Analogous forms of sensitivity are present at particular critical times during the development of motoneurons, so that paralysis of nerve-muscle transmission at a certain time allows survival of motoneurons that otherwise would have died (Pittman and Oppenheim, 1978). Paralysis of adult muscles induces sprouting from nerve terminals within the muscle (Brown et al., 1977; Brown and Ironton, 1977); this sprouting is prevented by direct stimulation of the muscle. These responses of motoneurons are conventionally supposed to reflect the existence of some form of message carried by retrograde axonal transport from periphery to cell body, but sensory feedback (or lack of it) may also be involved (Kuno et al., 1974; Clarke and Cowan, 1975). Lewis et al. (1977) suggested, as a result of changes seen to follow experimental cross-reinnervation of cat muscles, that the conduction velocity of motor axons is regulated by the type of muscle fiber they innervate. Conduction velocity of normal axons is related to the size of motor unit they control; the size of motor units in cross-reinnervated muscles was not examined in their experiments.

CONCLUSION

It is generally agreed that most but not all (Bray et al., 1976) of the components of the muscle reaction to denervation require a change in expression of the muscle genome. Thus, the final description of the mechanism of neurotrophic control of muscle properties will include a map of the pathway of control of transcription and translation in muscle cells, and all the points along that path which can be affected by nerve-released substances, hormones, products of muscle metabolism, and so on. Only then will it be possible to assess quantitatively the relative importance of all factors involved in the normal regulation of muscle properties while in the intact normal organism. Present knowledge allows us to list factors which affect muscle properties in various experimental circumstances but not the extent to which they affect these properties in normal, active adult muscle.

References

Abe, T., Limbrick, A. R., and Miledi, R.: Acute muscle denervation induced by β-bungarotoxin. Proc. R. Soc. Lond. [Biol.], *194*:545–553, 1976.

Albuquerque, E. X., and McIsaac, R. J.: Fast and slow mammalian muscles after denervation. Exp. Neurol., *26*:183–202, 1970.

Albuquerque, E. X., Schuh, F. T., and Kauffman, F. C.: Early membrane depolarisation of the fast mammalian muscle after denervation. Pfluegers Arch., *328*:36–50, 1971.

Albuquerque, E. X., Warnick, J. E., Tasse, J. R., and Sansone, F. M.: Effects of vinblastine and colchicine on neural regulation of the fast and slow skeletal muscles of the rat. Exp. Neurol., *37*:607–634, 1972.

Anderson, P., and Sears, T. A.: The mechanical properties and innervation of fast and slow motor units in the intercostal muscles of the cat. J. Physiol., *173*:114–129, 1964.

Axelsson, J., and Thesleff, S.: A study of supersensitivity in denervated mammalian skeletal muscle. J. Physiol. *147*:178–193, 1959.

Belmar, J., and Eyzaguirre, C.: Pacemaker site of fibrillation potentials in denervated mammalian muscle. J. Neurophysiol., *29*:425–441, 1966.

Bennett, M. R., Pettigrew, A. G., and Taylor, R. S.: The formation of synapses in reinnervated and cross-reinnervated adult avian muscle. J. Physiol., *230*:331–357, 1973.

Berg, D. K., and Hall, Z. W.: Loss of α-bungarotoxin from junctional and extrajunctional acetylcholine receptors in rat diaphragm muscle in vivo and in organ culture. J. Physiol., *252*:771–789, 1975.

Berg, D. K., Kelly, R. B., Sargent, P. B., Williamson, P., and Hall, Z. W.: Binding of α-bungarotoxin to acetylcholine receptors in mammalian muscle. Proc. Natl. Acad. Sci. U.S.A., *69*:147–151, 1972.

Bisby, M. A.: Inhibition of axonal transport in nerves chronically treated with local anesthetics. Exp. Neurol., *47*:481–489, 1975.

Braithwaite, A. W., and Harris, A. J.: Neural influence on acetylcholine receptor clusters in embryonic development of skeletal muscles. Nature, *279*:549–551, 1979*a*.

Braithwaite, A. W., and Harris, A. J.: Neurotoxins in the study of neuronal development. *In* Chubb, I., and Geffen, L. (eds.): Neurotoxins. Adelaide, University of Adelaide Press, 1979*b*, pp. 143–150.

Bray, J. J., and Harris, A. J.: Dissociation between nerve-muscle transmission and nerve trophic effects on rat diaphragm using type D botulinum toxin. J. Physiol., *253*:53–77, 1975.

Bray, J. J., Hawken, M. J., Hubbard, J. I., Pockett, S., and Wilson, L.: The membrane potential of rat diaphragm muscle fibres and the effect of denervation. J. Physiol., *255*:651–667, 1976.

Bray, J. J., Mills, R. G., and Hubbard, J. I.: The trophic influence of tetrodotoxin-inactivated nerves on normal and reinnervated rat skeletal muscles. J. Physiol., *297*:479–492, 1979.

Brockes, J. P., Berg, D. K., and Hall, Z. W.: The biochemical properties and regulation of acetylcholine receptors in normal and denervated muscle. Cold Spring Harbor Symp. Quant. Biol., *40*:253–262, 1975.

Brown, G. L.: The actions of acetylcholine on denervated mammalian and frog's muscle. J. Physiol., *89*:438–461, 1937.

TROPHIC EFFECTS OF NERVE ON MUSCLE

Brown, M. C., Goodwin, G. M., and Ironton, R.: Prevention of motor nerve sprouting in botulinum toxin-poisoned mouse soleus muscles by direct stimulation of the muscle. J. Physiol., *267*:42P, 1977.

Brown, M. C., and Ironton, R.: Suppression of motor nerve terminal sprouting in partially denervated mouse muscles. J. Physiol. *272*:70P, 1977.

Buller, A. J., Eccles, J. C., and Eccles, R. M.: Differentiation of fast and slow muscles in the cat hind limb. J. Physiol., *150*:399–416, 1960*a*.

Buller, A. J., Eccles, J. C., and Eccles, R. M.: Interactions between motoneurones and muscles in respect of the characteristic speeds of their responses. J. Physiol., *150*:417–439, 1960*b*.

Burden, S.: Development of the neuromuscular junction in the chick embryo: the number, distribution and stability of acetylcholine receptors. Dev. Biol., *57*:317–329, 1977.

Burden, S. J., Sargent, P. B., and McMahan, U. J.: Acethylcholine receptors in regenerating muscle accumulate at original synaptic sites in the absence of the nerve. J. Cell. Biol., *82*:412–429, 1979.

Burke, R. E., Levine, D. N., Zajac, F. E., Tsairis, P., and Engel, W. K.: Mammalian motor units: Physiological-histochemical correlation in three types of cat gastrocnemius. Science, *174*:709–712, 1971.

Byers, M. R., Fink, B. R., Kennedy, R. D., Middaugh, M. E., and Hendrickson, A. E.: Effects of lidocaine on axonal morphology, microtubules and rapid transport in rabbit vagus nerve *in vitro*. J. Neurobiol., *4*:125–143, 1973.

Cangiano, A., and Fried, J. A.: The production of denervation-like changes in rat muscle by colchicine, without interference with axonal transport or muscle activity. J. Physiol., *265*:63–84, 1977.

Cangiano, A., and Lutzemberger, L.: Partial denervation affects both denervated and innervated fibres in the mammalian skeletal muscle. Science, *196*:542–545, 1977.

Cangiano, A., Lutzemberger, L., and Nicotra, L.: Non-equivalence of impulse blockade and denervation in the production of membrane changes in rat skeletal muscle. J. Physiol., *273*:691–706, 1977.

Card, D. J.: Denervation: Sequence of neuromuscular degenerative changes in rats and the effect of stimulation. Exp. Neurol., *54*:251–265, 1977.

Carlson, B. M.: A quantitative study of muscle fibre survival and regeneration in normal, predenervated, and marcaine-treated free muscle grafts in the rat. Exp. Neurol., *52*:421–432, 1976.

Carlson, B. M., and Gutmann, E.: Contractile and histochemical properties of sliced muscle grafts regenerating in normal and denervated rat limbs. Exp. Neurol., *50*:319–329, 1976.

Clarke, P. G. H., and Cowan, W. M.: Ectopic neurons and aberrant connections during neural development. Proc. Natl. Acad. Sci. U.S.A., *72*:4455–4458, 1975.

Clausen, T., and Flatman, J. A.: The effect of catecholamines on Na-K transport and membrane potential in rat soleus muscle. J. Physiol., *270*:383–414, 1977.

Close, R.: Dynamic properties of fast and slow skeletal muscles of the rat after nerve cross-union. J. Physiol., *204*:331–346, 1969.

Dennis, M. J., and Ort, C. A.: The distribution of acetylcholine receptors on muscle fibres of regenerating salamander limbs. J. Physiol., *266*:765–776, 1977.

Dennis, M. J., and Sargent, P. B.: Loss of extrasynoptic acetylcholine sensitivity upon reinnervation of parasympathetic ganglion cells. J. Physiol., *289*:263–276, 1979.

Deshpande, S. S., Albuquerque, E. X., and Guth, L.: Neurotrophic regulation of prejunctional and post junctional membrane at the mammalian motor endplate. Exp. Neurol., *53*:151–165, 1976.

Devreotes, P. N., and Fambrough, D. M.: Turnover of acetylcholine receptors in skeletal muscle. Cold Spring Harbor Symp. Quant. Biol., *40*:237–251, 1975.

Drachman, D. B.: Is acetylcholine the trophic neuromuscular transmitter? Arch. Neurol., *17*:206–218, 1967.

Duchen, L. W., and Stefani, E.: Electrophysiological studies of neuromuscular transmission in hereditary 'motor end-plate disease' of the mouse. J. Physiol., *212*:535–548, 1971.

Eastlick, H. L.: Studies on transplanted embryonic limbs of the chick. J. Exp. Zool., *93*:27–45, 1943.

Eccles, J. C.: Disuse atrophy of skeletal muscle. Med. J. Aust., *2*:160–164, 1941.

Eccles, J. C.: Investigations on muscle atrophies arising from disuse and tenotomy. J. Physiol., *103*:253–266, 1944.

Eccles, J. C., Eccles, R. M., and Kozak, W.: Further investigations on the influence of motoneurones on the speed of muscle contraction. J. Physiol., *163*:324–339, 1962.

Edstrom, L., and Kugelberg, E.: Histochemical composition, distribution of fibres, and fatiguability of single motor units. J. Neurol. Neurosurg. Psychiatry, *31*:424–433, 1968.

Engel, W. K.: Fiber-type nomenclature of human skeletal muscle for histochemical purposes. Neurology, *24*:344–348, 1974.

Engel, W. K., Karpati, G.: Impaired skeletal muscle maturation following neonatal neurectomy. Dev. Biol., *17*:713–723, 1968.

Fambrough, D. M.: Acetylcholine sensitivity of muscle fiber membranes: Mechanism of regulation by motoneurons. Science, *168*:372–373, 1970.

Fambrough, D. M., and Devreotes, P. N.: Newly synthesized acetylcholine receptors are located in the Golgi apparatus. J. Cell Biol., *76*:237–244, 1978.

Fernandez, H. L.: Neurotrophic effects in relation to axoplasmic transport. Acta Fisologica (Lat. Am.), *23*:189–191, 1973.

Fernandez, H. L., and Ramirez, B. U.: Muscle fibrillation induced by blockage of axoplasmic transport in motor nerves. Brain Res., *79*:385–395, 1974.

Fischbach, G. D., and Robbins, N.: Changes in contractile

properties of disused soleus muscles. J. Physiol., *201*:305–320, 1969.

Fowler, T. J., Danta, G., and Gilliatt, R. W.: Recovery of nerve conduction after a pneumatic tourniquet: Observations on the hindlimb of the baboon. J. Neurol. Neurosurg. Psychiatry, *35*:638–647, 1972.

Frank, E., Nothmann, M., and Hirsch-Kauffmann, H.: Über die "tonische" Kontraktion des quergestreiften Säugetier muskels nach Ausschaltung des motorischen Nerven. Pfluegers Arch., *197*:270–287, 1922.

Gilliatt, R. W., Westgaard, R. H., and Williams, I. R.: Acetylcholine sensitivity of denervated and inactivated baboon muscle fibres. J. Physiol., *271*:21–22P, 1977.

Gilliatt, R. W., Westgaard, R. H., and Williams, I. R.: Extrajunctional acetylcholine sensitivity of inactive muscle fibers in the baboon during prolonged nerve pressure block. J. Physiol., *280*:499–514, 1978.

Goldberg, A. L.: Protein turnover in skeletal muscle. I. Protein catabolism during work-induced hypertrophy and growth induced with growth hormone. J. Biol. Chem., *244*:3217–3222, 1969*a*.

Goldberg, A. L.: Protein turnover in skeletal muscle. II. Effects of denervation and cortisone on protein catabolism in skeletal muscle. J. Biol. Chem., *244*:3223–3229, 1969*b*.

Grampp, W., Harris, J. B., and Thesleff, S.: Inhibition of denervation changes in skeletal muscle by blockers of protein synthesis. J. Physiol., *221*:743–754, 1972.

Guth, L.: "Trophic" influences of nerve on muscle. Physiol. Rev., *48*:645–687, 1968.

Gutmann, E. (ed.): The Denervated Muscle. Prague, Czech Academy of Sciences, 1962.

Gutmann, E.: Neurotrophic relations. Ann. Rev. Physiol., *38*:177–216, 1976.

Gutmann, E., and Hnik, P. (eds.): The Effect of Use and Disuse on Neuromuscular Functions. Amsterdam, Elsevier, 1963.

Hamburger, V., and Hamilton, H. L.: A series of normal stages in the development of the chick embryo. J. Morphol., *88*:49–92, 1951.

Harris, A. J.: Inductive functions of the nervous system. Ann. Rev. Physiol., *36*:251–305, 1974.

Harris, A. J., and Miledi, R.: A study of frog muscle maintained in organ culture. J. Physiol., *221*:207–226, 1972.

Harris, J. B., and Montgomery, A.: Some mechanical and electrical properties of dorsal hind limb muscles of genetically dystrophic mice (C57Bl/6J dy^{2J}/dy^{2J}). Exp. Neurol., *48*:569–585, 1975.

Harris, J. B., and Ribchester, R. R.: Neuromuscular transmission is adequate in identified abnormal dystrophic muscle fibres. Nature, *271*:362–364, 1978.

Hartzell, H. C., and Fambrough, D. M.: Acetylcholine receptors. Distribution and extrajunctional density in rat diaphragm after denervation correlated with acetylcholine sensitivity. J. Gen. Physiol., *60*:284–292, 1972.

Harvey, A. M., and Kuffler, S. W.: Motor nerve function with lesions of the peripheral nerves. Arch. Neurol. Psychiatry, (Chicago), 52:317–322, 1944a.

Harvey, A. M., and Kuffler, S. W.: Synchronization of spontaneous activity in denervated human muscle. Arch. Neurol. Psychiatry (Chicago), 52:495–498, 1944b.

Hayes, G. J., and Woolsey, C. N.: The unit of fibrillary activity and the site of origin of fibrillary contractions in denervated striated muscle. Fed. Proc., 1:38, 1942.

Hoffman, W. W., and Thesleff, S.: Studies of the trophic influence of nerve on skeletal muscle. Eur. J. Pharmacol., 20:256–260, 1972.

Holtzer, H., and Detwiler, S.: Induction of skeletogenous cells. J. Exp. Zool., 123:335–369, 1953.

Howe, P. R. C., Telfer, J. A., Livett, B. G., and Austin, L.: Extrajunctional acetylcholine receptors in dystrophic mouse muscles. Exp. Neurol., 56:42–51, 1977.

Jirmanová, I., and Thesleff, S.: Ultrastructural study of experimental muscle degeneration and regeneration in the adult rat. Z. Zellforsch, 131:77–97, 1972.

Johns, T. R., and Thesleff, S.: Effects of motor inactivation on the chemical sensitivity of skeletal muscle. Acta Physiol. Scand., 51:136–141, 1961.

Jones, R., and Vyskočil, F.: An electrophysiological examination of the changes in skeletal muscle fibres in response to degenerating nerve tissues. Brain Res., 88:309–317, 1975.

Kaufmann, F. C., Warnick,. J. E., and Albuquerque, E. X.: Uptake of [^{3}H] colchicine from silastic implants by mammalian nerves and muscles. Exp. Neurol., 44:404–416, 1974.

Kelly, A. M., and Zacks, S. I.: The fine structure of motor endplate morphogenesis. J. Cell Biol., 42:154–169, 1969.

Kidman, A. D., Dolan, L., and Sippe, H. J.: Blockade of fast axonal transport by diphtheritic demyelination in the chicken sciatic nerve. J. Neurochem., 30:57–62, 1978.

Konigsberg, I. R.: Clonal analysis of myogenesis. Science, 140:1273–1284, 1963.

Kuffler, S. W., and Yoshikami, D.: The distribution of acetylcholine sensitivity at the post-synaptic membrane of vertebrate skeletal twitch muscles; iontophoretic mapping in the micron range. J. Physiol., 244:703–730, 1975.

Kuno, M., Miyata, Y., and Muñoz-Martinez, E. J.: Properties of fast and slow alpha motoneurones following motor reinnervations. J. Physiol., 242:273–288, 1974.

Landmesser, L., and Morris, D. G.: The development of functional innervation in the hind limb of the chick embryo. J. Physiol., 249:301–326, 1975.

Langley, J. N.: The sympathetic and other related systems of nerves. In Schafer, E. A. (ed.): Textbook of Physiology. London, Pentland, 1900, pp. 616–696.

Langley, J. N.: Remarks on the cause and nature of the changes which occur in muscle after nerve section. Lancet, 191:6–7, 1916.

Langley, J. N., and Kato, T.: The physiological actions of physostigmine and its action on denervated skeletal muscle. J. Physiol., 49:410–431, 1915.

Lavoie, P. A., Collier, B., and Tenenhouse, A.: Comparison of α-bungarotoxin binding to skeletal muscles after inactivity or denervation. Nature, 260:349–350, 1976.

Lavoie, P. A., Collier, B., and Tenenhouse, A.: Role of skeletal muscle activity in the control of muscle acetylcholine sensitivity. Exp. Neurol., 54:148–171, 1977.

Lee, C. Y., Tseng, L. F., and Chiu, T. H.: Influence of denervation on localization of neurotoxins from Elapid venoms in rat diaphragm. Nature, 215:1177–1178, 1967.

Lee, J. C.: Electron microscopic observations on myogenic free cells of denervated skeletal muscle. Exp. Neurol., 12:123–135, 1965.

Lewis, D. M., Bagust, J., Webb, S. N., Westerman, R. A., and Finol, H. J.: Axon conduction velocity modified by reinnervation of mammalian muscle. Nature, 270:745–746, 1977.

Locke S., and Solomon, H. C.: Relation of resting potentials of rat gastrocnemius and soleus muscles to innervation, activity and the Na-K pump. J. Exp. Zool., 166:378–386, 1967.

Lømo, T.: Neurotrophic control of colchicine effects on muscle? Nature, 249:473–474, 1974.

Lømo, T., and Rosenthal, J.: Control of ACh sensitivity by muscle activity in the rat. J. Physiol., 221:493–513, 1972.

Lømo, T., and Westgaard, R. H.: Control of ACh sensitivity in rat muscle fibres. Cold Spring Harbor Symp. Quant. Biol., 40:263–274, 1975.

Mathews, M. R., and Raisman, G.: A light and electron microscopic study of the cellular response to axonal injury in the superior cervical ganglion on the rat. Proc. R. Soc. Lond. [Biol.], 181:43–79, 1972.

McArdle, J. J., and Albuquerque, E. X.: A study of the reinnervation of fast and slow mammalian muscles. J. Gen. Physiol., 61:1–23, 1973.

McArdle, J. J., and Sansone, F. M.: Reinnervation of rat fast and slow twitch muscle following nerve crush at birth. J. Physiol. 271:567–586, 1977.

Miledi, R.: The acetylcholine sensitivity of frog muscle fibres after complete or partial denervation. J. Physiol. Lond., 151:1–23, 1960a.

Miledi, R.: Properties of regenerating neuromuscular synapses in the frog. J. Physiol., 154:190–205, 1960b.

Miledi, R.: An influence of nerve not mediated by impulses. In Gutmann, E., and Hnik, P. (eds.): The Effect of Use and Disuse on Neuromuscular Functions. Amsterdam, Elsevier, 1963, pp. 35–40.

Miledi, R., and Potter, L. T.: Acetylcholine receptors in muscle fibres. Nature, 233:599–603, 1971.

Miledi, R., and Slater, C. R.: On the degeneration of rat neuromuscular junctions after nerve section. J. Physiol., 207:507–528, 1970.

Miledi, R., Stefani, E., and Steinbach, A. B.: Induction of the action potential mechanism in slow muscle fibres of the frog. J. Physiol., 217:737–754, 1971.

Miledi, R., and Trowell, O. A.: Acetylcholine sensitivity of rat diaphragm maintained in organ culture. Nature, 194:981–982, 1962.

217

Miledi, R., and Zelena, J.: Sensitivity to acetylcholine in rat slow muscle. Nature, *210*:855–856, 1966.

Mills, R. G., and Bray, J. J.: A slow-release technique for inducing prolonged paralysis by tetrodotoxin. Pfluegers Arch., *383*: 67–74, 1979.

Moravec, J., Melichar, I., Jansky, L., and Vyskocil, F.: Effect of hibernation and noradrenaline on the resting state of neuro-muscular junction of golden hamster (*Mesocricetus auratus*). Pfluegers Arch., *345*:93–106, 1973.

Neerunjun, J. S., Jones, D. A., and Dubowitz, V.: Functional properties of muscles transplanted between normal and dystrophic mice. Exp. Neurol., *52*:556–564, 1976.

Ochoa, J., Fowler, T. J., and Gilliatt, R. W.: Anatomical changes in peripheral nerves compressed by a pneumatic tourniquet. J. Anat., *113*:443–455, 1972.

Ochs, S.: Energy metabolism and supply of $\sim$P to the fast axoplasmic transport mechanism in nerve. Fed. Proc., *33*:1049–1058, 1974.

Parry, D. J.: A study of functional denervation in fast and slow muscles of dystrophic mice of various ages. Exp. Neurol., *55*:556–566, 1977.

Pestronk, A., Drachman, D. B., and Griffin, J. W.: Effect of muscle disuse on acetylcholine receptors. Nature, *260*:352–353, 1976.

Pittman, R. H., and Oppenheim, R. W.: Neuromuscular block-ade increases motoneurone survival during normal cell death in the chick embryo. Nature, *271*:364–365, 1978.

Pockett, S.: Clustering of acetylcholine receptors during neu-romuscular synapse formation in rat and chick embryos. Otago, New Zealand, University of Otago, PhD. thesis, 1977.

Purves, D., and Sakmann, B.: The effect of contractile activity on fibrillation and extrajunctional acetylcholine sensitivity of rat muscle maintained in organ culture. J. Physiol., *237*:157–182, 1974a.

Purves, D., and Sakmann, B.: Membrane properties underlying spontaneous activity of denervated muscle fibres. J. Physiol., *239*:125–153, 1974b.

Redfern, P., and Thesleff, S.: Action potential generation in denervated rat skeletal muscle. II. The action of tetrodotoxin. Acta Physiol. Scand., *82*:70–78, 1971.

Robbins, N.: Cation movements in normal and short-term den-ervated rat fast twitch muscle. J. Physiol., *271*:605–624, 1977.

Robbins, N., Antosiak, J., Gerding, R., and Uchitel, O. D.: Nonacceptance of innervation by innervated neonatal rat mus-cle. Dev. Biol. *61*:166–176, 1977.

Robert, E. D., and Oester, Y. T.: Nerve impulses and trophic effect. Arch. Neurol., *22*:57–63, 1970a.

Robert, E. D., and Oester, Y. T.: Absence of supersensitivity to acetylcholine in innervated muscle subjected to a prolonged pharmacologic nerve block. J. Pharmacol. Exp. Ther., *174*:133–140, 1970b.

Romanes, G. J.: Motor localization and the effects of nerve injury on the ventral horn cells of the spinal cord. J. Anat., *80*:117–131, 1946.

Salafsky, B., Bell, J., and Prewitt, M.: Development of fibrillation potentials in denervated fast and slow skeletal muscle. J. Physiol., *215*:637–643, 1968.

Sanes, J. R., and Hall, Z. W.: Antibodies that bind specifically to synaptic sites on muscle fiber basal lamina. J. Cell. Biol., *83*:357–370, 1979.

Sanes, J. R., Marshall, L. M., and McMahan, U. J.: Reinnervation of muscle fiber basal lamina after removal of myofibers. Differentiation of regenerating axons at original synaptic sites. J. Cell. Biol., *78*:176–198, 1978.

Schiff, M.: Ueber motorische laehmung der zunge. Tüb. Arch. Phys. Heilk, *10*:579–593, 1851.

Shellswell, G. B.: The formation of discrete muscles from the chick wing dorsal and ventral muscle masses in the absence of nerves. J. Embryol. Exp. Morphol., *41*:269–277, 1977.

Smith, J. W., and Thesleff, S.: Spontaneous activity in denervated mouse diaphragm muscle. J. Physiol., *257*:171–186, 1976.

Solandt, D. Y., Delury, D. B., and Hunter, J.: Effect of electrical stimulation on atrophy of denervated skeletal muscle. Arch. Neurol. Psychiatry, *49*:802–807, 1943.

Solandt, D. Y., and Magladery, J. W.: The relation of atrophy to fibrillation in denervated muscle. Brain, *63*:255–263, 1940.

Solandt, D. Y., and Magladery, J. W.: A comparison of effects of upper and lower motor neurone lesions on skeletal muscle. J. Neurophysiol., *5*:373–380, 1942.

Stewart, D. M.: Effect of age on the response of four muscles of the rat to denervation. Am. J. Physiol., *214*:1139–1146, 1968.

Stewart, D. M., Sola, O. M., and Martin, A. W.: Hypertrophy as a response to denervation in skeletal muscle. J. Physiol., *76*:146–167, 1972.

Studitsky, A., Zhenuskaya, R., and Rumyantseva, O.: The role of neurotrophic influences upon the restitution of structure and function of regenerating muscles. *In* Gutmann, E., and Hnik, P. (eds.): The Effect of Use and Disuse on Neuromuscular Functions. Amsterdam, Elsevier, 1963, pp. 71–81.

Thesleff, S., and Ward, M. R.: Studies on the mechanism of fibrillation potentials in denervated muscle. J. Physiol., *244*:313–323, 1975.

Tiedt, T. N., Albuquerque, E. X., and Guth, L.: Degenerating nerve fiber products do not alter physiological properties of adjacent innervated skeletal muscle fibers. Science, *198*:839–841, 1977a.

Tiedt, T. N., Wisler, P. L., and Youngkin, S. G.: Neurotrophic regulation of resting membrane potential and acetylcholine sensitivity in rat extensor digitorum longus muscle. Exp. Neurol., *57*:766–791, 1977b.

Tower, S. S.: The reaction of muscle to denervation. Physiol. Rev., *19*:1–48, 1939.

Tower, S. S., Howe, H., and Bodian, D.: Fibrillation in skeletal muscle in relation to denervation and to inactivation without denervation. J. Neurophysiol., *4*:398–401, 1941.

Warnick, J. E., Albuquerque, E. X., and Guth, L.: The demonstration of neurotrophic function by application of colchicine

219

or vinblastine to the peripheral nerve. Exp. Neurol., *57*:622–636, 1977.

Watson, W. E.: An autoradiographic study of the incorporation of nucleic-acid precursors by neurones and glia during nerve regeneration. J. Physiol., *180*:741–753, 1965.

Watson, W. E.: Observations on the nucleolar and total cell body nucleic acid of injured nerve cells. J. Physiol. *196*:655–676, 1968.

Watson, W. E.: Some metabolic responses of motor neurones to axotomy and to botulinum toxin after nerve transplantation. J. Physiol., *204*:138P, 1969.

Watson, W. E.: Some metabolic responses of axotomized neurones to contact between their axons and denervated muscle. J. Physiol., *210*:321–343, 1970.

Watson, W. E.: Cellular responses to axotomy and to related procedures. Br. Med. Bull., *30*:112–115, 1974.

Weddell, G., Feinstein, B., and Pattle, R. E.: The electrical activity of voluntary muscle in man under normal and pathological conditions. Brain, *67*:178–257, 1944.

Yaffe, D.: Retention of differentiation potentialities during prolonged cultivation of myogenic cells. Proc. Natl. Acad. Sci. U.S.A., *61*:477–483, 1968.

Zak, R., Grove, D., and Rabinowitz, M.: DNA synthesis in the rat diaphragm as an early response to denervation. Am. J. Physiol., *216*:647–654, 1969.

Zelena, J., and Hnik, P.: Absence of spindles in muscles of rats reinnervated during development. Physiol. Bohemoslov., *9*:373–381, 1960.

Ziskind, L., and Harris, A. J.: Reinnervation of adult muscle in organ culture restores tetrodotoxin sensitivity in the absence of electrical activity. Dev. Biol., *69*:388–399, 1979.

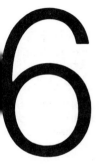

Axoplasmic Transport

David Pleasure

David Pleasure

INTRODUCTION Transport of macromolecules from sites of synthesis through cytosol to sites of function, or to plasma membrane for export, is a vital function of all cells. Agents which interfere with transport, such as colchicine and the vinca alkaloids, have profound effects upon the expression of specialized cellular functions. Thus, colchicine inhibits release of secretory materials from lacrimal glands (Chambaut-Guerin et al., 1978), fibrinogen from hepatocytes (Feldmann, et al., 1975), collagen from fibroblasts (Ehrlich and Bornstein, 1972; Harwood, et al., 1976), and peptide hormones from endocrine tissues (Bhattacharyya and Wolff, 1975; Sheterline et al., 1975).

Cytosolic transport is particularly prominent in neurons (Lubinska, 1964; Smith, 1971b; Weiss, 1972a, b; Jeffrey and Austin, 1973; Ochs, 1977). The mass of the axon relative to the neuronal perikaryon is immense, and axons are relatively poor in rough endoplasmic reticulum and Golgi apparatus, organelles required for synthesis and processing of proteins and lipids. Moreover, neurons are active secretory cells (Smith, 1971a, b), and most products are released at the axon terminal, often far removed from the cell body (Dahlstrom, 1971).

SLOW AXOPLASMIC TRANSPORT Transport of materials from neuronal perikaryon to axon terminal was postulated in 1906 (Scott, 1906), and studies of the phenomenon began during World War II (Weiss and Hiscoe, 1948). It was observed that when a constricting band was placed around a peripheral nerve, axons proximal to the constriction became folded and segmentally dilated. Distal to the constriction, axons were of reduced caliber. When the constricting band was released, axonal folding proximal to the constriction cleared and axons in the distal segment enlarged toward normal.

221

AXOPLASMIC TRANSPORT

To explain these findings, it was hypothesized that axoplasm is extruded by the nerve cell body like toothpaste from a tube, accumulates proximal to the "bottleneck" caused by the constricting band, and then moves distally when the obstruction is relieved. Based on the rate at which the redundant axonal segments appeared after the band was placed, and cleared after the constriction was removed, it was calculated that 1 to 2 mm of new axon is synthesized each day (Weiss and Hiscoe, 1948; Weiss, 1972a, b). This represents a mass of axonal cytoplasm considerably greater than the volume of the nerve cell body itself.

The neuronal perikaryon could not possibly exert sufficient force through a narrow axon to propel axoplasm many centimeters away. Some local process in the axon itself, or in its supporting cells, was hypothesized to provide such a force. Cinemicrographic observations of spontaneous, propagated axonal pulsations occurring at half-hourly intervals in organotypic dorsal root ganglion cultures were taken as visual evidence for such a local axonal process (Weiss, 1972a, b).

Later studies demonstrated that the original constriction experiments were somewhat misleading. Segmental axonal kinking above a nerve constriction reflected axonal transection and retraction. Segmental axonal dilatation in this nerve segment was usually due to the formation of axonal growth cones (Pinner-Poole and Campbell, 1969; Spencer, 1972). Thus, buckling and dilatation originally attributed to a "bottleneck" to flow in anatomically continuous axons was largely due, instead, to axonal disruption and regeneration. Many of the thin axons distal to the constriction, thought originally to represent axoplasm-starved continuations of segmentally constricted axons, were instead regenerating axonal sprouts (Spencer, 1972).

The development of in vitro techniques for serial observation of the process of axonal elongation by living neurons provided an opportunity for direct study of the axonal assembly process. It was noted that as bifurcated axons elongated the site of bifurcation remained stationary. When axonal plasma membrane was "tagged" with small adherent particles these particles did not move peripherally as the axon lengthened but rather remained stationary or, when near the growth cone, moved back toward neuronal perikaryon (Bray, 1970). Thus, new axonal segments appear to be assembled at the elongating axonal tip, not at the perikaryon as originally thought.

Although some of the conclusions drawn from the constriction experiments were incorrect, radiotracer experiments have confirmed the existence of bulk flow of axonal components from neuronal perikaryon into and through the axon (McEwen and Grafstein, 1968; Grafstein et al., 1970; Feit et al., 1971). Radioactive amino acids, injected into a dorsal root ganglion, anterior horn of the spinal cord, or posterior chamber of the eye, applied to the ventricular surface above brain stem motor nuclei, or injected intracellularly, are incorporated into proteins (Karlsson, 1977) and move toward the periphery within axons at the rate of a few millimeters/day. This is similar to the velocity of outgrowth of axonal sprouts in developing and regenerating neural tissue. Glycolytic enzymes and mitochondria are minor constituents of this slow flowing fraction (DiGiamberadino et al., 1973; Khan and Ochs, 1975). Resolution of the labelled flowing peptides by SDS-polyacrylamide gel electrophoresis indicated that more than 75 per cent of the total is made up of five peptides, two of which are the alpha and beta subunits of tubulin (Feit et al., 1971; Hoffman and Lasek, 1975; Luduena et al., 1977). The other three peptides have not been positively identified, but may be neurofilament components or myosin peptides (Blitz and Fine, 1974; Hoffman and Lasek, 1975; Gilbert et al., 1975). Recently, actin has been shown to be a minor component of the slow-flowing protein fraction (Black and Lasek, 1979).

Tubulin is the most abundant axonal protein (Bamburg et al., 1973; Blitz and Fine, 1974; Pleasure, 1975), and is important in the maintenance of neuronal shape (Daniels, 1972) and axoplasmic flow. Tubulin is polymerized into 25-nanometer diameter microtubules which form an internal cytoskeleton (Osborn et al., 1978). Tubulin polymerization is dependent upon hydrolysis of bound GTP (MacNeal and Purich, 1977) and is guided by a group of tubulin-associated "tau" proteins (Cleveland et al., 1977; Lockwood, 1978). Colchicine binds to tubulin and prevents its polymerization into microtubules (Luduena et al., 1977), thus causing microtubule dissociation and axonal retraction (Daniels, 1972). Vinca alkaloids (vincristine and vinblastine) also bind to tubulin, forming paracrystalline tubulin aggregates and thereby dissociating microtubules (Schlaepfer, 1971).

In unicellular organisms there is evidence for a large pool of cytosolic nonpolymerized tubulin (Weeks and Collis, 1976). Unicellular organisms draw upon this pool when called upon to synthesize new microtubules. In addition, during formation of flagellae, there is a rapid rise in the level of tubulin messenger RNA, with a consequent increase in synthesis of tubulin monomer (Weeks and Collis, 1976). A tubulin monomer pool is also available in neurons (Davison, 1975) and, during the "central chromatolysis" that follows axon section (Grafstein, 1975), induction of tubulin synthesis probably occurs to supplement this pool.

Two other neuronal cytoskeletal systems should be mentioned: 6-nanometer actin microfilaments (Buckley, 1974; Wolosewick and Porter, 1976) and 10-nanometer intermediate filaments (neurofilaments) (Metuzals and Mushynski, 1974; Lazarides and Hubbard, 1976). Actin microfilaments are abundant in nerve terminals (Blitz and Fine, 1974) and in the growth cones of developing and regenerating neurons (Yamada et al., 1970), where they insert into plasma membrane. Cytochalasin B disorganizes actin microfilaments (Buckley, 1974; Godman and Miranda, 1978) and causes axonal retraction and loss of axonal motility (Yamada et al., 1970; Wessells et al., 1971; Godman and Miranda, 1978). Although actin microfilaments have not been appreciated elsewhere in axons by usual electron microscopic methods, adult neural tissue contains considerable actin (Puszkin and Berl, 1972; Santerre and Rich, 1976), and recent high voltage electron microscopic and immunofluorescent studies suggest that most cells have a rich cytosolic network of actin microfilaments (Buckley, 1974; Wolosewick and Porter, 1976). It is conceivable that an actin network is present in axons and plays a role in bulk axoplasmic flow, perhaps by contributing to the "microperistaltic waves" previously described (Weiss, 1972a, b). The role of the 10-nanometer intermediate filaments in neuronal function has not been established, but these filaments accumulate in neuronal perikaryon and in axons when axoplasmic flow is interrupted (Hansson and Sjostrand, 1971; Schlaepfer, 1971; Fink et al., 1973; Friede and Ho, 1977). Filaments of similar dimensions accumulate in the cytoplasm of nonneural cells exposed to colchicine (Moellman and McGuire, 1975; Blose and Chacko, 1976).

If bulk axoplasmic flow were the only mechanism for transport of materials in neurons, chemical communication between perikaryon and axon would be unidirectional and require weeks or months. Other mechanisms than slow axoplasmic transport must exist to explain the rapid accumulation of dense core catecholamine-containing vesicles in the proximal stump of transected autonomic neurons, the profound metabolic changes induced in neuronal perikaryon within a few days after axon section many centimeters away, and the trophic effects of end-organs on neurons.

FAST AXOPLASMIC TRANSPORT

Fast axoplasmic transport provides a system by which neuronal perikarya can influence the metabolism of axon terminals on a day to day basis. Early evidence for fast axoplasmic transport, several orders of magnitude more rapid than bulk flow of axonal structural components, was provided by direct light microscopic observation of living axons (Lubinska, 1964). Particles near the limit of resolution of the microscope were in erratic movement, with net velocities many times that explicable by slow axoplasmic transport. Apparently anomalous results of autonomic nerve constriction experiments also suggested the existence of fast axoplasmic transport. Catecholamine-containing vesicles and vesicle-associated enzymes were noted to collect above a constriction or crush far more rapidly, given the concentration of these organelles in axoplasm, than could be explained by bulk axoplasmic flow (Dahlstrom and Haggendal, 1966; Dahlstrom, 1971).

Further evidence for fast axoplasmic transport was obtained by histochemical and radiochemical tracer experiments (Fukuda and Koelle, 1959; Kasa, 1968; McEwen and Grafstein, 1968). In the central nervous system radioactive amino acids are incorporated into neuronal proteins, and the labelled proteins appear in the synaptosomal fraction within hours (Barondes, 1968). In the PNS, although the bulk of labelled proteins moves through the axon at the rate of only a few mm/day, a small portion moves much more rapidly, with the radioactive crest passing distally in cat sciatic nerve, for example, at more than 400 mm/day (Ochs, 1972). SDS-polyacrylamide gel electrophoresis indicates that there are many labelled peptides in this fast flowing fraction, in contrast to the simpler pattern in the bulk flow fraction (Willard et al., 1974). Much of the rapidly transported fraction is particulate, made up in part of neurotransmitter vesicles and associated enzymes (McEwen and Grafstein, 1968; Karlsson and Sjostrand, 1971; DiGiamberardino et al., 1973; Anderson and McClure, 1973; Willard et al., 1974). Vesicles containing antidiuretic hormone and oxytocin, with associated carrier neurophysins, move at similar rates in the hypothalamohypophyseal tract (Dustin et al., 1975; Ochs, 1977).

Initial "packaging" of materials for fast axoplasmic transport (e.g., incorporation of radioactive amino acids into proteins in rough endoplasmic reticulum, posttranslational modifications in Golgi apparatus, assembly of vesicles) requires the neuronal perikaryon (Fukuda and Koelle, 1959; Kasa, 1968; Smith, 1971b), and this packaging takes an hour or more (Gross and Kreutzberg, 1978). If fast axoplasmic transport is blocked, perikaryal synthesis of materials normally destined for export to the axon continues, and these materials accumulate in perikaryon. For example, normally low concentrations of neurotransmitter synthetic enzymes in nerve cell body may increase considerably (Ribak et al., 1978). Once the material to be transported enters the axon, however, the neuronal perikaryon is no longer required, and fast axoplasmic transport proceeds for many hours in isolated nerve segments maintained in vitro in a well aerated medium (Lubinska, 1964; Ochs, 1972).

There is some evidence for an axonal "gating" control or "streamlining" of fast axoplasmic transport. For example, about twice as much material enters the peripheral axonal branch of dorsal root ganglion neurons as enters the branch to the central nervous system, and SDS-polyacrylamide gel electrophoresis of the radioactive material shows a different labelling pattern in the central and peripheral branches (Anderson and McClure, 1973). Further work is needed to establish whether this finding does indicate local axonal control over the direction of flow or, instead, a difference in rate of catabolism of labelled proteins in central and peripheral branches.

Fast axoplasmic transport proceeds at the same rate in large myelinated motor and sensory axons as in small unmyelinated sensory and autonomic fibers (Ochs, 1972, 1977). Fast axoplasmic transport is considerably more rapid in mammals than in fish, but this is the result of a marked temperature dependence of the transport process (Ochs, 1972; Edstrom and Hanson, 1973; Brimijoin, 1975; Gross and Kreutzberg, 1978). When transport is studied in axons of fish and mammals at the same temperature, fast axoplasmic transport proceeds at similar rates (Ochs, 1977).

Fast axoplasmic transport is dependent upon high energy phosphate compounds. Flow ceases if inhibitors of the citric acid cycle or uncouplers of mitochondrial oxidative phosphorylation are added to the medium, or oxygen is excluded (Ochs, 1972; Leone and Ochs, 1978). Fast axoplasmic transport also depends upon microtubules, and flow is blocked by colchicine, the vinca alkaloids (vincristine and vinblastine), and methylmercury in concentrations sufficient to cause microtubule dissociation (Banks et al., 1973; Fink et al., 1973; Abe et al., 1975; Goldman et al., 1976; Green et al., 1977; Schmidt and McDougal, 1978). Fast axoplasmic transport does not seem to require the involvement of actin microfilaments, for cytochalasin B in concentrations sufficient to impair the organization of this microfilament network (Godman and Miranda, 1978) does not block rapid transport (Banks et al., 1973). Fast transport is not dependent upon electrical excitability of axonal plasma membrane since it is not blocked by tetrodotoxin, a sodium channel inactivator which renders the axonal membrane unable to conduct action potentials (Ochs and Worth, 1975). However, batrachotoxin, which increases membrane sodium permeability and may alter axonal sodium-calcium exchange, does block flow (Ochs and Worth, 1975), as does papaverine, again possibly through an action on axonal calcium metabolism (Edstrom, 1977). Transport is blocked by oxalate (Ochs, 1972), a membrane-permeant anion that reduces cytosolic free calcium concentrations, but there is controversy as to the effects of omission of calcium from the medium on in vitro rapid transport in nerve (Edstrom, 1974; Dravid and Hammerschlag, 1975).

High resolution electron microscopy indicates that transmitter vesicles in axons frequently form rosette-like patterns around microtubules. The vesicles sometimes appear to be connected to the microtubules by cross-bridges (Smith, 1971a), but nothing is known about the composition and properties of these cross-bridges. However, bridges between adjacent microtubules are a common feature of flagellae and ciliae and are composed of an ATPase ("dynein") (McIntosh, 1974). In the presence of magnesium and ATP, dynein generates a sliding motion between adjacent microtubules (Warner, 1978). Similar cross-bridges between microtubules are present in mitotic spindles and sperm tails (McIntosh, 1974), and occasionally in axons as well (Smith, 1971a). Possibly the axonal neurotransmitter vesicle-microtubule cross-bridges have a similar mechanical function related to axoplasmic vesicle transport.

Labelled proteins reaching the nerve terminals by fast transport have short half-lives (Droz, 1973; Gross and Kreutzberg, 1978). Some may be catabolized in the terminal itself, but others are released into the synaptic cleft (Hines and Garwood, 1977; Younkin et al., 1978) and perhaps are taken up by the postsynaptic cell, either as intact peptides or after degradation to amino acids (Appeltauer and Korr, 1975; Griffin et al., 1976b). Fast axoplasmic transport is necessary for maintenance of the neurosecretory function of axon terminals. Focal application to a nerve of sufficient colchicine to block rapid axoplasmic transport results in denervation-like changes in the electrical properties of skeletal muscle fibers (Albuquerque et al., 1972; Hofmann and Peacock, 1973; Fernandez and Ramirez, 1974; Camerino and Bryant, 1976) and supersensitivity of extrajunctional muscle plasma membrane to acetylcholine (Albuquerque et al., 1972), despite maintenance of normal conduction of action potentials by the axons. Some of these alterations in muscle properties may, however, reflect a direct effect of colchicine, diffusing from the site of application, on the skeletal muscle fiber membrane itself (Cangiano and Fried, 1977).

REVERSE AXOPLASMIC TRANSPORT

Direct observation of living axons by light microscopy suggests the existence of retrograde axoplasmic transport (Lubinska, 1964). As many as 90 per cent of the moving particles in such axons pass from the distal portion toward the neuronal perikaryon (Forman et al., 1977a, b; Hammond and Smith, 1977). Both retrograde and anterograde particle movements are inhibited by colchicine and the vinca alkaloids (Hammond and Smith, 1977). Nerve constriction and transection experiments also suggest retrograde flow, for mitochondria and vesicles accumulate distal to as well as proximal to an axonal injury (Kasa, 1968; Griffin et al., 1977). Some of the

227

organelles passing retrograde within axons appear to be recycled neurotransmitter vesicles, perhaps destined for repair and reutilization in neurotransmission. In tissue culture, the leading edge of axon growth cones is particularly active in endocytosis of extracellular material. Much of this material is then transported within the axon toward perikaryon. Some material appears to be confined within tubular structures after endocytosis and throughout subsequent retrograde transport (Bunge, 1977).

Radiochemical and histochemical tracer techniques have confirmed the existence of retrograde axoplasmic transport. Labelled materials taken up by the nerve terminal, or by the cut ends of transected axons (DeVito et al., 1974; Olsson, Forsberg and Kristensson, 1978), move toward cell body at rates intermediate between fast and slow anterograde transport. Horseradish peroxidase (DeVito et al., 1974; Olsson et al., 1978), Evans blue-conjugated albumin (Kristensson and Sjostrand, 1972), and ^{125}I-labelled tetanus toxin (Stockel et al., 1975; Griffin et al.) have all been observed to move proximally within axons and to be accumulated by the neuronal cell body, although there is controversy concerning the retrograde transport of tetanus toxin (Hanson et al., 1975). Some experiments suggest that, while retrograde transport is itself nonspecific, specificity is conferred upon the process by selective uptake properties of certain nerve terminals (Max et al., 1978). Thus, sensory and autonomic terminals, but not motor endings, take up ^{125}I-labelled nerve growth factor (Stockel et al., 1975).

The significance of retrograde axoplasmic transport remains to be established. Retrograde flow may provide a route by which toxins and infectious agents penetrate the nervous system. For example, intradermally administered herpes simplex virus reaches the spinal cord via nerve, and local application of colchicine to the nerve serving the intradermal administration site prevents this transmission (Kristensson et al., 1970). The observation that nerve growth factor applied to autonomic terminals, transported retrograde in axons, and accumulated by cell body, produces the same morphological and biochemical changes (e.g., induction of tyrosine hydroxylase activity) as nerve growth factor applied directly to perikaryon (Hendry, 1977) suggests that retrograde axoplasmic transport may afford a mechanism for feedback control of neurons by end-organs (Price, 1974; Olsson et al., 1978). Also, chemical messages from the periphery conveyed by retrograde axoplasmic transport may stimulate the synthesis of neurotransmitter vesicles and inhibit the synthesis of structural axonal proteins (Watson, 1974). When an axon is severed, interrupting these messages from the periphery, there may be derepression of synthesis of axonal structural components, leading to the morphological and biochemical alterations in the neuronal perikaryon associated with axon regeneration (Grafstein, 1975). Evidence for this is provided by the observation that local administration of colchicine to axons of chick ciliary ganglion cells produces a perikaryal chromatolytic response mimicking that elicited by axotomy, even though the axon remains in continuity (Pilar and Landmesser, 1972; Purves, 1976).

AXOPLASMIC TRANSPORT IN NEUROPATHIES

Many inherited and acquired diseases of the central and peripheral nervous system are characterized by destruction of nerve terminals and distal axonal segments, with sparing of proximal axons and neuronal perikarya until late in the course. This pathological pattern has been termed "abiotrophy," "dying-back neuropathy," or "distal axonopathy" (Spencer and Schaumburg, 1977). Such selective terminal axonal degeneration might be the result of some selective vulnerability of this portion of the axon to a toxin or metabolic derangement. Alternatively, distal axonal degeneration might be the result of a quantitative or qualitative abnormality in axoplasmic transport of essential materials to the axon terminal from the site of synthesis in neuronal perikaryon.

A distinction ought to be made between axonal degenerative diseases *due* to an abnormality in axoplasmic transport and diseases in which axoplasmic transport is disturbed secondarily, as a result of some other pathogenetic process. In the first category, the defect in axoplasmic transport is the keystone leading to all other cellular events contributing to neurological deficits. In the much broader second category are processes in which disturbed axoplasmic transport is only an epiphenomenon of no pathogenetic significance and those in which an axoplasmic transport defect, itself secondary to some other cellular event, contributes to neuronal dysfunction (Bradley and Williams, 1973). In order to prove that an abnormality in axoplasmic transport belongs in the first category — that is, is primary in the causation of axonal degeneration — the following criteria should be met:

1. The flow abnormality should precede any demonstrable changes in nerve structure and function.

2. Perikaryal synthesis of the flowing material should be normal; one might expect that perikaryal levels of the flowing material be higher than in controls, because of the accumulation of untransported material.

3. If the observed abnormality in transport is one of rate, the temperature of the affected nerve must be identical with that of controls, or appropriate temperature corrections made (Brimijoin et al., 1979).

4. If the observed abnormality in transport is one of quantity of material moving through the axon, it must

229

be demonstrated that the rate of degradation of the material in the axon is the same as in controls. Moreover, if the quantity of material transported is calculated on the basis of extent of radioactive labelling, then the pool of endogenous unlabeled precursor in experimental and control nerves competing with the exogenous labelled precursor for incorporation must be the same. Otherwise, an apparent diminution in transport in a diseased nerve might merely reflect greater pool dilution in the affected nerve (Frizell and Sjostrand, 1974; Griffin et al., 1976*a*; Sidenius and Jakobsen, 1979).

Abnormalities in axoplasmic transport have been reported in inherited disorders such as mouse muscular dystrophy (McLane and McClure, 1977) and in acquired toxic and metabolic conditions such as colchicine, vincristine, methylmercury, and acrylamide neuropathies (Abe et al., 1975; Sumner et al., 1976; Green et al., 1977) and experimental diabetes mellitus in rats (Schmidt et al., 1975). Axoplasmic transport is impaired in the ischaemic retina, there responsible for "cotton-wool" exudates (Editorial, The Lancet, 1977). Various changes in anterograde and retrograde transport have been reported in regenerating nerves (Kristensson and Sjostrand, 1972; Frizell and Sjostrand, 1974; Frizell et al., 1976). Evidence sufficient to support the assertion that neural dysfunction is due to the abnormality in axoplasmic transport is available only in the case of colchicine-induced neuropathy, although it is likely that neuropathy resulting from administration of vincristine or vinblastine has a similar pathogenesis. Currently available optical, biochemical, and histochemical techniques, applied in studies similar to those already performed with colchicine, should permit a decision to be made as to whether axoplasmic transport is a major factor in the pathogenesis of axonal neuropathies.

References

Abe, T., Haga, T., and Kurokawa, M.: Blockage of axoplasmic transport and depolymerization of reassembled microtubules by methylmercury. Brain Res., *86*:504, 1975.

Albuquerque, E. X., Warnick, J. E., Tasse, J. R., and Sansone, F. M.: Effects of vinblastine and colchicine on neural regulation of the fast and slow skeletal muscles of the rat. Exp. Neurol., *37*:607, 1972.

Anderson, L. E., and McClure, W. O.: Differential transport of protein in axons: Comparison between the sciatic nerve and dorsal columns of cats. Proc. Natl. Acad. Sci. U.S.A., *70*:1521, 1973.

Appeltauer, G. S. L., and Korr, I. M.: Axonal delivery of soluble, insoluble and electrophoretic fractions of neuronal proteins to muscle. Exp. Neurol., *46*:132, 1975.

Bamburg, J. R., Shooter, E. M., and Wilson, L.: Developmental changes in microtubule protein of chick brain. Biochemistry, *12*:1476, 1973.

Banks, P., Mayor, D., and Mraz, P.: Cytochalasin B and the intra-axonal movement of noradrenaline storage vesicles. Brain Res., 49:417, 1973.

Barondes, S. H.: Further studies of the transport of protein to nerve endings. J. Neurochem., 15:343, 1968.

Bhattacharyya, B., and Wolff, J.: Membrane-bound tubulin in brain and thyroid tissue. J. Biol. Chem., 250:7639, 1975.

Black, M. M., and Lasek, R. J.: Axonal transport of actin: Slow component b is the principal source of actin for the axon. Brain Res., 171:401, 1979.

Blitz, A. L., and Fine, R. E.: Muscle-like contractile proteins and tubulin in synaptosomes. Proc. Natl. Acad. Sci. U.S.A., 71:4472, 1974.

Blose, S. H., and Chacko, S.: Rings of intermediate (100 angstrom) filament bundles in the perinuclear region of vascular endothelial cells. Their mobilization by Colcemid and mitosis. J. Cell Biol., 70:459, 1976.

Bradley, W. G., and Williams, M. H.: Axoplasmic flow in axonal neuropathies. I. Axoplasmic flow in cats with toxic neuropathies. Brain, 96:235, 1973.

Bray, D.: Surface movements during the growth of single explanted neurons. Proc. Natl. Acad. Sci. U.S.A., 65:905, 1970.

Brimijoin, S.: Stop-flow: A new technique for measuring axonal transport, and its application to the transport of dopamine-beta-hydroxylase. J. Neurobiol., 6:379, 1975.

Brimijoin, S., Olsen, J., and Rosenson, R.: Comparison of the temperature-dependence of rapid axonal transport and microtubules in nerves of the rabbit and bullfrog. J. Physiol. (Lond.), 287:303, 1979.

Buckley, I. K.: Subcellular motility: A correlated light and electron microscopic study using cultured cells. Tissue Cell, 6:1, 1974.

Bunge, M. B.: Initial endocytosis of peroxidase and ferritin by growth cones of cultured nerve cells. J. Neurocytol., 6:407, 1977.

Camerino, D., and Bryant, S. H.: Effects of denervation and colchicine treatment on the chloride conductance of rat skeletal muscle fibers. J. Neurobiol., 7:221, 1976.

Cangiano, A., and Fried, J. A.: The production of denervation-like changes in rat muscle by colchicine without interference with axonal transport or muscle activity. J. Physiol., 265:63, 1977.

Chambaut-Guerin, A. M., Muller, P., and Rossignol., B.: Microtubules and protein secretion in rat lacrimal glands. Relationship between colchicine binding and its inhibitory effect on the intracellular transport of proteins. J. Biol. Chem., 253:3870, 1978.

Cleveland, D. W., Hwo, S. Y., and Kirschner, M. W.: Purification of tau, a microtubule-associated protein that induces assembly of microtubules from purified tubulin. J. Mol. Biol., 116:207, 1977.

Dahlstrom, A.: Axoplasmic transport (with particular respect to adrenergic neurons). Philos. Trans. R. Soc. Lond. [Biol.], 261:325, 1971.

Dahlstrom, A., and Haggendal, J.: Studies on the transport and life-span of amine storage granules in a peripheral adrenergic neuron system. Acta Physiol. Scand., 67:278, 1966.

Daniels, M. P.: Colchicine inhibition of nerve fiber formation in vitro. J. Cell Biol., 53:164, 1972.

Davison, P. F.: Neuronal fibrillar proteins and axoplasmic transport. Brain Res., 100:73, 1975.

DeVito, J. L., Clausing, K. W., and Smith, O. A.: Uptake and transport of horseradish peroxidase by cut end of the vagus nerve. Brain Res., 82:269, 1974.

DiGiamberardino, L., Bennett, G., Koenig, H. L., and Droz, B.: Axonal migration of protein and glycoprotein to nerve endings. III. Cell fraction analysis of chicken ciliary ganglion after intracerebral injection of labelled precursors of proteins and glycoproteins. Brain Res., 60:147, 1973.

Dravid, A. R., and Hammerschlag, R.: Axoplasmic transport of proteins in vitro in primary afferent neurons of frog spinal cord: Effect of Ca^{2+}-free incubation conditions. J. Neurochem., 24:711, 1975.

Droz, B.: Renewal of synaptic proteins. Brain Res., 62:383, 1973.

Dustin, P., Hubert, J. P., and Flament-Durand, J.: Action of colchicine on axonal flow and pituicytes in the hypothalamopituitary system of the rat. Ann. N. Y. Acad. Sci., 253:670, 1975.

Editorial, The Lancet: Pathogenesis of cotton-wool spots. Lancet, 1:989, 1977.

Edstrom, A.: Effects of Ca^{2+} and Mg^{2+} on rapid axonal transport of proteins in vitro in frog sciatic nerves. J. Cell Biol., 61:812, 1974.

Edstrom, A.: Rapid axonal transport in vitro. Effects of derivatives of cyclic AMP and other agents acting on the cyclic AMP system. J. Neurobiol., 8:371, 1977.

Edstrom, A., and Hanson, M.: Temperature effects on fast axonal transport of proteins in vitro in frog sciatic nerves. Brain Res., 58:345, 1973.

Ehrlich, H. P., and Bornstein, P.: Microtubules in transcellular movement of procollagen. Nature [New Biol.], 238:257, 1972.

Feit, H., Dutton, G. R., Barondes, S. H., and Shelanski, M. L.: Microtubule protein. Identification in and transport to nerve endings. J. Cell Biol., 51:138, 1971.

Feldmann, G., Maurice, M., Sapin, C., and Benhamou, J. P.: Inhibition by colchicine of fibrinogen translocation in hepatocytes. J. Cell Biol., 67:237, 1975.

Fernandez, H. L., and Ramirez, B.: Muscle fibrillation induced by blockage of axoplasmic transport in motor nerves. Brain Res., 79:385, 1974.

Fink, B. R., Byers, M. B., and Middaugh, M. E.: Dynamics of colchicine effect on rapid axonal transport and axonal morphology. Brain Res., 56:299, 1973.

Forman, D. S., Padjen, A. L., and Siggins, G. R.: Axonal transport of organelles visualized by light microscopy: Cinemicrographic and computer analysis. Brain Res., 136:197, 1977a.

Forman, D. S., Padjen, A. L., and Siggins, G. R.: Effect of temperature on the rapid retrograde transport of microscopically visible intra-axonal organelles. Brain Res., *136*:215, 1977*b*.

Friede, R. L., and Ho, K. C.: The relation of axonal transport of mitochondria with microtubules and other axoplasmic organelles. J. Physiol., *265*:507, 1977.

Frizell, M., McLean, W. G., and Sjostrand, J.: Retrograde axonal transport of rapidly migrating labelled proteins and glycoproteins in regenerating peripheral nerves. J. Neurochem., *27*:191, 1976.

Frizell, M., and Sjostrand, S.: The axonal transport of slowly migrating (^{3}H) leucine-labelled proteins and the regeneration rate in regenerating hypoglossal and vagus nerves of the rabbit. Brain Res., *81*:267, 1974.

Fukuda, T., and Koelle, G. B.: The cytological localization of intracellular neuronal acetylcholinesterase. J. Biophys. Biochem. Cytol., *5*:433, 1959.

Gilbert, D. S., Newby, B. J., and Anderton, B. H.: Neurofilament disguise, destruction and discipline. Nature, *256*:586, 1975.

Godman, G. C., and Miranda, A. F.: Cellular contractility and the visible effects of cytochalasin. *In* Tanenbaum, S. W. (ed.): Cytochalasins — Biochemical and Cell Biological Aspects. Amsterdam, Elsevier, 1978, pp. 277–429.

Goldman, J. E., Kim, K. S., and Schwartz, J. H.: Axonal transport of (^{3}H) serotonin in an identified neuron of *Aplysia californica*. J. Cell Biol., *70*:304, 1976.

Grafstein, B.: The nerve cell response to axotomy. Exp. Neurol., *48* (No. 3, Part 2):32, 1975.

Grafstein, B., McEwen, B., and Shelanski, M. L.: Axonal transport of neurotubule protein. Nature, *277*:289, 1970.

Green, L. S., Donoso, J. A., Heller-Bettinger, I. E., and Samson, F. E.: Axonal transport disturbances in vincristine-induced peripheral neuropathy. Ann. Neurol., *1*:255, 1977.

Griffin, J. W., Drachman, D. B., and Price, D. L.: Fast axonal transport in motor nerve regeneration. J. Neurobiol., *7*:355, 1976*a*.

Griffin, J. W., Price, D. L., Drachman, D. B., and Engel, W. K.: Axonal transport to and from the motor nerve ending. Ann. N. Y. Acad. Sci., *274*:31, 1976*b*.

Griffin, J. W., Price, D. L., and Engel, W. K.: The pathogenesis of reactive axonal swellings: Role of axonal transport. J. Neuropathol. Exp. Neurol., *36*:214, 1977.

Gross, G., and Kreutzberg, G. W.: Rapid axoplasmic transport in the olfactory nerve of the pike: I. Basic transport parameters for proteins and amino acids. Brain Res., *139*:65, 1978.

Hammond, G. R., and Smith, R. S.: Inhibition of the rapid movement of optically detectable axonal particles by colchicine and vinblastine. Brain Res., *128*:337, 1977.

Hanson, M., Tonge, D., and Edstrom, A.: Tetanus toxin and axonal transport. Brain Res., *100*:462, 1975.

Hansson, H. A., and Sjostrand, J.: Ultrastructural effects of colchicine on the hypoglossal and dorsal vagal neurons of the rabbit. Brain Res., *35*:379, 1971.

Harwood, R., Grant, M. E., and Jackson, D. S.: The route of secretion of procollagen. Biochem. J., *156*:81, 1976.

Hendry, I. A.: The effect of retrograde axonal transport of nerve growth factor on the morphology of adrenergic neurones. Brain Res., *134*:213, 1977.

Hines, J. W., and Garwood, M. M.: Release of protein from axons during rapid axonal transport: An in vitro preparation. Brain Res., *125*:141, 1977.

Hoffman, P. N., and Lasek, R. J.: The slow component of axonal transport. Identification of major structural polypeptides of the axon and their generality among mammalian neurons. J. Cell Biol., *66*:351, 1975.

Hoffman, W. W., and Peacock, J. H.: Postjunctional changes induced by partial interruption of axoplasmic flow in motor nerves. Exp. Neurol., *41*:345, 1973.

Jeffrey, P. L., and Austin, L.: Axoplasmic transport. Neurobiology, *2*:207, 1973.

Karlsson, J. O.: Is there axonal transport of amino acids? J. Neurochem., *29*:615, 1977.

Karlsson, J. O., and Sjostrand, J.: Characterization of the fast and slow components of axonal transport in retinal ganglion cells. J. Neurobiol., *2*:135, 1971.

Kasa, P.: Acetylcholinesterase transport in the central and peripheral nervous tissue: The role of tubules in the enzyme transport. Nature, *218*:1265, 1968.

Khan, M. A., and Ochs, S.: Slow axoplasmic transport of mitochondria (MAO) and lactic dehydrogenase in mammalian nerve fiber. Brain Res., *96*:267, 1975.

Kristensson, K., Lycke, E., and Sjostrand, J.: Transport of herpes simplex virus in peripheral nerves. Acta Physiol. Scand. [Suppl.], *357*:13, 1970.

Kristensson, K., and Sjostrand, J.: Retrograde transport of protein tracer in the rabbit hypoglossal nerve during regeneration. Brain Res., *45*:175, 1972.

Lazarides, E., and Hubbard, B. D.: Immunological characterization of the subunit of the 100 angstrom filaments from muscle cells. Proc. Natl. Acad. Sci. U.S.A., *73*:4344, 1976.

Leone, J., and Ochs, S.: Anoxic block and recovery of axoplasmic transport and electrical excitability in nerve. J. Neurobiol., *9*:229, 1978.

Lockwood, A. H.: Tubulin assembly protein: Immunochemical and immunofluorescent studies on its function and distribution in microtubules and cultured cells. Cell, *13*:613, 1978.

Lubinska, L.: Axoplasmic streaming in regenerating and in normal nerve fibres. Prog. Brain Res., *13*:1, 1964.

Luduena, R. F., Shooter, E. M., and Wilson, L.: Structure of the tubulin dimer. J. Biol. Chem., *252*:7006, 1977.

MacNeal, R. K., and Purich, D. L.: On the role of the tubulin non-exchangeable GTP site in bovine neurotubule assembly. J. Biol. Chem., *252*:4440, 1977.

Max, S. R., Schwab, M., Dumas, M., and Thoenen, H.: Retrograde axonal transport of nerve growth factor in the ciliary ganglion of the chick and the rat. Brain Res., *159*:411, 1978.

McEwen, B. S., and Grafstein, B.: Fast and slow components in axonal transport of protein. J. Cell Biol., *38*:494, 1968.

McIntosh, J. R.: Bridges between microtubules. J. Cell Biol., *61*:166, 1974.

McLane, J., and McClure, W. O.: Rapid axoplasmic transport in dystrophic mice. J. Neurochem., *29*:865, 1977.

Metuzals, J., and Mushynski, W. E.: Electron microscope and experimental investigations of the neurofilamentous network in Deiters' neurons. Relationship with the cell surface and nuclear pores. J. Cell Biol., *61*:701, 1974.

Moellman, G., and McGuire, J.: Correlation of cytoplasmic microtubules and 10-nm filaments with the movement of pigment granules in cutaneous melanocytes of *Rana pipiens*. Ann. N. Y. Acad. Sci., *253*:711, 1975.

Ochs, S.: Fast transport of materials in mammalian nerve fibers. Science, *176*:252, 1972.

Ochs, S.: Axoplasmic transport in peripheral nerve and hypothalamo-neurohypophyseal systems. Adv. Exp. Med. Biol., *87*:13, 1977.

Ochs S., and Worth, R.: Batrachotoxin block of fast axoplasmic flow in mammalian nerve fibers. Science, *187*:1087, 1975.

Olsson, T. P., Forsberg, I., and Kristensson, K.: Uptake and retrograde axonal transport of horseradish peroxidase in regenerating facial motor neurons of the mouse. J. Neurocytol., *7*:323, 1978.

Osborn, M., Webster, R. E., and Weber, K.: Individual microtubules viewed by immunofluorescence and electron microscopy in the same PtK2 cell. J. Cell Biol., *77*:R27, 1978.

Pilar, G., and Landmesser, L.: Axotomy mimicked by localized colchicine application. Science, *177*:1116, 1972.

Pinner-Poole, B., and Campbell, J. B.: Effect of low temperature and colchicine on regenerating sciatic nerve. Exp. Neurol., *25*:603, 1969.

Pleasure, D.: The structural proteins of peripheral nerve. *In* Dyck, P. J., Thomas, P. K., and Lambert, E. H. (eds.): Peripheral Neuropathy. Philadelphia, W. B. Saunders, 1975, pp. 231–252.

Price. D. L.: The influence of the periphery on spinal motor neurons. Ann. N. Y. Acad. Sci., *228*:355, 1974.

Purves, D.: Functional and structural changes in mammalian sympathetic neurones following colchicine application to post-ganglionic nerves. J. Physiol., *259*:159, 1976.

Puszkin, S., and Berl, S.: Actomyosin-like protein from brain. Separation and characterization of the actin-like component. Biochim. Biophys. Acta, *256*:695, 1972.

Ribak, C. E., Vaugn, J. E., and Saito, K.: Immunocytochemical localization of glutamic acid decarboxylase in neuronal somata following colchicine inhibition of axonal transport. Brain Res., *140*:315, 1978.

Santerre, R. F., and Rich, A.: Actin accumulation in developing chick brain and other tissues. Dev. Biol., *54*:1, 1976.

Schlaepfer, W. W.: Vincristine-induced axonal alterations in rat peripheral nerve. J. Neuropathol. Exp. Neurol., *30*:488, 1971.

235

Schmidt, R. E., Matschinsky, F. M., Godfrey, D. A., Williams, A. D., and McDougal, D. B., Jr.: Fast and slow axoplasmic flow in sciatic nerve of diabetic rats. Diabetes. *24*:1081, 1975.

Schmidt, R. E., and McDougal, D. B., Jr.: Axonal transport of selected particle-specific enzymes in rat sciatic nerve in vivo and its response to injury. J. Neurochem., *30*:527, 1978.

Scott, F. H.: On the relation of nerve cells to fatigue of their nerve fibres. J. Physiol., *34*:145, 1906.

Sheterline, P., Schofield, J. G., and Mira, F.: Colchicine binding to bovine anterior pituitary slices and inhibition of growth-hormone release. Biochem. J., *148*:453, 1975.

Sidenius, P., and Jakobsen, J.: Axonal transport in early experimental diabetes. Brain Res., *173*:315, 1979.

Smith, D. S.: On the significance of cross-bridges between microtubules and synaptic vesicles. Philos. Trans. R. Soc. Lond. [Biol.], *261*:395, 1971*a*.

Smith, D. S.: Summing up: Some implications of the neuron as a secreting cell. Phils. Trans. R. Soc. Lond. [Biol.], *261*:423, 1971*b*.

Spencer, P. S.: Reappraisal of the model for "bulk axoplasmic flow." Nature [New Biol.], *240*:283, 1972.

Spencer, P. S., and Schaumburg, H. H.: Central-peripheral distal axonopathy—the pathology of dying-back polyneuropathies. Prog. Neuropathol., *3*:253, 1977.

Stockel, K., Schwab, M., and Thoenen, H.: Comparison between the retrograde axonal transport of nerve growth factor and tetanus toxin in motor, sensory and adrenergic neurons. Brain Res., *99*:1, 1975.

Sumner, A., Pleasure, D., and Cieilka, K.: Slowing of fast axoplasmic transport in acrylamide neuropathy. J. Neuropathol. Exp. Neurol., *35*:319, 1976.

Warner, F.: Cation-induced attachment of ciliary dynein cross-bridges. J. Cell Biol., *77*:R19, 1978.

Watson, W. E.: Cellular responses to axotomy and to related procedures. Br. Med. Bull., *30*:112, 1974.

Weeks, D. P., and Collis, P. S.: Induction of microtubule protein synthesis in *Chlamydomonas reinhardi* during flagellar regeneration. Cell., *9*:15, 1976.

Weiss, P. A.: Neuronal dynamics and axonal flow: Axonal peristalsis. Proc. Natl. Acad. Sci. U.S.A., *69*:139, 1972*a*.

Weiss, P. A.: Neuronal dynamics and axonal flow, V. The semisolid state of the moving axonal column. Proc. Natl. Acad. Sci. U.S.A., *69*:620, 1972*b*.

Weiss, P. A., and Hiscoe, H. B.: Experiments on the mechanism of nerve growth. J. Exp. Zool., *107*:315, 1948.

Wessells, N. K., Spooner, B. S., Ash, J. F., Bradley, M. O., Luduena, M. A., Taylor, E. L., Wrenn, J. T., and Yamada, K. M.: Microfilaments in cellular and developmental processes. Science, *171*:135, 1971.

Willard, M., Cowan, W. M., and Vagelos, P. R.: The polypeptide composition of intra-axonally transported proteins: Evidence for four transport velocities. Proc. Natl. Acad. Sci. U.S.A., *71*:2183, 1974.

Wolosewick, J. J., and Porter, K. R.: Stereo high-voltage electron microscopy of whole cells of the human diploid line, WI-38. Am. J. Anat., *147*:303, 1976.

Yamada, K. M., Spooner, B. S., and Wessells, N. K.: Axon growth: Roles of microfilaments and microtubules. Proc. Natl. Acad. Sci. U.S.A., *66*:1206, 1970.

Younkin, S. G., Brett, R. S., Davey, B., and Younkin, L. H.: Substances moved by axonal transport and released by nerve stimulation have an innervation-like effect on muscle. Science, *200*:1292, 1978.

Neuromuscular Transmission

7

Jackson B. Pickett

The 50-nm step from nerve to muscle is usually a sure one, beginning with the conduction of a nerve impulse into its terminals. These depolarized nerve terminals release acetylcholine which diffuses across the synaptic cleft and interacts with acetylcholine receptors, leading to an end-plate potential (Fig. 7–1). When the muscle fiber depolarization produced by an end-plate potential (EPP) is large enough, a muscle fiber action potential (MAP) is produced (Fig. 7–1D) which then causes the muscle fiber to contract. Reviews of neuromuscular transmission can be found in Katz (1966), Kuffler and Nicholls (1976), and Kandel (1977).

COMPOUND MUSCLE ACTION POTENTIAL

Clinical testing of neuromuscular transmission typically starts with surface-recorded compound muscle action potentials (CMAPs) evoked by nerve stimulation. CMAPs are a measure of muscle fiber activation, and are used to make inferences about the earlier steps. The relationship between muscle fiber action potentials (Fig. 7–1D) and compound muscle action potentials (Fig. 7–2 and 7–3) is not a simple one. An intracellularly recorded human intercostal MAP is a monophasic positive potential of about 85 mV in amplitude and 15 msec in duration (Elmqvist et al., 1964). An extracellularly recorded volume-conducted MAP is di- or triphasic (positive onset), and can be up to about 1 to 3 mV in amplitude and 3 msec in duration (Håkansson, 1957). The volume-conducted MAP amplitude falls rapidly with distance from the muscle fiber, and varies with muscle fiber diameter. Monophasic recording with surface electrodes sums the volume-conducted MAPs, and its amplitude should be proportional to the number of active muscle fibers (Katz, 1966). CMAP amplitude and configuration vary with electrode placement. Over the zone where muscle fibers are innervated CMAPs have a negative onset, reflecting the initial depolarization of muscle

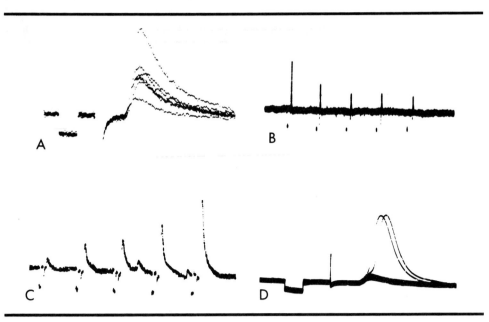

Figure 7–1 End-plate potentials after various treatments. *A,* End-plate potentials evoked by 1-Hz repetitive stimulation after increasing extracellular magnesium concentration which reduces the number of acetylcholine quanta released by a nerve stimulus. Clearly, end-plate potentials vary in quantal steps. Similar findings may occur in Lambert-Eaton syndrome and botulism. *B,* End-plate potentials evoked by 3-Hz repetitive stimulation after adding curare, which reduces the postsynaptic response to a quanta. The decrement in end-plate potential amplitude reflects depletion of the "immediately available" store of vesicles in the presynaptic nerve terminal. Similar findings are seen in myasthenia gravis. *C,* End-plate potentials evoked by 50-Hz repetitive stimulation after increasing extracellular magnesium concentration. Facilitation of end-plate potential amplitude is due to an increase in calcium concentration in the presynaptic nerve terminal. *D,* End-plate potentials which occasionally activate the muscle fiber, causing a muscle fiber action potential. Slight variations in muscle fiber threshold or end-plate potential rise time cause the muscle fiber to fire at slightly different times. (Calibration: Horizontal, 1 msec; vertical, *A, B, C,* — 1 mV, *D,* — 5 mV.)

fibers at the innervation zone. The duration of the negative portion of the CMAP is often 4 to 10 msec and is much longer than a single MAP because of the asynchronous activation of muscle fibers and the conduction of MAPs across the innervation zone. In clinical practice, the peak amplitude of the negative portion of the CMAP is often used as a measure of the number of active muscle fibers. A more accurate measure of the number of active muscle fibers would be the area under the negative portion of the CMAP. These simple assumptions have been questioned by Slomic et al. (1968), who found that the "inactive" electrode lowered CMAP amplitude by as much as 30 to

40 per cent with differential recording. Thus, a simple direct relationship between the proportion of active muscle fibers and CMAP amplitude or area may only be a useful fiction.

CMAP Amplitude

Myasthenia gravis can usually be separated from botulism and Lambert-Eaton syndrome by CMAP amplitude (Table 7–1; Figs. 7–2 and 7–3). CMAP amplitude is usually normal in patients with myasthenia gravis, and is reduced in patients with botulism and Lambert-Eaton syndrome. Mean CMAP amplitude is reduced by 15 to 30 per cent (Desmedt, 1973; Johns et al, 1956; Lambert et al., 1961) in myasthenic patients, but only 3 to 15 per cent fall below the normal range. This suggests that most myasthenic muscle fibers are activated by a single nerve stimulus, and this is supported by recordings in human intercostal muscle (Elmqvist et al., 1964). CMAP amplitude in patients with Lambert-Eaton syndrome and severe botulism is often reduced to a fraction of the lower limit of normal (Cherington, 1973; Lambert et al., 1961). Small CMAP amplitude is due to subthreshold EPPs in the majority of intercostal muscle fibers from patients with Lambert-Eaton syndrome and botulism (Lambert and Elmqvist, 1971; Lambert et al., 1974). While a reduced CMAP amplitude would help separate patients with botulism and Lambert-Eaton syndrome from myasthenic patients, a small CMAP amplitude can be seen in patients with any disorder causing a loss of function of motor axons, neuromuscular junctions, or muscle fibers.

Paired Stimuli

Paired stimuli may give more direct evidence of a neuromuscular junction disorder. The test involves giving paired supramaximal stimuli at fixed intervals, and comparing the amplitude of the second and first CMAP. A plot of the interval between paired stimuli vs. the ratio of the amplitude of the second CMAP to the first is called a transmission curve. In a normal transmission curve the second CMPA is equal to the first for intervals more than about 15 to 20 msec (Desmedt, 1973; Johns et al., 1956; Lambert et al., 1961). For intervals less than 15 to 20 msec the second CMAP is less than the first, due to the relative refractory period of neuromuscular transmission. A transmission curve in patients with myasthenia gravis shows two abnormalities: (1) during the relative refractory period, the second CMAP is larger than expected when compared with the first and can be larger than the first (Desmedt, 1973; Lambert et al., 1961; Takamori and Gutmann, 1971); and (2) at longer intervals between paired stimuli, about 100 to 1000 msec (Desmedt, 1973; Johns et al., 1956; Lambert et al., 1961), the second CMAP is smaller than the first. The transmission curve abnormalities in patients with Lambert-Eaton syndrome and botulism are similar to those in myasthenic

Table 7-1 Effects on CMAP Amplitude

Disorder	Abnormality	Single Stimulus	Paired Stimuli		Repetitive Stimulation	
			Short Intervals (20-40 msec)	Long Intervals (200-1000 msec)	2-3 Hz	10-25 Hz
Normal	—	—	First CMAP is equal to second CMAP		Decrement up to 8-10%	May increase up to 40%
Myasthenia gravis	Reduced quantal response	Normal or slightly reduced	Second CMAP may be slightly larger than first	Second CMAP often smaller than first	Decrement more than 10%	May have small increment, rarely large increment
Lambert-Eaton syndrome; botulism	Reduced quantal content	Very small	Second CMAP often larger	Second CMAP may be smaller	May decrease more than 10%	Often increment more than 100%

patients, but the increase in the second CMAP amplitude relative to the first at short intervals (3 to 20 msec) is more prominent. Conversely, the decrease in the second CMAP relative to the first at longer intervals (200 to 1000 msec) is less (Cherington, 1973; Lambert et al., 1961).

Abnormal transmission curves should reflect changes in the proportion of active muscle fibers. If the stimulus is supramaximal, the recording is monophasic and electrode movement can be prevented; then the CMAP amplitude changes should reflect changes in the proportion of active muscle fibers. Thus, the increase of the second CMAP relative to the first at short intervals between paired stimuli suggests that a larger proportion of muscle fibers are activated by the second stimulus than the first. A decrease in the proportion of active muscle fibers would explain the decrease in the second CMAP relative to the first, with longer intervals between paired stimuli.

The activation of muscle fibers is the result of a complex sequence of events. First, motor axons are activated by the stimulus and action potentials are conducted into the presynaptic terminals (Katz and Miledi, 1965). This causes calcium permeability to increase in a voltage-dependent fashion (Llinas et al., 1976), which is thought to increase calcium concentration near the sites where vesicles are released. The number of vesicles released by an activated presynaptic terminal is a third or fourth power function of extracellular $[Ca^{++}]$ (Bennett et al., 1975: Dodge and Rahamimoff, 1967; Hubbard et al., 1968). Iontophoretic injection of calcium into a presynaptic squid synapse increases the frequency of spontaneous quantal release (Miledi and Slater, 1966). After the nerve terminal action potential ends, the increment in $[Ca^{++}]$ (and possibly sodium) near the sites where vesicles are released slowly returns to normal, due to nerve terminal buffers such as mitochondria (Rahamimoff et al., 1976) and calcium-sodium exchange across the nerve terminal membrane (Baker, 1975). An increased sodium concentration in the nerve terminal may release calcium from mitochondria (Silbergeld, 1977) and indirectly increase nerve terminal $[Ca^{++}]$.

The number of vesicles normally released by a nerve stimulus produces an EPP which is much greater than the 7 to 20 mV (Elmqvist et al., 1964) required to activate a muscle fiber. The small CMAP amplitude in patients with Lambert-Eaton syndrome and botulism is the result of a large proportion of muscle fibers with subthreshold EPPs. EPP amplitude is a function of the number of quanta released, quantal size, and nonlinear summation of quantal responses (Martin, 1955). Both Lambert-Eaton syndrome and botulism are characterized by a reduced number of quanta released by a nerve terminal action potential (Figure 7–1A) with normal nerve-evoked quantal response (Lambert and Elmqvist, 1971; Lambert et al., 1974). The quantal response is the amplitude of the postsynaptic depolarization produced by a single quantum (Figure 7–1A). In myasthenia gravis, the reverse is true; the quantal response is reduced while the number of quanta released by a nerve terminal action potential, or quantal content, is normal (Elmqvist et al., 1964). Thus, the reason muscle fibers fail to fire in patients with Lambert-Eaton syndrome and botulism is a reduced quantal content (m), and in myasthenia gravis is decreased quantal response (q).

With paired stimuli at short intervals, the increments in nerve terminal $[Ca^{++}]$ are greater than with either single stimulus. This increase in $[Ca^{++}]$ near the sites where vesicles are released is thought to increase m (Magleby, 1973). EPP amplitude increases as m increases, and the second stimulus could fire some subthreshold muscle fibers. Thus, the second CMAP evoked by paired stimuli would be larger than the first if the first stimulus produced a small average m, and if the interval between the two stimuli was short. The increase in EPP amplitude by the second of two stimuli is called facilitation. Facilitation decays with time and, at the frog neuromuscular junction, this decay can be described as the sum of two exponential curves with time constants of 50 msec and 300 msec (Magleby, 1973). To avoid confusion, increases in CMAP amplitude will be called increments (Özdemir and Young, 1976), and the term facilitation will be restricted to increases in EPP amplitude. With paired stimuli at longer intervals, the second CMAP is smaller than the first in myasthenic patients, and to a smaller degree in patients with Lambert-Eaton syndrome and botulism. A decrease in the second CMAP amplitude suggests that a larger proportion of end-plate potentials are subthreshold, and that on the average the second EPP is smaller than the first. Microelectrode studies on muscles from normal experimental animals have confirmed the decrease of the second EPP relative to the first at long intervals between paired stimuli, and demonstrate that it is due to a reduction in m (Hubbard et al., 1963). Depression of the second m is thought to reflect depletion of an "immediately available" store of vesicles in the presynaptic terminal. Depletion would be explained by assuming that: (1) only a fraction of the total number of vesicles in the nerve terminal, the "immediately available" store, is likely to be released by a nerve stimulus; (2) each vesicle in the "immediately available" store (n) has an equal probability (p) of release; (3) the replacement of released vesicles, mobilization, is slow relative to the rate of stimulation; and (4) $m = np$ (Hubbard et al., 1969). For example, if n = 500, p = 0.2 and is unchanged by stimulation and mobilization is negligible, then the first stimulus produces a value for m of 100 and the second stimulus results in a value for m of 80. Thus, the first stimulus depletes n by 100 and depresses the second EPP by 20 quanta. This analysis ignores changes in p

$m = np$

caused by the first stimulus (Elmqvist and Quastel, 1965). With long intervals between stimuli depletion is usually more prominent than the decaying remnant of facilitation, which is usually insignificant 100 msec after a stimulus.

Repetitive Stimulation Changes in CMAP amplitude with repetitive stimulation (Figs. 7–2 and 7–3) are those that would be expected from the changes seen with paired stimuli. The reciprocal of the interval between paired stimuli would equal the frequency of stimulation. As expected, CMPA amplitude

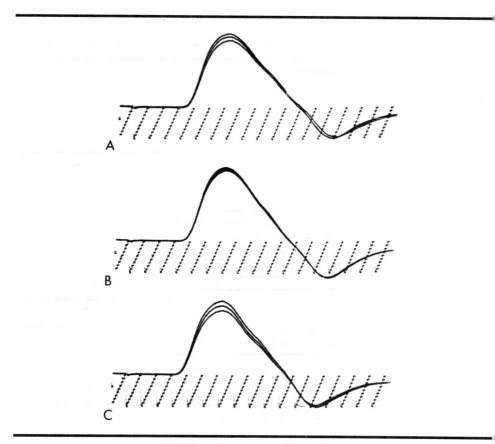

Figure 7–2 Repetitive stimulation in myasthenia gravis. *A*, Compound muscle action potentials evoked by 2-Hz stimulation repeated three times. A significant, (greater han 10 per cent decrement) is seen. First CMAP is largest and third CMAP is smallest in each tracing. *B*, Identical repetitive stimulation 3 seconds after 1 minute of exercise. Decrement is smaller after exercise owing to "pseudofacilitation" and a true facilitation of vesicle release. *C*, Identical repetitive stimulation 240 seconds after exercise. Postactivation exhaustion has increased the decrement. Calibration: Height of time lines = 5 mV, ramp of time lines = 1 msec. Median nerve was stimulated.

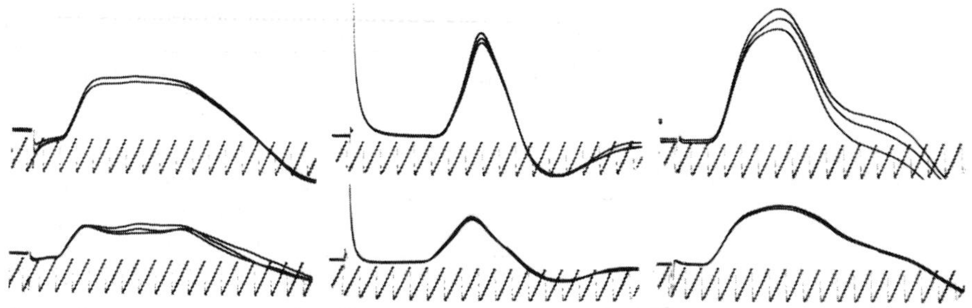

Figure 7–3 Repetitive stimulation in botulism. *Lower tracings:* Compound muscle action potentials evoked by 2-Hz repetitive stimulation. *Upper tracings:* Compound muscle action potentials evoked by 2-Hz repetitive stimulation 3 seconds after 50-Hz stimulation for 10 seconds. Musculocutaneous *(A)*, ulnar *(B)*, and peroneal *(C)* nerve stimulation. Calibration: Height of time lines = 1 mV; ramp of time lines = 1 msec. From Pickett et al., 1976. Reprinted by permission from the New England Journal of Medicine 295:770, 1976.)

increases with high frequency stimulation (20 to 40 Hz) in disorders where m is small, such as Lambert–Eaton syndrome and botulism (Figures 7–1C and 7–3). Slow repetitive stimulation (2 to 3 Hz) produces decrements more marked in myasthenia gravis (Figs. 7–1B and 7–2) than in disorders with a low m (Fig. 7–3, *upper right*). Decrements can be calculated by 1−(third or fifth CMAP/first CMAP) and expressed as a percentage by multiplying by 100. Repetitive stimulation in normal subjects shows decrements up to 8 to 10 per cent with 2 to 3 Hz stimulation (Desmedt, 1973; Özdemir and Young, 1976), and increments up to 40 per cent with rapid (10 to 35-Hz) stimulation (Özdemir and Young, 1976). Increments with rapid repetitive stimulation in Lambert-Eaton syndrome and botulism would result from minimal depletion of the "immediately available" store since initial m is small and maximal facilitation of vesicle release by stimulating at short intervals. Decrements in CMAP amplitude with slow repetitive stimulation in myasthenia gravis are caused by a fall in EPP amplitude (Fig. 7–1B), which reflects depletion of the "immediately available" store of vesicles. Depletion is more marked the larger the initial m, and facilitation of vesicle release would be small at long intervals between stimuli. While decrements are characteristic of neuromuscular transmission disorders, they may be seen with motor neuron disease (Mulder et al., 1959), myotonic disorders (Aminoff et al., 1977), other nerve and muscle diseases (Simpson, 1966), and central disorders (Patten et al., 1972).

Patients with myasthenia gravis may show a triphasic response to repetitive stimulation (Johns et al., 1956;

245

Lambert et al., 1961). Here the CMAP amplitude declines with repetitive stimulation for the first four to eight stimuli, then increases toward its initial value, and later decreases again. Similar changes in EPP amplitude have been seen in normal curare-treated human intercostal muscle (Elmqvist and Quastel, 1965). EPP amplitude decreases until the number of vesicles entering the "immediately available" store, or mobilization, equals the number of vesicles leaving the "immediately available" store of vesicles. The rate of mobilization is a function of the rate of stimulation and the degree of depletion. If depletion is large then mobilization might overshoot, and EPP amplitude would be transiently increased.

Exercise and Tetanic Stimulation

Exercise and tetanic stimulation may accentuate changes in CMAP amplitude seen with repetitive stimulation (Desmedt, 1973; Johns et al., 1956; Lambert et al., 1961). Typical testing would include a train of three to five stimuli at 2 to 3 Hz before and 3, 30, 60, 120, 180, and 240 seconds after exercise or tetanic stimulation. Normal subjects show little change in CMAP amplitude (5 to 10 per cent) with repetitive stimulation after exercise (Desmedt, 1973; Johns et al., 1956; Lambert et al., 1961). In neuromuscular transmission disorders there may occur a variable increase in CMAP amplitude a few seconds after exercise. This increment in CMAP amplitude is due to: (1) "pseudofacilitation" (Desmedt, 1973), which is the result of a more synchronous activation of muscle fibers due to an increase in muscle fiber conduction velocity which decreases CMAP duration and increases CMAP amplitude; and (2) an increased proportion of active muscle fibers due to a reduced proportion of subthreshold EPPs. In patients with Lambert-Eaton syndrome or botulism, CMAP amplitude may double immediately after exercise (Fig. 7–3). The mechanism of this postexercise increment is unknown, but it is probably similar to posttetanic potentiation in which calcium accumulates in the presynaptic nerve terminal (Martin, 1977). At frog neuromuscular junctions where EPP amplitude is made subthreshold by increasing the magnesium/calcium concentration ratio, which reduces m, tetanic stimulation (20 Hz × 10 sec) is followed by an increase in EPP amplitude which decays over seconds to a few minutes (Magleby and Zengel, 1976).

Thus, the slow decay of posttetanic potentiation may explain the postexercise increments seen in patients with Lambert-Eaton syndrome and botulism, where m is small and depletion would be slight. When m is normal, EPP amplitude after exercise is determined by posttetanic potentiation of vesicle release, depletion of the "immediately available" store of vesicles (Elmqvist and Quastel, 1965), and reduction in postsynaptic sensitivity to re-

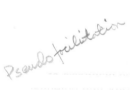

Pseudofacilitation

leased acetylcholine due to acetylcholine receptor desensitization (Nastuk and Wolfson, 1976). With appropriate stimulation parameters, EPP amplitude in human intercostal muscle is increased for 10 to 60 sec after a tetanus (Elmqvist et al., 1964). Therefore, even with a normal m, posttetanic potentiation dominates over depletion and desensitization immediately after a tetanus. If posttetanic potentiation decays more rapidly than depletion (Desmedt, 1973) and desensitization, then EPP amplitude would be reduced at longer intervals after a tetanus. When slow (2 to 3 Hz) stimulation is applied for three to five stimuli before and after exercise in patients with myasthenia gravis (Fig. 7–2), the following changes are seen: immediately after a tetanus, CMAP amplitude may increase with a reduction in the decrement and, 3 to 5 minutes after exercise, CMAP amplitude may decrease with a larger decrement (Desmedt, 1973; Lambert et al., 1961). These changes in CMAP amplitude after exercise can be explained by assuming that mean EPP amplitude is near threshold, and an increase or decrease in EPP amplitude would cause an appropriate change in the proportion of active muscle fibers and CMAP amplitude. Decrements of CMAP amplitude immediately after exercise would be lessened by increasing EPP amplitude, so that EPP amplitude in a larger proportion of muscle fibers would stay above threshold even after decrementing with repetitive stimulation. Larger decrements several minutes after exercise would reflect a lower EPP amplitude which rapidly becomes subthreshold in a larger proportion of muscle fibers with repetitive stimulation.

Electromyography
Variation in motor unit potential amplitude (Fig. 7–4) seen on electromyography may aid the diagnosis of neuromuscular junction disorders. Motor unit potential amplitude is a function of the number of muscle fibers active at a given time and their distance from the recording electrode. As some EPPs become subthreshold, some muscle fibers will fire intermittently (Fig. 7–1D) and the motor unit potential will vary in amplitude and configuration. While variation in amplitude is characteristic of neuromuscular junction disorders, it can also be seen in neurogenic (Lambert, 1969) and myopathic (Pickett, 1977b) disorders. With severe reduction in the number of active muscle fibers, motor unit potentials may become small and short, as seen in Fig. 7–4.

Single fiber electromyography is very sensitive to neuromuscular junction disorders (Stålberg et al., 1976). Single fiber electromyography allows measurement of the interval between the onset of two muscle fiber action potentials in the same motor unit. Jitter (Fig. 7–5), or the variation of this interval, is increased in neuromuscular junction disorders. Jitter probably reflects differences in EPP rise time and muscle fiber threshold (Fig. 7–1D). The time it takes for an EPP to reach threshold for muscle

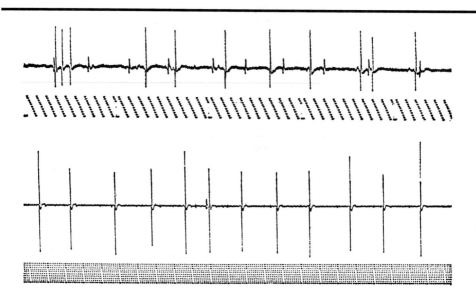

Figure 7–4 Motor unit potentials in neuromuscular transmission disorders. *A,* Small and short motor unit potentials in botulism. *B,* Variation in motor unit potential amplitude in myasthenia gravis. (Calibration: Ramp of time lines — 10 msec; height of time lines — *A,* 100 μV, *B,* 200 μV.)

fiber activation varies with its amplitude; a large EPP would activate the muscle fiber before a small EPP. EPP amplitude varies because m varies from stimulus to stimulus (Martin, 1977). Any disorder which reduces EPP amplitude or increases muscle fiber threshold would increase jitter. As the severity of neuromuscular junction disorders increases, increased jitter is associated with blocking of either of the two muscle fiber action potentials. Blocking implies that the EPP is subthreshold for firing the muscle fiber (Fig. 7–1D). Increased jitter and blocking may be found in neurogenic and myopathic disorders, as well as in disorders of neuromuscular transmission (Stålberg and Ekstedt, 1973).

DISORDERS OF NEUROMUSCULAR TRANSMISSION

Myasthenia Gravis

Myasthenia gravis is a disorder of neuromuscular transmission characterized by fluctuating weakness which often improves with the administration of anticholinesterase drugs. The success of thymectomy, corticosteroids, and plasmapheresis in the treatment of myasthenia gravis has placed a premium on accurate diagnosis. Current diagnostic tests include acetylcholine receptor antibody titers, repetitive stimulation, and electromyography, bulb ergogram to record rapid exhaustion in myasthenic muscles, Tensilon tomography (Wray and

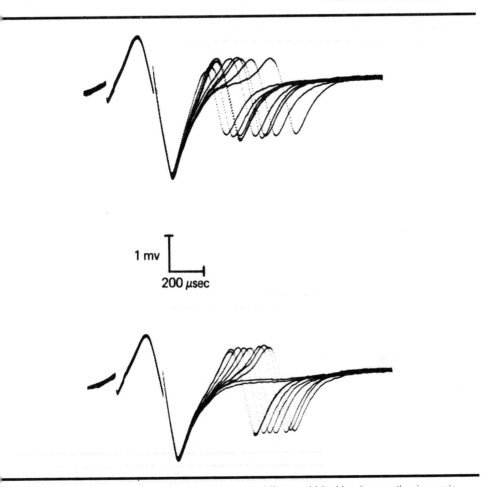

1 mv

200 μsec

Figure 7–5 Increased jitter and blocking in myasthenia gravis. Two muscle fiber action potentials from the same motor unit can be recorded with a single fiber electrode. The first muscle fiber action potential triggers the oscilloscope sweep, and the variability in time of occurrence, or jitter, or the second muscle fiber action potential can be measured. In normal muscles jitter is less than 100 μsec. Both the upper and lower tracing show increased jitter. The lower tracing also shows an occasional absence, or blocking, of the second muscle fiber action potential. (Photography courtesy of Charles K. Jablecki, M. D., Department of Neurosciences, University of California, San Diego.)

NEUROMUSCULAR TRANSMISSION

Pavan-Langston, 1971), optokinetic electronystagmography (Spector and Daroff, 1976), ocular velocity recordings (Baloh and Keesey, 1976), ocular electromyography (Sears et al., 1960), and tympanometry to document enhanced transmission of sound in the 1000 to 4000-Hz range, possibly due to weakness of the stapedius muscle (Morioka et al., 1976). This discussion will focus on the first two diagnostic methods.

Typical electrodiagnostic findings (Fig. 7–2) in myasthenia gravis include:

1. Normal CMAP amplitude with 3 to 15 per cent of the potentials below the normal range (Desmedt, 1973; Johns et al., 1956; Lambert et al., 1961; Slomic et al., 1968).

2. Decrements greater than 8 to 10 per cent (Desmedt, 1973; Lambert et al., 1961) in 95 per cent of myasthenic patients (Özdemir and Young, 1976), and a reduction in the second CMAP amplitude with paired stimuli at 0.2 to 1.0-sec intervals (Desmedt, 1973; Johns et al., 1956; Lambert et al., 1961).

3. Increments in CMAP amplitude with paired or repetitive stimulation which are usually small, 15 to 35 per cent (Lambert et al., 1961), but rarely may be more than 100 per cent (Schwartz and Stålberg, 1975; Takamori and Gutmann, 1971).

4. Decrements are less 3 to 5 sec after exercise or tetanic stimulation, and are increased 3 to 5 min after exercise or tetanic stimulation.

5. Motor unit potentials which vary in amplitude (Fig. 7–4).

If slow (2 to 3-Hz) repetitive stimulation before and after exercise is normal in a patient suspected of having myasthenia gravis, the incidence of positive tests may be increased by stimulating proximal muscles (Desmedt, 1973; Özdemir and Young, 1976), warming the muscles (Desmedt, 1973), ischemia (Desmedt and Borenstein, 1976a), regional infusion of curare (Brown and Charlton, 1975; Horowitz et al., 1976), single fiber electromyography (Stålberg et al., 1976), or acetylcholine receptor antibody titers (Lindstrom et al., 1976b). At present, no study has compared these methods of diagnosing myasthenia gravis, and laboratories have tended to use methods most familiar to them.

The pathophysiology of myasthenia gravis has slowly been unravelled. Microelectrode studies on intercostal muscles from patients with myasthenia gravis reveal miniature end-plate potentials (MEPPs) which are one fifth of the normal size, while the number of quanta released by a nerve impulse is normal (Elmqvist et al., 1964). Measurement of MEPP amplitude is a simple way to estimate the postsynaptic response to a single quantum of acetylcholine. The amount of acetylcholine released by nerve stimulation in muscle from patients with myasthenia gravis is normal (Ito et al., 1976), making a presynaptic disorder unlikely. Assay of the number of acetylcholine receptor (AChR) molecules on the postsynaptic membrane is possible by using α-bungarotoxin, which binds specifically and irreversibly with AChR. Using α-bungarotoxin, the number of AChRs in muscle from patients with myasthenia gravis was found to be about one fifth of normal (Fambrough et al., 1973).

This reduction in the number of AChRs per end-plate is probably a significant factor in reducing the size of MEPPs seen in myasthenia gravis. When acetylcholine is applied to an end-plate, the depolarization produced is associated with an increase in voltage noise. Statistical analysis of this acetylcholine noise provides estimates of the changes produced by the interaction of a single acetylcholine molecule and its receptor. Each AChR activation produces a 0.3-μV depolarization lasting about 1 msec, with a conductance change of $10^{-10}\ \Omega^{-1}$ (Katz and Miledi, 1972). Acetylcholine noise has a square wave configuration when recorded directly (Neher and Sakmann, 1976). A MEPP is the sum of about 1000 acetylcholine-AChR interactions. Each acetylcholine molecule has only about one chance of interacting with an AChR before it is hydrolyzed by acetylcholinesterase or diffuses away from the end-plate (Katz and Miledi, 1973). Thus, as the number of AChRs per end-plate decreases, more acetylcholine molecules will be hydrolyzed by acetylcholinesterase or diffuse away from the end-plate before they can depolarize the postsynaptic membrane by interacting with AChRs.

A reduction in number of functional AChRs per end-plate could be due to the binding of antibodies to AChR, destruction of the AChR containing postsynaptic membrane, or increased turnover of AChR. Evidence for each of these possibilities has been found. Serum from patients with myasthenia gravis caused a 50 per cent reduction in MEPP amplitude when it is injected into mice for 1 to 14 days (Toyka et al., 1977). The fraction of serum causing this reduction in MEPP amplitude is IgG (Fig. 7–6), and its effect is increased by the third component (C3) of the complement system. While most AChR antibodies are not directed at the acetylcholine binding site (Lindstrom et al., 1976a), they do reduce the time the AChR is open by 20 per cent (Heinemann et al., 1977). This may reflect an allosteric effect. That antibodies to AChR are a factor in the pathogenesis of myasthenia gravis is suggested (see Drachman, 1978) by the presence of AChR antibodies in about 90 per cent of patients with myasthenia gravis (Appel et al., 1975; Lindstrom and Lambert, 1978) and

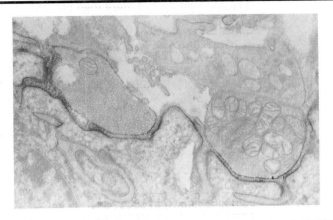

Figure 7–6 Presence of IgG at myasthenic end-plates. IgG was identified at end-plates from patients with myasthenia gravis using a peroxidase conjugated with staphylococcal protein A, which binds to human IgG. The postsynaptic membrane lacks the usual folds. (From Engel et al., 1977.)

rapid improvement in strength after plasmapheresis (Dau et al., 1977). While antibodies to AChR may alter its function, there also is clear evidence of abnormalities in the AChR-containing postsynaptic AChR membrane. These include simplification of the postsynaptic membrane with degeneration of some postsynaptic folds (Engel and Santa, 1971) and a positive linear relationship between MEPP amplitude and the amount of postsynaptic AChR surface (Engel et al., 1977c). These findings are consistent with the idea that binding of antibodies to AChRs are a stage in destruction of the postsynaptic membrane. When IgG from patients with myasthenia gravis is added to muscle fibers in tissue culture, the rate of degradation of AChR increases (Kao and Drachman, 1977; Heinemann et al., 1977). This suggests that increased AChR turnover may also be a factor in the decreased number of AChRs.

Blockade of acetylcholine receptors with α-bungarotoxin or the α-toxin of the Formosan cobra reproduces electrical findings that qualitatively resemble those seen in patients with myasthenia gravis (Satyamurti et al., 1975; Takamori and Iwanaga, 1976). After administering α-bungarotoxin or the cobra α-toxin intravenously, the following abnormalities developed: (1) CMAP amplitude was reduced by about 20 per cent; (2) a 10 to 90 per cent decrement in CMAP amplitude was seen with 2–3 Hz stimulation; (3) 5 to 40 seconds after tetanic stimulation, the decrement produced by 2 to 3 Hz stimulation was less than before tetanic stimulation; and (4) 4 to 20 minutes after tetanic stimulation, the decrement produced by 2 to

3 Hz stimulation was more than that before tetanic stimulation. Also, animals immunized with AChR develop an illness which has many of the electrical and clinical findings of myasthenia gravis (Seybold et al., 1976).

Botulism The most lethal toxin on a weight basis is botulinal toxin. Four of the eight toxins produced by Clostridium botulinum — A, B, E, and F — cause paralysis in man (Smith, 1977). One third of the 21 cases of botulism reported to the Center for Disease Control each year are fatal (U.S. Department of Health, Education, and Welfare, 1974). When the toxin type can be identified, which occurs in two thirds of the cases, 70 per cent are caused by type A, 20 per cent by type B, and 10 per cent by type E. The toxin source is known in about one third of cases; it is often home-canned vegetables, such as beans and peppers.

Symptoms of botulism typically develop 12 to 36 hours after exposure to the toxin. The earliest symptoms are usually nausea and vomiting, postural dizziness, and blurred vision (Koenig et al., 1967). These symptoms are followed by weakness and impaired autonomic function in structures innervated by cranial nerves, and then by paralysis of respiratory and somatic muscles. Electron microscopic examination of botulinal toxin-poisoned muscle and neuromuscular junctions is normal (Harris and Miledi, 1971), or shows increased postsynaptic folds and retraction of atrophic nerve terminals (Gutmann et al., 1973). While electrical testing may suggest botulism, more direct evidence can be obtained by identification of the toxin in serum or stool (Dowell et al., 1977).

Usual electrodiagnostic findings in botulism are (Oh, 1977) (Figs. 7–3 and 7–4):

1. Normal to low normal motor conduction velocity with normal sensory conduction studies.

2. Small CMAP amplitudes.

3. Decrements with slow repetitive stimulation.

4. Increments with rapid repetitive stimulation, or after tetanic stimulation or exercise.

5. Small and short motor unit potentials and fibrillation on needle examination.

These electrodiagnostic findings should differentiate botulism from myasthenia gravis. The following parameters help to separate botulism from the Lambert-Eaton syndrome: (1) the response to electrical stimulation does not vary from limb to limb in Lambert-Eaton syndrome (Cherington, 1974); and (2) the increment in CMAP amplitude after tetanic stimulation may last for minutes in

253

botulism (Gutmann and Pratt, 1976; Pickett et al., 1976), while it usually only lasts for seconds in Lambert-Eaton syndrome. It is important to remember that some cases of botulism may not have an increment or decrement with paired stimuli, rapid or slow repetitive stimulation, or slow repetitive stimulation before and after tetanic stimulation. Thus, findings that would suggest a neuromuscular junction defect are lacking, and the only abnormalities are small CMAP amplitudes and small-short motor unit potentials (Pickett, 1977a).

Botulinal toxin blocks acetylcholine release from peripheral cholinergic nerve terminals without altering impulse conduction in nerves or acetylcholine sensitivity in the end-plate region. The number of acetylcholine quanta released by a nerve stimulus, the quantal content (m), is markedly reduced (Fig. 7–1A), while the response to a quantum released by nerve stimulation is normal (Cull-Candy et al., 1976). The average quantal content in an intercostal muscle from a patient with botulism was 0.07 in comparison to a normal value of 60 (Lambert et al., 1974). In experimental animals, this marked reduction in quantal content may persist during 4 hours of 16-Hz stimulation. The marked reduction in quantal content would produce subthreshold EPPs in most muscle fibers, and produce a small CMAP amplitude. The absence of an increase in m, or facilitation, after repetitive stimulation probably explains the absence in some cases, of an increment in CMAP amplitude with paired, repetitive or after tetanic stimulation. EPP amplitude is larger if the dose of botulinal toxin is small or if recovery, which involves formation of new neuromuscular junctions (Duchen, 1971), is in progress (Bray and Harris, 1975). When EPP amplitude is larger, facilitation (Fig. 7–1C) may increase the number of muscle fibers activated and result in a clinically evident increment in CMAP amplitude with paired, repetitive, or after tetanic stimulation (Fig. 7–3). The marked reduction in m in botulism may be due to an irreversible blockade of calcium entry during depolarization of the presynaptic nerve terminal, or to a reduced sensitivity of the release sites to calcium (Cull-Candy et al., 1976; Kao et al., 1976).

Guanidine may increase limb strength and improve extraocular movement, but has less effect on respiratory or autonomic function (Oh, 1977). Guanidine probably acts by increasing the nerve terminal calcium concentration, perhaps by blocking calcium uptake by mitochondria (Lundh et al., 1977).

Lambert-Eaton Syndrome

The combination of easy fatigability of proximal muscles, dry mouth, peripheral paresthesias, impotence, aching of limbs, absent stretch reflexes, mild proximal weakness, and delayed onset of maximal strength during a contraction in a man over 40 years of age suggests a diagnosis of

Lambert-Eaton syndrome. About two thirds of the cases initially have or develop a bronchogenic carcinoma (Elmqvist and Lambert, 1968). Electron miscroscopic examination of neuromuscular junctions from patients with Lambert-Eaton syndrome shows a markedly enlarged postsynaptic membrane with a greatly increased number of folds (Engel and Santa, 1971). An acetone extract of lung cancer tissue from a patient with Lambert-Eaton syndrome reduces the number of quanta released by nerve stimuli in a frog neuromuscular preparation (Ishikawa et al., 1977).

Typical electrodiagnostic findings (Lambert et al., 1961) in Lambert-Eaton syndrome include:

1. Small CMAP amplitude:

2. An increment in CMAP amplitude with rapid repetitive stimulation, or with paired stimuli separated by a short interval.

3. An increase in CMAP amplitude after a brief exercise or tetanic stimulation, which decays over 1 to 2 min.

4. Decrement in CMAP amplitude with slow repetitive stimulation or paired stimuli at an interval of 0.2–1 sec.

5. Normal nerve conduction studies.

6. An increase in motor unit potential amplitude during a volitional contraction.

The Lambert-Eaton syndrome can be differentiated from most cases of myasthenia gravis by low CMAP amplitude which approaches normal during rapid repetitive stimulation or after exercise, and from botulism by the larger increments in CMAP amplitude during rapid repetitive stimulation.

A marked reduction in the number of quanta (m) released by a nerve stimulus (Fig. 7–1A) is the main physiological abnormality in the Lambert-Eaton syndrome (Elmqvist and Lambert, 1968; Lambert and Elmqvist, 1971). Microelectrode studies of intercostal muscle from patients with Lambert-Eaton syndrome show a quantal content of three to nine in comparison with a normal quantal content of 50 to 60. Miniature end-plate potential (MEPP) amplitude is normal. With rapid repetitive stimulation, the m in muscle fibers from patients with the Lambert-Eaton syndrome increases (Fig. 7–1C). This facilitation is more prominent in fibers with a low initial m, and is absent in fibers with a high initial m. The net result of this facilitation is that the number of muscle fibers activated during rapid repetitive stimulation or after exercise increases, and an increment in CMAP amplitude is seen. A decrement is seen with slow repetitive stimulation, which reflects a reduction in m due to depletion of the "immediately available" store of vesicles that is not compensated by facilitation. Guanidine increases m two to four times, which probably explains its clinical effectiveness.

Diseases Involving Motor Neurons

Patients with diseases involving motor neurons frequently have weakness, atrophy, and fasciculation on physical examination. Electrical testing shows fibrillation, fasciculation, and a reduced number of motor unit potentials which are long, large, and polyphasic (Lambert, 1969). Occasionally, patients with diseases involving motor neurons have excessive muscular fatigability and decrements in CMAP amplitude with slow repetitive stimulation (Mulder et al., 1959). A few seconds after a brief exercise, the decrement may be less or absent, and 2 to 4 minutes after exercise it may be larger than before exercise (Fig. 7–2). In addition to the usual abnormalities seen with neurogenic processes, needle examination may show motor unit potentials which vary (Fig. 7–4) or decline in amplitude. These findings in isolation might suggest myasthenia gravis but, when combined with a reduced number of motor units and the presence of large and long motor unit potentials, a neurogenic disorder is likely. Increased jitter and blocking may be seen with single fiber electromyography in neurogenic and myopathic disorders (Stålberg and Ekstedt, 1973), and motor unit potentials may vary in amplitude in myopathic disorders (Pickett, 1977b).

Decrements with repetitive stimulation, variation in motor unit potential amplitude, and increased jitter and blocking suggest a disorder of neuromuscular transmission in neurogenic and myopathic disorders. These abnormalities could reflect subthreshold end-plate potentials or conduction block in distal nerve terminals. When anterior horn cells or their motor axons are destroyed, surviving motor axons in the muscle sprout and reinnervate the denervated muscle fibers (Wohlfart, 1958). Collateral sprouting also occurs in myopathic disorders (Desmedt and Borenstein, 1976b). Recently reinnervated muscle fibers from rabbit diaphragm (Bennett et al., 1973) have a small end-plate potential quantal content (Fig. 7–1A), which increases as the newly formed neuromuscular junctions mature. Similar findings are seen when minced muscle fibers regenerate and are reinnervated (Bennett et al., 1974). These newly formed neuromuscular junctions attain normal function in 1 to 2 months. Thus, clinical evidence of abnormal neuromuscular transmission in neurogenic and myopathic disorders may be due to small end-plate potentials in recently formed neuromuscular junctions resulting from collateral sprouting.

Conduction block can occur along axons supplying newly formed neuromuscular junctions (Miledi, 1960) at frequencies as low as 0.1 Hz. Evidence of a conduction block in distal nerve terminals has been seen in neurogenic (Stålberg and Ekstedt, 1973) and myopathic (Pickett, 1978) disorders. If impulse conduction is blocked to a sufficient number of muscle fibers, motor unit potential amplitude varies, and a disorder of neuromuscular transmission is simulated.

Tick Paralysis

The occurrence of incoordination followed by an ascending flaccid paralysis and absent stretch reflexes in a child should suggest the diagnosis of tick paralysis (Stanbury and Huyck, 1945). Complete recovery usually follows if the tick is removed before signs of bulbar paralysis develop. Electrodiagnostic studies in tick paralysis (Cherington and Snyder, 1968; Swift and Ignacio, 1975) show:

1. Small CMAP amplitude.

2. Normal to low normal motor conduction velocities.

3. Normal sensory conduction studies or mildly prolonged sensory distal latencies.

4. Normal repetitive stimulation before and after exercise.

Tick paralysis is thought to be due to a toxin; the mechanism of action of this toxin is unknown. Microelectrode studies have shown a temperature-dependent reduction in the number of acetylcholine quanta released by a nerve stimulus (Cooper and Spence, 1976), suggesting a presynaptic abnormality.

Antibiotic Paralysis

The occurrence of apnea after surgery in a patient with renal failure is sometimes the result of antibiotic paralysis. Other physical findings include dilated and fixed pupils, impaired eye movements, dysphagia, flaccid paralysis, and paresthesias (Wright and McQuillen, 1971). Severe weakness can be seen with lincomycin and three groups of antibiotics: aminoglycosides, polypeptides, and tetracyclines. Electrical testing on patients given antibiotics (McQuillen et al., 1968; Wright and McQuillen, 1971) shows:

1. Small CMAP amplitude

2. Decrements with slow and rapid repetitive stimulation.

3. No increments in CMAP amplitude with repetitive stimulation before or after tetanic stimulation.

257

4. Slowed conduction velocity.

Antibiotics such as neomycin and colistin (McQuillen and Engback, 1975) decrease the number of quanta released by a nerve stimulus (m), decrease quantal response (q), and slow mobilization, or the rate at which vesicles in the "immediately available" store are replaced, at the end of a train of stimuli. A reduction in m, q, and slowed mobilization probably explains the small CMAP amplitude and decrements in CMAP amplitude with repetitive stimulation. Slowed mobilization may mask facilitation of acetylcholine release, and explain the absence of increments in CMAP amplitude.

Myasthenic Syndrome with End-Plate Acetylcholinesterase Deficiency

End-plate acetylcholinesterase was decreased in a 16-year-old boy with: (1) weakness and fatigability of muscles innervated by cranial and somatic nerves; and (2) hyporeflexia (Engel et al., 1977a). Electrical findings include:

1. A decrement in CMAP amplitude with stimulation at high and low frequencies.

2. Repetitive muscle action potentials to a single nerve stimulus.

3. A small increase in CMAP amplitude seen immediately after exercise, with decrements increasing a few minutes after exercise.

4. Motor unit potentials which vary in amplitude.

5. Normal conduction studies.

Microelectrode studies of intercostal muscle reveal low normal miniature end-plate potential (MEPP) amplitude with an increased duration and a reduced MEPP frequency, a reduced number of quanta released by a nerve stimulus (m), and a reduced number of quanta "immediately available" for release (n). Muscle biopsy demonstrates small presynaptic nerve terminals, postsynaptic folds with focal degeneration and membranous networks, and an absence of a 16S species of end-plate acetylcholinesterase. A reduction in m and n probably explains the decrements observed, and repetitive muscle action potentials to a single nerve stimulus reflect the absence of acetylcholinesterase.

References

Aminoff, M. J., Layzer, R. B., Satya-Murti, S., et al.: The declining electrical response of muscle to repetitive nerve stimulation in myotonia. Neurology (Minneap.), 27:812, 1977.

Appel, S. H., Almon, R. R., and Levy, N.: Acetylcholine receptor antibodies in myasthenia gravis. N. Engl. J. Med., 293:760, 1975.

NEUROMUSCULAR TRANSMISSION

Baker, P. F.: Transport and metabolism of calcium ions in nerve. *In* Baker, P. F. and Reuter, H. (eds.): Calcium Movement in Excitable Cells. Elmsford, N.Y., Pergamon Press, 1975, p. 7.

Baloh, R. W., and Keesey, J. C.: Saccade fatigue and response to edrophonium for the diagnosis of myasthenia gravis. Ann. N.Y. Acad. Sci., *274*:631, 1976.

Bennett, M. R., Florin, T., and Woog, R.: The formation of synapses in regenerating mammalian striated muscle. J. Physiol. (Lond.), *238*:79, 1974.

Bennett, M. R., Florin, T., and Hall, R.: The effect of calcium ions on the binomial statistic parameters which control acetylcholine release at synapses in striated muscle. J. Physiol. (Lond.), *247*:429, 1975.

Bennett, M. R., McLachlan, E. M., and Taylor, R.: The formation of synapses in reinnervated mammalian striated muscle. J. Physiol. (Lond.), *233*:481, 1973.

Bray, J. J., and Harris, A. J.: Dissociation between nerve-muscle transmission and nerve trophic effects on rat diaphragm using type D botulinum toxim. J. Physiol. (Lond.), *253*:53, 1975.

Brown, J. C., and Charlton, J. E.: A study of sensitivity to curare in myasthenic disorders using a regional technique. J. Neurol. Neurosurg. Psychiatry, *38*:27, 1975.

Cherington, M.: Botulism: Electrophysiologic and therapeutic observations. *In* Desmedt, J. E. (ed.): New Developments in Electromyography and Clinical Neurophysiology, Vol. 1. Basel, S. Karger, 1973, p. 375.

Cherington, M.: Botulism. Arch. Neurol., *30*:432, 1974.

Cherington, M., and Snyder, R. D.: Tick paralysis. Neurophysiologic studies. N. Engl. J. Med., *278*:95, 1968.

Cooper, B. J., and Spence, I.: Temperature-dependent inhibition of evoked acetylcholine release in tick paralysis. Nature, *263*:693, 1976.

Cull-Candy, S. G., Lundh, H., and Thesleff, S.: Effects on botulinum toxin on neuromuscular transmission in the rat. J. Physiol. (Lond.), *260*:177, 1976.

Dau, P. C., Lindstrom, J. M., Cassel, C. K., et al.: Plasmapheresis and immunosuppressive drug therapy in myasthenia gravis. N. Engl. J. Med., *297*:1134, 1977.

Desmedt, J. E.: The neuromuscular disorder in myasthenia gravis. *In* Desmedt, J. E. (ed.): New Developments in Electromyography and Clinical Neurophysiology, Vol. 1. Basel, S. Karger, 1973, p. 241.

Desmedt, J. E., and Borenstein, S.: Diagnosis of myasthenia gravis by nerve stimulation. Ann. N.Y. Acad. Sci., *274*:174, 1976*a*.

Desmedt, J. E., and Borenstein, S.: Regeneration in Duchenne muscular dystrophy. Electromyographic evidence. Arch. Neurol., *33*:642, 1976*b*.

Dodge, F. A., and Rahamimoff, R.: Co-operative action of calcium ions in transmitter release at the neuromuscular junction. J. Physiol. (Lond.), *193*:419, 1967.

Dowell, V. R., McCroskey, L. M., Hatheway, C. L., et al.: Coproexamination for botulinal toxin and *Clostridium botulinum*. J.A.M.A., *238*:1829, 1977.

Drachman, D. B.: Myasthenia gravis. N. Engl. J. Med., 298 136, 1978.

Duchen, L. W.: An electron microscopic study of the changes induced by botulinum toxin in the motor end-plates of slow and fast skeletal muscle fibers of the mouse. J. Neurol. Sci., *14*:47, 1971.

Elmqvist, D., Hoffman, W. W., Kugelberg, J., et al.: An electrophysiological investigation of neuromuscular transmission in myasthenia gravis. J. Physiol. (Lond.), *174*:417, 1964.

Elmqvist, D., and Lambert, E. H.: Detailed analysis of neuromuscular transmission in a patient with the myasthenic syndrome sometimes associated with bronchogenic carcinoma. Mayo Clin. Proc., *43*:689, 1968.

Elmqvist, D., and Quastel, D. M. J.: A quantitative study of end-plate potentials in isolated human muscle. J. Physiol. (Lond.), *178*:505, 1965.

Engel, A. G., Lambert, E. H., and Gomez, M. R.: A new myasthenic syndrome with end-plate acetylcholinesterase deficiency, small nerve terminals, and reduced acetylcholine release. Ann. Neurol., *1*:315, 1977*a*.

Engel, A. G., Lambert, E. H., and Howard, F. M., Jr.: Immune complexes (IgG and C3) at the motor end-plate in myasthenia gravis: Ultrastructural and light microscopic localization and electrophysiologic correlations. Mayo Clin. Proc., *52*:267, 1977*b*.

Engel, A. G., Lindstrom, J. M., Lambert, E. H., et al.: Ultrastructural localization of the acetylcholine receptor in myasthenia gravis and in its experimental autoimmune model. Neurology (Minneap.), *27*:307, 1977*c*.

Engel, A. G., and Santa, T.: Histometric analysis of the ultrastructure of the neuromuscular junction in myasthenia gravis and in the myasthenic syndrome. Ann. N.Y. Acad. Sci., *183*:46, 1971.

Fambrough, D. M., Drachman, D. B., and Satyamurti, S.: Neuromuscular junction in myasthenia gravis: Decreased acetylcholine receptors. Science, *182*:293, 1973.

Gutmann, L., Oguchi, K., and Chou, S. M.: Neuromuscular junction in human botulism. Neurology (Minneap.), *23*:424, 1973.

Gutmann, L., and Pratt, L.: Pathophysiologic aspects of human botulism. Arch. Neurol. *33*:175, 1976.

Håkansson, C. H.: Action potentials recorded intra- and extracellularly from the isolated frog muscle fibre in Ringer's solution and in air. Acta Physiol. Scand., *39*:291, 1957.

Harris, A. J., and Miledi, R.: The effect of type D botulinum toxin on frog neuromuscular junctions. J. Physiol. (Lond.), *217*:497, 1971.

Heinemann, S., Bevan, S., Kullberg, R., et al.: Modulation of acetylcholine receptor by antibody against the receptor. Proc. Natl. Acad. Sci. U.S.A., *74*:3090, 1977.

Horowitz, S. H., Genkins, G., Kornfeld, P., et al.: Electrophysiologic diagnosis of myasthenia gravis and the regional curare test. Neurology (Minneap.), *26*:410, 1976.

NEUROMUSCULAR TRANSMISSION

Hubbard, J. I.: Repetitive stimulation at the mammalian neuro-muscular junction, and the mobilization of transmitter. J. Physiol. (Lond.), *169*:641, 1963.

Hubbard, J. I., Llinás, R., and Quastel, D. M. J.: Electrophysiological Analysis of Synaptic Transmission. Baltimore, Williams and Wilkins, 1969.

Hubbard, J. I., Jones, S. F., and Landau, E. M.: On the mechanism by which calcium and magnesium affect the release of transmitter by nerve impulses. J. Physiol. (Lond.), *196*:75, 1968.

Ishikawa, K., Engelhardt, J. K., Fujisawa, T., et al.: A neuromuscular transmission block produced by a cancer tissue extract derived from a patient with the myasthenic syndrome. Neurology (Minneap.), *27*:140, 1977.

Ito, Y., Miledi, R., Molenaar, P. C., et al.: Acetylcholine in human muscle. Proc. R. Soc. Lond. [Biol.], *192*:475, 1976.

Johns, R. J., Grob, D., and Harvey, A. M.: Studies in neuromuscular function. II. Effects of nerve stimulation in normal subjects and in patients with myasthenia gravis. Bull. Johns Hopkins Hosp., *99*:125, 1956.

Kandel, E. R. (ed.): Cellular Biology of Neurons, Vol. 1, Part I; Handbook of Physiology, Section 1, The Nervous System. Baltimore, Williams and Wilkins, 1977.

Kao, I., and Drachman, D. B.: Myasthenic immunoglobulin accelerates ACh receptor degradation. Neurology (Minneap.), *27*:364, 1977.

Kao, I., Drachman, D. B., and Price, D. L.: Botulinum toxin: Mechanism of presynaptic blockade. Science, *193*:1256, 1976.

Katz, B.: Nerve, Muscle and Synapse. New York, McGraw-Hill, 1966.

Katz, B., and Miledi, R.: Propagation of electrical activity in motor nerve terminals. Proc. R. Soc. Lond. [Biol.], *161*:453, 1965.

Katz, B., and Miledi, R.: The statistical nature of the acetylcholine potential and its molecular components. J. Physiol. (Lond.), *244*:665, 1972.

Katz, B., and Miledi, R.: The binding of acetylcholine to receptors and its removal from the synaptic cleft. J. Physiol. (Lond.), *231*:549, 1973.

Koenig, M. G., Drutz, D. J., Mushlin, A. I., et al.: Type B botulism in man. Am. J. Med., *42*:208, 1967.

Kuffler, S. W., and Nicholls, J. G.: From Neuron to Brain. Sunderland, Mass., Sinauer Associates, 1976.

Lambert, E. H.: Electromyography in amyotrophic lateral sclerosis. *In* Norris, F. H., and Kurland, L. T. (eds.): Motor Neuron Diseases: Research on Amyotrophic Lateral Sclerosis and Related Disorders. New York, Grune and Stratton, 1969, p. 135.

Lambert, E. H., and Elmqvist, D.: Quantal components of end-plate potentials in the myasthenic syndrome. Ann. N.Y. Acad. Sci., *183*:183, 1971.

Lambert, E. H., Engel, A. G., and Cherington, M.: End-plate potentials in human botulism. *In* Bradley, W. G., Gardner-Medwin, D., and Walton, J. N. (eds): Third International Congress on Muscle Disease. Amsterdam, Excerpta Medica, 1974, Series No. 334, p. 65.

Lambert, E. H., Rooke, E. D., Eaton, L. M., et al.: Myasthenic syndrome occasionally associated with bronchial neoplasm: Neurophysiologic studies. *In* Viets, H. R. (ed.): Myasthenia Gravis. Springfield, Ill., Charles C Thomas, 1961, p. 362.

Lindstrom, J. M., and Lambert, E. H.: Content of acetylcholine receptor and antibodies bound to receptor in myasthenia gravis, experimental autoimmune myasthenia gravis, and Eaton-Lambert syndrome. Neurology (Minneap.) 28:130, 1978.

Lindstrom, J. M., Lennon, V. A., Seybold, M. E., et al.: Experimental autoimmune myasthenia gravis and myasthenia gravis: Biochemical and immunochemical aspects. Ann. N.Y. Acad. Sci., 274:254, 1976a.

Lindstrom, J. M., Seybold, M. E., Lennon, V. A., et al.: Antibody to acetylcholine receptor in myasthenia gravis: Prevalence, clinical correlates and diagnostic value. Neurology (Minneap.), 26:1054, 1976b.

Llinás, R., Steinberg, I. Z., and Walton, K.: Presynaptic calcium currents and their relation to synaptic transmission: Voltage clamp study in squid giant synapse and theoretical model for the calcium gate. Proc. Natl. Acad. Sci. U.S.A., 73:2918, 1976.

Lundh, H., Leander, S., and Thesleff, S.: Antagonism of the paralysis produced by botulinum toxin in the rat. The effects of tetraethylammonium, guanidine and 4-aminopyridine. J. Neurol. Sci., 32:29, 1977.

Magleby, K. L.: The effect of repetitive stimulation on facilitation of transmitter release at the frog neuromuscular junction. J. Physiol. (Lond.), 234:327, 1973.

Magleby, K. L., and Zengel, J. E.: Stimulation-induced factors which affect augmentation and potentiation of transmitter release at the neuromuscular junction. J. Physiol. (Lond.), 260:687, 1976.

Martin, A. R.: A further study of the statistical composition of the end-plate potential. J. Physiol. (Lond.), 130:114, 1955.

Martin, A. R.: Junctional transmission. II. Presynaptic mechanisms. *In* Kandel, E. R. (ed.): Cellular Biology of Neurons, Vol. 1, Part I; Handbook of Physiology, Section 1, The Nervous System. Baltimore, Williams and Wilkins, 1977, p. 329.

McQuillen, M. P., Cantor, H. E., and O'Rourke, J. R.: Myasthenic syndrome associated with antibiotics. Arch. Neurol., 18:402, 1968.

McQuillen, M. P., and Engback, L.: Mechanism of colistin-induced neuromuscular depression. Arch. Neurol., 32:235, 1975.

Miledi, R.: Properties of regenerating neuromuscular synapses in the frog. J. Physiol. (Lond.), 154:190, 1960.

Miledi, R.: Transmitter release by injection of calcium into nerve terminals. Proc. R. Soc. Lond. [Biol.], 183:421, 1973.

Miledi, R., and Slater, C. R.: The action of calcium on neuronal synapses in the squid. J. Physiol. (Lond.), 184:473, 1966.

Morioka, W. T., Neff, P. A., Boisseranc, T. E., et al.: Audiotympanometric findings in myasthenia gravis. Arch. Otolaryngol., 102:211, 1976.

Mulder, D. W., Lambert, E. H., and Eaton, L. M.: Myasthenic syndrome in patients with amyotrophic lateral sclerosis. Neurology (Minneap.), 9:627, 1959.

Nastuk, W. L., and Wolfson, C. H.: Cholinergic receptor desensitization. Ann. N.Y. Acad. Sci., 274:130, 1976.

Neher, E., and Sakmann, B.: Single-channel currents recorded from membrane of denervated frog muscle fibers. Nature, 260:799, 1976.

Oh, S. J.: Botulism: Electrophysiologic studies. Ann. Neurol., 1:481, 1977.

Özdemir, C., and Young, R. R.: Electrical testing in myasthenia gravis. Ann. N.Y. Acad. Sci., 183:287, 1971.

Özdemir, C., and Young, R. R.: The results to be expected from electrical testing in the diagnosis of myasthenia gravis. Ann. N.Y. Acad. Sci., 274:203, 1976.

Patten, B. M., Hart, A., and Lovelace, R.: Multiple sclerosis associated with defects in neuromuscular transmission. J. Neurol. Neurosurg. Psychiatry, 35:385, 1972.

Pickett, J. B.: Severe botulism with motor unit potentials resembling fibrillation. Electroencephalogr. Clin. Neurophysiol., 43:114, 1977a.

Pickett, J. B.: Unpublished observation in a patient with polymyositis. 1977b.

Pickett, J. B.: Late components of motor unit potentials in a patient with myoglobinuria. Ann. Neurol., 3:461, 1978.

Pickett, J. B., Berg, B., Chaplin, E., et al.: Syndrome of botulism in infancy: Clinical and electrophysiologic study. N. Engl. J. Med., 295:770, 1976.

Rahamimoff, R., Erulkar, S. D., Alnaes, E., et al.: Modulation of transmitter release by calcium ions and nerve impulses. Cold Spring Harbor Symp. Quant. Biol., 40:107, 1976.

Rash, J. E., Albuquerque, E. X., Hudson, C. S., et al.: Studies of human myasthenia gravis: Electrophysiological and ultrastructural evidence compatible with antibody attachment to the acetylcholine receptor complex. Proc. Natl. Acad. Sci. U.S.A., 73:4584, 1976.

Satyamurti, S., Drachman, D. B., and Slone, F.: Blockade of acetylcholine receptors: A model of myasthenia gravis. Science, 187:955, 1975.

Schwartz, M. S., and Stålberg, E.: Myasthenia gravis with features of the myasthenic syndrome. An investigation with electrophysiologic methods including single-fiber electromyography. Neurology (Minneap.), 25:80, 1975.

Sears, M. L., Walsh, F. B., and Teasdall, R. D.: The electromyogram from ocular muscles in myasthenia gravis. Arch. Ophthalmol., 63:791, 1960.

Seybold, M. E., Lambert, E. H., Lennon, V. A., et al.: Experimental autoimmune myasthenia: Clinical, neurophysiologic and pharmacologic aspects. Ann. N.Y. Acad. Sci., 274:275, 1976.

Silbergeld, E. K.: Sodium regulates release of calcium sequestered in synaptosomal mitochondria. Biochem. Biophys. Res. Commun., 77:464, 1977.

Simpson, J. A.: Disorders of neuromuscular transmission. Proc. R. Soc. Med., 59:993, 1966.

Slomic, A., Rosenfalck, A., and Buchthal, F.: Electrical and mechanical responses of normal and myasthenic muscle. Brain Res., 10:1, 1968.

Smith, L. D.: Botulism — the Organism, Its Toxins, the Disease. Springfield, Ill., Charles C Thomas, 1977.

Spector, R. H., and Daroff, R. B.: Edrophonium infrared optokinetic nystagmography in the diagnosis of myasthenia gravis. Ann. N.Y. Acad. Sci., 274:642, 1976.

Stålberg, E., and Ekstedt, J.: Single fiber EMG and microphysiology of the motor units in normal and diseased human muscle. In Desmedt, J. E. (ed.): New Developments in Electromyography and Clinical Neurophysiology, Vol. 1. Basel, S. Karger, 1973, p. 113.

Stålberg, E., Trontelj, J. V., and Schwartz, M. S.: Single-muscle-fiber recordings of the jitter phenomenon in patients with myasthenia gravis and members of their families. Ann. N.Y. Acad. Sci., 274:189, 1976.

Stanbury, J. B., and Huyck, J. H.: Tick paralysis: A critical review. Medicine (Baltimore), 24:219, 1945.

Swift, T. R., and Ignacio, O. J.: Tick paralysis: Electrophysiologic studies. Neurology (Minneap.), 25:1130, 1975.

Takamori, M., and Gutmann, L.: Intermittent defect of acetylcholine release in myasthenia gravis. Neurology (Minneap.), 21:47, 1971.

Takamori, M., and Iwanaga, S.: Experimental myasthenia due to alpha-bungarotoxin. Neurology (Minneap.), 26:844, 1976.

Toyka, K. V., Drachman, D. B., Griffin, D. E., et al.: Myasthenia gravis. Study of humoral immune mechanisms by passive transfer to mice. N. Engl. J. Med., 296:125, 1977.

U.S. Dept. of Health, Education, and Welfare: Botulism in the United States. Review of Cases, 1899–1973, and Handbook for Epidemiologists, Clinicians and Laboratory Workers. Washington, D.C., U.S. Government Printing Office, June, 1974.

Wohlfart, G.: Collateral regeneration in partially denervated muscles. Neurology, 8:175, 1958.

Wray, S. H., and Pavan-Langston, D.: A re-evaluation of edrophonium chloride (Tensilon) tonography in the diagnosis of myasthenia gravis. Neurology (Minneap.), 21:586, 1971.

Wright, E. A., and McQuillen, M. P.: Antibiotic-induced neuromuscular blockade. Ann. N.Y. Acad. Sci., 183:358, 1971.

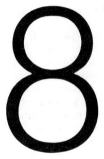

Physiological Consequences of Demyelination*

W. I. McDonald

INTRODUCTION Demyelination is a common pathological finding in peripheral neuropathy. Investigation of its physiological consequences has led not only to a greater comprehension of the role of the myelin sheath in conduction but to improved diagnostic methods and to an increased understanding of the origin of symptoms in peripheral nerve disease. In this chapter the various abnormalities of conduction produced by demyelination, their mechanisms and, finally, their roles in symptom production will be described.

Conduction Block Complete conduction block was first inferred by Erb (1876) from the observation that, in certain patients with complete paralysis of a muscle due to traumatic peripheral nerve lesion, muscular contraction could be obtained by electrical stimulation of the nerve below the lesion but not from above. Although Gombault (1881), within 5 years of Erb's work, demonstrated segmental demyelination in local traumatic lesions of human peripheral nerve, it was not until Denny-Brown and Brenner (1944 a,b,c) made their systematic experimental observations on compression lesions that the association between demyelination and interference with conduction was established. They showed that, as in Erb's patients, apparently full contraction of a muscle could be obtained by stimulation below a lesion induced some days earlier in the cat by tourniquet or local compression, at a time when no contraction was obtained by stimulation above the lesion.

The first direct demonstration of conduction block was made in the diphtheria toxin lesion. Parenteral administration of diphtheria toxin in the cat results in focal

---

*I have had many useful discussions with Dr. K. J. Smith concerning the effects of remyelination on conduction.

demyelination in the region of the dorsal root ganglion (McDonald, 1963*a*). Figure 8–1 shows antidromic compound action potentials elicited by stimulation of the peripheral end of a dorsal root cut close to the spinal cord (McDonald, 1963*b*). The records were obtained with a mobile electrode from multiple sites on the dorsal root, dorsal root ganglion, and mixed spinal nerve root. Figure 8–1 (*left*) shows records from a normal animal; on the right are records from an animal with demyelination in the dorsal root ganglion. There is an abrupt loss of the negative component of the action potential and a relative increase in the initial positive wave where the demyelination commences. These are the electrical signs of conduction block.

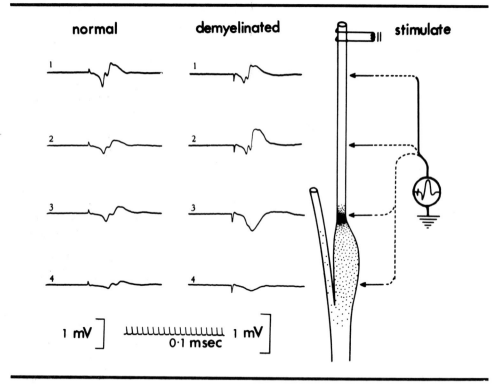

Figure 8–1 Evidence for conduction block in a demyelinating lesion. (From McDonald, 1963b.)

Conduction block has been demonstrated in demyelinating lesions produced in a wide variety of ways, including tourniquet (Mayer and Denny-Brown, 1964; Ochoa et al., 1973), experimental allergic neuritis (Cragg and Thomas, 1964; Hall, 1967), compression (Gilliatt, Chapter 10 of this volume), and the local injection of lysophosphatidyl choline (Smith, 1979).

Slowed Conduction Experiments on the diphtheria toxin lesion also showed that complete conduction block is not an inevitable consequence of demyelination (McDonald, 1961, 1962*a*, 1963*b*; Kaeser and Lambert, 1962). The maximum conduction velocity of peripheral nerve determined by recording the compound action potential either directly from the nerve trunk (Fig. 8–2) or from the muscle action potential after stimulation of the nerve is reduced in the diphtheria toxin lesion. The delay occurs in the demyelinated region (Fig. 8–3). These observations were subsequently confirmed for demyelinating lesions produced by allergic, mechanical, inflammatory, and other toxic mechanisms (Cragg and Thomas, 1964; Mayer and Denny-Brown, 1964; Lehmann and Ule, 1964; Fullerton, 1966; Hall, 1967), and it is clear that the slow conduction in certain acute human neuropathies is attributable to demyelination (Bannister and Sears, 1962; Gilliatt, 1973; Kurdi and Abdul-Kader, 1979).

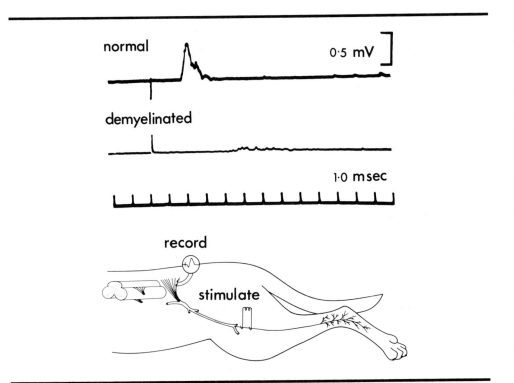

Figure 8–2 Compound action potentials recorded from a cut dorsal root after stimulation of the sural nerve. *Upper record:* Normal cat. *Lower record:* Cat with demyelination in the dorsal root ganglion. The conduction distance was the same in both experiments; experimental arrangements are shown diagrammatically. (From McDonald, 1963*b*.)

267

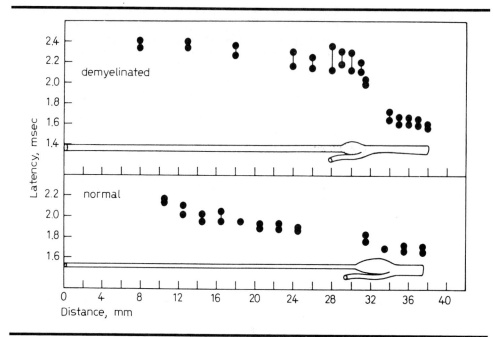

Figure 8–3 Relationship between latency and conduction distance for compound action potentials recorded directly with a mobile recording electrode from successive sites on the surface of the mixed spinal nerve root, dorsal root ganglion, and dorsal root after stimulation of the sural nerve in the leg. The approximate distribution of demyelination is shown by the stippling in the upper diagram. (From McDonald, 1962a.)

ORIGIN OF SLOWED CONDUCTION In principle, two possible mechanisms might contribute to the decrease in maximum conduction velocity observed in demyelinated nerve — block of conduction of the fastest fibers and slowing of conduction in individual fibers. Evidence for slowing of conduction in individual fibers was first obtained by recording from isolated skin and muscle afferent fibers in diphtheritic neuritis in the cat and experimental allergic neuritis in the guinea pig (McDonald 1961, 1962b, 1963b; Hall, 1967). McDonald and Gilman (1968) recorded from dorsal root filaments in cats with diphtheria toxin-induced demyelination in the dorsal root ganglia. By stimulating at two separate sites in the conduction pathway they showed that the reduction in velocity in a given single fiber occurs in the portion of the pathway containing the lesion, and that the conduction velocity in the histologically intact nerve is normal.

A new dimension was added to the analysis of conduction defects in demyelinated nerve by the experiments of Rasminsky and Sears (1972), who developed a method enabling them to record from successive internodes on single undissected larger diameter ventral root fibers in the rat. This method avoided possible damage to the fibers by teasing. Using a pair of electrodes separated by approximately 500 μm, they recorded the longitudinal action currents from multiple sites within each internode. (Fig. 8–4). The latency of the action currents shows a stepwise increase at approximately 1-mm intervals, corresponding with the normal internodal length of these fibers. The membrane current was derived from the records and it was shown that there is a net inward current flow only where the latency increases — i.e., at the presumed location of the nodes. These observations on the undissected root closely resemble those of Huxley and Stämpfli (1949) on isolated single fibers.

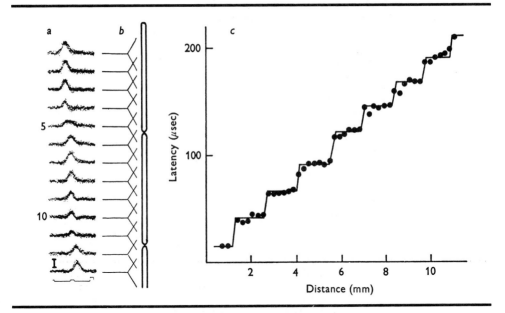

Figure 8–4 Normal single fiber from intact rat ventral root. *A,* Successive records of external longitudinal current recorded from a single fiber as electrodes were moved along ventral root in steps of 0.2 mm. Time scale, 100 μsec/division; vertical bar, 100 μV. Upward deflection here and in Figure 8–5 represents current flowing opposite to the direction of propagation. *B,* Lines from each record indicate positions of electrodes with respect to diagrammatic fiber. Sites of nodes of Ranvier inferred from records. *C,* Latency to peak of external longitudinal current as a function of distance along the fiber. Zero time and latency are arbitrary; temperature, 30° C. (From Rasminsky and Sears, 1972.)

In fibers demyelinated by diphtheria toxin, Rasminsky and Sears (1972) showed that the slowing of conduction is due to increases in internodal conduction time and that the magnitude of the changes varies from segment to segment (Fig. 8–5), in keeping with the variety and distribution of the pathological changes known to occur in this type of lesion.

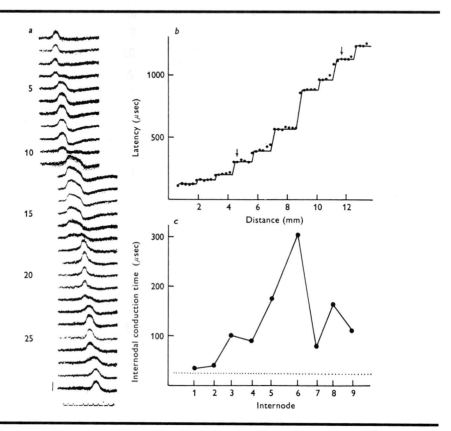

Figure 8–5 Single fiber from demyelinated ventral root. A, Successive records of external longitudinal current recorded as electrodes were moved along ventral root in steps of 0.2 mm. Time scale, 100 μsec./small division; vertical bar, 100 μV. B, Latency to initial peak of external longitudinal current as a function of distance along the fiber. Zero time and distance are arbitrary. Arrows indicate first and last records illustrated in A. C, Data of B replotted, and internodal conduction time for each of the nine successive internodes examined. Dotted line indicates normal internodal conduction time; temperature, 30° C. (From Rasminsky and Sears, 1972.)

NATURE OF SLOW CONDUCTION Recently the technique has been refined and it has been possible to record from a greater number of sites within each internode, using more closely spaced electrodes (120 to 140 μm) (Bostock and Sears, 1976, 1978). The new experiments on the diphtheria toxin lesion have confirmed the findings of the earlier experiments and have revealed a new phenomenon in some fibers — continuous conduction over lengths corresponding approximately to an internode. A typical example is shown in Figure 8–6, in which longitudinal action current averages (n = 1024, current calibration 1.5 nA) are plotted against distance along the root. Diphtheria toxin had been applied to the root 9 days previously. Conduction

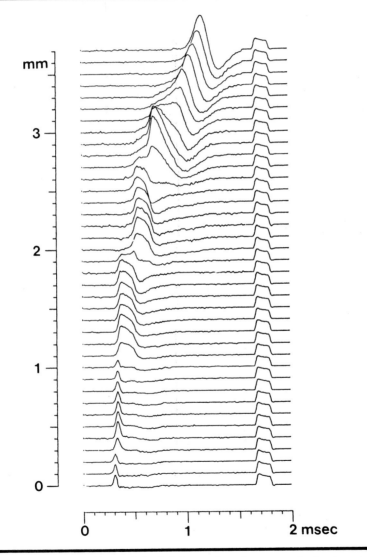

Figure 8–6 Saltatory and continuous conduction in a single ventral root fiber 9 days after diphtheria toxin injection. (From Bostock and Sears, 1978.)

from the first to the second nodes (the site of which is indicated by the stepwise increase in latency) is relatively normal, whereas from the second to the third nodes and the third to the fourth it is grossly delayed. The internodal conduction times, measured between points of current reversal, are 30, 160, and 110 μsec, respectively. When the fourth node is excited outward current is drawn most strongly from the next internode, indicating internodal demyelination. The internodal current then reverses, indicating excitation on the internodal axon. There is then a steady increase in latency between each successive recording site, indicating continuous conduction. The local velocity in this segment was approximately 2 meters per second. Figure 8–7 shows a comparable set of records from a smaller fiber (mean internodal length 515 μm) with a 6-day lesion, which resumes saltatory conduction after a stretch of continuous conduction. In eight fibers the mean velocity in the segment of continuous conduction was in the range for normal unmyelinated fibers (1.1 to 2.3 m/sec) representing one sixteenth to one forty-third of the normal estimated velocity for the fibers concerned.

Continuous conduction has also been observed in the dystrophic mouse in the midportion of the ventral root where there is a congenital defect in myelin formation, resulting in the persistence of lengthy amyelinated gaps (Raminsky et al., 1978). Bostock et al. (1977) have reported a phase of continuous conduction in the regenerating tips of crushed dorsal root fibers in the rat.

The significance of continuous conduction in demyelinating peripheral neuropathy cannot yet be assessed fully. Neither the frequency with which it appears in diphtheritic demyelination nor the time course of its development in relation to the evolution of demyelination has been determined. The occurrence of continuous conduction in demyelinating lesions produced in other ways also needs to be investigated. There is indirect evidence for its occurrence in experimental allergic neuritis (Cragg and Thomas, 1964). The fact remains, however, that extensive demyelinating lesions, both experimental and clinical, are regularly associated with conduction block. The factors determining the development of continuous conduction and its role in producing the clinical and electrophysiological characteristics of human peripheral neuropathy have still to be elucidated.

The observations described thus far have the important physiological implication that the internodal axon membrane is excitable in the absence of a myelin sheath in diphtheritic demyelination and in the congenital neuropathy of the dystrophic mouse. The findings also imply the presence of sodium channels in the

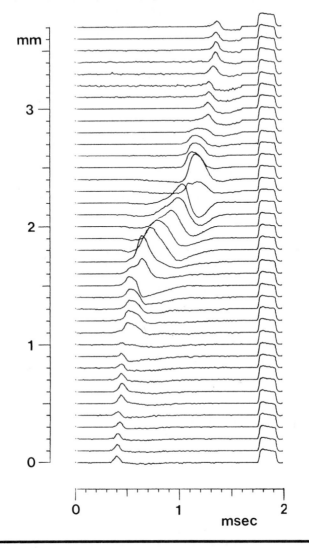

Figure 8–7 Saltatory and continuous conduction in small mye-linated fiber 6 days after diphtheria toxin injection. Note that saltatory conduction is resumed after the segment of continuous conduction. (From Bostock and Sears, 1978.)

internodal axon. Ritchie and Rogart (1977) failed, how-ever, to find any significant differences between the ^{3}H-saxitoxin uptake of intact and homogenized rabbit sciatic nerves, and concluded that the sodium channels were normally confined to the nodes. If this is the case, there must be a redistribution of sodium channels in the demyelinated fibers. The mechanism and the fac-tors governing the occurrence of such a change are quite unknown.

273

Intermittent Conduction Block

The slow conduction in demyelinated nerve fibers is more vulnerable than normal. The refractory period determined in the conventional way by stimulation of the whole nerve trunk is prolonged in experimental allergic neuritis (Lehmann et al., 1971*a*), diphtheritic polyneuritis (Lehmann et al., 1971*b*), and circumscript (granulomatous) neuritis (Lehmann and Tackmann, 1970). A more sensitive index of the function of demyelinated nerve fibers is the refractory period of transmission (RPT), which denotes the longest interval at which the second of two impulses enters but does not traverse a region of demyelination (McDonald and Sears, 1970). The RPT of individual fibers is prolonged in the experimental diphtheria (Rasminsky and Sears, 1972) and lysophosphatidyl choline lesions (Smith and Hall, 1978; Smith, 1979) and, as a consequence, the ability of the fibers to transmit long trains of impulses faithfully at physiological frequencies is impaired. Intermittent conduction failure has been observed at frequencies as low as 1 Hz (McDonald, 1980). Prolonged stimulation of demyelinated fibers may lead to the accumulation of refractoriness (posttetanic depression) and complete although reversible conduction block may supervene (McDonald and Sears, 1970; Rasminsky and Sears, 1972).

Effect of Temperature

The fact that small rises in temperature may increase neurological deficit in patients with multiple sclerosis led Davis and Jacobson (1971) to investigate the effect of temperature on conduction in peripheral nerve fibers demyelinated by experimental allergic neuritis in the guinea pig. They found that the blocking temperature in the pathological nerve is lowered from 46° to 38° C. Rasminsky (1973) examined conduction in individual undissected fibers and showed that increases of as little as 0.5° C within the physiological range can block conduction in critically demyelinated internodes. Figure 8–8 shows action currents from four different fibers recorded at the same site. When the temperature was raised from 36° to 36.5° C the latency in internode b became erratic and, after a further rise of 0.5° C, fiber b was blocked altogether. The process was reversed as the temperature was lowered. The internodal conduction time was *decreased* with rising temperature — i.e., the conduction velocity was *increased*.

Spontaneous Activity and Interaction Between Nerve Fibers

It has often been suggested that certain symptoms of peripheral neuropathy such as paresthesias might arise from spontaneous activity and/or interaction between damaged nerve fibers. Until recently, there has been no direct evidence that such phenomena occur under physiological conditions. Matteucci (1847) showed that it is possible to excite a motor nerve trunk by the electric current developed by a contracting muscle. Cross-excitation from nerve fiber to nerve fiber *within* a nerve

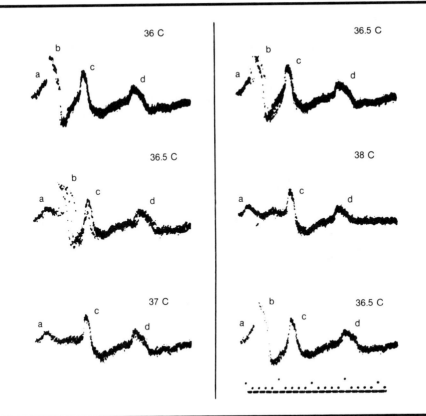

Figure 8–8 Effect of changes in temperature on conduction in four single fibers from a demyelinated ventral root. All external longitudinal current records are from the same postion on the fibers. Time scale 100 μsec/small division. (From Rasminsky, 1973.)

trunk does not, however, occur under normal conditions. Subthreshold changes in excitability nevertheless occur in inactive fibers when a synchronous volley of impulses is transmitted by adjacent fibers (Katz and Schmitt, 1940). Granit et al. (1944); Granit and Skoglund (1945) reported ephaptic activation of nerve fibers at the site of a crush or section of nerve trunks but Wall et al. (1974) were unable to confirm these observations.

Important new observations have been made on the granulomatous demyelinating lesion (circumscript neuritis) described by Lehmann and Ule (1964) and on the roots of the dystrophic mouse which contain stretches of amyelinated or incompletely myelinated axon. Howe et al. (1977) observed spontaneous activity in single units in cat and rabbit arising with granulomatous lesions of not less than 10 days duration. The discharge frequency was low, 0.25 to 1.5 Hz (Fig. 8–9). Rasminsky (1978), recording

275

from undissected single fibers, demonstrated convincingly that impulses may arise spontaneously in the amyelinated portion of the dystrophic mouse root. The impulses occur singly or in short bursts, with a frequency up to 100 Hz. Occasionally, continuous firing for up to 30 minutes is observed. The spontaneous activity is particularly prominent when the temperature of the preparation is low (26° to 28° C) but, although the discharges tended to decrease as the temperature is raised, some spontaneous activity persists at 37° C.

In these experiments Rasminsky (1978) also obtained evidence for cross-excitation between single fibers in the amyelinated portion of the roots where the naked axons frequently come into close contact with each other (Bray and Aguayo, 1975) (Fig. 8–10). These observations provide the first clear evidence of cross-excitation at the single fiber level in chronically abnormal nerve fibers.

Abnormal Irritability

Another well-known aspect of the function of abnormal nerves is their increased susceptibility to excitation by mechanical means — for example, Tinel's sign and the paresthesias induced by percussion at the wrist in the carpal tunnel syndrome. Howe et al. (1977) showed that, whereas acute static compression of normal peripheral nerve produces a burst of impulses lasting only a few msec, the same stimulus applied to a focal experimental granuloma of nerve produces a train of impulses usually lasting some 30 seconds but occasionally up to 3 minutes (Fig. 8–11.)

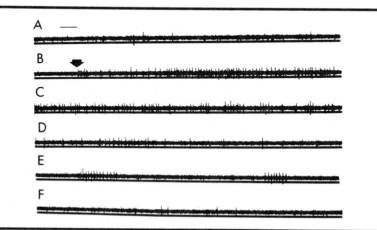

Figure 8–9 Single fiber recording from an Aδ fiber from a chronically injured dorsal root. *A,* Spontaneous activity (root section proximal to lesion site, nerve section distal to recording site). *B* through *F,* Response to acute compression at the site of the chronic injury. Each line represents the first 3 seconds of activity of successive 1-min intervals. Mechanical stimulus delivered at arrow and maintained. Response lasted over 3 minutes. Time bar = 200 msec. (From Howe et al., 1977.)

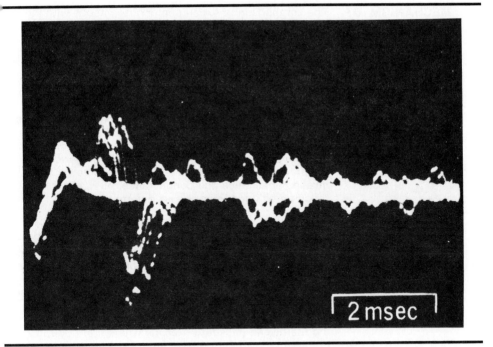

Figure 8–10 Variable latency of cross-talk between two dystrophic ventral root fibers. A centrifugal impulse *(downward deflection)* triggering an oscilloscope sweep is succeeded at an inconstant latency or not at all by a centrifugal impulse *(upward deflection)*. (From Rasminsky, 1978.)

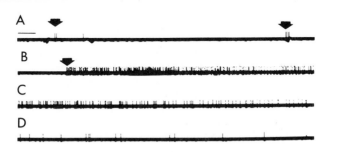

Figure 8–11 Single dorsal root fiber recording of a chronically injured $A\beta$ axon. *A*, Response to acute static compression of root at a site *remote* from the lesion. Each arrow marks a compression trial. *B, C,* and *D* show the first 3 sec of each successive 10-sec interval following a single acute, static compression of the chronic lesion itself, in the same chronically injured dorsal root as in *A*. The compression occurs at the arrow and was maintained throughout the recording (a 5-g weight was gently rested on the injured root). Time bar = 200 msec. (From Howe et al., 1977.)

277

MECHANISM OF CONDUCTION ABNORMALITIES

The comparison of experimental observations with the results of computer simulations of conduction has suggested mechanisms for a number of the abnormalities produced by demyelination. Tasaki (1953) demonstrated an increase in conduction time culminating in conduction block in the single frog internode treated with a lipid solvent (saponin). The internodal membrane capacitance and conductance were derived from the records, and they were found to increase as the properties of conduction changed. Rasminsky and Sears (1972) inferred from the form of the records of longitudinal current obtained from demyelinated mammalian fibers that the increase in internodal conduction time is due to an increase in myelin capacitance and conductance, but technical limitations precluded their precise determination.

Koles and Rasminsky (1972) investigated a computer model of conduction in nerve. The effects of demyelination were simulated by increasing internodal capacitance and conductance. The resulting form of the action potentials and the magnitude of the changes in internodal conduction time are reasonable approximations of those actually observed in the experimental situation (Rasminsky and Sears, 1972). In the computer model, reducing the myelin thickness over the whole internode to 2.7 per cent of normal (probably equivalent to leaving three bilayers of myelin intact) increases internodal conduction time 12.5-fold. A further reduction to 2.4 per cent of normal myelin thickness results in complete conduction block. This is in broad agreement with the experimental results, although increases of internodal conduction time of up to 25 times have been observed. The reason for the discrepancy is uncertain but may be related to the fact that much of the data used in the computer model was derived from amphibian nerve.

It is of interest to note that, in the computer model, paranodal demyelination is more effective in slowing impulse conduction than is uniform demyelination of the entire internode, with an equivalent rise in overall internodal capacitance and conductance. This result is in accord with the slowing of conduction observed in the tourniquet lesion of the baboon, which is characterized by paranodal as opposed to segmental demyelination (Rudge et al., 1974).

Posttetanic Depression

Rasminsky and Sears (1972) showed that the progressive increase in internodal conduction time and the accumulation of refractoriness with prolonged stimulation encountered in demyelinated nerve fibers is accompanied by a progressive reduction in the amplitude of the external longitudinal current. They thought it unlikely that such rapid, reversible changes would be reflecting changes in myelin conductance and capacitance. Also, since the membrane E.M.F. driving the axial currents is the sodium diffusion potential, the most likely explanation of the *progressive* decline in the external longitudinal current during repetitive conduction is a progressive decrease in the sodium diffusion potential, presumably due to an increase in the internal concentration of sodium. Simulation of these conditions in the computer model produces the predicted changes in internodal conduction time, culminating in conduction block.

Effect of Temperature

The mechanism of the temperature effect has been discussed authoritatively by Rasminsky (1973). In normal nerve fibers the time integral of inward nodal current decreases as the temperature rises (Tasaki and Fujita, 1948) — i.e., the current available for local excitation diminishes. This is the consequence of the more rapid initial increase of outward potassium current and decrease of inward nodal sodium current (Frankenhaeuser and Moore, 1963). In the normal fiber the safety factor is such (five for amphibian nerve) that the nodal current does not fall below the level necessary for excitation with temperature rises in the physiological range. In demyelinated fibers there are substantial resistive and capacitative current losses through the thinned myelin sheath. It seems likely, therefore, that conduction block with increasing temperature occurs as a result of the combination of these two factors reducing the available current below the threshold level.

Spontaneous Activity and Cross-Excitation

Rasminsky (1978) has pointed out that the existence of spontaneous activity in the dystrophic fibers provides evidence for hyperexcitability of the axon membranes. Cross-excitation has been demonstrated in artificially opposed normal invertebrate axons in metabolic conditions which enhance nerve activity. Rasminsky therefore suggests that, in the circumstances of his experiments, the close proximity of hyperexcitable naked axons to each other permits cross-excitation instead of merely the usual subthreshold interaction observed between normal adjacent active and inactive fibers. The factors leading to hyperexcitability are uncertain. It has been suggested that following a train of impulses there is hyperexcitability at the junction between myelinated and unmyelinated portions of the normal mammalian motor axon (Standaert, 1963). It is conceivable that a similar state of heightened excitability might develop at the junction of myelinated and amyelinated axon in the dystrophic root (Rasminsky, 1978).

REMYELINATION

The small number of studies devoted to the changes of conduction produced by remyelination contrasts with the large number of investigations of the physiological effects of demyelination. On the basis of the slowed conduction found in patients with acute or chronic

279

neuropathies, in which biopsy reveals evidence of newly formed myelin sheaths, it is often assumed that conduction velocity is persistently lowered after remyelination. However, Kaeser (1962) and Morgan-Hughes (1968) have shown clearly that after experimental diphtheritic polyneuritis the conduction velocity ultimately approaches normal values. This observation has been confirmed for human diphtheritic polyneuritis by McDonald and Kocen (1975) and Kurdi and Abdul-Kader (1979), who found that normal velocities are reached 9 months after the acute paralytic phase.

In an important new study of the properties of nerve fibers remyelinating in the lysophosphatidyl choline lesion, Smith (1979) and Smith and Hall (1978, and unpublished observations) have again confirmed that conduction velocity approaches normal values. Of particular interest is their finding that security of conduction, as measured by the refractory period of transmission, is normal 60 days after inducing the lesion. At this stage electron microscopy and teased single fiber preparations show that the new internodes are still inappropriately thin and short for the diameter of the axons.

The explanation for the differences between the findings in many human neuropathies (but not diphtheria) and experimental neuropathies so far investigated probably lies in the time course of the demyelinating and remyelinating phases. In the experimental lesions demyelination is relatively short-lived. This is particularly striking with the lysophosphatidyl choline lesion in which there is a clear separation of the two phases, the majority of affected fibers being clearly demyelinated within 4 days and remyelination commencing at the end of the first week — facts which have permitted a more precise correlation of the morphological and physiological changes than has been possible hitherto (Smith, 1979; Smith and Hall, unpublished). On the other hand, in the human neuropathies showing persistent conduction deficits (e.g., idiopathic polyneuritis, diabetes, chronic hypertrophic neuropathy) the histological changes are mixed and both demyelination and remyelination are found together.

RELATION OF CONDUCTION ABNORMALITIES TO SYMPTOMS

When discussing the pathogenesis of clinical features it is important to bear in mind that each neural function is subserved by many more nerve fibers than the minimum necessary for its performance. Impairment of a particular function occurs when the proportion of fibers conducting normally is reduced below a critical level. Each of the abnormalities of conduction described — block, slowing, and impairment of the ability to transmit long trains of impulses faithfully — is likely to contribute to the clinical deficit, although the influence of each will vary in different functions. Since similar conduction abnormalities have been described in all forms of experimental demyelinating polyneuropathy, it is probable that the same basic mechanisms operate in the different features of human demyelinating neuropathy.

Complete conduction block in large numbers of nerve fibers is almost certainly the major factor in the production of the severe paralysis or sensory loss seen in the acute stages of a demyelinating neuropathy. Less severe deficits probably arise from conduction block in a smaller proportion of the relevant groups of fibers, and from the failure of a significant proportion of the impulses initiated in incompletely blocked fibers to reach their terminations. The accumulation of refractoriness of transmission culminating in complete — although reversible — conduction block is plausible as a factor contributing to the increasing weakness observed in sustained muscular contraction and during exercise.

Slowing of conduction is probably of relatively little importance in producing symptoms but, when severe and of unequal degree in different fibers subserving the same function, it is likely to interfere with clinical tests that depend upon the delivery of synchronized bursts of impulses at particular sites in the nervous system. It is noteworthy that two of the most common and persistently abnormal signs in peripheral neuropathy, depression of the tendon jerks and impairment of vibration sense, belong to this category (cf. Gilliatt and Willison, 1962).

It seems likely that the spontaneous discharges and cross-excitation observed in demyelinated and amyelinated fibers contribute to some of the abnormal sensations reported by patients with peripheral neuropathy. Waxman et al. (1976) have suggested, on the basis of an investigation of a computer model of peripheral neuropathy, that randomly distributed axonal dysfunction (such as would be produced by patchy demyelination) could provide a sufficient although not necessary explanation for both the proximodistal gradient of sensory loss and paresthesias, the latter being a result of weak interactions between nerve fibers.

There has so far been no detailed analysis of the relationship between clinical recovery and serial changes in conduction, either in experimental animals or in man. There is no doubt that a necessary first step in recovery must be restoration of conduction across the completely blocked portions of demyelinated nerve fibers. It is, however, well known that in the later stages of recovery, in both human and experimental neuropathy, there are discrepancies between performance on the one hand and conduction velocity and action potential size on the other. The same is true of the chronic polyneuropathies.

Some of the difficulties may be more apparent than real. There are two important points to be made in relation to action potential size. As already stressed, there are more fibers subserving each function than are necessary for satisfactory performance as judged by clinical testing. Second, the amplitude of the electrically evoked compound action potential is a reliable guide only to conduction in large diameter fibers. It would not be surprising, therefore, if in some cases functions mediated by small diameter fibers were still intact when the size of the compound action potential was reduced.

As far as conduction velocity is concerned, the tests that depend most critically upon accurate timing of impulse volleys do indeed remain abnormal for considerable periods. Yet it is not surprising that muscle strength may be normal in the presence of persistent slowing of conduction. Sustained powerful contraction requires the maintenance of a tetanus in many motor units. In turn the development of a tetanus depends upon the frequency of the nerve impulses setting up muscle action potentials, not upon the absolute velocity of individual impulses. Moreover, smoothness of contraction depends on asynchronous contraction in different motor units. Thus, provided the damaged fibers have recovered sufficiently to transmit impulses at approximately 25 per second (cf. Allum et al., 1978), slowing of conduction in individual fibers is probably of little importance. The experiments of Smith (1979) and Smith and Hall (unpublished) suggest that such security of conduction for a *short* burst of impulses returns when the new internodes are still quite thin. The ability to transmit longer trains would require thicker sheaths. The details of the relationship between the time courses of remyelination, restoration of conduction, and behavioral recovery have yet to be explored.

There are insufficient data to be certain whether all the apparent discrepancies between recovery of conduction and recovery of function can be accounted for in the ways suggested. If some discrepancies do remain, it is possible that they may be explained by another mechanism that may contribute to recovery once conduction has been restored in a proportion of the blocked fibers. This is the development of adaptive changes in the central nervous system that would help to compensate for the distorted input from skin and muscle (McDonald, 1963b). Such changes obviously underlie the recovery which follows central lesions that break the continuity of nerve fibers — for example, capsular hemorrhage in man and experimental partial degeneration of the optic nerves in the cat (Jacobson et al, 1979) — and it would be surprising if similar mechanisms did not operate following peripheral lesions. There is as yet no detailed information available about the nature of such central mechanisms, but it is known that considerable functional and anatomical reorganization can occur at central synapses when one of several imputs is removed (Wall and Egger, 1971).

This discussion has been restricted deliberately to a consideration of the clinical features of polyneuropathy in view of the established special properties of demyelinated nerve fibers. This is not to imply that other factors, such as changes in blood supply or alterations of the electrical properties of extracellular fluid, are irrelevant. In the final analysis, such abnormalities would be expressed through alterations in conduction, but further discussion here is inappropriate without additional factual information.

CONCLUSION The major gap remaining in our knowledge of the properties of demyelinated nerve fibers concerns the *necessary* morphological and physiological conditions for the development of each class of conduction defect. The clear separation of the demyelinating and remyelinating phases in the lysophosphatidyl choline lesion has led to some progress, but much of the information required to close the gap will need physiological observations on identified abnormal fibers which are then examined microscopically. The technical problems involved in achieving this have yet to be overcome.

References Allum, J. H. J., Dietz, V., and Freund, H.-J.: Neural mechanisms underlying physiological tremor. J. Neurophysiol., *41*:557, 1978.

Bannister, R. G., and Sears, T. A.: The changes of nerve conduction in acute idiopathic polyneuritis. J. Neurol. Neurosurg. Psychiatry, *25*:321, 1962.

Bostock, H., Feasby, T. E., and Sears, T. A.: Continuous conduction in regenerating myelinated nerve fibres. J. Physiol., *269*:88P, 1977.

Bostock, H., and Sears, T. A.: Continuous conduction in demyelinated mammalian nerve fibers. Nature, *263*:786, 1976.

Bostock, H., and Sears, T. A.: The internodal axon membrane: Electrical excitability and continuous conduction in segmental demyelination. J. Physiol. (Lond.), *280*:273, 1978.

Bray, G. M., and Aguayo, A. J.: Quantitative ultra-structural studies of the axon-Schwann cell abnormality in spinal nerve roots from dystrophic mice. J. Neuropathol. Exp. Neurol., *34*:517, 1975.

Cragg, B. G., and Thomas, P. K.: Changes in nerve conduction in experimental allergic neuritis. J. Neurol. Neurosurg. Psychiatry, *27*:106, 1964.

Davis, F. A., and Jacobson, S.: Altered thermal sensitivity in injured and demyelinated nerve: A possible model of temperature effects in multiple sclerosis. J. Neurol. Neurosurg. Psychiatry, *34*:551, 1971.

Denny-Brown, D., and Brenner, C.: Paralysis of nerve induced by direct pressure and by tourniquet. Arch. Neurol. Psychiatry (Chicago) *51*:1, 1944*a*.

283

Denny-Brown, D., and Brenner, C.: Lesion in peripheral nerve resulting from compression by spring clip. Arch. Neurol. Psychiatry (Chicago), 52:1, 1944b.

Denny-Brown D., and Brenner, C.: The effect of percussion on nerve. J. Neurol. Neurosurg. Psychiatry, 7:76, 1944c.

Erb, W. H.: Diseases of the cerebro-spinal nerves. In von Ziemssen, H. (ed.): Cyclopaedia of the Practice of Medicine. London, Sampson, Lowe, Marston, Searle and Rivington, 1876.

Frankenhaeuser, B., and Moore, L. E.: The effect of temperature on the sodium and potassium permeability changes in myelinated nerve fibers of Xenopus laevis. J. Physiol. (Lond.), 169:431, 1963.

Fullerton, P. M.: Chronic peripheral neuropathy produced by lead poisoning in guinea pigs. J. Neuropathol. Exp. Neurol., 25:214, 1966.

Gilliatt, R. W.: Recent advances in the pathophysiology of nerve conduction. In Desmedt, J. E. (ed.): New Developments in Electromyography and Clinical Neurophysiology, Vol 2. Basel: S. Karger, 1973.

Gilliatt, R. W., and Willison, R. G.: Peripheral nerve conduction in diabetic neuropathy. J. Neurol. Neurosurg. Psychiatry, 25:11, 1962.

Gombault, M.: Contribution à l'étude anatomique de la nevrite parenchymateuse subaique et chronique — nevrite segmentaire peri-axile. Arch. Neurol. (Paris), 1:11, 1881.

Granit, R., Leksell, K., and Skoglund, C. R.: Fiber interaction in injured or compressed region of nerve. Brain, 67:125, 1944.

Granit, R., and Skoglund, C. R.: Facilitation, inhibition and depression at the 'artificial synapse' formed by the cut end of a mammalian nerve. J. Physiol. (Lond.), 103:435, 1945.

Hall, J. I.: Studies on demyelinated peripheral nerves in guinea pigs with experimental allergic neuritis. A histological and electrophysiological study. II. Electrophysiological observations. Brain, 90:313, 1967.

Howe, J. F., Loeser, J. D., and Calvin, W. H.: Mechanosensitivity of dorsal root ganglia and chronically injured axons: A physiological basis for the radicular pain of nerve root compression. Pain, 3:25, 1977.

Huxley, A. M., and Stämpfli, R.: Evidence for saltatory conduction in peripheral myelinated nerve fibres. J. Physiol. (Lond.), 108:315, 1949.

Jacobson, S. G., Eames, R., and McDonald, W. I.: Optic nerve fibre lesions in adult cats: Pattern of recovery of spatial vision. Exp. Brain Res., 36:491, 1979.

Kaeser, H. E.: Funktionsprüfungen peripherer Nerven bei experimenteller Polyneuritiden und bei der Wallerschen Degeneration. Dtsch. Z. Nervheilkd., 183:268, 1962.

Kaeser, H. E. and Lambert, E. H.: Nerve function studies in experimental polyneuritis. Encephalogr. Clin. Neurophysiol., 22:29, 1962.

Katz, B., and Schmitt, O. H.: Electric interaction between two adjacent nerve fibers. J. Physiol. (Lond.), 97:471, 1940.

Koles, Z. J., and Rasminsky, M.: A computer simulation of conduction in demyelinated nerve fibers. J. Physiol. (Lond.), *227*:351, 1972.

Kurdi, A., and Abdul-Kader, M.: Clinical and electrophysiological studies of diphtheritic neuritis in Jordan. J. Neurol. Sci., *42*:243, 1979.

Lehmann, H. J., Lehmann, G., and Tackmann, W.: Refraktärperiode und Übermittlung von Serienimpulsen im N. tibialis des Meerschweinchens bei experimenteller allergischer Neuritis. Z. Neurol., *199*:67–85, 1971a.

Lehmann, H. J., and Tackmann, W.: Die Übermittlung frequenter Impulsserien in demyelinisierten und in degenerierenden Nervenfasern. Arch. Psychiatr. Nervenkr., *213*:215–227, 1970.

Lehmann, H. J., Tackmann, W., and Lehmann, G.: Fünktionsanderung markhaltiger Nervenfasern im N. tibialis des Meerschweinchens bei postdiptherischer Polyneuritis. Z. Neurol. *199*:86–104, 1971b.

Lehmann, H. J., and Ule, G.: Electrophysiological findings and structural changes in circumscript inflammation of peripheral nerves. Prog. Brain. Res., *6*:169, 1964.

Matteucci, C.: Electrophysiological researches — fifth series. Part 1. Upon induced contractions. Philos. Trans. R. Soc. Lond. [Biol.]. *137*:231, 1847.

Mayer, R. F., and Denny-Brown, D.: Conduction of velocity in peripheral nerve during experimental demyelination of the cat. Neurology (Minneap.), *14*:714, 1964.

McDonald, W. I.: Conduction velocity of cutaneous afferent fibres during experimental demyelination. Proc. Univ. Otago Med. School, *39*:29, 1961.

McDonald, W. I.: The effects of experimental demyelination on conduction in peripheral nerve. A histological and electrophysiological study. Ph.D. Thesis, University of New Zealand, 1962a.

McDonald, W. I.: Conduction in muscle afferent fibres during experimental demyelination in cat nerve. Acta Neuropathol. (Berl.), *1*:425, 1962b.

McDonald, W. I.: The effects of experimental demyelination on conduction in peripheral nerves: A histological and electrophysiological study: I. Clinical and histological observations. Brain, *86*:481, 1963a.

McDonald, W. I.: The effects of experimental demyelination on conduction of peripheral nerve: A histological and electrophysiological study: II. Electrophysiological observations. Brain, *86*:501, 1963b.

McDonald, W. I., and Gilman, S.: Demyelination and muscle spindle function. Effect of diphtheritic polyneuritis on nerve conduction and muscle spindle function in the cat. Arch. Neurol., *18*:508, 1968.

McDonald, W. I., and Kocen, R. S.: Diphtheritic neuropathy. *In* Dyck, P. J., Thomas, P. K., and Lambert, E. H. (eds.): Peripheral Neuropathy, Vol. 2. Philadelphia, W. B. Saunders, 1975.

McDonald, W. I., and Sears, T. A.: The effects of experimental demyelination on conduction in the central nervous system. Brain, *93*:583, 1970.

PHYSIOLOGICAL CONSEQUENCES OF DEMYELINATION

Morgan-Hughes, J. A.: Experimental diphtheritic neuropathy. A pathological and electrophysiological study. J. Neurol. Sci., 7:157, 1968.

Ochoa, J., Fowler, T. J., and Gilliatt, R. W.: Changes produced by a pneumatic tourniquet. *In* Desmedt, J. E. (ed.): New Developments in Electromyography and Clinical Neurophysiology, Vol. 2. Basel, S. Karger, 1973.

Rasminsky, M.: The effects of temperature on conduction in demyelinated single nerve fibres. Arch. Neurol., 28:287, 1973.

Rasminsky, M.: Ectopic generation of impulses and cross-talk in spinal nerve roots of 'dystrophic' mice. Ann. Neurol., 3:351, 1978.

Rasminsky, M., Kearney, R. E., Aguayo, A. J., and Bray, G. M.: Conduction of nervous impulses in spinal roots and peripheral nerves of dystrophic mice. Brain Res., 143:71, 1978.

Rasminsky, M., and Sears, T. A.: Internodal conduction in undissected demyelinated nerve fibers. J. Physiol. (Lond.), 227:323, 1972.

Ritchie, J. M., and Rogart, R. B.: Density of sodium channels in mammalian myelinated nerve fibers and nature of the axonal membrane under the myelin sheath. Proc. Natl. Acad. Sci. U.S.A., 74:211, 1977.

Rudge, P., Ochoa, J., and Gilliatt, R. W.: Acute peripheral nerve compresion in the baboon. J. Neurol. Sci., 23:403, 1974.

Smith, K. J.: Impulse conduction during demyelination and remyelination in central and peripheral nerve fibres. Ph.D. Thesis, University of London, 1979.

Smith, K. J., and Hall, S. M.: Nerve conduction during demyelination and remyelination. Abstract, IVth International Congress on Neuromuscular Diseases, Montreal, 1978.

Smith, K. J., and Hall, S. M.: Nerve conduction during peripheral demyelination and remyelination, unpublished, 1980.

Standaert, F. G.: Post-tetanic repetitive activity in the cat soleus nerve: Its origin, cause and mechanism of generation. J. Gen.Physiol., 47:53, 1963.

Tasaki, I.: Nervous transmission. Springfield, Ill., Charles C Thomas, 1953.

Tasaki, I., and Fujita, M.: Action currents of single nerve fibres as modified by temperature changes. J. Neurophysiol., 11:311, 1948.

Wall, P. D., and Egger, M. D.: Formation of new connections in adult rat brains after partial deafferentation. Nature, 232:542, 1971.

Wall, P. D., Waxman, S., and Basbaum, A. I.: Ongoing activity in peripheral nerve: Injury discharge. Exp. Neurol., 45:576, 1974.

Waxman, S. G., Brill, M. H., Geschwind, N., Sabin, T. D., and Lettvin, J. Y.: Probability of conduction deficit as related to fibre length in random-distribution models of peripheral neuropathies. J. Neurol. Sci., 29:39, 1976.

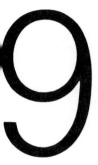

Acute Compression Block*

R. W. Gilliatt

When a peripheral nerve is subjected to acute compression, the three grades of injury shown in Table 9–1 may be recognized.

Table 9–1   Effects of Acute Peripheral Nerve Compression

Rapidly reversible physiological block (Lewis et al., 1931)
Local demyelinating block (Denny-Brown and Brenner, 1944)
Wallerian degeneration

Our understanding of the first category is largely derived from the classical studies of Sir Thomas Lewis and his colleagues before World War II. *Rapidly reversible physiological block* is the condition from which everyone suffers when a leg or arm "goes to sleep," and then recovers when posture is altered and blood supply to the nerve is restored. Lewis et al. (1931) used a sphygmomanometer cuff or a special clamp lined with a pneumatic pad to reproduce this phenomenon. When these were inflated they found that conduction is blocked by a pressure just sufficient to occlude the small blood vessels supplying the compressed nerve. When the clamp is used, a pressure of 60 or 70 mm Hg over the radial or median nerve is found to be sufficient, the blood supply to the rest of the limb being preserved. When a pneumatic cuff which encircles the arm is used, a higher pressure is needed to occlude the main artery to the limb and to prevent venous distention in its distal part. It was shown, however, that with a cuff pressure of 150 mm Hg sensory loss and paralysis develop in the hand at the same rate as when a pressure of 300 mm Hg is used.

*I am most grateful to Drs. T. J. Fowler, J. Ochoa, P. Rudge, and Professor W. I. McDonald for permission to include unpublished data. I wish to thank Miss M. Jenkyns and Mr. H. Long for assistance in the preparation of this manuscript.

ACUTE COMPRESSION BLOCK

Additional evidence that these changes are due to ischemia of the compressed nerve fibers and not to direct mechanical distortion came from another experiment (Lewis et al., 1931). A sphygmomanometer cuff is inflated around the arm to greater than arterial pressure, and maintained until sensory loss is present in the hand. If, at this stage, a second cuff is inflated proximal to the first and the latter released, sensation in the hand does not recover until blood is readmitted to the previously compressed region.

These experiments do not mean that a pneumatic cuff, inflated in this way, acts only upon the blood vessels immediately underlying it. By preventing blood flow to the periphery of the limb it causes conduction failure in the peripheral nerves throughout their length, but the changes in nerves distal to the cuff occur later than in those immediately beneath it, probably due to the complete occlusion of the vasa nervorum at the actual site of the compression.

The failure of impulse conduction in myelinated nerve fibers during ischemia, either beneath a compressing cuff or distal to it, has led some authors to conclude that the structural damage which results from more severe nerve compression is also due to ischemia and that, in these cases too, the compressing force acts by occluding neural blood vessels rather than by producing mechanical distortion of nerve fibers. Recent studies have, however, failed to support the postulated role of ischemia in acute compression neuropathy, and have accumulated some evidence against it (summarized below).

PROLONGED CONDUCTION BLOCK AFTER ACUTE COMPRESSION

Sustained paresis following a single episode of compression may, in severe cases, be associated with Wallerian degeneration of the underlying nerve fibers. More commonly the nerve fibers sustain local damage, insufficient to cause Wallerian degeneration, from which recovery is relatively rapid. For this intermediate degree of injury the term *acute demyelinating block* has been used (Table 9–1), since it is now known that there is local demyelination at the site of injury. This was first shown by Denny-Brown and Brenner in 1944, and it was an observation of the greatest importance. The concept of a local conduction block persisting after nerve injury and causing paralysis without Wallerian degeneration had been accepted for many years, but its pathological basis remained unknown until Denny-Brown and Brenner's experimental study. For example, Erb (1876), in his excellent clinical description of sustained conduction block after peripheral nerve compression, referred to " a change in the molecular constitution of the motor nerves so as to abolish their power of conduction." Nearly 70 years later Seddon (1943), reviewing this type of nerve injury (for which he coined the term *neurapraxia*), was forced to admit "neurapraxia is as yet insecure morpho-logically."

To produce the demyelination Denny-Brown and Bren-ner (1944) used a narrow rubber tourniquet around the knee of a cat. When a pressure of 800 to 1200 mm Hg is maintained on the skin for 2 hours, the underlying nerve damage is sufficient to cause paralysis of the hind limb; this lasts for several weeks and then recovers without Wallerian degeneration. Longitudinal sections of the compressed region showed that the axons remained in continuity, but that defects were present in the myelin sheaths which were thought to be similar to those origi-nally seen in lead neuropathy by Gombault in 1880, described under the title of *névrite segmentaire peri-axile.* It was, in fact, a remarkably imaginative step by Dr. Denny-Brown to have related the conduction block in his pressure lesions to the presence of segmental demyelin-ation, as this was some years before the concept was taken up in relation to generalized peripheral neuropa-thy.

In 1968 our own group in London set out to repeat Denny-Brown and Brenner's experiment. At that time we were particularly interested in the time course of remye-lination and regeneration in primate nerves, and our original intention was to study this aspect of Denny-Brown's lesion. Working with baboons, we used a small sphygmomanometer cuff with a rubber bag (5 × 10 cm) to make the lesions. When this is inflated around the knee to a pressure of approximately 1000 mm Hg and maintained for 90 to 180 minutes, satisfactory conduc-tion blocks are obtained, but the demyelination which is found shows interesting differences from that described by Denny-Brown and Brenner (1944). It rarely affects complete internodal segments but is confined to the regions of the nodes of Ranvier, with as many as 12 or 15 consecutive nodes sometimes being affected in single teased fibers (Fig. 9–1). This is in itself an interesting finding, suggesting that these paranodal defects are sufficient to cause conduction block without demyelina-tion of complete internodal segments (Ochoa et al., 1973). With the relatively wide cuff another finding was made which had not been obvious in the earlier ex-periments of Denny-Brown and Brenner (1944). It be-came clear that the demyelination occurs towards the edges of the compressed region, with sparing of the myelin in the center. With a cuff 5 cm wide the demyelin-ating lesions might extend for 1 to 2 cm inwards from each end of the compressed zone, but there remains a region of similar length in the center in which only occasional abnormalities are seen (Ochoa et al., 1971, 1972).

This curious distribution of nerve damage under the cuff is confirmed by electrophysiological studies performed a

289

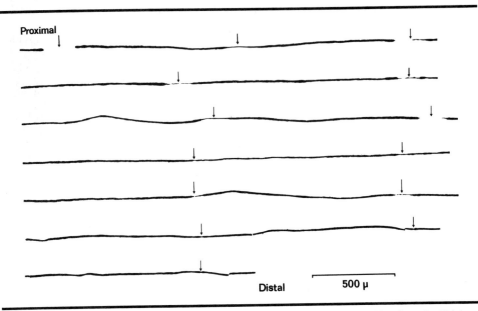

Proximal

Distal   500 μ

Figure 9–1 Consecutive lengths of a single fiber from the tibial nerve of a baboon, 50 days after compression at 1000 mm Hg for 2 hours. Demyelination extending for up to 200 μm can be seen in the region of the nodes of Ranvier *(arrows)*. A further seven nodes were affected proximal to those shown. (From Fowler, 1975.)

few days after the acute compression, when a severe conduction block is still present. When the previously compressed nerve is examined by direct stimulation and recording in a paraffin pool, two distinct zones of abnormality can be demonstrated, with relatively normal nerve between them (Gilliatt et al., 1974). In the example shown in Figure 9–2 it can be seen that the muscle action potential recorded from the abductor hallucis muscle is approximately 12 mV in amplitude when the tibial nerve is stimulated with single shocks distal to the compressed region. The stimulus intensity is 50 per cent supramaximal and is unchanged as the stimulating electrodes are moved proximally. Approximately 40 mm from the distal end of the exposed nerve the site of the distal conduction block is signalled by an abrupt fall in response amplitude. The stimulus threshold is also raised in this region for the less severely damaged fibers. This abnormal zone extends for approximately 2 cm, beyond which 20 per cent of the fibers recover their normal electrical excitability and are able to conduct impulses through the block. When the stimulating electrodes are moved further proximally and approach the upper end of the compressed zone, there is a further abrupt decrease in response amplitude, indicating conduction block in some of the fibers, accompanied by a locally raised electrical threshold

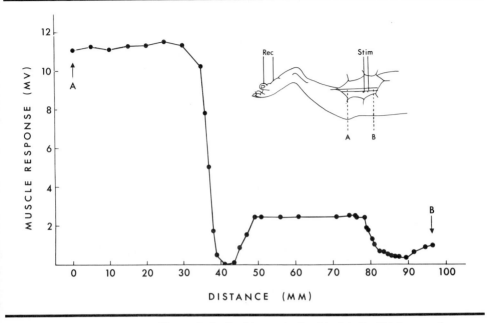

Figure 9–2 Double conduction block in the tibial nerve of a baboon after a compressing cuff. Ten days previously a 5-cm cuff had been inflated to 1000 mm Hg around the knee and maintained for 1 hour. *Vertical scale:* Muscle response amplitude, mV. *Horizontal scale:* Distance of stimulating cathode from distal end of popliteal fossa. (Unpublished data reproduced courtesy of Professor W. I. McDonald and Dr. P. Rudge.)

in others. It may be concluded that nearly 80 per cent of the large motor fibers to the abductor hallucis muscle fail to conduct impulses through the distal block, and that approximately 60 per cent of the remainder fail to conduct impulses through the proximal block. Out of four animals examined in this way, two showed conduction blocks which appeared to be rather more severe at the distal than the proximal end of the compressed region, whereas in the other two animals the block was more severe at the proximal end.

At first it was thought that the concentration of myelin damage near the edges of the cuff might be due to angulation of the nerve fibers. However the true explanation, as revealed by the careful electron microscopy of Dr. Ochoa, was much more interesting than this (Ochoa et al., 1971). When single teased fibers are examined within a few hours or days of compression — that is to say, before demyelination has occurred — the nodes of Ranvier are seen to be distorted or occluded, similar to those shown in Figure 9–3. To assess the significance of this it was necessary to cut longitudinal sections of single teased fibers for electron microscopy, a consider-

291

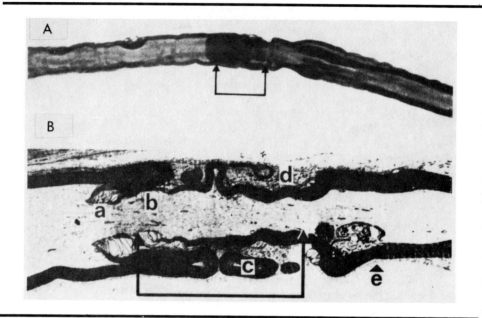

Figure 9–3 *A,* Part of a single nerve fiber teased in Epon, showing an abnormal node. The length enclosed by the arrows shows the depth of penetration. *B,* Electron micrograph (longitudinal section) of nodal region shown in *A.* a = terminal myelin loops of ensheathing paranode; b = terminal myelin loops of ensheathed paranode; c = myelin fold of ensheathing paranode cut tangentially; d = Schwann cell cytoplasm; e = microvilli indicating site of Schwann cell junction. Large arrows show length of ensheathed paranode (approx. 20 μm). (From Ochoa et al., 1971.)

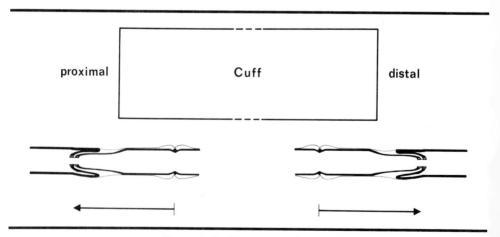

Figure 9–4 Diagram showing the direction of displacement of the nodes of Ranvier in relation to a compressing cuff. (From Ochoa et al., 1972.)

able technical feat, but when this was done Ochoa was able to observe that there had been movement of the nodes of Ranvier which had been displaced along each fiber, so that the paranodal myelin was stretched on one side of the node and invaginated on the other. The force displacing the node appears to be the pressure gradient within the axon between its compressed and uncompressed portions, the displacement in each case being away from the region of high pressure towards the uncompressed region beyond the edge of the cuff (Fig. 9–4).

In the example shown at the top of Figure 9–5 the node of Ranvier has been displaced for approximately 120 microns, but displacements of more than 300 microns are sometimes observed. The Schwann cells themselves are not displaced, so that the Schwann cell junctions, instead of overlying the nodes of Ranvier, are found in

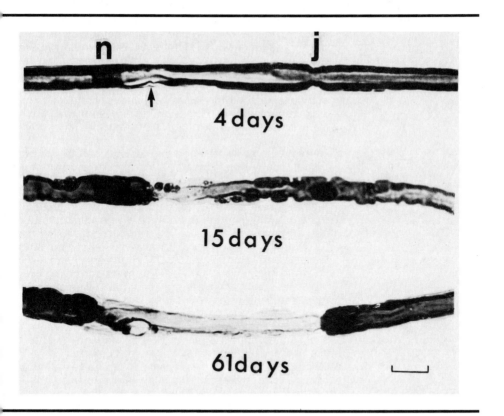

Figure 9–5 Single myelinated fibers showing suggested sequence after compression. Nodal displacement is apparent for a few days after injury and is then followed by paranodal demyelination and remyelination. j = Schwann cell junction; n = new position of node. Rupture of stretched myelin at arrow. Scale 20 μm. (Modified from Ochoa et al., 1972.)

electron micrographs to be overlying internodal myelin, thus marking the original positions of the nodes. The attachment of the terminal loops of the myelin sheaths to the axolemma is such that the compact myelin adjacent to a node is dragged from its own Schwann cell and carried into an adjacent one, with rupture of its own mesaxon. In addition, the stretched and distorted lamellae sometimes rupture or become separated from each other by swollen Schwann cell cytoplasm (Ochoa et al., 1972). Degeneration of the damaged myelin appears to follow, giving rise to the classic appearance of paranodal demyelination (middle fiber of Fig. 9–5) followed by remyelination (Fig. 9–5, *bottom*).

In considering the effect of these changes on conduction, it is of some interest to speculate on the nature of the conduction block during the first few hours or days before demyelination occurs. Do the buried nodes of Ranvier behave like the locally anesthetized nodes in Tasaki's (1953) classic experiments? Would one expect the compression of the axon and increased core resistance to be important in reducing the safety factor of conduction, as suggested by McComas (1977)? Partial rupture of the myelin sheath as a result of distortion, reducing its transverse resistance and allowing current leakage through this portion of the compact myelin, might be an additional factor. Unfortunately, a study of conduction in single fibers after compression has not yet proved possible, so these theoretical questions remain unanswered.

However, some information may be obtained from studying minimal lesions made by a much narrower compressing force than that exerted by the pneumatic cuff. If, in the baboon, a narrow weighted nylon cord is placed over the deep peroneal (anterior tibial) nerve on the dorsum of the ankle long enough to produce a persistent conduction block, the nerve lesion is so circumscribed that the full extent of the structural damage can be seen in single teased fibers (Rudge et al., 1974). Figures 9–6 and 9–7 illustrate such an experiment. The nylon cord lying on the skin at right angles to the nerve has a diameter of 1.6 mm, and is weighted with 1.0 kg, maintained for 2 hours; this is sufficient to produce a mild lesion in the deep peroneal (anterior tibial) nerve. Single supramaximal shocks are applied to the nerve proximal and distal to the site of compression to test the motor fibers to the extensor digitorum brevis muscle. It can be seen that 24 hours after compression the muscle response is both delayed and reduced in amplitude compared with that obtained beforehand. From the reduction in both the height and area of the negative deflection it seems that approximately 40 per cent of the motor fibers to the test muscle are blocked by the lesion, with the remainder showing a slightly increased conduction time through the damaged zone.

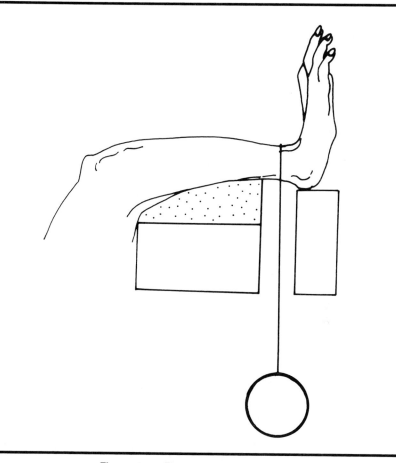

Figure 9–6 The deep peroneal (anterior tibial) nerve of the baboon can be compressed against the tibia by a loop of nylon cord placed around the ankle, with a suitable weight attached. (Courtesy Dr. P. Rudge.)

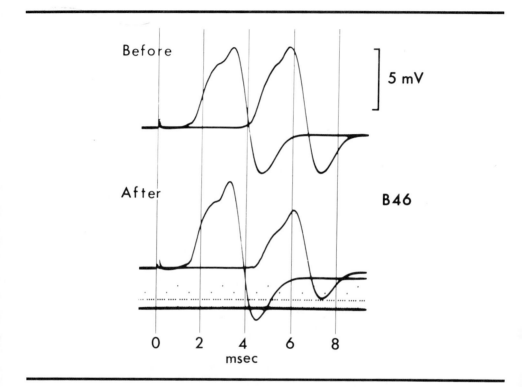

Figure 9–7 Compression of the deep peroneal (anterior tibial) nerve with 1 kg for 120 min. Muscle responses to distal and proximal stimulation superimposed before compression and on the following day. Stimuli at zero time in each case. The post-compression response to distal stimulation is unchanged, whereas proximal stimulation evokes a small muscle action potential with increased latency. (From Rudge et al., 1974.)

ACUTE COMPRESSION BLOCK

Typical paranodal changes in a single fiber from this nerve are shown in Figure 9–8; successive nodal regions are mounted one below the other, most of the internodal myelin being omitted. The nerve was examined 8 days after compression and nodal invagination is no longer recognizable, the pathological appearances being those of early demyelination. The proximal node (Fig. 9–8, *top*), is normal; below it are five successive nodal regions showing varying degrees of damage to the paranodal myelin. In the center are one or two unaffected nodes and below them a further five abnormal ones, showing degeneration of paranodal myelin. The node at the bottom is normal, as are those further distally (not shown).

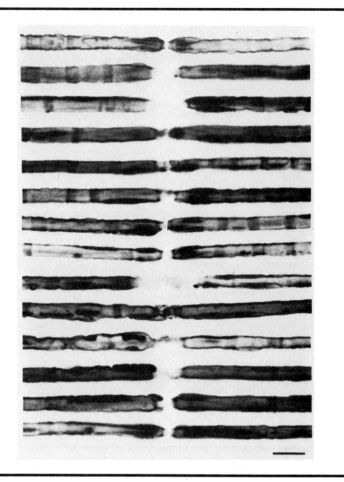

Figure 9–8 Successive nodes from a single fiber in the compressed portion of the nerve from which the recordings in Figure 9–8 were made. The nerve was removed for histology 8 days after compression. Early demyelination is present. Note normal nodes at center and at each edge of lesion. Bar, 20 μm. (From Rudge et al., 1974.)

ACUTE COMPRESSION BLOCK

This fiber, with paranodal defects extending for up to 40 microns, and with five consecutive nodes affected on either side of the center, may be contrasted with one from another animal shown in Figure 9–9. In this case compression of the deep peroneal nerve was produced by the same nylon cord but with a weight of only 750 g, continued for 90 minutes. Postoperative conduction studies carried out after 24 hours showed no evidence of either block or a significant conduction delay as a result of this procedure, but histological examination revealed

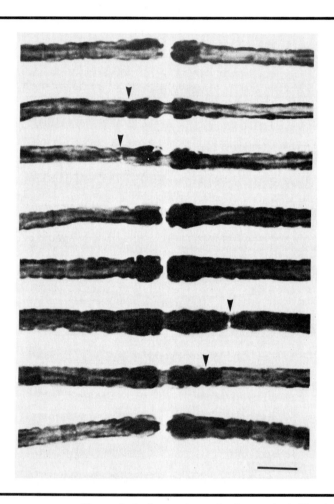

Figure 9–9 Successive nodes from a single fiber in the deep peroneal (anterior tibial) nerve 24 hours after compression by a loop of nylon cord weighted with 750 g for 90 min, to show the extent of the lesion. The proximal end of the fiber is at the top. Note two normal nodes in the center of the lesion and nodal displacement on either side (the new positions of the nodes are marked by arrows). Beyond these the nodes are again normal. Bar, 20 μm. (From Rudge et al., 1974.)

minimal changes in teased fibers; an example is shown in the figure. At the top is a normal node and below it two nodes which have been displaced for a distance of about 20 microns; the new position of the node in each case is marked by an arrow. In the center are two normal nodes and below them two nodes which have been displaced in the opposite direction. At the bottom of the figure there is a normal node and others (not shown) are normal distal to this.

A number of the large myelinated fibers in this nerve showed histological changes similar to those illustrated in Figure 9–9, and it is interesting that these were not associated with any change in the amplitude or area of the muscle action potential, such as would be expected if conduction had been blocked in a proportion of the motor fibers. The changes are therefore those of a minimal or subclinical lesion. Other examples of subclinical compression are described in Chapter 10.

THE EFFECT OF ACUTE COMPRESSION ON CONDUCTION VELOCITY

The effect of acute compression on conduction velocity is best studied by direct recording from the exposed nerve. Figures 9–10 and 9–11 show results from the same experiment as that illustrated in Figure 9–2 (unpublished), in which 60 to 80 per cent of the motor fibers were blocked near the edges of a length of nerve previously compressed by a 5-cm cuff around the knee. In this part of the experiment single supramaximal shocks were delivered to the tibial nerve at the ankle, and the ascending action potential was recorded through a platinum wire electrode which could be moved along the exposed nerve in the popliteal fossa, with a remote electrode placed on subcutaneous tissue at the proximal end of the exposure.

Illustrative tracings are shown in Figure 9–10; those from the distal end of the exposed nerve are at the top of the figure. Between 30 and 40 mm from the distal end there is an abrupt change in the shape of the action potential, with an increase in the initial positive deflection and a reduction in the negative phase. In the center of the compressed region the amplitude of the negative deflection remains constant for 20 to 30 mm, after which there is a further decrease, with an increase in the initial positive deflection. These changes confirm the presence of two separate regions in which conduction is blocked in a proportion of the fibers. Latency measurements to the peak of the negative deflection are shown in Figure 9–11, from which it can be calculated that velocity decreases from 54 m/sec in the distal part of the nerve to 12 to 14 m/sec in the region of the distal block. Proximal to this region, velocity in unblocked fibers recovers to 44 m/sec; a second abrupt reduction occurs at the site of the proximal block.

299

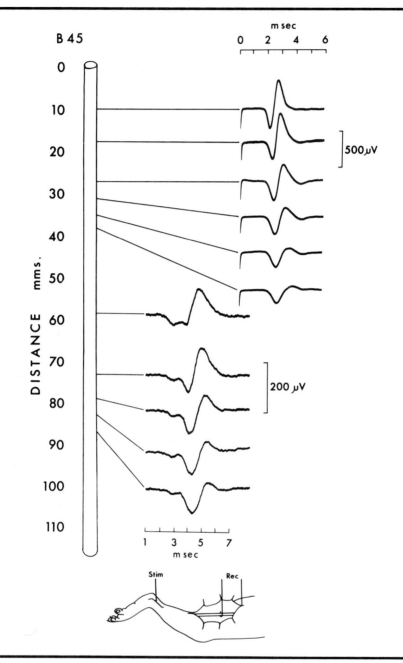

Figure 9–10 Action potentials recorded from the tibial nerve in the popliteal fossa, with stimulation at the ankle. Distance from the distal end of the exposed nerve is in mm. Two sites of conduction block are shown by the increased initial positivity and loss of negative deflection of the nerve action potential, occurring at 40 and 80 mm. Results from the same experiment as in Figure 9–2. (Unpublished data reproduced courtesy of Professor W. I. McDonald and Dr. P. Rudge.)

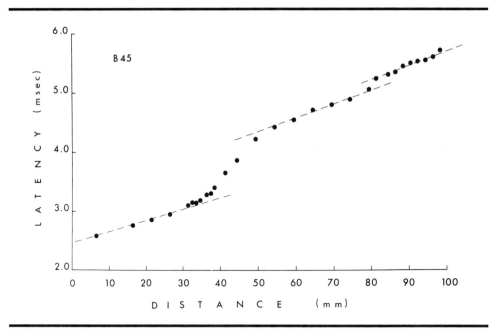

Figure 9–11 Two sites of slow conduction of the tibial nerve action potential shown by abrupt latency increases at 40 and 80 mm from the distal end of the exposure. Stimulating and recording conditions as in Figure 9–10. Latency was measured to the peak of the negative deflection of the action potential. Temperature of paraffin pool, 36° C. (Unpublished data reproduced courtesy of Professor W. I. McDonald and Dr. P. Rudge.)

Findings in the other animals studied in this way were similar, with peak velocity of the nerve action potential in the regions of partial block ranging from 10 to 14 m/sec, compared with 50 to 65 m/sec for the distal part of the nerve and 30 to 49 m/sec for the portion which had been under the center of the cuff (Gilliatt et al., 1974). The slightly reduced velocity in the center of the lesions could have been due to mild paranodal damage extending into this region but there was little histological evidence for this; selective large fiber block at the distal edge of the lesion is a more probable explanation (cf. Trojaborg, 1978).

The results described above, which were obtained by direct recording from the nerve, may be contrasted with those obtained when motor conduction is studied by percutaneous stimulation at sites proximal and distal to a block, with recording from a distal muscle. Results from 11 animals studied by Fowler et al. (1972) are shown in Figure 1–12, and it can be seen that there were some severely affected nerves in which there was no conduction through the block for several weeks after compression.

ACUTE COMPRESSION BLOCK

The first latency measurements (with proximal stimulation) shown in Figure 9–12 for these severely affected nerves were obtained at a time when only one or two motor fibers were capable of conducting impulses through the block. Response latency for these units was markedly increased (9 to 11 msec compared with 5 to 7 msec in controls), the increase being much more than would be expected from direct recordings such as those shown in Figures 9–10 and 9–11 (which indicated that the additional conduction delay through the block was 1.0 to 1.5 msec). The difference is probably due to the fact that the first motor fibers to recover are small alpha fibers with velocities at the lower end of the normal range, since it is known from previous work that such fibers have velocities 30 to 40 per cent less than those of the fastest fibers supplying the same muscles (Gilliatt et al., 1976).

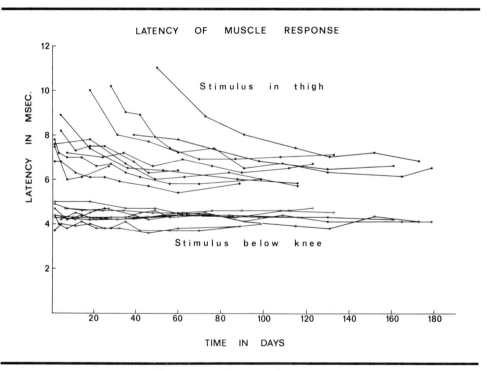

Figure 9–12 Recovery of velocity in the motor fibers to the abductor hallucis muscle after nerve compression at the knee in baboons. Data from 11 nerves studied by Fowler et al. (1972). Motor latency was unchanged after compression when the tibial nerve was stimulated distal to the site of the compressing cuff. With proximal stimulation motor latency was initially increased and subsequently fell towards normal over several weeks or months. (From Fowler, 1975.)

This example emphasizes a general point which arises when different populations of motor units are activated by stimulation at two levels. If the two evoked muscle action potentials show a marked difference in height and area, the difference in latency between them will provide no information about velocity changes in individual fibers.

FIBER SIZE AND SUSCEPTIBILITY TO DAMAGE DURING COMPRESSION

It was found by Ochoa et al. (1972) that displacement of the nodes of Ranvier during compression, with associated damage to the paranodal myelin, tends to occur in the large myelinated fibers, with sparing of smaller fibers having an external diameter of less than 5 μm. Two points were made to explain this. In the first place it is known that in the large fibers there is normally narrowing of the axon at the node (Hess and Young, 1952; Berthold, 1968) which could form an obstacle to the free movement of axoplasm, the result being displacement of the nodal axolemma and of the myelin attached to it. In small myelinated fibers the axons are not narrowed at the nodes, so that movement of axoplasm along the fibers could occur without nodal displacement. Alternatively, it is possible that little if any movement of axoplasm along small myelinated fibers occurs under a compressing cuff, since cuff pressures which are adequate to produce massive axoplasmic movement in large fibers might be insufficient to do so in small ones.

The observation that compression produces structural damage in large myelinated fibers but not in small ones may explain one of the characteristic clinical features of compression block — namely, the relative sparing of sensation which is so commonly found. This was first described by Erb (1876) who commented, "Experience teaches that motor nerves offer less resistance to such lesions than the sensory ones." As a clinical observation this is undoubtedly true, and has been confirmed by many subsequent authors (see, for example, Seddon, 1943). However, the preservation of appreciation of pin prick and light touch is more likely to be due to the sparing of small myelinated fibers than to a difference in susceptibility between large efferent and afferent fibers of comparable size, since Fowler et al. (1972) were unable to demonstrate any consistent difference between the two after mild or moderate compression in the baboon.

Structural damage to nonmyelinated fibers was reported by Fowler and Ochoa (1975) as occurring only in those baboons in whom compression with a pneumatic tourniquet was continued for long enough to produce severe damage to myelinated fibers, including Wallerian degeneration in a proportion of them. In such cases histological examination, carried out some weeks after compression, showed evidence of fine axonal sprouts in the

303

Schwann cells of the nonmyelinated fibers, the number of such sprouts being sufficient to alter the shape of the diameter histogram of the nonmyelinated axons. In the tibial nerve of the baboon the diameter of nonmyelinated axons normally ranges from 0.2 to 1.8 μm, with a peak at 1.0 μm, but histograms from two nerves which had been severely damaged by compression were bimodal, with a second peak at 0.2 μm. In the baboon no physiological studies were carried out to detect any vasomotor disturbance which might have been present, but in a human case of tourniquet paralysis Bolton and McFarlane (1977, 1978) described loss of sweating which recovered after 4 weeks and was followed by a severe causalgic syndrome with hyperhidrosis. Many peripheral nerve surgeons would regard warm, dry skin in a paralyzed limb as indicative of either complete nerve section or the most severe type of lesion in continuity, but the interesting case report of Bolton and McFarlane suggests that transient disturbances of vasomotor and sudomotor function can occur with milder lesions. Further studies of this aspect of acute compression block would be of considerable interest.

ISCHEMIA AND ACUTE COMPRESSION

Until a few years ago it was believed that the prolonged conduction block caused by acute compression was due to nerve ischemia rather than to direct mechanical deformation of nerve fibers. This misconception arose in part from the experiments of Grundfest and Cattell (1935), in which it was shown that a portion of excised frog sciatic nerve placed in a pressure vessel could be subjected to pressures of up to 1000 atmospheres before conduction failed (see also Grundfest, 1936). It is now known that this experiment was irrelevant; since there was no pressure gradient between one part of the nerve and another, there was no movement of axoplasm such as occurs with localized compression in vivo. The Grundfest and Cattell experiment is more comparable to the situation of a deep sea diver who can tolerate a pressure of several atmospheres without paralysis, since this is distributed uniformly throughout the tissues without a gradient between one part and another.

In our recent studies of tourniquet paralysis in baboons (see above) both the nature of the anatomical lesion and the pressure required to produce it make an ischemic etiology unlikely. For example, Fowler et al. (1972) found that with a standard 5-cm pneumatic cuff inflated around the knee for 2 hours, a cuff pressure of 500 mm Hg produced a minimal lesion with conduction delay, whereas 1000 mm Hg produced a block. The systolic blood pressure of the baboons was in the region of 120 mm Hg but a cuff pressure of 250 mm Hg for 2 hours produced no anatomical lesion or persistent physiological deficit. These results were not due to a lower pressure being developed in the tissues around the nerve than in the encircling cuff, since the tissue pressure was measured in a few animals and found to be within 20 per cent of the cuff pressure (Rudge, unpublished observations).

These findings do not, of course, exclude the possibility that ischemia during a period of compression might exaggerate or potentiate the direct effect of the compressive force. Before considering this possibility, a brief review of the effects of ischemia alone is in order.

It is generally agreed that when the large myelinated fibers of mammalian nerves are deprived of oxygen, they cease to conduct impulses within ½ to 1 hour (for references see Fox and Kenmore, 1967). Conduction in human limb nerves during ischemia produced by a pneumatic tourniquet has been studied by a number of authors (Magladery et al., 1950; Gilliatt and Willison, 1963; Fullerton, 1963; Cathala and Scherrer, 1963; Castaigne et al., 1972; Seneviratne and Peiris, 1968; Caruso et al., 1973; Nielsen and Kardel, 1974). In the ischemic human limb distal to an arterial cuff, changes in the conduction velocity, refractory period, and nerve threshold of the large myelinated fibers can be demonstrated within a few minutes of arterial occlusion, and complete conduction failure occurs within 30 to 40 minutes.

From the rapid failure of conduction in ischemic nerve it might be thought that continuation of the ischemia would soon lead to structural damage. However, it seems likely that mammalian nerve fibers can withstand 4 to 6 hours of ischemia without the development of structural damage. In our own work on baboons arterial arrest in the hind limb, by means of a cuff inflated to 300 mm Hg around the thigh for 4 hours, did not result in either demyelination or degeneration of nerves distal to the knee. This period of ischemia, however, was in some animals sufficient to produce a change in capillary permeability, resulting in postcompression edema of muscle and subcutaneous tissue which took several days to subside (Williams et al., 1977, 1980). In experiments by Lundborg (1970) on the rabbit, it was noted that after arterial arrest by a cuff around the thigh for 6 hours the nerve action potential could still be recorded from the tibial nerve below the knee 24 hours later; this was not the case after ischemia for 8 hours. Leone and Ochs (1978) described recovery of axoplasmic transport after nerve ischemia for 6 hours in the cat. No recovery was seen after ischemia for 8 hours.

In view of these findings the recent claim by Mäkitie and Teräväinen (1977) that ischemia can produce structural damage to nerve fibers within two or three hours is rather surprising. These authors used a pneumatic tourniquet to produce hind limb ischemia in the rat and attempted to avoid direct nerve compression by using a relatively low cuff pressure. However, it is possible that they were not

305

successful in this and that some of their results were due to the effect of direct compression rather than ischemia (Leone and Ochs, 1978).

In man, such evidence as we have on the duration of ischemia necessary to produce structural damage in peripheral nerve fibers comes from case reports of patients with emboli in major limb arteries, who subsequently underwent embolectomy. In such a patient it is, of course, unlikely that occlusion of the brachial or femoral artery is sufficient to arrest the blood supply to the distal part of the limb completely, and the contribution of collateral flow must always be taken into account. However, in cases with sufficiently profound ischemia to produce paralysis and sensory loss within a few minutes, it seems that the peripheral nerves withstand a further period of several hours' ischemia relatively well, often better than muscles at the same level in the limb. There are good examples of this in the older literature, in which single cases of successful embolectomy were reported in detail (see, for example, Jefferson, 1925; Learmonth, 1948; Burt et al., 1952). The view of Sir Thomas Lewis, expressed in his monograph, is as follows:

The nerves of the limbs lose their function under ischaemic conditions long before muscle becomes inexcitable; but long-continued ischaemia kills muscle more readily than it kills nerve. The times are not precisely known, but the death of muscle fibres is probably assured when in the warm limb they are deprived of blood for 6 to 8 hours. . . . Nerves recover after being ischaemic for 12 or even 20 hours, but longer periods lead to degeneration of their fibers and recovery is then a slow process and dependent upon regeneration.[*]

That muscle fibers are more susceptible than nerve fibers to structural damage during ischemia is not, however, universally true. For example, Wilbourn and Hulley (1977) have described examples of acute ischemic nerve damage without muscle necrosis in patients with sudden occlusions of major limb arteries. Their results may be contrasted with those of animal experiments in which arterial ligation is used. Both Korthals and Wisniewski (1975) in the cat and Hess et al. (1979) in the rabbit found that arterial ligations adequate to produce neural damage in the hind limb also cause muscle necrosis.

From what has been said earlier it is doubtful whether one should expect nerve ischemia during acute compression to influence the result, at least within 4 to 6 hours, unless it is postulated that this makes the nerve more susceptible to mechanical damage. This possibility was tested directly in the baboon by making a mild pressure lesion in the anterior tibial nerve on both sides

---

[*]Lewis, 1946, p. 21.

with a weighted nylon cord. On one side the blood supply to the distal part of the limb was cut off by a tourniquet inflated to 300 mm Hg around the thigh for a period of 3 or 4 hours; the local compression by the nylon cord was maintained during the last hour of the ischemic period. In the small number of animals in which this was done, no difference could be detected between pressure lesions made in an ischemic nerve and control lesions made in the opposite hind limb (Williams et al., 1977, 1980). There is thus no evidence, at least in this experimental animal, that ischemia for 4 hours exaggerates the effect of mechanical pressure on peripheral nerves.

RECOVERY FROM COMPRESSION BLOCK

Recovery from compression block is easily followed by serial studies in which motor fibers to a distal muscle are stimulated percutaneously at sites proximal and distal to that of the injury, and action potentials from an appropriate distal muscle recorded through belly-tendon electrodes. By plotting the amplitude of the response to a proximal stimulus as a percentage of the response to a distal one, a recovery curve for the motor fibers is obtained. This method has the advantage that the percentage recovery will be unaffected by the absolute size of the muscle responses, which may vary from one examination to another according to the exact placement of the recording electrodes. Furthermore, if any fibers have undergone Wallerian degeneration as a result of compression they will not contribute to these action potentials so that the curve provides rather precise information about the behavior of the local block itself.

Measurements of this kind allow the time course of recovery to be related to the duration of the initial compression. Data from Fowler et al. (1972) are shown in Figure 9–13, in which the results of compression in 11 nerves are shown, the size of the pneumatic cuff and cuff pressure being constant but the duration varying in different nerves, from 75 to 180 minutes. In spite of some random variation it can be seen that long compression times are in general associated with slow recovery. When the time to 50 per cent recovery is matched with the duration of compression, using Spearman's ranking test, this correlation is significant at the 0.01 level (r = 0.82). Another factor which appears to influence the duration of the conduction block is the length of nerve compressed. For example, the weighted nylon cord used with some of the baboons never produced as long-lasting blocks as a wide pneumatic cuff, even when the weight on the cord was sufficient to produce Wallerian degeneration in a large proportion of the compressed fibers (Rudge et al., 1974).

The duration of conduction block after a single episode of compression shows a similar variation in man. This is illustrated in Figure 9–14, which shows recovery curves

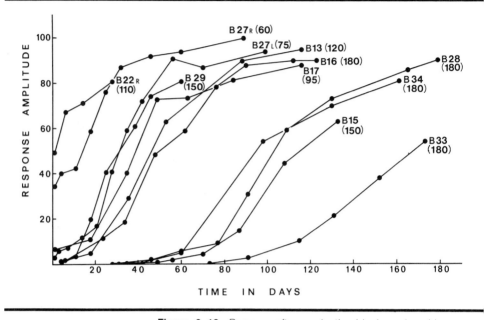

Figure 9–13 Recovery after conduction block produced by a tourniquet in 11 nerves. Muscle action potentials recorded from abductor hallucis muscle, with motor nerve stimulation in thigh and at ankle. *Vertical scale:* Amplitude of muscle response to proximal stimulation as percentage of response to distal stimulation. *Horizontal scale:* Time in days after tourniquet. Animal number and duration of tourniquet in minutes shown for each nerve. (From Fowler et al., 1972.)

from two patients. Case A was a patient studied by Trojaborg (1970) who had a classic Saturday night palsy affecting his radial nerve, acquired when he slept for an hour while intoxicated with alcohol. Recovery began within 3 weeks and was complete within 6 weeks. Case B was a patient studied by Rudge (1974), a man who had put his hand through a plate glass window and cut some tendons at the wrist. These were sutured in a bloodless field with a pneumatic tourniquet inflated around the arm; unfortunately, tourniquet paralysis followed, affecting the median, ulnar, and radial nerves. It can be seen from Figure 9–14 that the median and ulnar conduction blocks did not begin to recover for 10 weeks, reaching only 50 per cent recovery at 4 months (after which time the patient was not available for follow-up studies). An even longer-lasting conduction block was reported in a patient by Trojaborg (1977). As might be expected, cases of this severity show conduction block in some fibers and Wallerian degeneration in others. In the animal experiments of Fowler et al. (1972) an attempt was made to assess the amount of Wallerian degeneration by comparing the amplitude of the muscle response

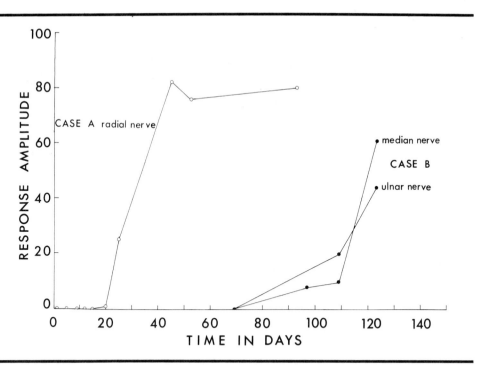

Figure 9–14 Recovery from conduction block after compression injury in man. *Vertical Scale:* Amplitude of muscle response on stimulation proximal to the block, expressed as a percentage of response on distal stimulation. *Horizontal scale:* Time in days. (From Rudge, 1974.)

to distal stimulation before compression with that recorded 1 to 2 weeks after compression, by which time any fibers undergoing Wallerian degeneration would have become electrically inexcitable. In the 11 examples illustrated in Figure 9–13 it was estimated that the proportion of fibers undergoing Wallerian degeneration varied from 0 per cent in the least affected nerves to 30 per cent in severely affected ones. A recent histological study of the ulnar nerve after compression in the forearm gave similar results (Gilliatt et al., 1978).

The pathological basis of these long-lasting conduction blocks is a point of some interest. The original histological data of Ochoa et al. (1972) suggests that axons do not remain without myelin for long periods. In fact, the reverse seems to be true; while thinly remyelinated fibers are commonly found persistent demyelination is relatively rare, even in nerves examined histologically at a time when a persistent conduction block is present in most or all of the motor fibers tested physiologically. There is, however, a change that precedes demyelination which seems more likely to be associated with the continued

309

conduction block, as it is both persistent and widespread in severely affected nerves. This is the presence of swollen Schwann cell cytoplasm, either within the myelin sheath or splitting the lamellae of the compact myelin at the major dense line. An example is shown in Figure 9–15 from a nerve examined 6 weeks after compression, at which time swollen edematous fibers were plentiful in transverse sections. The low power electron micrograph in Figure 9–15A shows a grossly swollen fiber with an external diameter of approximately 25 microns; the compact myelin is intact but the axon itself is shrunken and suspended in a finely granular matrix, which almost completely separates it from the myelin sheath. The arrowed portion is shown at higher magnification in Figure 9–15B, and it can be seen that the axon is still suspended by its mesaxon. The abnormal material which surrounds the axon is thus within the inner tongue of Schwann cell cytoplasm, and probably represents intracellular Schwann cell edema similar to that which can be produced by certain toxic agents such as 6-aminonicotinamide (Friede and Bischhausen, 1978).

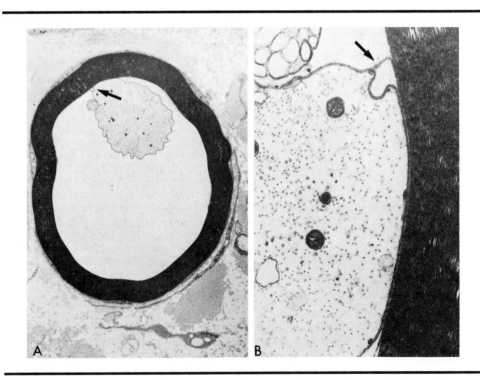

Figure 9–15 A, Low power electron micrograph of a swollen fiber showing distention of myelin sheath and shrunken eccentric axon (× 3000). B, Enlargement of region arrowed in A, showing the mesaxon (arrow) passing through a finely granular matrix suggestive of edema fluid. (× 44,000). (From Ochoa et al., 1972.)

It was suggested by Ochoa et al. (1972) that these changes might be responsible for the persistent conduction block in severely damaged nerves and that, once the distended myelin has been removed by macrophages, remyelination and resumption of conduction occur relatively rapidly. It was also suggested that the damage to any one fiber should be regarded as a series of separate paranodal lesions, each of which might recover at a different rate; conduction will only be resumed when the last of these has recovered. This point has been made by Rasminsky (1973) in another context: "Just as a chain is only as strong as its weakest link, a remyelinated fiber is only as functional as its most severely affected internode." Accepting this, the probability of delayed recovery of conduction would be higher in the pneumatic tourniquet lesion, in which 20 to 30 nodes might be damaged, than in that made by the weighted nylon cord, in which a maximum of eight to ten nodes would be affected (Rudge et al., 1974).

TROPHIC CHANGES DISTAL TO A COMPRESSION BLOCK

Recent work has emphasized the importance of an intact nerve supply in maintaining the normal physiological properties of a muscle fiber — for example, its resting membrane potential and the acetylcholine (ACh) sensitivity of the membrane. As described in Chapter 5, the resting membrane potential falls after denervation and the number of extrajunctional ACh receptors rises, with a marked increase in the sensitivity of the extrajunctional membrane to locally applied ACh and the appearance of spontaneous fibrillation. These changes are seen to a lesser degree distal to nerve blocks produced in a variety of ways, such as by local anesthetics, local application of tetrodotoxin (TTX), or compression (Lomo and Rosenthal, 1972; Lavoie et al., 1976, 1977; Pestronk et al., 1976; Cangiano et al., 1977; Gilliatt et al., 1977, 1978).

In none of the experiments have the changes been as marked as those which follow denervation; the reason for this difference is of some interest. If inactivity of the muscle fibers were the only factor operating, one might expect the changes distal to a nerve block to be equal in intensity to those which follow section of a motor nerve. One suggested explanation of the difference is that the intact but inactive motor nerve fibers distal to a conduction block exert a trophic influence upon the muscle fibers which is insufficient to prevent some change in the muscle membrane, but which prevents the full development of the changes seen after denervation. An alternative interpretation has been that the presence of degenerating terminals following nerve section exaggerates the effect of inactivity alone. Nerve block by means of TTX can only be maintained in an experimental animal for 5 to 7 days and local anesthetic block for up to 14 days; in neither case is the experimental period long enough to distinguish with certainty between the two possible explanations offered above. An acute compression block may, however, last for many weeks, and recent studies in the baboon have shown that the difference in extrajunctional ACh sensitivity of denervated and nerve-blocked muscle fibers is one which persists for at least 9 weeks (Gilliatt et al., 1977, 1978). It is not, therefore, a short-lived effect caused by the presence of degenerating nerve terminals after nerve section. There is thus good evidence of a trophic effect of intact but inactive nerve fibers upon the muscle membrane.

In the baboon experiments of Gilliatt et al. (1978) spontaneous fibrillation was found to be virtually absent from muscles rendered inactive by a prolonged compression block, the only abnormality being a slight increase in muscle fiber activity caused by needle movement (insertion activity). This is in accord with the original description by Weddell et al. (1944) of electromyographic findings in patients with muscle paralysis due to conduction block. The authors commented that, in such cases, "Fibrillation action potentials are absent or few in number and may be confined to discrete positions in the affected muscles."

Subsequently some doubt has arisen among clinical electromyographers as to whether fibrillation might not occur as a result of a nerve block alone (see, for example, Trojaborg, 1970, 1978). However, the recent findings in the baboon make it more likely that, when sustained fibrillation is found in patients with paralysis due to nerve compression, it means that some of the motor fibers have undergone Wallerian degeneration. In this respect there may well be a genuine species difference between primates and lower mammals since Cangiano et al. (1977), in their experiments on the rat, recorded from single muscle fibers distal to a compression block with intracellular electrodes, and were able to demonstrate fibrillation in nerve-blocked muscle fibers which still responded to distal nerve stimulation.

References

Berthold, C. H.: Ultrastructure of the node-paranode region of mature feline ventral lumbar spinal-root fibres. Acta Soc. Med. Upsaliensis, 73(Suppl. 9):36, 1968.

Bolton, C. F., and McFarlane, R. M.: Pneumatic tourniquet paralysis in man. Electroencephalogr. Clin. Neurophysiol., 43:599, 1977.

Bolton, C. F., and McFarlane, R. M.: Human pneumatic tourniquet paralysis. Neurology (Minneap.), 28:787, 1978.

Burt, C. C., Learmonth, J. R., and Richards, R. L.: On occlusion of the abdominal aorta. Part III. Aortic embolism. Edin. Med. J., 59:113, 1952.

Cangiano, A., Lutzemberger, L., and Nicotra, L.: Non-equivalence of impulse blockade and denervation in the production of membrane changes in rat skeletal muscle. J. Physiol., 273:691, 1977.

ACUTE COMPRESSION BLOCK

Caruso, G., Labianca, O., and Ferrannini, E.: Effect of ischaemia on sensory potentials of normal subjects of different ages. J. Neurol. Neurosurg. Psychiatry, *36*:455, 1973.

Castaigne, P., Cathala, H.-P., Beaussart-Boulengé, L., and Petrover, M.: Effect of ischaemia on peripheral nerve function in patients with chronic renal failure undergoing dialysis treatment. J. Neurol. Neurosurg. Psychiatry, *35*:631, 1972.

Cathala, H.-P., and Scherrer, J.: Modifications du potentiel de nerf, sous l'influence d'un brassard ischémiant chez l'homme. Rev. Neurol. (Paris) *108*:201, 1963.

Denny-Brown, D., and Brenner, C.: Paralysis of nerve induced by direct pressure and by tourniquet. Arch. Neurol., *51*:1, 1944.

Erb, W.: Diseases of the peripheral cerebro-spinal nerves. *In* von Ziemssen, H. (ed.): Cyclopaedia of the Practice of Medicine, Vol. XI. London, Samson Low, Marston, Searle and Rivington, 1876.

Fowler, T. J.: Tourniquet paralysis. D.M. Thesis, University of Oxford, 1975.

Fowler, T. J., Danta, G., and Gilliatt, R. W.: Recovery of nerve conduction after a pneumatic tourniquet: Observations on the hind limb of the baboon. J. Neurol. Neurosurg. Psychiatry, *35*:638, 1972.

Fowler, T. J., and Ochoa, J.: Unmyelinated fibers in normal and compressed peripheral nerves of the baboon: A quantitative electron microscopic study. Neuropathol. Appl. Biol., *1*:247, 1975.

Fox, J. L., and Kenmore, P. I.: The effect of ischaemia on nerve conduction. Exp. Neurol., *17*:403, 1967.

Friede, R. L., and Bischhausen, R.: How do axons control myelin formation? The model of 6-aminonicotinamide neuropathy. J. Neurol. Sci., *35*:341, 1978.

Fullerton, P. M.: The effect of ischaemia on nerve conduction in the carpal tunnel syndrome. J. Neurol. Neurosurg. Psychiatry, *26*:385, 1963.

Gilliatt, R. W., Hopf, H. C., Rudge, P., and Baraitser, M.: Axonal velocities of motor units in the hand and foot muscles of the baboon. J. Neurol. Sci., *29*:249, 1976.

Gilliatt, R. W., McDonald, W. I., and Rudge, P.: The site of conduction block in peripheral nerves compressed by a pneumatic tourniquet. J. Physiol., *238*:31P, 1974.

Gilliatt, R. W., Westgaard, R. H., and Williams, I. R.: Acetylcholine-sensitivity of denervated and inactivated baboon muscle fibers. J. Physiol., *271*:21P, 1977.

Gilliatt, R. W., Westgaard, R. H., and Williams, I. R.: Extrajunctional acetylcholine sensitivity of inactive muscle fibers in the baboon during prolonged nerve pressure block. J. Physiol., *280*:499, 1978.

Gilliatt, R. W., and Willison, R. G.: The refractory and supernormal periods of the human median nerve. J. Neurol. Neurosurg. Psychiatry, *26*:136, 1963.

Gombault, A.: Contribution à l'étude anatomique de la névrite parenchymateuse subaigue et chronique — névrite segmentaire péri-axile. Arch. Neurol. (Paris), *1*:11, 1880.

Grundfest, H.: Effects of hydrostatic pressures upon the excitability, the recovery, and the potential sequence of frog nerve. Cold Spring Harbor Symp. Quant. Biol., 4:179, 1936.

Grundfest, H., and Cattell, M.: Some effects of hydrostatic pressure on nerve action potentials. Am. J. Physiol., 113:56P, 1935.

Hess, K., Eames, R. A., Darveniza, P., and Gilliatt, R. W.: Acute ischaemic neuropathy in the rabbit. J. Neurol. Sci., 44:19, 1979.

Hess, A., and Young, J. Z.: The nodes of Ranvier. Proc. R. Soc. Lond. [Biol.], 140:301, 1952.

Jefferson, G.: A successful case of embolectomy. Br. Med. J., 2:985, 1925.

Korthals, J. K., and Wisniewski, H. M.: Peripheral nerve ischaemia. J. Neurol. Sci., 24:65, 1975.

Lavoie, P. A., Collier, B., and Tenenhouse, A.: Comparison of alpha-bungarotoxin binding to skeletal muscles after inactivity or denervation. Nature, 260:349, 1976.

Lavoie, P. A., Collier, B., and Tenenhouse, A.: Role of skeletal muscle activity in the control of muscle acetylcholine sensitivity. Exp. Neurol., 54:148, 1977.

Learmonth, J. R.: Arterial embolism. Edin. Med. J., 55:449, 1948.

Leone, J., and Ochs, S.: Anoxic block and recovery of axoplasmic transport and electrical excitability of nerve. J. Neurobiol., 9:229, 1978.

Lewis, T.: Effects of circulatory arrest. In Vascular Disorders of the Limbs, 2nd ed. London, Macmillan, 1946, p. 21.

Lewis, T., Pickering, G. W., and Rothschild, P.: Centripetal paralysis arising out of arrested blood flow to the limb, including notes on a form of tingling. Heart, 16:1, 1931.

Lømo, T., and Rosenthal, J.: Control of ACh-sensitivity by muscle activity in the rat. J. Physiol., 221:493, 1972.

Lundborg, G.: Ischaemic nerve injury. Scand. J. Plast. Reconstr. Surg., Suppl. 6:1, 1970.

Magladery, J. W., McDougal, D. B., and Stoll, J.: Electrophysiological studies of nerve and reflex activity in normal man. II. The effects of peripheral ischemia. Bull. Johns Hopkins Hosp., 86:291, 1950.

Mäkitie, J., and Teräväinen, H.: Peripheral nerve injury and recovery after temporary ischemia. Acta Neuropathol. (Berl.), 37:55, 1977.

McComas, A. J.: Neuromuscular Function and Disorders. London, Butterworth, 1977.

Nielsen, V. K., and Kardel, T.: Decremental conduction in normal human nerves subjected to ischemia. Acta Physiol. Scand., 92:249, 1974.

Ochoa, J., Danta, G., Fowler, T. J., and Gilliatt, R. W.: Nature of the nerve lesion caused by a pneumatic tourniquet. Nature, 233:265, 1971.

Ochoa, J., Fowler, T. J., and Gilliatt, R. W.: Anatomical changes in peripheral nerves compressed by a pneumatic tourniquet. J. Anat., 113:433, 1972.

ACUTE COMPRESSION BLOCK

Ochoa, J., Fowler, T. J., and Gilliatt, R. W.: Changes produced by a pneumatic tourniquet. *In* Desmedt, J. E. (ed.): New Developments in Electromyography and Clinical Neurophysiology, Vol. 2. Basel, S. Karger, 1973, p. 174.

Pestronk, A., Drachman, D. B., and Griffin, J. W.: Effect of muscle disuse on acetylcholine receptors. Nature, *260*:352, 1976.

Rasminsky, M.: The effects of temperature on conduction in demyelinated single nerve fibers. Arch. Neurol., *28*:287, 1973.

Rudge, P.: Tourniquet paralysis with prolonged conduction block: An electrophysiological study. J. Bone Joint Surg. [Br.], *56B*:716, 1974.

Rudge, P., Ochoa, J., and Gilliatt, R. W.: Acute peripheral nerve compression in the baboon. J. Neurol. Sci., *23*:403, 1974.

Seddon, H. J.: Three types of nerve injury. Brain, *66*:237, 1943.

Seneviratne, K. N., and Peiris, O. A.: The effect of ischaemia on the excitability of human sensory nerve. J. Neurol. Neurosurg. Psychiatry, *31*:338, 1968.

Tasaki, I.: Nervous Transmission. Springfield, Ill., Charles C Thomas, 1953.

Trojaborg, W.: Rate of recovery in motor and sensory fibres of the radial nerve: Clinical and electrophysiological aspects. J. Neurol. Neurosurg. Psychiatry, *33*:625, 1970.

Trojaborg, W.: Prolonged conduction block with axonal degeneration. An electrophysiological study. J. Neurol. Neurosurg. Psychiatry, *40*:50, 1977.

Trojaborg, W.: Early electrophysiological changes in conduction block. Muscle Nerve, *1*:400, 1978.

Weddell, G., Feinstein, B., and Pattle, R. E.: The electrical activity of voluntary muscle in man under normal and pathological conditions. Brain, *67*:178, 1944.

Wilbourn, A. J., and Hulley, W.: Monomelic ischemic neuropathies; Report of six cases. Neurology, *27*:363, 1977.

Williams, I. R., Gilliatt, R. W., and Jefferson, D.: Limb ischaemia and acute nerve compression. Electroencephalogr. Clin. Neurophysiol., *43*:592, 1977.

Williams, I. R., Jefferson, D., and Gilliatt, R. W.: Acute nerve compression during limb ischaemia: An experimental study. J. Neurol. Sci., 1980 (in press).

Chronic Nerve Compression and Entrapment*

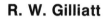

R. W. Gilliatt

The term *entrapment neuropathy* is used to describe isolated peripheral nerve lesions occurring at certain specified sites where the nerve is distorted by a fibrous band or constricted in a fibrous or fibro-osseous tunnel. At some sites the nerve may be damaged by direct compression, at others angulation or stretch may be more important, and the possibility of further damage due to impairment of blood supply must also be considered. Regardless of the exact mechanism of nerve damage, however, entrapment is a useful term for all these conditions, as it implies that surgical intervention to release the nerve is likely to be required.

Some common examples of entrapment lesions are shown in Table 10–1. In the carpal tunnel and cubital tunnel syndromes the most common finding at operation is constriction of the nerve within the tunnel, with mild swelling proximal to it (Tanzer, 1959; Feindel and Stratford, 1958; Osborne, 1959). In the tardy ulnar palsy which follows fractures of the elbow joint the nerve may be grossly thickened over several centimeters, and may sometimes be adherent to the medial aspect of the disorganized joint (McGowan, 1950; Jensen, 1959). In patients with a cervical rib and band the C8 and T1 roots may be sharply angulated over the band and flattened into a broad ribbon at this point. In one case described by Gilliatt et al. (1970) the change was so extreme that the T1 root was described in the operation note as a "broad pinkish-grey film spread over the band and adherent to it."

The conditions shown in group 3 of Table 10–1 are different again. These are examples of recurrent compression, such as occur in people who regularly rest the inner side of the elbow on a hard surface. These cases

*I particularly wish to thank Miss M. Jenkyns and Mr. H. Long for their assistance in the preparation of this manuscript.

Table 10–1   Examples of Chronic Nerve Entrapment
and Compression*

1. Compression in a fibro-osseous tunnel:
   a. Carpal tunnel syndrome.
   b. Cubital tunnel syndrome.
2. Angulation and stretch:
   a. Ulnar lesions associated with gross deformity of the elbow joint ("tardy ulnar palsy").
   b. Cervical rib syndrome.
3. Recurrent compression by external forces:
   a. Some ulnar lesions at the elbow.
   b. Lesions of deep branch of ulnar nerve in the hand.

*From Gilliatt, 1975, p. 155.

may sometimes have a sudden onset but, because the compression is repeated, the lesion persists or gradually worsens, a situation intermediate between acute and chronic compression (cf. Payan, 1970). Cumulative damage also occurs in the rarer condition in which the deep branch of the ulnar nerve in the palm is repeatedly compressed by some implement which is used at work or in the house (Ebeling et al., 1960).

ANIMAL MODELS OF CHRONIC COMPRESSION

With lesions as varied as those in Table 10–1 it may be asked whether one should even expect to find common pathological mechanisms. Unfortunately, our knowledge of the histological changes and of the mechanism of nerve damage is still fragmentary and incomplete, mainly owing to the rarity of human pathological material. However, several animal models have been developed (Table 10–2) which have proved helpful in the interpretation of human material.

Brief comments may be made on the models listed in Table 10–2. Weiss and his colleagues (for references see Weiss and Hiscoe, 1948) developed a technique in the rat by which the tibial or peroneal nerve is divided at the knee, and a cuff made from a small ring of artery is slipped up the nerve to lie just below its origin from the sciatic. The sciatic nerve itself is crushed with forceps and allowed to regenerate. The model is thus a rather complex one, in which the nerve is not only divided distally but is crushed proximally and then allowed to regenerate through the constriction.

Duncan (1948) placed "snug but non-constricting" ligatures and bands around the sciatic nerves of young rats and kittens so that constriction would develop gradually with the growth of the animal. Aguayo et al. (1971) used a similar technique; they placed a siliconized rubber tube around the tibial nerve of young rabbits, allowing gradual constriction to occur during normal growth.

The guinea pig model studied by Fullerton and Gilliatt (1967b), Anderson et al. (1970), Ochoa and Marotte

317

Table 10–2   Animal Models of Chronic or Recurrent Peripheral Nerve Compression

Reference	Animal	Method
Chronic progressive:		
Weiss and Hiscoe (1948)	Rat	Compression of the tibial or peroneal nerve by a ring of artery
Duncan (1948)	Rat	Ligatures placed around sciatic nerve to produce compression
	Kitten	during growth
Fullerton and Gilliatt (1967*b*)	Guinea pig	Naturally occurring median nerve compression with increasing age
Aguayo et al. (1971)	Rabbit	Silastic cuff around tibial nerve to produce compression during growth
Recurrent:		
Dyck (1969)	Rat	Inflatable cuff placed round sciatic nerve
Fullerton and Gilliatt (1967*a*)	Guinea pig	Compression of plantar nerves in animals caged on wire mesh flooring
Hopkins and Morgan-Hughes (1969)	Guinea pig	Compression of plantar nerves on wire mesh or solid flooring in animals also given diphtheria toxin

(1973), and Marotte (1974) is an interesting one in that it is not an experimental but a naturally occurring lesion. Guinea pigs, as they grow older, may develop entrapment lesions of both the median and ulnar nerves under the transverse carpal ligament and the cartilaginous bar which overlies it at the wrist. In elderly animals this may sometimes be severe enough to result in complete denervation of the small muscles of the forepaw.

The models in the second part of Table 10–2 are concerned with recurrent compression. Dyck (1969) placed a very small pneumatic cuff around the sciatic nerve in the rat, bringing the pressure tubing out through the skin so that the cuff could be inflated periodically at intervals of several days or weeks, as part of a chronic experiment. The guinea pig plantar nerve preparation of Fullerton and Gilliatt (1967*a*) made use of the fact that, if these animals are caged on wire mesh flooring for many months, they develop a localized plantar neuropathy in the hind foot, presumably due to recurrent compression of the plantar nerves against the wire mesh bars of the cage floor. The lesion is avoided if the animals are kept in cages with solid floors covered by sawdust. When the guinea pigs are given small parenteral doses of diphtheria toxin, animals kept on solid floors also develop plantar nerve damage which can only be prevented by stopping the hind foot from weight-bearing altogether (Hopkins and Morgan-Hughes, 1969).

In the continuously constricted nerves studied by Weiss and Hiscoe (1948), Duncan (1948) and Aguayo et al. (1971), reduction in caliber of the whole nerve at the site of constriction was commonly seen. In some of Duncan's animals the cross-sectional area of the nerve was reduced at this point to less than one quarter of the normal, with bulbous swelling immediately proximal to this and less marked swelling distal to it. These swellings were shown to be due to an increase in the endoneurium, with separation of the nerve fibers. In addition, there is axonal swelling proximal to the site of constriction, interpreted by Weiss and Hiscoe (1948) as evidence of obstruction to axoplasmic flow, whereas Duncan (1948) considered that the swelling occurs in the proximal ends of fibers which degenerate completely at the site of constriction. This question has been reinvestigated by Spencer (1972), who found that axonal swelling occurs in regenerating fibers just proximal to the point where they are constricted, but that in mature nerves changes are seen only in fibers which have already degenerated as a result of the constriction, and then regenerated.

In the naturally occurring median nerve entrapment syndrome of guinea pigs, endoneurial swelling proximal to the lesion is only seen in severely affected cases. In more mildly affected nerves endoneurial changes are inconspicuous, and the characteristic feature is local demyelination with recovery of myelination distally. Examination of single teased fibers shows that segmental and paranodal demyelination are present, the appearances being similar to those seen in acute compressive or inflammatory lesions (cf. Lehmann and Ule, 1964; Lehmann, 1973) or in generalized demyelinating neuropathy. Characteristic of the guinea pig lesions, and of the rabbit lesions studied by Aguayo et al. (1971) is the presence of short, thinly remyelinated internodes, indicating attempted repair during continued compression or constriction.

Onion bulb formations consisting of concentric cuffs of Schwann cell processes around fibers which had probably been repeatedly demyelinated were seen by Dyck (1969) after recurrent compression in the rat, but these were not found in the guinea pig lesions listed in Table 10–2, either in compressed median nerves (Marotte, 1974) or in plantar nerves in the hind foot (Eames, unpublished observations).

PATHOLOGICAL FEATURES OF HUMAN CASES

Neuromatous thickening in a human ulnar nerve lesion studied by Neary and Eames (1975) is shown in Figure 10–1. It can be seen that the enlargement is mainly due to increased endoneurial area, with only slight perineurial thickening. At higher magnification (Fig. 10–2) the sections confirm that the nerve fiber density is correspondingly reduced. The occurrence of demyelination at level C in Figure 10–2 is indicated by the presence of large, thinly

319

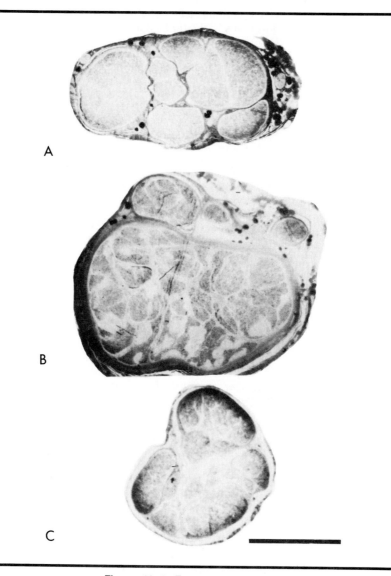

Figure 10–1 Transverse sections of the ulnar nerve from a patient, aged 68, with a chronic lesion at the elbow. *A,* In upper arm. *B,* In ulnar groove at level of upper border of tendinous arch of flexor carpi ulnaris (f.c.u.), to show fascicular enlargement and numerous Renaut bodies. *C,* 5 cm distal to *B.* Scale, 2 mm. (From Neary and Eames, 1975.)

remyelinated axons in the transverse section. Teasing of individual fibers subsequently confirmed this. The occurrence of degeneration at the same level is indicated by the small cluster of regenerating fibers which can be seen near the right-hand margin of section *C.* As might be expected, regenerating clusters are more conspicuous as the nerve passes distally; an example from the distal part is shown in Fig. 10–3.

The fiber diameter histograms in Figure 10–2 reflect the presence of both demyelination and degeneration at

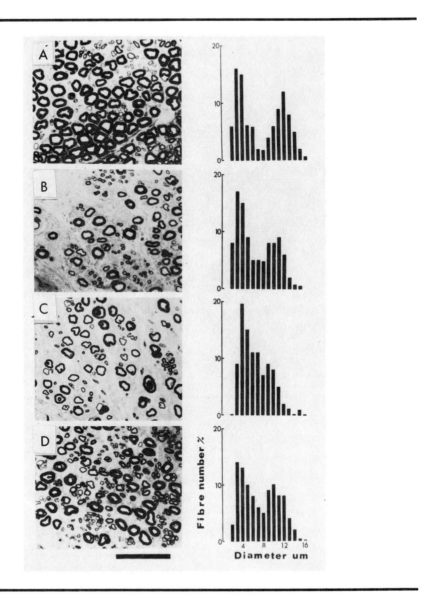

Figure 10–2 Portions of sections shown in Figure 10–1 at higher magnification, and with one additional level, *B.* Percentage histograms of fiber diameter for each level are shown on the right. *A,* Upper arm. *B,* 5 cm above upper border of tendinous arch of f.c.u. *C,* Upper border of tendinous arch of f.c.u. *D,* 5 cm distal to *C.* Scale, 50 μm. (From Neary and Eames, 1975.)

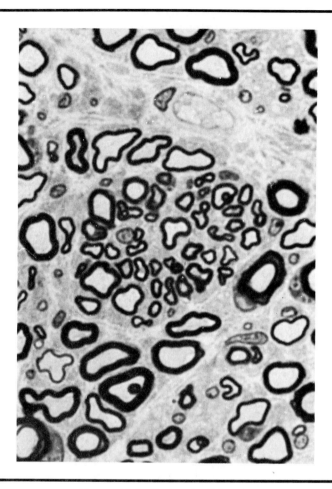

Figure 10–3 Further detail from the transverse section at level C in Figure 10–1. There is a regenerating cluster with a diameter of 20 to 30 μm in the center of the field, containing many small fibers and a few larger ones. (From Neary and Eames, 1975.)

level C where there is an excess of 2 to 4-μm fibers, which is characteristic of regeneration. The decreased number of large diameter fibers at this level is presumably due to demyelination as well as to degeneration, as there is partial recovery distally, shown in the histogram below.

In a study of subclinical entrapment lesions in routine autopsy material, Neary et al. (1975) noted that connective tissue changes such as neuromatous thickening and a local excess of Renault bodies might occur in the ulnar nerve at the elbow or the median nerve at the wrist in the absence of significant nerve fiber changes. Similar observations have recently been made by Jefferson and

Eames (1979) on the lateral cutaneous nerve of the thigh. Thus, it seems that in mild lesions the connective tissue and nerve fiber changes can be largely independent of each other.

THE CAUSE OF NERVE DAMAGE IN CHRONIC ENTRAPMENT

As in acute compression, the question can be asked whether the demyelination and degeneration seen in chronic lesions is due to direct mechanical damage or to ischemia of the entrapped nerve fibers. This question would be answered easily if the morphological change which precedes demyelination in acute compression, namely displacement of the nodes of Ranvier with distortion of paranodal myelin, were also present in chronic lesions. However, although this has been looked for carefully in single teased fibers from chronic entrapment lesions, it has only rarely been found (for example, Case 5 of Neary et al., 1975). The characteristic morphological change which appears to lead to demyelination in chronic entrapment implies a different mechanism of nerve damage. As described below, this change was first seen in the entrapped median nerve of the guinea pig, and its presence has now been confirmed in a variety of human lesions.

In the median nerve of the guinea pig, single fibers immediately proximal to the site of entrapment at the wrist show a consistent asymmetry of the myelin sheath which appears to be thinned at one end of the internodal segment and thickened or swollen at the other (Anderson et al., 1970).

When very mildly affected animals were examined by Ochoa and Marotte (1973), this change was found on either side of the entrapment site but with reversed polarity, so that the thin myelin was always at the end of the internodal segment closer to the center of the lesion. Electron micrographs such as those shown in Figure 10–4 suggest that the terminal loops of the inner lamellae of the myelin sheath have become detached from the axolemma at the node, with retraction of the myelin along the internode. There is a corresponding excess of myelin at the other end of the internode, with purse-like folding. The change appears to be a progressive one, starting with detachment of the inner lamellae but proceeding gradually to retraction of the whole of the myelin sheath from one end of the internode, leaving a length of bared axon. In an individual fiber the changes affect several consecutive internodes on either side of the lesion, becoming increasingly severe towards the center (Fig. 10–5). In the center completely demyelinated internodal segments are present. In many cases this change is only seen on the proximal side of the lesion, with degeneration of the axon occurring distal to this.

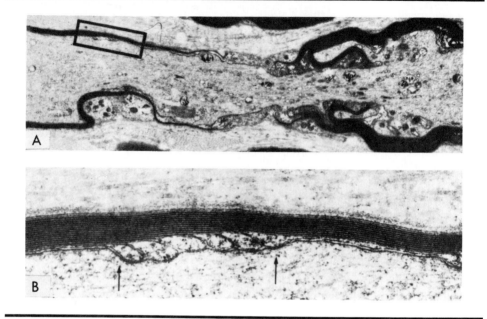

Figure 10–4 Guinea pig median nerve at the proximal edge of a compression lesion at the wrist. *A,* Low power electron micrograph of a node of Ranvier showing tapering of the paranodal myelin on the proximal side of the node *(left)* and purse-like folding of the myelin on the distal side of the node *(right)* (× 7000). *B,* Enlargement of the area enclosed in the rectangle in *A.* The detached terminal loops of the innner myelin lamellae are arrowed (× 48,000). (From Ochoa and Marotte, 1973.)

The sequence of events postulated by Ochoa is shown diagrammatically in Figure 10–6. The initial stage is asymmetry of the myelin sheath, leading to retraction from one end and thus to paranodal demyelination. At a later stage myelin loss from the complete internodal segment will occur or, in the most severe cases, complete degeneration of the fiber. Single teased fibers undergoing these changes have been seen not only in the median nerve of the guinea pig but also in the plantar nerves when these animals are kept on wire mesh floors to produce a plantar neuropathy (Eames, unpublished observations). In man, they have been found in median nerve fibers at the wrist and ulnar nerve fibers at the elbow (Neary et al., 1975; Neary and Eames, 1975; Harriman, 1977), and in the lateral cutaneous nerve of the thigh at the anterior end of the inguinal ligament (Jefferson and Eames, 1979).

These changes are of considerable theoretical interest as they suggest that the demyelination and nerve fiber degeneration are the result of mechanical deformation rather than ischemia. However, this interpretation is by no means generally accepted (see Sunderland, 1976), and other factors such as altered capillary permeability and endoneurial pressure clearly require further study.

CONDUCTION BLOCK AND CONDUCTION DELAY

The presence of conduction block in chronic entrapment is less often demonstrable by nerve stimulation than in acute compression lesions. For example, a study by Brown et al. (1976), in which entrapped nerves were stimulated directly while exposed at operation, demonstrated conduction block in only one third of the ulnar nerves examined, and in one quarter of the median nerves, although locally reduced velocity was present in all of them. This implies that in the majority of the patients muscular weakness is due to degeneration of motor axons and loss of motor units, since the reduced conduction velocity in surviving motor axons would not be expected to affect muscle power.

The most marked slowing of motor conduction was seen by Brown et al. (1976) in a diabetic patient with the carpal

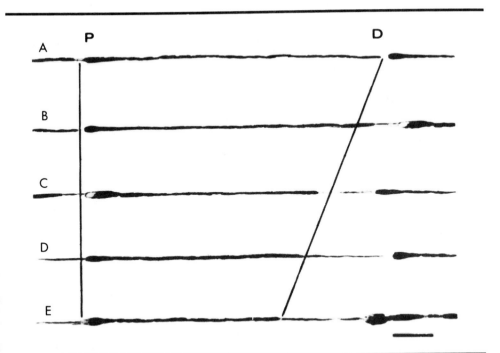

Figure 10–5 Guinea pig median nerve showing five consecutive internodes (a through e) from a single fiber at the proximal edge of a compressive lesion. P = proximal, D = distal. The oblique line illustrates the increasing extent of the demyelination at the tapered end of each internode as the center of the lesion is approached. Scale, 100 μm. (From Ochoa and Marotte, 1973.)

325

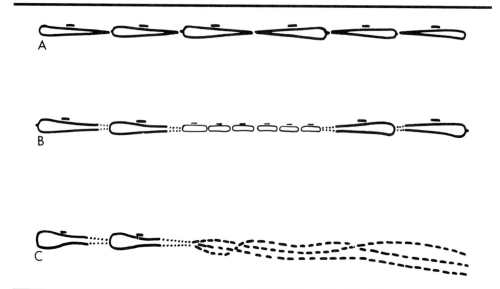

Figure 10–6 The sequence of changes in chronic compression suggested by Ochoa. *A,* Distorted internodal segments in a minimal entrapment lesion, with reversal of polarity at the center. *B,* A more severe lesion with paranodal demyelination affecting the distorted internodes at the edges, and complete demyelination followed by remyelination in the center. *C,* More marked distortion of the internodes on the proximal side of the lesion, with Wallerian degeneration distally. (From Ochoa, 1980.)

tunnel syndrome, in whom the motor latency with stimulation just proximal to the wrist was 11 msec. The muscle responses to stimulation of the exposed nerve in this case are shown in Figure 10–7, from which it can be seen that there is also a substantial conduction block; the area of the negative deflection of the muscle action potential in response to distal nerve stimulation is approximately three times that obtained by proximal stimulation.

In another study of patients with the carpal tunnel syndrome, direct evidence of conduction block in sensory fibers was obtained by Hongell and Mattsson (1971) from recordings made at the time of operation, using an intraneural microelectrode (Vallbo and Hagbarth, 1968) placed in the median nerve just above the wrist. In this way, it is possible to demonstrate that sensory fibers which have previously been blocked begin within a few minutes of decompression to respond both to physiological stimulation by receptors in the finger pads and to electrical stimulation of the digital nerve trunks.

From the studies of Brown et al. (1976) and Hongell and Mattsson (1971) it can be concluded that conduction block does occur in chronically compressed or entrapped nerves, although it is a less common finding than in acute entrapment. If we accept that conduction block is due to demyelination (Chapter 8) this suggests that in the time scale of chronic entrapment the demyelination is a short-lived phenomenon, either proceeding to complete degeneration of the axon or being succeeded by local repair, leading to conduction delay without block.

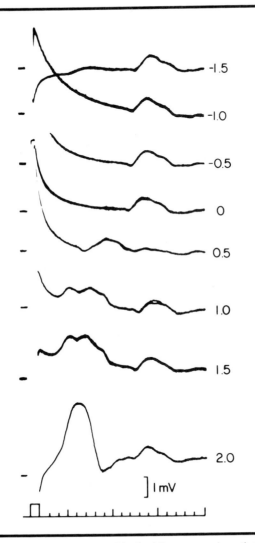

Figure 10–7 Maximal thenar muscle action potentials evoked by stimulation of the exposed median nerve at 0.5-cm intervals through the site of compression at the wrist, in a diabetic patient with pain and numbness of the fingers. At operation the nerve was observed to be markedly constricted along the length of the carpal tunnel. The numbers to the right of each trace indicate the position of the stimulating electrodes in cm proximal (−) or distal to the upper border of the flexor retinaculum. Time scale msec. (From Brown et al., 1976.)

Recovery After Relief of Chronic Compression

A particularly interesting aspect of Hongell and Mattsson's (1971) findings is the rapidity with which recovery of conduction can occur after decompression. Sensory fibers which have hitherto been inactive are seen to resume conduction within a few minutes of division of the flexor retinaculum (Fig. 10–8). That the compressed motor fibers in carpal tunnel patients are also sometimes extremely sensitive to metabolic changes was shown by Fullerton (1963). She found that in some patients ischemia produced by a pneumatic cuff around the arm blocks conduction at the wrist in a much shorter time than in control subjects, the block being rapidly reversible once the cuff is released. Of particular interest is the fact that nerves showing this increased sensitivity to local ischemia are not those with severe or long-standing lesions, as indicated by the amount of wasting or conduction delay in routine tests. On the contrary, an increased sensitivity of the motor fibers to ischemia is seen in patients who are having frequent spontaneous attacks of pain at the time of the test, regardless of the duration of the clinical history. In some of them ischemia of the arm not only blocks motor conduction but produces an intense attack of pain in the limb, as originally described by Gilliatt and Wilson (1953).

In this context it should be remembered that patients with the carpel tunnel syndrome nearly always obtain relief of pain from the time of the operation, although the conduction delay in motor fibers resolves much more slowly, taking weeks or months to return to normal (Goodman and Gilliatt, 1961). From this and the cuff experiments cited above, it seems that ischemia of the compressed nerve fibers is important in relation to the attacks of pain which occur in carpal tunnel patients, and that it may also be responsible for the rapidly reversible conduction block seen by Hongell and Mattsson (1971) in some of the large myelinated fibers.

Conduction Velocity Proximal to Chronic Entrapment

It has been known since the work of Kiraly and Krnjevic (1959) and Cragg and Thomas (1961) that after transection of a peripheral nerve, the conduction velocity and diameter of axons proximal to the site of injury are reduced and do not recover until regeneration occurs. If the reinnervation of muscle is prevented, velocity continues to decrease. Kuno and his colleagues (1974a; 1974b) showed that in the large motor fibers to the gastrocnemius and soleus muscles of the cat, velocity (recorded in single fibers) may fall by as much as 20 per cent within 1 or 2 months of nerve section. If reinnervation is prevented, velocity may be reduced by 35 to 40 per cent at the end of 3 or 4 months (Table 10–3).

Comparable data for conduction in single axons proximal to a compression block are not available. In chronic

NORMAL

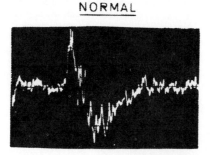

MEDIAN NERVE COMPRESSION

1. Immediately before section of the volar carpal ligament.

2. 4 minutes after section of the ligament.

3. 30 minutes after section of the ligament.

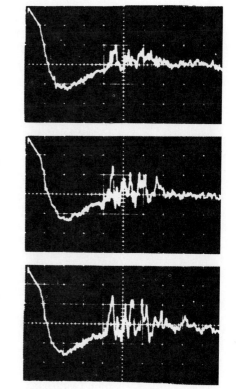

1 msec.

Figure 10–8 Recording of the complex compound potential evoked by electrical stimulation of a finger nerve and recorded with a microelectrode in the corresponding skin nerve fascicle of the median nerve. Normal potential is recorded percutaneously; potentials from the patient with median nerve compression are recorded from the exposed nerve. There is improvement in amplitude and complexity of the compound evoked potential 4 and 30 min after sectioning of the transverse carpal ligament. (From Hongell and Mattsson, 1971.)

Table 10-3 Conduction Velocity in Single Axons Proximal to Nerve Section to Show the Effect of Axotomy on Fast and Slow Twitch Motoneurons in the Cat*
(Data of Kuno et al., 1974a, 1974b)

	Medial Gastrocnemius (fast twitch)†	Soleus (slow twitch)†
Control	94 (100)	74 (100)
Axotomy		
Before reinnervation		
(14 to 52 days)	76 (81)	58 (78)
After reinnervation		
After reinnervation		
(139 to 144 days)	81 (86)	67 (91)
Reinnervation prevented		
(110 to 119 days)	58 (62)	49 (66)

*From Gilliatt and Westgaard, 1978, p. 549. Note that the difference between values for fast and slow twitch motoneurons remains statistically significant throughout.

†Mean values, in m/sec. Values in parentheses are mean velocities expressed as percentages of controls

compression and entrapment most studies are carried out by stimulating whole nerve trunks at sites proximal and distal to that of the entrapment, and recording from a distal muscle, so that proximal velocity is measured for motor fibers still capable of conducting through the lesion, although with a distal delay. Illustrative data are shown in Figure 10–9 (Thomas, 1960). In patients with the carpal tunnel syndrome and in healthy controls the median nerve was stimulated just above the wrist and elbow and in the axilla; the muscle recordings were made with a coaxial needle from the abductor pollicis brevis. It can be seen that between one third and one half of the carpal tunnel patients had reduced velocities in the forearm and upper arm, this change being most marked in those with prolonged distal latencies.

Even in the worst affected patients studied by Thomas (1960), proximal velocity is not more than 30 per cent below the lower limit of the normal range. Could this result be explained by selective blocking of the largest and fastest conducting fibers in the lesion, with velocity then being measured in (normal) fibers of smaller diameter and lower velocity? There is good evidence from animal models that both acute and chronic compression affect the large diameter fibers first (Aguayo et al., 1971; Ochoa et al., 1972; Marotte, 1974).

However, selective large fiber block is unlikely to explain results of the type shown in Figure 10–10. These are records from the hind limb of a guinea pig kept for many months on wire mesh flooring in order to produce a localized plantar neuropathy. This is a partial lesion in

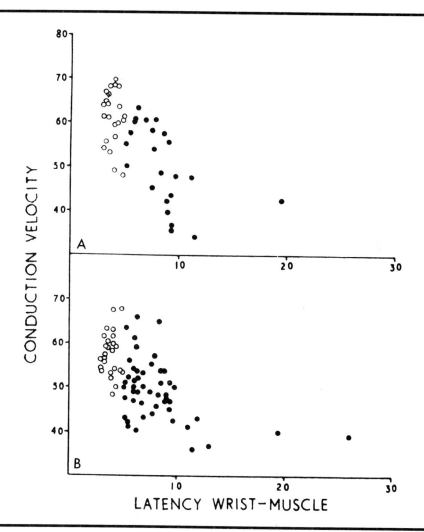

Figure 10–9 Relationship between maximal motor nerve conduction velocity (m/sec) in upper arm *(A)* and forearm *(B)* and distal latency (msec). Recordings from abductor pollicis brevis in patients with carpal tunnel syndrome *(filled circles)* and in control series *(open circles)*. (From Thomas, 1960.)

which some of the motor fibers appear to be unaffected, whereas others show a long distal delay. In the experiment shown in Figure 10–10 a bipolar needle electrode was used to identify a single motor unit with a long distal delay and with a slightly higher electrical threshold than the motor units with normal distal latencies. This allows direct comparison of the conduction times in the proximal part of the limb for affected and unaffected motor axons supplying the same muscle in the foot. The results of this and similar experiments are shown in Figure

331

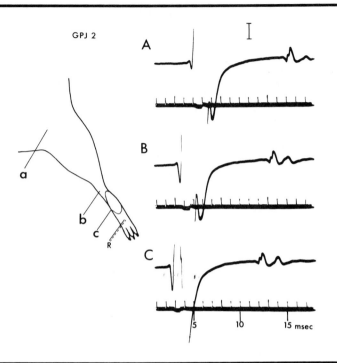

Figure 10–10 Muscle action potentials from a guinea pig with plantar neuropathy, recorded from the foot through a bipolar needle electrode, with stimulation (1 msec before the commencement of the sweep) at levels a, b, and c. Stimulus intensity was adjusted to excite a late component with a constant wave form and with a slightly higher threshold than the earlier components of the muscle response. Calibration, 500 μV. (From Fullerton and Gilliatt, 1967a.)

10–11, from which it can be seen that conduction time is consistently slightly increased in the proximal segments of motor axons which have been compressed distally, compared with those which are unaffected. The possibility must therefore be accepted that in chronic or recurrent compression there is a retrograde change in the proximal motor axon, similar to that which is known to occur after nerve section.

A recent study of muscle afferent fibers in the cat by Czéh et al. (1977) has shown that after peripheral nerve transection there is a fall in axonal velocity both distal and proximal to the dorsal root ganglion. This suggests that the large afferent fibers from muscle behave like motor fibers when separated from their end-organs. In human entrapment syndromes, however, no definite evidence of reduced velocity in afferent fibers proximal to a compressive lesion has been obtained (Buchthal and Rosenfalck, 1971; Buchthal et al. 1974). Further studies on a suitable experimental model would be helpful in clarifying this problem.*

Conduction Velocity Distal to Chronic Entrapment

In the carpal tunnel patient studied by Brown et al. (1976) (Fig. 10–7), the greater part of the prolonged motor latency can be attributed to the reduced velocity at the site of compression, conduction distal to this point being relatively normal. However, it cannot be assumed that this is always the case, as we know that in the ulnar nerve

*Since this paper was submitted, a valuable study by Kimura (1979) has been published, establishing that in patients with the carpal tunnel syndrome a significant reduction in sensory conduction velocity is present proximal to the wrist (Kimura J., Brain, *102*:619, 1979).

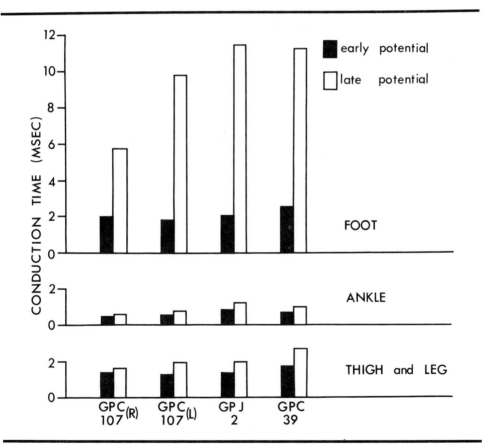

Figure 10–11 Conduction times in different segments of the motor axons responsible for early and late motor unit potentials recorded from guinea pigs with plantar neuropathy. Stimulating and recording arrangements as in Figure 10–10. (From Fullerton and Gilliatt, 1967a.)

a severe entrapment lesion at the elbow may be associated with a markedly reduced velocity throughout the distal part of the nerve. For example, in the series of ulnar nerve lesions at the elbow described by Gilliatt and Thomas (1960), there are several cases in which the increase in motor latency was too great to be accounted for by local slowing at the level of the lesion. In one patient with a grossly deformed elbow joint following an old fracture, conduction time from just above the elbow to a hand muscle was 36 msec; in another it was 23 msec. In both cases there was considerable wasting of ulnar-supplied hand muscles, and the possibility arises that the few motor fibers which were still excitable were already regenerating, since the lesions were of long standing. In one of the patients a stimulus strong enough to excite motor fibers at the wrist could not be tolerated owing to pain, but in the other patient wrist stimulation revealed distal slowing of conduction similar to that in the forearm and elbow segment. This latter finding supports the possibility that regenerating fibers are responsible for the prolonged latency.

In the carpal tunnel syndrome the examination of motor conduction does not usually include stimulation distal to the carpal ligament, but several relevant studies have been made of distal afferent conduction. McLeod (1966) used a mechanical stimulus to the nail bed to excite a digital afferent volley, and recorded velocities as low as 17 m/sec from digital fibers in the fingers of patients with unoperated carpal tunnel compression; the normal range in control subjects is 40 to 67 m/sec. Other studies in which electrical stimulation of digital afferents has been used in such patients have produced similar results (Buchthal and Rosenfalck, 1971; Casey and LeQuesne, 1972; Buchthal et al. 1974).

Recovery of digital afferent velocity after surgical division of the flexor retinaculum in one of McLeod's (1966) cases is shown in Figure 10–12, from which it can be seen that velocity remained unchanged at 21 m/sec for the first 4 weeks after operation but subsequently improved slowly, reaching 38 m/sec at 42 weeks. The effect of operation on digital afferent velocity has recently been studied systematically by LeQuesne and Casey (1974), who found no significant change after 6 to 8 weeks and a small but significant increase in velocity after 12 to 18 weeks, the improvement being most marked in those patients who had the lowest preoperative values.

The nature of this change in afferent fibers distal to the site of entrapment deserves comment. The only relevant anatomical study is that of Thomas and Fullerton (1963) who obtained the median nerve and its digital branches from a patient with a carpal tunnel syndrome who subsequently developed a cerebral glioma from which he died. In this patient there was a marked reduction in the

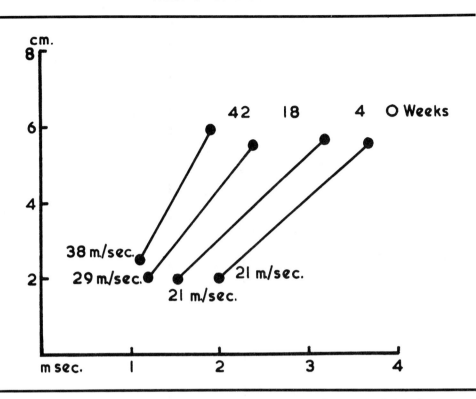

Figure 10–12 Graph showing the increase in digital afferent velocity in a carpal tunnel patient re-examined 4, 18, and 42 weeks after surgical division of the flexor retinaculum. Latency to the peak of action potential evoked by mechanical stimulation (nail tap) is plotted against conduction distance along the finger. Conduction velocity is represented by the slope of the line. (From McLeod, 1966.)

number of large fibers in the digital nerves on the more severely affected side, with less than 2 per cent of the myelinated fibers having an external diameter greater than 10 μm, as compared with 20 per cent on the less affected side.

Possible causes of the reduction in fiber diameter and conduction velocity are discussed by LeQuesne and Casey (1974). Degeneration of the largest and fastest conducting fibers, leaving a population of (normal) small myelinated fibers, is rejected by these authors as it does not explain the recovery of velocity commencing within 3 to 4 months of surgery, at a time when regeneration from the level of the wrist to the finger cannot be a relevant factor. It is therefore argued that if degeneration of the large myelinated fibers is responsible it must be followed by regeneration, with impairment of the normal matura- tion of the regenerated fibers. The release of compres- sion will then allow this latter process to proceed. Such

335

an explanation is in accord with the conclusions of Weiss and Hiscoe (1948); in their experimental model regenerating fibers passing through a constricting ring failed to achieve a normal diameter distal to the constriction.

Also discussed by LeQuesne and Casey (1974) is the possibility that there might be a reduction in fiber diameter in the distal parts of fibers which are compressed proximally but which do not degenerate completely. Weiss and Hiscoe (1948) claimed that this could occur, and the term *axonocachexia* was suggested by Bauwens (1961) to describe the phenomenon. However, in the animal model studied by Aguayo et al. (1971), in which a Silastic tube is used in growing animals to compress the tibial nerve just below its origin, mean fiber diameter at the ankle remained normal in spite of the proximal compression. They specifically commented that:

> ...there was no detectable arrest of nerve growth even though the constriction was applied in early stages of postnatal neural maturation and myelination. That normal growth did indeed take place was substantiated by the normal fiber diameters and the preservation of internodal distance in the distal portions of the constricted nerves.*

These findings make it more likely that the reduced velocity of motor and sensory conduction which is sometimes observed distal to an entrapment site is the result of degeneration followed by regeneration in the untreated lesion. This may be accompanied by a failure of maturation of the regenerated fibers, which is corrected by surgical decompression of the entrapped nerve, accounting for the relatively rapid postoperative recovery of distal velocity.

References

Aguayo, A., Nair, C. P. V., and Midgley, R.: Experimental progressive compression neuropathy in the rabbit. Arch. Neurol., *24*:358, 1971.

Anderson, M. H., Fullerton, P. M., Gilliatt, R. W., and Hern, J. E. C.: Changes in the forearm associated with median nerve compression at the wrist in the guinea-pig. J. Neurol. Neurosurg. Psychiatry, *33*:70, 1970.

Bauwens, P.: Electrodiagnosis revisited: Tenth John Stanley Coulter Memorial Lecture. Arch. Phys. Med. Rehabil., *42*:6, 1961.

Brown, W. F., Ferguson, G. G., Jones, M. W., and Yates, S. K.: The location of conduction abnormalities in human entrapment neuropathies. Can. J., Neurol. Sci., *3*:111, 1976.

Buchthal, F., and Rosenfalck, A.: Sensory conduction from digit to palm and from palm to wrist in the carpal tunnel syndrome. J. Neurol. Neurosurg. Psychiatry, *34*:243, 1971.

---

*Aguayo, et al., p. 364.

Buchthal, F., Rosenfalck, A., and Trojaborg, W.: Electrophysiological findings in entrapment of the median nerve at the wrist and elbow. J. Neurol. Neurosurg. Psychiatry, 37:340, 1974.

Casey, E. B., and LeQuesne, P. M.: Digital nerve action potentials in healthy subjects and in carpal tunnel and diabetic patients. J. Neurol. Neurosurg. Psychiatry, 35:612, 1972.

Cragg, B. G., and Thomas, P. K.: Changes in conduction velocity and fibre size proximal to peripheral nerve lesions. J. Physiol., 157:315, 1961.

Czéh, G., Kudo, N., and Kuno, M.: Membrane properties and conduction velocity in sensory neurones following central or peripheral axotomy. J. Physiol., 270:165, 1977.

Duncan, D.: Alterations in the structure of nerves caused by restricting their growth with ligatures. J. Neuropathol. Exp. Neurol., 7:261, 1948.

Dyck, P. J.: Experimental hypertrophic neuropathy. Arch. Neurol., 21:73, 1969.

Ebeling, P., Gilliatt, R. W., and Thomas, P. K.: A clinical and electrical study of ulnar nerve lesions in the hand. J. Neurol. Neurosurg. Psychiatry, 23:1, 1960.

Feindel, W., and Stratford, J.: The role of the cubital tunnel in tardy ulnar palsy. Can. J. Surg., 1:287, 1958.

Fullerton, P. M. : The effect of ischaemia on nerve conduction in the carpal tunnel syndrome. J. Neurol. Neurosurg. Psychiatry, 26:385, 1963.

Fullerton, P. M., and Gilliatt, R. W.: Pressure neuropathy in the hind foot of the guinea-pig. J. Neurol. Neurosurg. Psychiatry, 30:18, 1967a.

Fullerton, P. M., and Gilliatt, R. W.: Median and ulnar neuropathy in the guinea pig. J. Neurol. Neurosurg. Psychiatry, 30:393, 1967b.

Gilliatt, R. W.: Peripheral nerve compression and entrapment. In Lant, A. F. (ed.): Eleventh Symposium on Advanced Medicine, Royal College of Physicians of London. London, Pitman Medical Publishing, 1975.

Gilliatt, R. W., LeQuesne, P. M., Logue, V., and Sumner, A. J.: Wasting of the hand associated with a cervical rib or band. J. Neurol. Neurosurg. Psychiatry, 33:615, 1970.

Gilliatt, R. W.,and Thomas, P. K.: Changes in nerve conduction with ulnar lesions at the elbow. J. Neurol. Neurosurg. Psychiatry, 23:312, 1960.

Gilliatt, R. W., and Westgaard, R. H.: Nerve-muscle interactions: Some clinical aspects. In Cobb, W. A., and Van Duijn, H. (eds.): Contemporary Clinical Neurophysiology. Electroencephalogy. Clin. Neurophysiol., Suppl. 34:547, 1978.

Gilliatt, R. W., and Wilson, T. G.: A pneumatic-tourniquet test in the carpal-tunnel syndrome. Lancet, 2:595, 1953.

Goodman, H. V., and Gilliatt, R. W.: The effect of treatment on median nerve conduction in patients with the carpal tunnel syndrome. Ann. Phys. Med., 6:137, 1961.

Harriman, D. G. F.: Ischemia of peripheral nerve and muscle. J. Clin. Pathol., 30, Suppl. (R. Coll. Pathol.) 11:94, 1977.

Hongell, A., and Mattsson, H. S.: Neurographic studies before, after, and during operation for median nerve compression in the carpal tunnel. Scand. J. Plast. Reconstr. Surg., 5:103, 1971.

Hopkins, A. P. and Morgan-Hughes, J. A.: The effect of local pressure in diphtheritic neuropathy. J. Neurol. Neurosurg. Psychiatry, 32:614, 1969.

Jefferson, D., and Eames, R. A.: Subclinical entrapment of the lateral femoral cutaneous nerve: An autopsy study. Muscle Nerve, 2:145, 1979.

Jensen, E.: Ulnar perineuritis. Acta Psychiatr. Neurol. Scand., 34:205, 1959.

Kiraly, J. K., and Krnjevic, K.: Some retrograde changes in function of nerves after peripheral section. Q. J. Exp. Physiol., 64:244, 1959.

Kuno, M., Miyata, Y., and Muñoz-Martinez, E. J.: Differential reaction of fast and slow alpha motoneurones to axotomy. J. Physiol., 240:725, 1974a.

Kuno, M., Miyata, Y., and Muñoz-Martinez, E. J.: Properties of fast and slow alpha motoneurones following motor reinnervation. J. Physiol., 242:273, 1974b.

Lehmann, H. J.: Segmental demyelination and changes in nerve conduction in experimental circumscribed neuropathy. In Desmedt, J. E. (ed.): New developments in Electromyography and Clinical Neurophysiology, Vol. 2. Basel, S. Karger, 1973, p. 145.

Lehmann, H. J., and Ule, G.: Electrophysiological findings and structural changes in circumscript inflammation of peripheral nerves: In Bargmann, W., and Schadé, J. (eds.): Topics in Basic Neurology. Amsterdam, Elsevier, Prog. Brain Res., 6:169, 1964.

LeQuesne, P. M., and Casey, E. B.: Recovery of conduction velocity distal to a compressive lesion. J. Neurol. Neurosurg. Psychiatry, 37:1346, 1974.

Marotte, L. R.: An electron microscope study of chronic median nerve compression in the guinea-pig. Acta Neuropathol. (Berl.), 27:69, 1974.

McGowan, A. J.: The results of transposition of the ulnar nerve for traumatic ulnar neuritis. J. Bone Joint Surg. [Br.], 32B:293, 1950.

McLeod, J. G.: Digital nerve conduction in the carpal tunnel syndrome after mechanical stimulation of the finger. J. Neurol. Neurosurg. Psychiatry, 29:12, 1966.

Neary, D., and Eames, R. A.: The pathology of ulnar nerve compression in man. Neuropathol. Appl. Neurobiol., 1:69, 1975.

Neary, D., Ochoa, J., and Gilliatt, R. W.: Sub-clinical entrapment neuropathy in man. J. Neurol. Sci., 24:283, 1975.

Ochoa, J.: Nerve fiber pathology in acute and chronic compression. In Omer, G. E., and Spinner, M. (eds): Management of Peripheral Nerve Problems. Philadelphia, W. B. Saunders, 1980.

Ochoa, J., Fowler, T. J., and Gilliatt, R. W.: Anatomical changes in peripheral nerves compressed by a pneumatic tourniquet. J. Anat., 113:433, 1972.

Ochoa, J. and Marotte, L.: The nature of the nerve lesion caused by chronic entrapment in the guinea-pig. J. Neurol. Sci., 19:491, 1973.

Osborne, G. V.: Ulnar neuritis. Postgrad. Med. J., *35*:392, 1959.

Payan, J.: Anterior transposition of the ulnar nerve: An electromyographical study. J. Neurol. Neurosurg. Psychiatry, *33*:157, 1970.

Spencer, P. S.: Reappraisal of the model for "bulk axoplasmic flow." Nature [New Biol.], *240*:283, 1972.

Sunderland, S.: The nerve lesion in the carpal tunnel syndrome. J. Neurol. Neurosurg. Psychiatry *39*:615, 1976.

Tanzer, R. C.: The carpal tunnel syndrome. J. Bone Joint Surg. [Am.], *41A*:626, 1959.

Thomas, P. K.: Motor nerve conduction in the carpal tunnel syndrome. Neurology, *10*:1045, 1960.

Thomas, P. K., and Fullerton, P. M.: Nerve fibre size in the carpal tunnel syndrome. J. Neurol. Neurosurg. Psychiatry, *26*:520, 1963.

Vallbo, A. B., and Hagbarth, K. E.: Activity from skin mechanoreceptors recorded percutaneously in awake human subjects. Exp. Neurol., *21*:270, 1968.

Weiss, P., and Hiscoe, H. B.: Experiments on the mechanism of nerve growth. J. Exp. Zool., *107*:315, 1948.

Axonal Polyneuropathies*

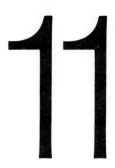

A. J. Sumner

INTRODUCTION In many conditions a generalized primary axonal degeneration of peripheral nerves, which is essentially similar to Wallerian degeneration, occurs in the absence of focal nerve damage. The polyneuropathies associated with chronic alcoholism, uremia, multiple myeloma, carcinoma, diabetes, malnutrition, heavy metal poisoning, and many toxic chemicals and drugs are generally accepted as examples of axonal neuropathies. Recent experimental morphological and electrophysiological studies employing certain neurotoxins, especially acrylamide, triorthocresyl phosphate, (TOCP) and the hexacarbons (2, 5-hexanedione, *n*-hexane, methylbutyl ketone), have resulted in the accumulation of much new information. By contrast, the human axonal neuropathies encountered in clinical practice have not been studied as thoroughly because of limitations associated with nerve biopsy and postmortem morphological techniques, and because routine EMG and nerve conduction studies often fail to address important questions about the pathophysiology of these neuropathies.

Because axonal degeneration is believed to begin in the distal portions of axons and in time to spread slowly more proximally, the term *dying-back reaction* is often used to describe this pattern of peripheral nerve pathology (Cavanaugh, 1964). More recently Schaumburg and Spencer (1979) introduced the term *distal axonopathy* in preference to *dying back*. Largely on the basis of morphological studies of the experimental hexacarbon neuropathies, they concluded that the pathological change begins, not at the terminals, but rather in a multifocal manner in the distal portion of axons. With continued intoxication the proximal spread of degeneration is not seriate but again multifocal, with *short lengths* of terminal axon appearing

*Much of the work reviewed in this chapter was supported by U.S. Public Health Service Grants, NS121301 and NS08075.

to undergo simultaneous degenerative *changes* distal to nodal points at which giant axonal swellings had occurred.

In most distal axonopathies the fact that degeneration is concentrated in parts of the nerve fiber furthest removed from the perikaryon has led to the assumption that an effect on the cell body itself results in a failure to maintain the integrity of the most distant portions of the cell, but the many studies undertaken to demonstrate abnormalities in perikaryon synthesis or axoplasmic transport have not revealed a plausible explanation for the pathology. Most distal axonopathies — for example, acrylamide, TOCP, and thiamine deficiency — show a clear nerve *fiber length susceptibility*. In others — for instance the neuropathy associated with acute intermittent porphyria — the distal parts of all the larger fibers appear to degenerate irrespective of the length of axons (Ridley, 1975).

ELECTRO-PHYSIOLOGICAL STUDIES OF EXPERIMENTAL AXONAL NEUROPATHIES

Following the observation made in Lambert's laboratory at the Mayo Clinic in the early 1950's that nerve impulse propagation occurs at greatly reduced velocity in certain patients with polyneuropathy (Henriksen, 1956), nerve conduction velocity testing has played an important role in the assessment of clinical and experimental peripheral nerve diseases. Marked slowing of conduction velocity was shown to be characteristic of those neuropathies such as diphtheric neuropathy (McDonald, 1962, 1963), or experimental allergic neuropathy (Cragg and Thomas, 1964), which display prominent segmental demyelination. By contrast, in the distal axonopathies, conduction velocity slowing is not a prominent feature and conduction velocities usually remain normal, or are mildly slowed. This was first studied by Kaeser and Lambert (1962) in guinea pigs with acute thallium poisoning. In appropriate dosage thallium produces an acute axonal neuropathy with a rapid fall in the amplitude of the muscle response to nerve stimulation occurring over 3 to 4 days but, even when the muscle response is reduced to almost zero, conduction velocity is virtually unchanged. Thallium neuropathy is not very suitable for laboratory study because many animals either fail to develop peripheral nerve disease or develop an acute illness, followed by death.

The discovery by Fullerton and Barnes (1966) that acrylamide ($CH_2CHCONH_2$) readily produces a pure axonal neuropathy in rats which otherwise remain generally well represented a considerable advance, and experimental acrylamide neuropathy was rapidly adopted as the prototypical laboratory model for the study of the dying back type of peripheral nerve disease. In their original electrophysiological and pathological study Fullerton and Barnes (1966) observed that as clinical neuropathy ad-

341

vances in severity there is a progressive decline in maximum motor conduction velocities to approximately 80 per cent of control values. When the administration of acrylamide is stopped, animals recover from their disabilities and motor conduction velocities return to normal values. Essentially similar results were obtained in later studies of acrylamide neuropathy in the baboon (Hopkins and Gilliatt, 1971). Both groups of investigators showed histological evidence of a selective large diameter fiber loss, and were inclined to conclude that the slowed conduction velocities are the result of selective axonal degeneration of the fastest conducting axons rather than slowed conduction in individual axons. It is interesting to contrast these findings in acrylamide neuropathy with those obtained in experimental organophosphorus neuropathy in the baboon where no reduction in maximal velocity occurs even when weakness is severe (Hern, 1971, 1973). Although these two toxic axonal neuropathies are superficially similar, fiber diameter histograms of affected nerves in organophosphorus neuropathy indicate that in spite of generalized axonal loss some large diameter fibers are spared, in contrast to acrylamide neuropathy in which there appears to be selective loss of the largest diameter fibers (LeQuesne, 1978).

An important exception to the general rule that nerve conduction velocities are not greatly reduced in axonal neuropathies is provided by hexacarbon neuropathy, in which conduction velocities may be substantially decreased. In a patient who developed n-hexane neuropathy as a result of glue sniffing, motor nerve conduction velocities of 33.5 m/sec in the median nerve and 25 m/sec in the peroneal nerve were recorded (Korobkin et al., 1975). A sural nerve biopsy from this patient demonstrated prominent axonal degeneration. Many fibers, however, contained giant axonal swellings, which were associated with thinning of the overlying myelin, and retraction of the myelin sheath in the region of nodes of Ranvier. Although hexacarbon solvents produce a primary axonal neuropathy, secondary changes in the myelin probably explain the observed slowing of conduction.

The Distal Lesion Although nerve conduction velocity studies have proved to be useful in routine electrophysiological evaluation of axonal neuropathies, they do not provide direct evidence of a distal lesion or demonstrate its physiological consequences. Such direct evidence that physiological responsiveness fails in the distal axon has depended upon single unit studies carried out in cats with experimental acrylamide neuropathy.

MUSCLE STRETCH AFFERENTS IN ACRYLAMIDE NEUROPATHY After daily administration of acrylamide (10 mg/kg) animals develop moderately severe hind limb ataxia, weakness, loss of deep tendon reflexes, and distal sensory impairment. In spite of these obvious clinical deficits, medial gastrocnemius nerve action potentials recorded in the whole L7 dorsal root often do not differ significantly in amplitude or conduction velocity from those of control animals. Single unit response of stretch receptor afferents in nerve were studied in finely teased dorsal root filaments and it was immediately apparent that a large number of these afferents respond abnormally. Many axons which are electrically excitable in the medial gastrocnemius nerve, and which conduct at velocities which indicate that they innervate muscle stretch receptors, fail to discharge to appropriate physiological stimulation by muscle stretch or contraction of medial gastrocnemius muscle (Sumner and Asbury, 1975). It was concluded that nonresponsive units are a consequence of a failure of function along the distal intramuscular axon. "Early discharge," which is thought to be due to ephaptic excitation of intramuscular afferents by the synchronous compound muscle action potential, is preserved in these nonresponsive axons (Sumner, 1975). There does not appear to be any difference in susceptibility among the large axons subserving different receptors (e.g., tendon organs and primary spindle endings) but it is clear that these largest fibers fail before those of smaller diameter — that is, those innervating secondary spindle endings.

The question of whether receptor responses were abnormal prior to complete inactivation was not answered in this study. Units were classified as functional if any receptor discharge could be elicited by physiological stimulation, and nonfunctional if no response was elicitable. No gross abnormalities in stretch receptor responses before complete inactivation were noted, and it seems that receptor failure is an abrupt all-or-nothing event, rather than a graded qualitative failure. Lowndes et al. (1978a), on the other hand, found an elevation in stretch receptor threshold and diminished discharge frequencies of both primary and secondary endings of muscle spindles as an early abnormality in cats intoxicated with higher daily doses of acrylamide (15 to 30 mg/kg). The dynamic responses of primary endings are particularly affected (Lowndes et al., 1978b). These latter findings, if confirmed, indicate an early receptor abnormality and would not be compatible with the current view that the terminal axonal lesion is a simultaneous Wallerian degeneration occurring over several internodes. Such a lesion would be expected to result in an abrupt and complete disconnection between axon and receptor.

CUTANEOUS AFFERENTS IN ACRYLAMIDE NEUROPATHY The sural cutaneous nerve offers certain advantages for experimental study. It contains some of the longest cutaneous afferent axons and should be affected early in the "fiber length-dependent" dying-back reaction. It is also the nerve most commonly studied by electrophysiological and biopsy techniques in human neuropathy. This nerve innervates skin on the lateral aspect of the lower leg and foot. It has previously been studied in detail by single unit techniques in normal cats (Hunt and McIntyre, 1960). Most of the myelinated axons in this nerve innervate either mechanoreceptors or hair receptors. Hair receptors are rapidly adapting, have large overlapping receptive fields, and are innervated by axons that vary in size over the entire myelinated fiber spectrum and that separate into two groups, the Aα afferents (5 to 16 μ) with conduction velocities ranging from 24 to 96 m/sec, and the Aδ afferents (1 to 4 μ) with conduction velocities ranging from 4 to 24 m/sec. Most "touch" receptors, on the other hand, have very discrete receptive fields, are slowly adapting, and are innervated by a unimodal range of large myelinated axons with conduction velocities restricted to the Aα group. A small number of mechanoreceptors have large and continuous receptive fields.

Single cutaneous afferent responses were studied in four animals with acrylamide neuropathy. In teased S1 dorsal root filaments 246 single unit responses were identified by electrical stimulation of the sural nerve; this pooled population is illustrated as a histogram in Figure 11–1, showing the typical bimodal distribution found in normal animals. The fastest conducting myelinated axons found in normal animals have velocities up to 96 m/sec, and are absent from this population, in which the fastest axons conduct at only 78 m/sec. Maximum conduction velocity of the sural sensory action potential (SAP) is 76.7 $\pm$ S.D. 9.4 m/sec compared with the value in six control animals of 89.5 $\pm$ S.D. 2.4 m/sec. The shaded area within this population histogram represents those single units which can be activated by appropriate skin stimulation, and are thus physiologically responsive. Note that almost 80 per cent of the Aα fibers are nonresponsive, including all of the fastest conducting axons. Within the Aδ group the percentage of nonresponsive units is much lower, especially when allowance is made for the 15 per cent nociceptor units normally present in this group (Burgess and Perl, 1967). These units are not identified in these experiments because the vigorous skin pinching required to activate them blocks mechanoreceptor responses. As in the case of muscle stretch receptors, it is apparent that when a population of axons is excited in a peripheral nerve trunk the compound action potential is composed of responses from many axons that are nonfunctional because of terminal disconnection, and is not a sensitive measure of the extent of early neuropathy. Mixed nerve action potential amplitudes may be normal at a time when terminal axonal failure is

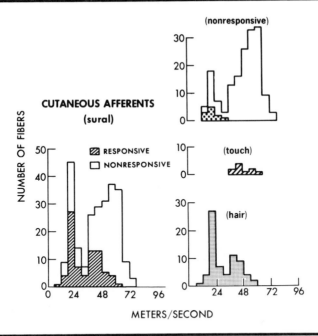

Figure 11–1 Physiological histograms of sural cutaneous afferent fibers in cats with acrylamide neuropathy. *Left:* The solid line represents the conduction velocity distribution of the total population of units. The enclosed shaded portion represents those units which were capable of responding to the skin stimulation. *Right:* The population has been subdivided into nonresponsive units *(above),* touch units *(center),* and hair units *(below).* The nonresponsive group is presumed to contain some nonreceptor afferents *(checked).* (From Sumner, 1978, by permission.)

present in a considerable percentage of fibers. The explanation for the slowing of maximum conduction velocity again seems to be selective loss of the largest diameter axons, as indicated by the histograms which show selective large fiber loss, while surviving fibers fall within a normal bimodal distribution. Note that mechanoreceptor afferents are still unimodally distributed and restricted to the Aδ group, and surviving hair receptors still show the same bimodal distribution as is found in normal animals. In both instances these findings provide no evidence of slowed conduction in individual axons, in which case histograms would show a distribution shift to the left, as seen in experimental demyelinative neuropathy (McDonald, 1963).

Selective Vulnerability of Sensory Compared to Motor Axons

Although it is a consistent finding that large diameter long axons are more susceptible to the neurotoxic effects of acrylamide, fiber size and length are not the only determinants of neurotoxic susceptibility. When the responses of single motor axons from medial gastrocnemius are compared with those of sensory afferents of similar size and length from the same muscle, it is apparent that sensory axons are much more susceptible to distal axonopathy than motor axons. Sensory responses to physiological stimulation were assessed as previously described, while motor responsiveness was determined by recording the tension produced in medial gastrocnemius by stimulating single ventral root efferents. The histograms of populations of stretch afferent, cutaneous afferent, and motor efferent fibers are compared in Figure 11–2. Of 201 alpha motor fibers only 10 per cent were nonfunctional at a time when sensory fibers of comparable length and diameter were 80 per cent nonresponsive.

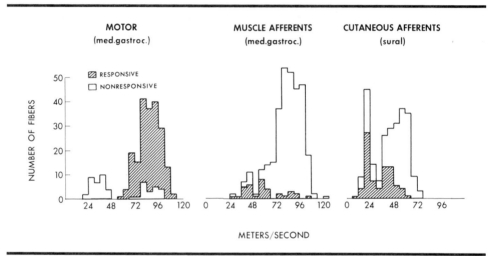

Figure 11–2 A comparison of the physiological histograms of single muscle afferents, muscle afferents, and cutaneous afferents in acrylamide neuropathy. Units showing normal physiological responses are enclosed in the shaded areas. (From Sumner, 1978, by permission.)

One possible explanation for this unexpected finding may reside in the concept of toxin vulnerability and total cell size. Sensory axons have, of course, both peripheral and central extensions. In the case of lumbosacral dorsal root ganglion cells, the central extensions are of considerable length. It is speculated that the total cytoplasmic volume of the cell in some way determines toxic susceptibility of the cell, with a consequent failure of the most distal peripheral and central axonal extensions.

Incidentally, an ultrastructural study of actylamide neuropathy by Schaumburg et al. (1974) claimed that the earliest degeneration occurs in the pacinian corpuscles of the cat's hind paw. Now, although the peripheral axons innervating those receptors are smaller than those supplying the primary endings of stretch receptors, it turns out that the central extensions of these foot pad receptor axons are the largest in the dorsal columns (Brown, 1968). Schaumburg et al. (1974) also provided morphological support for the physiological findings. They showed that primary endings of muscle spindles reveal degenerative changes before secondary endings, and those both occur before there is any ultrastructural evidence of involvement of adjacent motor end-plates.

Centripetal Degeneration It is a prediction of the dying back hypothesis that with continued intoxication axonal degeneration which begins in the terminal axon should progress centripetally. Casey and LeQuesne (1972) developed a technique for recording potentials from the digital nerves and compared the findings with potentials obtained from recording from the median nerve at the wrist after stimulating the tip of the index finger. They studied alcoholic subjects who had minimal or no clinical evidence of peripheral neuropathy, and were able to demonstrate abnormalities in the distal sensory nerve trunks in 7 of 16 subjects, only one of whom had an abnormal sensory potential of the wrist. Whereas these studies are consistent with axonal degeneration progressing centripetally, more direct demonstration is possible in experimental animals.

EXPERIMENTAL ARRANGEMENT The sural nerve in the cat runs a long unbranched course from the lower thigh to at least midcalf before dividing into branches that innervate the lateral aspect of the lower leg and hind paw. Using the experimental arrangement illustrated in Figure 11–3 it is possible to record the sural SAP

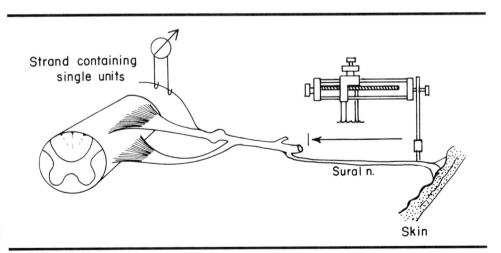

Strand containing single units

Sural n.

Skin

Figure 11-3 Stimulating and recording arrangement used in these studies of dying-back axons.

in whole S1 dorsal root, or to record individual unit responses in teased dorsal root filaments as previously described. The site of stimulation of the sural nerve trunk can be precisely positioned from distal to proximal along the unbranched portion of the nerve. Figure 11–4 illustrates typical recordings of the sural SAP evoked by stimulation at progressively more distal sites along the nerve. Distance in mm from the recording site is found in the right-hand corner, while the calculated conduction velocity of the response is found at the left-hand corner of each recording. A striking progressive decrease in response amplitude is seen which cannot be accounted for by increased dispersion of response. This is not seen in control animals in whom the size of response is identical at proximal and distal sites of stimulation. The progressive decrease in amplitude is associated with a progressive slowing of the maximum conduction velocity of the response. The explanation for these findings becomes clear when unitary responses are studied.

SINGLE UNIT STUDIES Recordings from a fine dorsal root filament are illustrated in Figure 11–5. When the exposed sural nerve, immersed in paraffin oil, is stimulated at a point 235 mm from the dorsal root recording site, stimulus strength up to 50 times that of threshold produces the single unit response illustrated. As the stimulus site is moved more proximal additional units respond as their excitable tips are approached. Thus, at 215 mm a second unit is excited, at 170 mm a third, and at 150 mm a fourth and fifth unit. Note that in each instance the new unit excited conducts at a faster velocity than those that could be excited at more distal points along the nerve trunk. It has been concluded that these pathophysiological findings are due to the presence of axons undergoing progressive centripetal degeneration. The degenerating tip of a dying back axon is located by this technique at the most distal point along a nerve trunk at which electrical stimulation elicits a response in the axon, with progressive latency increase. The increasing latency indicates that the point of initiation of the impulse is also moving distally, and is not simply the result of forward spread of the stimulus current (stimulus escape).

This method can be used to compare the extent of centripetal degeneration of different axons in a nerve trunk. For instance, Figure 11–6 shows the locations of the most distal excitable points in a sampling of single axons from the sural nerve plotted against their conduction velocities. It graphically illustrates that the largest myelinated sensory axons show a much greater extent of centripetal degeneration than those of smaller diameter. The vulnerability of large sensory fibers shows that early distal axonal failure is accompanied by a more rapid and extensive degree of centripetal

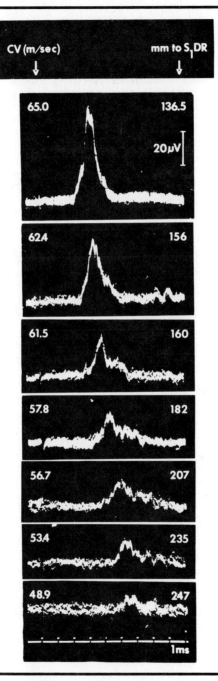

Figure 11–4 Sural sensory action potential recorded from whole S1 dorsal root following supramaximal stimulation of the peripheral nerve trunk at different points along its length. The distance from recording to stimulating sites is displayed at the top left-hand corner of each recording, while the maximum conduction velocity is displayed at the top right-hand corner.

349

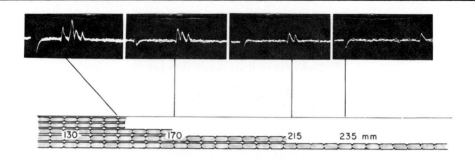

Figure 11–5 Recordings from an S1 dorsal root filament after supramaximal stimulation of sural nerve at 150, 170, 215, and 235 mm distance along the nerve, respectively.

degeneration in these same axons, and highlights the importance of axon size and length in relation to the dying-back response. A more direct demonstration of the sparing of the slower conducting axons is illustrated in Figure 11–7. The slowly conducting Aδ fibers are

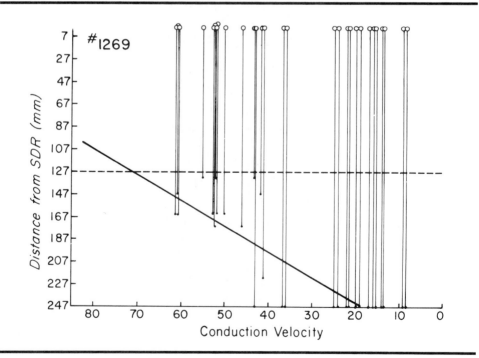

Figure 11–6 Graph illustrating the relationship between axon size (conduction velocity) and the extent of centripetal degeneration in acrylamide neuropathy.

seen to be present at each point of stimulation along the same nerve trunk, whereas more and more Aα units become excitable as the stimulation site is moved proximally. Although large sensory axons are selectively vulnerable, it is important to point out that this is a relative effect and, with chronic acrylamide intoxication, eventually peripheral nerve fibers of all sizes, including autonomic fibers, show some degree of degeneration (Post and McLeod, 1977).

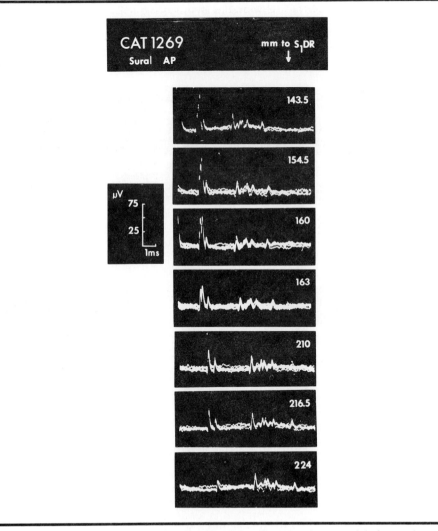

Figure 11–7 Recordings of sural action potentials from a dorsal root filament containing multiple units. These show that A delta units are excitable at each point along the exposed length of the nerve, whereas A alpha units appear in increasing numbers as the stimulation site is moved proximally.

Electrical Properties of Dying-back Axons

The electrical threshold in the region of the degenerating tip of dying-back axons is abnormally elevated. In Figure 11–8 these properties are illustrated by comparing the electrical threshold of a dying-back axon with that of an intact neighboring axon. Again the stimulating electrode is moved in increments of a few millimeters, and the threshold of the neuropathic axon expressed as a ratio of *its intact neighbor (T1).* In the proximal portions of the sural nerve the two excitable axons have a relatively constant threshold ratio (0.7 to 0.8 T1) but, as the inexcitable termination of the dying-back axon is approached, the relative threshold increases sharply to 12.8 T1. Moving the stimulus site still further distally results in a response at very high stimulus strength (59 T1) but *without* further latency increase which, as was previously stated, is taken to mean that the site of impulse initiation is unchanged and excitation is due to stimulus escape.

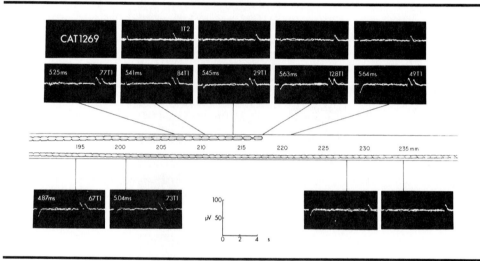

Figure 11–8 A series of recordings to illustrate the electrical properties of a dying-back axon in the region of its tip. Stimulus strengths are related to the threshold of an intact axon T₁ *(top left);* unit response latency in milliseconds *(top right).*

This increase in electrical threshold is restricted to the terminal 5 mm or so of excitable axons and is thought to be due to paranodal demyelination, which in teased single axons occurs just proximal to the terminal axonal degeneration. These same electrical properties can be demonstrated in a number of dying-back axons in a nerve whose tips are located more proximally (Fig. 11–9).

The conduction velocity also may be altered in the terminal region of some dying-back axons, as illustrated in Figure

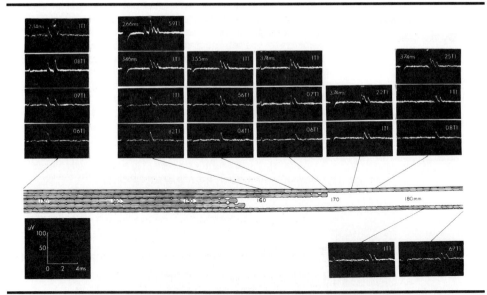

Figure 11-9 Electrical properties of further single dying-back axons studied at more proximal levels in the same nerve as in Figure 11-8. The effects of increasing stimulus strengths at different points along the nerve can be observed. In each instance stimulus strength is expressed relative to the threshold of unit 1 (T_1).

11-10 where conduction in the terminal 10 mm is abnormally slow over the same region in which the threshold is abnormally elevated. This terminal slowing has been found in approximately 20 per cent of fibers studied.

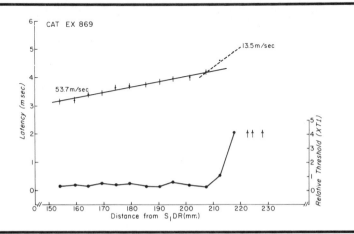

Figure 11-10 Graph illustrating slowed conduction in the terminal region of a single dying-back axon. The relative electrical threshold of the axon is also shown. *Ordinates:* Latency in milliseconds *(right);* relative threshold *(left). Abscissa:* Distance from dorsal root recording site (mm).

353

AXONAL POLYNEUROPATHIES

One practical electrophysiological consequence of these altered properties of dying-back axons is an altered recruitment order of axons within a mixed nerve trunk in response to graded electrical stimulation. A paradoxical situation may arise such as illustrated in Figure 11–11, in which the slowest conducting axons respond at threshold, and *gradually increasing strength of stimulation* results in faster and faster conducting fibers being excited. Here the fastest conducting fiber has an electrical threshold 3.21 times that of the slowest.

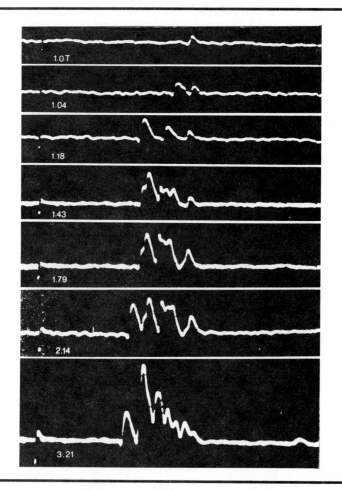

Figure 11–11 Paradoxical recruitment of axons to increasing strengths of nerve stimulation as a consequence of dying-back neuropathy.

Regeneration in Distal Axonopathy

Upon stopping acrylamide administration to experimental animals neuropathy may progress for 1 to several weeks, depending upon the duration of intoxication, and

354

then animals recover, often completely. Motor conduction velocities return to normal, in contrast to regeneration following nerve section. Even though there is very effective regeneration after withdrawal of the toxin, the regeneration process is abnormal during the period of administration. Morgan-Hughes et al. (1974) studied regeneration following nerve crush in rats with acrylamide neuropathy. The pattern of peripheral nerve regeneration is quite abnormal. In some fibers regeneration is completely inhibited, whereas in others the rate of growth is delayed and fibers remain immature. In spite of this a proportion of fibers do succeed in establishing functional contact with their end-organs, but this takes twice as long as in control animals. Regenerative motor fibers are hypoplastic, and motor conduction velocities are lower than those recorded in regenerating fibers of normal animals. This altered pattern of nerve regeneration is compatible with the hypothesis of either a defect in the synthesis of axoplasmic protein by the neuron, or a defect in protein transport along the fiber. Evidence of a defect in rate of transport in either fast or slow flow has not been forthcoming (Bradley and Williams, 1973). Many fibers end in bulbous axonal swellings concentrated over a segment of sciatic nerve immediately above the site of crush. Griffin et al. (1976) have shown that these terminal bulbs are heavily labelled by transported radioactively labelled proteins, and have concluded that impaired regeneration is the result of failure of utilization rather than failure of delivery of transported materials.

CONCLUSIONS Recent knowledge obtained from neurophysiological studies of one experimental model of a distal axonopathy has been reviewed. Although many examples of this type of peripheral nerve disease are encountered in clinical practice, routine electrophysiological testing is of limited value in detecting the earliest lesion in the terminal sensory fibers, or even distinguishing between distal axonopathy and other causes of axonal degeneration.

Acrylamide neuropathy has become widely accepted as a model for the variety of distal axonopathies encountered in clinical practice, but a note of caution must be sounded about extrapolating too readily from this model. The superficial clinical similarities between the different axonal polyneuropathies encountered in a wide variety of toxic and metabolic states often prove to be associated with quite distinctive pathophysiological and ultrastructural differences when studied in detail. There is a need to study other models in addition to acrylamide in order to ascertain those pathophysiological features that are shared and those that prove to be unique to this toxin. One would speculate that the pattern of selective fiber vulnerability may be unique to acrylamide, whereas the physiological properties of dying-back axons are likely to be common to the whole group of distal axonopathies.

355

AXONAL POLYNEUROPATHIES

There is increasing emphasis on electrophysiological techniques for the early detection of subclinical neuropathy resulting from industrial and environmental exposure to potential neurotoxic hazards (LeQuesne, 1978). On the basis of the pathophysiological studies reviewed in this chapter, early detection of the distal axonal lesion is likely to depend upon techniques for eliciting sensory action potentials by physiological stimulation of the skin receptors (McLeod, 1966; Buchthal, 1979).

REFERENCES

Bradley, W. C., and Williams, M. H.: Axoplasmic flow in axonal neuropathies. I. Axoplasmic flow in cats with toxic neuropathies. Brain, 96:235, 1973.

Brown, A. G.: Cutaneous afferent fiber collaterals in the dorsal column of the cat. Exp. Brain Res., 5:293, 1968.

Buchthal, F.: Action potentials in the sural nerve evoked by tactile stimuli. Mayo Clin. Proc. 55:223, 1980.

Buchthal, F., and Behse, F.: Electrophysiology and nerve biopsy in men exposed to lead. Br. J. Ind. Med., 36:135, 1979.

Burgess, P. R., and Perl, E. R.: Myelinated afferent fibers responding specifically to noxious stimulation of the skin. J. Physiol. (Lond.), 190:541, 1967.

Casey, E. B., and LeQuesne, P. M.: Evidence for a distal lesion in alcoholic neuropathy. J. Neurol. Neurosurg. Psychiatry, 35:624, 1972.

Cavanaugh, J. B.: The significance of the "dying-back" process in experimental and human neurological disease. Int. Rev. Exp. Pathol., 3:219, 1964.

Cragg, B. G., and Thomas, P. K.: The conduction velocity of regenerated peripheral nerve fibers. J. Physiol., 171:164, 1964.

Fullerton, P. M., and Barnes, J. M.: Peripheral neuropathy in rats produced by acrylamide. Br. J. Ind. Med., 23:210, 1966.

Griffin, J. W., Price, D. L., and Drachman, D. B.: Impaired regeneration in acrylamide neuropathy: Role of axoplasmic transport. Neurology (Minneap.), 26:350, 1976.

Henriksen, J. D.: Conduction velocity of motor nerves in normal subjects and patients with neuromuscular disorders. M.S. Thesis, University of Minnesota, 1956.

Hern, J. E. C.: Some effects of experimental organophosphorus intoxication in primates. D.M. Thesis, Oxford University, 1971.

Hern, J. E. C.: Tri-ortho cresyl phosphate neuropathy in the baboon. In Desmedt, J. E. (ed.): New Developments in Electromyography and Clinical Neurophysiology, Vol. 2, Basel, S. Karger, 1973, p. 181.

Hopkins, A. P., and Gilliatt, R. W.: Motor and sensory nerve conduction velocity in the baboon: Normal values and changes during acrylamide neuropathy. J. Neurol. Neurosurg. Psychiatry, 34:415, 1971.

AXONAL POLYNEUROPATHIES

Hunt, C. C., and McIntyre, A. K.: Analysis of fiber diameter and receptor characteristics of myelinated cutaneous afferent fibers in the cat. J. Physiol. (Lond.), *153*:99, 1960.

Kaeser, H. E., and Lambert, E. H.: Nerve function studies in experimental polyneuritis. Electroencephalogr. Clin. Neurophysiol. (Suppl.), *22*:29, 1962.

Korobkin, R., Asbury, A. K., Sumner, A. J., and Nielsen, S. L.: Glue-sniffing neuropathy. Arch. Neurol., *32*:158, 1975.

LeQuesne, P. M.: Neurophysiological investigation of subclinical and minimal toxic neuropathies. Muscle Nerve, *1*:392, 1978.

Lowndes, H. E., Baker, T., Cho, E., and Jortner, B. S.: Position sensitivity of de-efferented muscle spindles in experimental acrylamide neuropathy. J. Pharmacol. Exp. Thera., *205*:40, 1978*a*.

Lowndes, H. E., Baker, T., Michelson, L. P., Vincent-Ablazey, M.: Attenuated dynamic responses of primary endings of muscle spindles: A basis for depressed tendon responses in acrylamide neuropathy. Ann. Neurol., *3*:433, 1978*b*.

McDonald, W. I.: Conduction in muscle afferent fibers during experimental demyelination in cat nerve. Acta Neuropathol. (Berl.), *1*:425, 1962.

McDonald, W. I.: The effects of experimental demyelination in conduction in peripheral nerve: A histological and electrophysiological study. II. Electrophysiological observations. Brain, *86*:501, 1963.

McLeod, J. G.: Digital nerve conduction in the carpal tunnel syndrome after mechanical stimulation of the finger. J. Neurol. Neurosurg. Psychiatry, *29*:12, 1966.

Morgan-Hughes, J., Sinclair, S., and Durston, J. H. H.: The pattern of peripheral nerve regeneration induced by crush in rats with severe acrylamide neuropathy. Brain, *92*:232, 1974.

Post, E. J., and McLeod, J. G.: Acrylamide autonomic neuropathy in the cat. Part 1. Neurophysiological and histological studies. J. Neurol. Sci., *33*:375, 1977.

Ridley, A.: Porphyric neuropathy. *In* Dyck, P. J., Thomas, P. K., and Lambert, E. H. (ed.): Peripheral Neuropathy. Philadelphia, W. B. Saunders, 1975, Chapter 64.

Schaumburg, H. H., and Spencer, P. S.: Toxic neuropathies. Neurology, *29*:429, 1979.

Sumner, A. J.: Early discharge of muscle afferents in acrylamide neuropathy. J. Physiol. (Lond.), *246*:277, 1975.

Sumner, A. J.: The physiology of dyingback neuropathies. *In* Waxman S. G. (ed.): Physiology and Pathobiology of Axons. New York, Raven Press, 1978.

Sumner, A. J., and Asbury, A. K.: Physiological studies of the dying-back phenomenon. I. Effects of acrylamide on muscle stretch afferents. Brain, *98*:91, 1975.

Regeneration of Peripheral Nerve

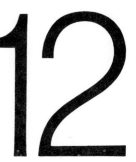

Michael E. Selzer

INTRODUCTION

Following a lesion of a peripheral nerve in vertebrates there occurs a sequence of distal degeneration of axons (Wallerian degeneration) combined with temporary changes in the proximal nerve cells. These include retraction of the axons for short distances proximal to the lesion, disruption of Nissl substance (chromatolysis), and other alterations in the somata of neurons (known collectively as central chromatolysis or retrograde axon reaction). These changes are followed either by cell death or by a variable amount of regeneration of axons into the distal stump and to the end-organs. The purpose of this chapter is twofold: first, to describe the usual sequence of events, in order to provide the foundation for the diagnostic evaluation of nerve injury; second, to discuss more recently acquired knowledge of the factors which modify the rate and effectiveness of regeneration. The latter is stressed because it is this work which will provide clues whereby nerve injuries might be treated more effectively in the future.

DEGENERATION

Wallerian Degeneration

HISTOLOGY The light microscopic features of the degeneration of axons distal to a transection were described by Waller in 1850; his account has since been confirmed and elaborated upon many times. Useful reviews of the subject may be found in Young (1942), Guth (1956), Sunderland (1978), and Allt (1976). The sequence of events is similar in all species, although there is considerable variation in the time course. With electron microscopy the earliest intra-axonal changes following nerve transection can be seen in the first 24 hours. They include a focal swelling adjacent to the transection site, with fragmentation of endoplasmic reticulum and an accumulation of mitochondria and other organelles (Vial, 1958; Honjin et al., 1959; Lee, 1963; Holtzman and Novikoff, 1965; Webster, 1965; Zelena et al., 1968; Donat and Wisniewski, 1973). This is followed shortly by a loss of longitudinal orientation and a fragmentation of neurotubules and neurofilaments throughout the axon. The rapid breakdown of neurofilament protein appears to be mediated by calcium influx into the damaged axon (Schlaepfer and Bunge, 1973; Schlaepfer, 1974). Mitochondria swell and the axolemma becomes discontinuous in places. By about the third day the axon shows areas of swelling (varicosities) and narrowing, giving the beaded appearance which was the first degenerative change noted in early light microscopic studies. This beading progresses to fragmentation, generally at first between nodes of Ranvier, and is earliest in the smallest fibers (Weddell and Glees, 1941). The beading is a process intrinsic to the axon and independent of Schwann cell or myelin, since it can be seen in degenerating axons of the lamprey spinal cord which contains no myelin (Tang and Selzer, 1979).

Changes in the myelin sheath generally lag behind those in the axon. However, observations on mouse nerve fibers in vivo have shown that within 2 minutes following a crush injury the nodes widen and Schmidt-Lanterman incisures, which appear to increase in number (Webster, 1965), dilate in the 5 mm adjacent (distal) to the crush (Williams and Hall, 1971a). These changes progress either simultaneously along the entire distal stump or, as some believe, centrifugally over the next 36 hours, affecting small fibers earlier than large. Both the centrifugal progression of the degenerative changes and their earlier appearance in small fibers may be intrinsic properties of axons in general, since they are seen in the unmyelinated axons of the lamprey spinal cord (Tang and Selzer, 1979). As axons degenerate their fragments are surrounded by myelin which also breaks up by pinching off at the incisures (Williams and Hall, 1971b). The result is the formation of rows of ellipsoids, which then subdivide into progressively smaller spheres. The end products are finally degraded by proliferating Schwann cells and macrophages, beginning around the fifth day. The process of digestion of these globules seems to continue for more than a month, during which time the globule-containing cells increase in number and migrate outward within the endoneurial spaces to positions just behind the perineurium. The resulting longitudinal arrays of Schwann cells are sometimes called bands of Büngner. The endoneurial tube begins to shrink and will collapse unless it is invaded by a regenerating axon (Sunderland and Bradley, 1950). After 30 days the population of globule-filled cells decreases. These degenerative changes are similar regardless of whether the injury to the nerve is a crush or a complete sectioning. However, the nature of the injury does affect the nature of the regenerative response and the prognosis for recovery. For this reason Seddon (1943) classified mechanical nerve injury into three categories: (1) the complete severing of the nerve is called *neurotmesis;* (2) *axonotmesis* is a lesion (such as crush) which severs the axon, causing distal degeneration, but which leaves the endoneurium intact; and (3) *neurapraxia* is an injury which causes interruption of nerve function without subsequent Wallerian degeneration (e.g., temporary nerve compression). The effect of the nature of the lesion on the process of regeneration, which develops simultaneously with degenerative changes, will be discussed later.

ELECTROPHYSIOLOGY In contrast to the morphological changes, which many but not all observers believe to progress centrifugally, the earliest electrophysiological changes following axotomy are seen in the nerve terminals. In motor axons of baboons there is a failure of neuromuscular transmission by 4 to 5 days (Gilliatt and Hjorth, 1972), with subsequent axonal conduction block which develops centripetally. Conduction block, at least in the largest fibers, would seem to occur in an all-or-none fashion, since the maximal conduction velocities of both motor and sensory fibers do not decrease during degeneration. Similar conclusions have been drawn from studies on other species, although the sequence of events tends to be faster in lower mammals (see Gilliatt and Hjorth, 1972, for review).

Proximal Axonal Changes Although not as extensively studied, histological changes in nerve fibers just proximal to injury are similar to those in the distal nerve. The degenerative effects extend only a few millimeters proximal to the lesion in mild injuries, such as a clean crush, but may extend several centimeters in cases of severe injuries (see Sunderland, 1978, Chapter 7). In addition, several investigators have reported a decrease in conduction velocity in nerves proximal to injury (Kiraly and Krnjevic, 1959; Cragg and Thomas, 1961; Kuno et al., 1974a; Mendell et al., 1976). The basis for this is not clear, but it may be due in part to reduction in fiber diameter (Cragg and Thomas, 1961). In humans and other primates evidence for reduction in conduction velocity proximal to a lesion is questionable. This issue is of importance for clinical electromyography and will be discussed later.

Neuronal Reaction to Axon Injury **HISTOLOGY** Increasingly the retrograde changes seen in the cell bodies of injured nerves have been interpreted as primarily regenerative in nature. That is, the histological changes known as central chromatolysis represent the metabolic preparation of the neuron for the demands placed upon it by the regenerating fiber. The biochemical changes of chromatolysis will therefore be presented later, when nerve regeneration is discussed. Only the histological and physiological aspects of chromatolysis will be considered here. The retrograde neuronal changes vary in time course and morphological detail among different cell types. The classical changes are best seen in spinal and brain stem motoneurons, dorsal root ganglion cells, pyramidal cells, and Clark's column neurons. Since these changes are varied and complex they are best called collectively the "retrograde axon reaction," reserving the name "chromatolysis" for the dispersal of Nissl substance. This is especially true because many neurons do not have a distinct collection of Nissl granules or, if they do, may never show chromatolysis, although they do show other distinct retrograde cellular changes. The retrograde reaction, first described by Nissl in 1892, was carefully quantified for the sciatic motoneurons of the cat by Barr and Hamilton (1948), and in several other species by others (for an extensive review see Lieberman, 1971). In some cases, within 24 hours of a nerve injury the basophilic Nissl substance, which is composed of the ribonucleoprotein of the rough endoplasmic reticulum, begins to break up into smaller granules and disperses into the cytoplasm. The cisternae of the rough endoplasmic reticulum vesiculate. At the same time the cell body swells, and the nucleus enlarges and moves toward the outer cell membrane. The nucleolus also enlarges. The Golgi complexes and lysosomes proliferate according to some accounts and fragment according to others, and electron micrographs show swelling of mitochondria. These changes become maximal over a period of 2 to 3 weeks, and are followed either by cell death or by a gradual reversal which may take several months to be completed. The electron microscopic appearance of the chromatolytic response in ventral horn cells is well demonstrated in the work of Price and Porter (1972). The severity of the chromatolytic changes depends not only upon the cell type but also upon the severity of the injury and proximity of the site of injury to the perikaryon. The closer the lesion is to the cell body, the greater the volume of axoplasm removed and the greater the axon reaction (Marinesco, 1909; Geist, 1933; Bodian, 1947). The rate and degree of axon reaction and the tendency to cell death are also greater in young than old animals (see Sunderland, 1978).

ELECTROPHYSIOLOGICAL MANIFESTATIONS OF THE RETROGRADE REACTION

The effects of axotomy on the electrophysiological properties of neurons are less well known than the morphological effects. Axotomy of spinal motoneurons is known to reduce the strength of their monosynaptic reflex discharge to muscle nerve stimulation (Campbell, 1944; Downman et al., 1953; Thulin, 1961). This is accompanied by a reduc-

361

tion in the size and rate of rise of the monosynaptic excitatory postsynaptic potential (EPSP) (Eccles et al., 1958; McIntyre et al., 1959; Kuno and Llinas, 1970b; Mendell et al., 1976). However, the mechanism of this effect on EPSPs is not known, and attempts to measure the effects of axotomy upon passive and active properties of neuronal membranes have yielded inconsistent results. Eccles et al. (1958) stated that resting membrane potentials, membrane capacitances, membrane resistances, spike amplitudes, and afterpotentials of chromatolyzed spinal motoneurons are comparable with those of control neurons, but that there is a tendency toward more rapid deterioration in resting potentials and spike amplitudes following penetration by microelectrodes. They also found that chromatolyzed motoneurons have lower voltage thresholds than normal for spike activation, and that the neurons show partial all-or-none responses (not found by Mendell et al., 1976), which the authors interpreted as representing patches of unusually excitable membrane in the soma and dendrites. These last features would tend to enhance rather than reduce reflex activity. Thus Eccles et al. (1958) concluded that the reduced reflex activity is due to the decrease in amplitude and rate of rise of EPSPs, but whether this is due to pre- or postsynaptic changes is not clear. Similar conclusions were drawn by Kuno and Llinas (1970a, b). On the other hand, Kuno et al. (1974a; also see Huizar et al., 1977) found an increase in spike overshoots and a decrease in axonal conduction velocities in chromatolyzed motoneurons. They also found that the effects of axotomy on passive and active membrane properties could depend upon the type of muscle innervated (Kuno et al., 1974a). Axotomy of motoneurons to soleus, a slow twitch muscle, produces a decrease in the duration of the postspike hyperpolarization but no change in resting potential (a decrease is seen in the subsequent study of Huizar et al., 1977) or membrane resistance, while motoneurons to the medial gastrocnemius, a fast twitch muscle, show a decrease in membrane potential and an increase in resistance but no change in afterhyperpolarization. The changes in these and other parameters are always in a direction which reduces the differences between fast and slow twitch motoneurons. Thus, the effects of axotomy could be interpreted as a dedifferentiation, in agreement with the observation of Bodian (1947), that all morphological, physiological, and biochemical changes observed up to that time in axotomized neurons were in the direction of reversion toward the embryonic state. In any case, physiological studies have failed to demonstrate changes in the electrical properties of axotomized neurons which would adequately explain their reduced susceptibility to synaptic activation.

REGENERATION OF PERIPHERAL NERVE

During the past few years it has been found that axotomized neurons lose many of their afferent boutons (Blinzinger and Kreutzberg, 1968; Hamberger et al., 1970; Kerns and Hinsman, 1973; Sumner and Sutherland, 1973; Cull, 1974). Recent electron microscopic observations have shown that, during the retrograde axon reaction, there is a gradual retraction of synaptic boutons away from the chromatolyzed neuron's surface membrane (Sumner, 1975) which is reversed only if the nerve is allowed to re-establish neuromuscular junctions (Cull, 1974; Sumner, 1976). The resulting decrease in the density of synaptic boutons, and the increase in the size of the synaptic clefts which has been seen, may well explain why synaptic excitation of these neurons is reduced (Matthews and Nelson, 1975; Purves, 1975), even with excitation of peripherally axotomized spinal motoneurons by activation of synergistic type Ia afferents whose peripheral processes have not been cut (Eccles et al., 1959). Rotter et al. (1977) have demonstrated a reduction in muscarinic acetylcholine receptors in axotomized hypoglossal neurons during the period of loss of synaptic contacts. However, whether there is a causal relationship between the two phenomena is not known.

THE SIGNAL FOR THE RETROGRADE REACTION The mechanism by which axotomy induces retrograde neuronal changes has been the subject of much speculation. The chromatolytic change (dispersal of Nissl substance) can be prevented by the application of actinomycin D, an inhibitor of RNA synthesis, onto the soma within a few hours after axotomy (Torvik and Heding, 1967, 1969). This finding suggests the possibility that the chromatolytic changes are induced by an effect of some substance upon the transcription process between the genetic material DNA and messenger RNA, and that some of the retrograde changes may be mediated by certain enzymes whose production would be blocked by the inhibition of messenger RNA production. Indirect as this reasoning may be, evidence for the involvement of particular substances, involvement of retrograde axoplasmic transport on the delivery of such substances to the soma, or role of loss of contact of the axon with its end-organ in the induction of retrograde changes is even more circumstantial. Some aspects of this problem will be discussed further in relation to control of regeneration (detailed consideration of this question can be found in Cragg, 1970; Lieberman, 1974; Grafstein and McQuarrie, 1978).

Summary of Degenerative Changes The most prominent anatomical and physiological changes which occur in a neuron and its axon following axotomy are illustrated for the mammalian motoneuron in Figure 12–1. Wallerian degeneration consists of beading and fragmentation of axons surrounded by myelin fragments distal to the transection. These are taken up by Schwann cells (and possibly macrophages) which are multiplying and lining up along the edge of the shrinking endoneurial tube. Similar changes occur just proximal to the transection. By mechanisms which are still unclear the injury is detected by the cell body, which swells. The rough-surfaced endoplasmic reticulum (Nissl substance) in the center of the soma breaks up into individual ribosomes and polysomes (see below). What rough-surfaced endoplasmic reticulum remains migrates into the proximal dendrites (Fig. 12–1B). The nucleus migrates to the lateral margin of the soma and, along with the nucleolus, may increase in size. Presynaptic terminals, such as those from Ia afferents, gradually withdraw from the soma and dendrites. This correlates with a reduction in the effectiveness of synaptic transmission to the point where dorsal root stimulation fails to elicit action potentials in the motoneuron, and thus fails to evoke a reflex discharge in the ventral root.

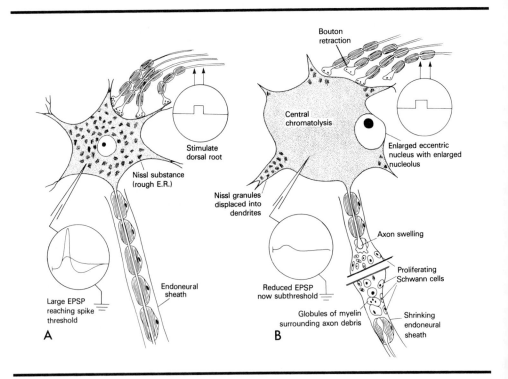

Figure 12–1 Summary of the most prominent morphological and physiological changes in axotomized mammalian spinal motoneurons. A, Normal motoneuron. B, After ventral root transection.

REGENERATION

**Axonal
Regeneration**

HISTOLOGY AND RATE OF REGENERATION Experimental evidence for regeneration of peripheral nerves has accumulated over two centuries; the early literature has been reviewed by West (1978). The modern era of nerve regeneration research began with the work of Ramón y Cajal (1914, 1928), who demonstrated definitively that viable nerve fibers in a previously degenerated peripheral nerve originate by outgrowth from the proximal stump and not by autoregeneration of the degenerated distal portion. Ramón y Cajal's histological observations on silver-stained nerve fibers of rabbits, cats, and dogs suggest that following injury there is a variable latent period of about 6 hours for the appearance of the earliest sprouting fibers and, in most cases, 30 to 36 hours before outgrowth of the cut axon tips. The latent period is somewhat shorter in younger than in older animals. Thereafter the tips swell into "cones of growth." Forward growth occurs by advancement of the tip, sprouting of collaterals from the tip, or sprouting of collaterals from the nodes of Ranvier up to several segments proximal to the tip. By about 24 hours some sprouts have reached the area of injury. They penetrate the scar from the second or third day on. Growth through the scar is slow (about 0.25 mm per day), so that in severed nerves invasion of the distal stump does not occur until the tenth to fifteenth day. Thereafter the rate of regeneration for most fibers is 2 to 3 mm per day, but as much as 4 mm per day in some fibers. It is remarkable that, despite the many theoretical considerations raised to cast doubt upon the validity of Ramón y Cajal's observations, and the application of numerous other techniques for the demonstration of regeneration (e.g., electrical stimulation of nerves, behavioral testing to demonstrate functional reinnervation of muscles, light pinching of nerve growth tips which are hyperexcitable to elicit reflexes, labelling regenerated axons by radioactively labelled protein precursors transported from the soma, and extrapolation of distance measurements obtained by all these techniques at varying times after injury back to the transection site), the figures determined by subsequent studies have basically confirmed those of Ramón y Cajal for both the latent period and the rate of regeneration in the distal stump (cf. Forman and Berenberg, 1978, for recent data and a literature review). While initial electron microscopic studies suggested a latent period of 36 hours (Morris et al., 1972), some electron microscopic observations showed sprouting in some fibers within a few (4 to 6) hours of injury (Zelena et al., 1968; Duce et al., 1976; Grafstein and McQuarrie, 1978), thus confirming the observations of Ramón y Cajal and his contemporaries. However, the last two references suggested that the early sprouts may degenerate, so that permanent regeneration does not occur in most fibers before 24 hours (Grafstein and McQuarrie, 1978).

REGENERATION OF PERIPHERAL NERVE

A further observation of Ramón y Cajal's (which was at first denied; Gutmann et al., 1942) is that the rate of regeneration through the distal stump decreases with time. Ramón y Cajal believed that a quantification of this effect would require excessively tedious experiments, so his observation was qualitative. As pointed out by Sunderland (1978), animal experiments seem to contradict this notion because the nerves studied were too short to distinguish linear from nonlinear growth rates. However, studies of the longer nerves of human patients following nerve injuries (Fig. 12–2) suggest that the rate of regeneration does indeed diminish with the distance of regeneration (Seddon et al., 1943; interpreted by Sunderland, 1947; Sunderland, 1946, 1947; Napier, 1949; Sunderland and Bradley, 1952). These studies employed sequential observations in individual patients of the furthest distance from a lesion at which Tinel's sign (Tinel, 1915) could be elicited. This sign is produced by tapping the skin over a damaged nerve gently with a hammer. The region of the growing tip is hyperexcitable, and its mechanical stimulation in sensory axons produces a shock-like or tin-

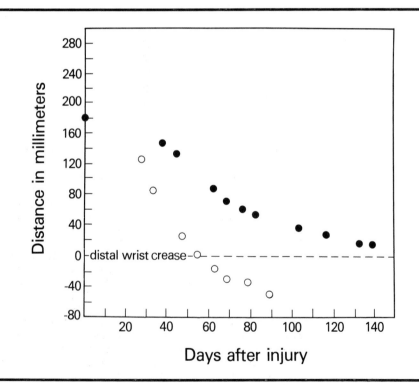

Figure 12–2 Advance of Hoffmann-Tinel's sign following a median nerve crush injury *(open circles)* and ulnar nerve suture *(filled circles)* 358 and 180 mm above the distal wrist crease, respectively. (Adapted from Sunderland, 1978.)

gling sensation in the region of normal distribution of the nerve. Sunderland (1947) determined that rates of regeneration across any given segment of nerve are constant regardless of the level of the lesion. He found that the rate of regeneration decreases with distance from the soma and therefore only secondarily with time following a lesion or cumulative distance of regeneration. Detailed consideration to the various methods of assessing the rate of regeneration is given by Sunderland (1978) who concluded that, in the human patient with a severed nerve repaired by simple suture of the cut ends, the average rate of nerve regeneration is 2.5 mm/day in the upper forearm, 2 mm/day in the lower forearm, and 1 mm/day in the wrist and hand.

Still another principle enunciated by Ramón y Cajal which has been consistently reaffirmed is that the rate of regeneration is greater the less disruptive the lesion. This is especially true of the rate at which fibers approach and cross the transection scar. Thus, the time required for reinnervation to begin in the distal stump in a crush injury which does not disrupt the endoneurial tube (axonotmesis) may be about 3 days, as compared to 10 to 15 days for a severed nerve. Intermediate values are obtained by procedures which lessen the thickness of the scar, such as hemisection of nerve so that the cut ends remain apposed, or suturing the two ends together. While less marked, the rate of regeneration within the distal stump also seems to be faster following a crush lesion than after complete severance. For example, Sunderland (1978) reported regeneration rates in human crush injured nerves as 8.5+ mm per day in the upper arm, 6 mm per day in the upper forearm, 1 to 2 mm per day at the wrist, and 1 to 1.5 mm per day in the hand. The reason for this difference in regeneration rate in the distal stump between crush and cut injured axons is not definitely known, but it is widely assumed that regeneration is facilitated by the presence of the endoneurial tube to guide the advancing axon (Young, 1942). When the nerve crush spares the endoneurial tube, regeneration of each axon proceeds within the tube. Generally only one of the sprouts formed at the axon tip survives and regenerates within the endoneurial tube (Denny-Brown and Brenner, 1944). This is in contrast to the situation in severed nerve in which numerous sprouts survive from each axon tip, cross the scar, and several sprouts may enter and regenerate within each endoneurial tube in the distal stump. The presence of multiple sprouts per endoneurial tube has been thought to increase the resistance to growth. In addition, the increased time required for invasion of the distal stump by severed as opposed to crushed nerve fibers results in an increase in the amount of endoneurial shrinkage. This may also slow distal regeneration.

367

REGENERATION OF PERIPHERAL NERVE

It was Ramón y Cajal's impression that regeneration was more complete in younger than in older animals. Evidence from studies of both the central nervous system (CNS) and peripheral nervous system (PNS) has borne this out. It is therefore not surprising that Black and Lasek (1979) suggested that the rate of regeneration of crushed motor axons of rats decreases with age. They estimated the distance of regeneration by following the front of radioactively labelled proteins transported into the axon. Since they began their observations at a time (4 days) when the front was already beyond the crush site, it can be assumed that their results reflect differences in rates of regeneration and not in latency of regeneration or delays in crossing the site of injury. In an earlier study using the reinnervation of denervated muscle as a measure of regeneration, Gutmann et al. (1942) also claimed that motor axons of young rabbits regenerate more rapidly than those of older rabbits. However, they found no differences in the rates of regeneration of sensory axons, as measured by the distance at which pinching a lesioned nerve elicits a reflex muscle contraction. Black and Lasek (1979) proposed that the differences in rates of regeneration at different ages are due to differences in the rates of a slow component of axonal transport (see below).

The structure of the growth cone of regenerating axons is similar to that of growing axons in tissue culture and in the embryo, and has often been studied by electron microscopy (cf. Estable et al., 1957; Wettstein and Sotelo, 1963; Lampert, 1967; Lentz, 1967; Tennyson, 1970; Yamada et al., 1971; Morris et al., 1972; Bunge, 1973). The cone itself is a region of axoplasmic enlargement from which several fine sprouts or filopodia may extend. The classical experiments of Weiss suggested that the elongation may be assisted by outward streaming of axoplasm, and that the shape and direction of the growing tip is influenced by mechanical factors in its path (Weiss, 1941, 1944; see below). These features are diagrammed in Figure 12–3. The cone is characteristically rich in smooth-surfaced endoplasmic reticulum, microtubules, microfilaments, mitochondria (often unusually large), lysosomes, and a variety of other vacuolar and vesicular structures. The latter are mostly large and clear, but some are small, dense-cored, or coated. The filopodia are less complex, usually containing only microfilaments and small amounts of membranous structures (Fig. 12–4). Although the nature and purpose of the vesicular structures in the growth cone are not known, it has been widely assumed that they are not synaptic vesicles, which appear only when synaptic contacts are made (Yamada et al., 1971; Bunge, 1973; Rees et al., 1976). However, Landis (1978) has demonstrated that small dense-cored vesicles in growth cones of cultured sympathetic neurons probably contain cate-

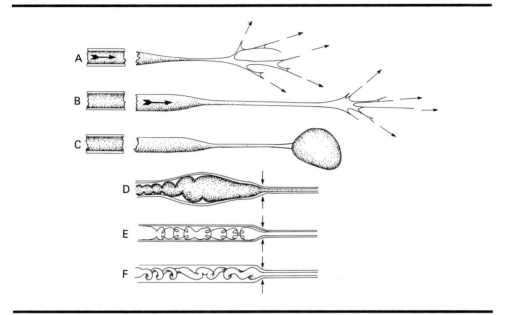

Figure 12–3 Diagrams illustrating normal and impeded outgrowth of axons. *A, B,* Two successive stages of outgrowth showing progressive elongation by interfacial tensions *(simple arrows),*
which draw out the transitory terminal filopodia to fine points,
followed by lateral enlargement resulting from centrifugal con-
vection of axonal substance by intra-axonal pressure *(feathered
arrows). C,* Terminal bulb, produced by the damming up of axonal
substance in front of an unsurmountable obstacle. *D, E, F,* Bal-
looning, telescoping, and coiling of the axonal substance just
proximal to a constriction which reduces the diameter of the
tubes (level of constriction indicated by arrows). Centrifugal
growth pressure in the axon continues to move axonal substance
distad, and the damming up of this substance in front of the
"bottleneck" leads to the various forms of contortion shown in
these schematic reproductions from photomicrographs. (From
Weiss, 1944.)

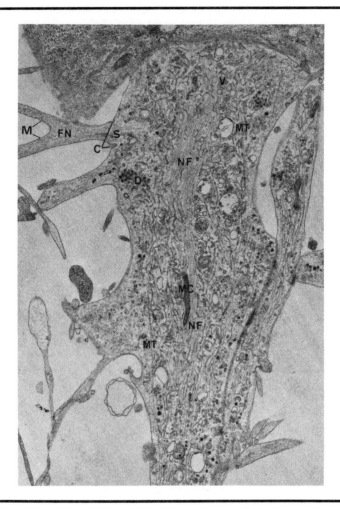

Figure 12–4 The growth cone of a dorsal root ganglion cell. The filamentous network (FN) of microfilaments is the predominant organelle within the microspikes (M). Smooth endoplasmic reticulum (S) extends into the base of one microspike, and coated vesicles (C) arise near its base. A bundle of neurofilaments (NF) occupies the core of the growth cone, and few microtubules (MT) extend into this region of the nerve cell. Near the top of the figure, the growth cone abuts against a glial cell. Smooth-walled vesicles V; dense-core granules D; mitochondrion, MC. (× 13, 500.) (Generously supplied by Dr. K. Yamada.)

cholamines; this raises the possibility that, at least in tissue culture, growth cones do contain synaptic vesicles before contacts with postsynaptic cells are made. By analogy with the vesicle recirculation hypothesis at normal neuromuscular junctions (Heuser and Reese, 1972), the presence of coated vesicles, combined with the observation of what appear to be invaginations from the membranous tip of severed nerve (Wettstein and Sotelo, 1963), suggests that some of these vesicles are of axolemmal origin.

To summarize the histological features of nerve regeneration, injured nerve fibers form terminal enlargements similar to the growth cones of embryonic nerve. Elongation occurs by the sending out of fine extensions, called filopodia, from the growth cone, and sprouts from nodes of Ranvier proximal to the lesion. Growth cones contain numerous membranous structures such as vacuoles, vesicles, smooth-surfaced endoplasmic reticulum, and mitochondria, as well as microtubules and microfilaments. Forward growth occurs by amoeboid movement of fine filopodia. The driving forces behind this forward movement are still not clear, although peristaltic streaming of axoplasm may be a factor. When possible, axons regenerate within pre-existing endoneurial tubes which facilitate and speed regeneration. Thus, the less traumatic the injury the shorter the distance between proximal cut axon tip and distal endoneurial tubes and the more rapid the regeneration. The most rapid regeneration occurs after nerve crush which leaves the endoneurium intact.

THE BEHAVIOR OF SCHWANN CELLS DURING REGENERATION It has been mentioned that during Wallerian degeneration there is a proliferation of cellular elements of peripheral nerve, especially the Schwann cells. By the use of autoradiographic labelling of incorporated ^{3}H-thymidine, Bradley and Asbury (1970) demonstrated that in the mouse Schwann cell division begins within 19 hours of nerve section. Labelling reaches a peak at 3 days, when 15.5 per cent of Schwann cells are dividing, and rapidly decreases thereafter. These cells are instrumental in degrading the globules of degenerated myelin and axonal debris. As they proliferate within the basement membrane of the endoneurial connective tissue sheath the Schwann cells form distinct rows called bands of Büngner. These cells are then available to remyelinate the advancing axon. While there is a tendency at first for distal portions of severed nerves to show partial dissolution of the endoneurial sheaths (Glees, 1943; Thomas, 1964a), electron microscopic observations show that during regeneration, at between 28 and 35 days following a lesion, there is a thickening of the endoneurium by deposition of a third layer of collagen

371

(Thomas, 1964b). Therefore an advancing axon, if properly oriented after traversing the scar, is welcomed by a strengthened though narrowing endoneurial tube within which proliferated Schwann cells have cleared a path by migrating to the inner surface of the basement membrane. Despite the fact that in transected nerves a single endoneurial tube may be invaded by more than one sprout of a regenerating fiber, the total number of axons in the distal stump is reduced (Gutmann and Sanders, 1943). This is presumably due to the death of some chromatolytic neurons and to failure of many axons to cross the transection and enter the distal stump. However, the number of Schwann cells is increased, and the number of Schwann cells per axon is greater following regeneration than before the injury. The number of nodes of Ranvier is therefore increased and the internodal length is reduced (Hiscoe, 1947; Vizoso and Young, 1948; Cragg and Thomas, 1964). Following a crush lesion, the number of axons in the regenerated distal stump is the same as in the central stump (Gutmann and Sanders, 1943) but the proliferation of Schwann cells still results in a shortening of the internodal length. The significance of this for the electrical conduction properties will be discussed below.

The ultrastructural sequence of events during remyelination has been described by Nathaniel and Pease (1963). The advancing axon forms an indentation in the Schwann cells which are lined up along the edge of the endoneurial tube. The process of remyelination is basically the same as the initial myelination. Remyelination of regenerating rat dorsal roots has been noted as early as 7 days after crush. Following nerve section the delay is predictably longer (Terry and Harkin, 1957).

REGENERATION OF UNMYELINATED FIBERS The processes of degeneration and regeneration of unmyelinated fibers have been less well studied than those of myelinated fibers, despite the fact that unmyelinated fibers far outnumber myelinated fibers in mammalian peripheral nerves. Nevertheless, as a result of recent use of autonomic nerves as a source of relatively pure unmyelinated fibers, some differences have been described. It is now widely suggested that regeneration of unmyelinated fibers is particularly rapid (Bray et al., 1972; Hopkins and Lambert, 1972; Dyck and Hopkins, 1972; Aguayo et al., 1973; Allt, 1976). However, these studies do not concentrate on distinguishing the various early phases of regeneration, and it appears that the most striking aspect of the rapid regeneration of unmyelinated fibers is the short latent period between injury (either crush or transection) and the entry of axons into the distal stump. Where a specific rate of regeneration is mentioned as the result of observations of regeneration over several millimeters of nerve (Gutmann et al., 1942; Evans and Murray, 1954), or when it can be roughly calculated from the data (Hopkins and Lambert, 1972), regeneration times suggest rates of between 1 and 2 mm per day, which are similar to those for myelinated nerves. It might be thought surprising that unmyelinated fibers show such a strong regenerative capacity; a single Schwann cell can enfold several unmyelinated fibers. In unmyelinated nerves injury results in much less Schwann cell proliferation than in myelinated nerves (Abercrombie et al., 1959; Joseph, 1947; King and Thomas, 1971), with most of this proliferation restricted to the site of the lesion (Romine et al., 1976). Thus, bands of Büngner are probably less well formed and the effect of Schwann cell encouragement of axon regeneration might be less marked (King and Thomas, 1971). Typical growth cones have not been seen in regenerating unmyelinated fibers in situ (Dyck and Hopkins, 1972; Bray et al., 1972; Aguayo et al., 1973). However, growth cones are a prominent feature of axonal growth in unmyelinated sympathetic neurons in tissue culture (Bunge, 1973).

Another difference between myelinated and unmyelinated nerve fibers is that in the case of the latter multiple sprouts from a single injured fiber not only invade the distal stump but regenerate for long distances within it (Bray et al., 1973), while in myelinated nerves usually only a single sprout survives among several which may invade the endoneurial space of a single degenerated axon. This sprouting, combined with the paucity of Schwann cell proliferation, results in a marked increase in the number of unmyelinated axons per Schwann cell in electron micrographs (Bray et al., 1972; Dyck and Hopkins, 1972; Aguayo et al., 1973). These axons are about half the diameter of normal unmyelinated axons. In a prolonged study (up to 6 months) of crushed cervical sympathetic trunks in rat, Bray and Aguayo (1974) found a progressive decrease in the number of surviving fibers in the distal stump and an increase in the proportion of fibers with diameters in the normal range (i.e., greater than 0.9 μm). While fiber numbers revert to normal by the end of 6 months, the average fiber diameter remains about one half that of normal nerves. In this regard unmyelinated fibers show less tendency toward maturation following regeneration than do myelinated nerve fibers (Gutmann and Sanders, 1943).

ELECTROPHYSIOLOGY During the phase of Wallerian degeneration the conduction velocities of axons in the proximal stump decrease, which correlates with a decrease in axon diameter. In later stages these changes are at least partially reversed. Cragg and Thomas (1961) found that for both crushing and cutting injuries

373

conduction velocities of rabbit peroneal nerves proximal to the lesion are reduced by about 10 per cent after 25 to 30 days and by 20 per cent after 50 to 100 days. Between 150 and 200 days, however, conduction velocities return to normal and remain so beyond 400 days. Axon diameters and total fiber diameters also show concomitant reversible reductions (to 85.9 and 89.8 per cent, respectively) as compared to nonlesioned nerves. In man reports suggesting that conduction slowing develops proximal to a compressive or section lesion (Ebeling et al., 1960; Thomas, 1960; Gilliatt, 1961) must be interpreted with caution because they depend upon recording differences in the distal latencies of muscle responses to stimulation at two different proximal sites along the course of the injured nerve. It has been pointed out that apparent slowing might be due to selective block of the fastest fibers at the lesion site leaving muscle responses only to slower fibers conducting at their normal rates (Thomas, 1960). In fact, in the carpal tunnel syndrome, Sumner (1978) has stated that ascending nerve action potential velocities are normal. Normal ascending action potential velocities were found by Gilliatt and Hjorth (1972) in severed nerves of baboon. Apparently an adequate test of the hypothesis that slowing of conduction proximal to a nerve lesion in man has not been performed.

Regenerating nerve fibers occupy shrunken endoneurial tubes and are remyelinated by an increased number of Schwann cells, resulting in a narrower axon with a shorter internodal length. These factors should work to reduce the conduction velocity of regenerating fibers in the distal nerve stump. Although the fiber diameter may eventually return almost to normal the internodal length remains constant and, according to Sanders and Whitteridge (1946), of relatively uniform size, as opposed to normal axons in which internodal distance increases with axon diameter. Thus, it is not surprising that most studies in both humans and experimental animals show an enduring reduction by 20 to 40 per cent in conduction velocities of regenerating nerves distal to a lesion (Berry et al., 1944; Erlanger and Schoepfle, 1946; Hodes et al., 1948; Cragg and Thomas, 1964; Jacobson and Guth, 1965). However, some studies in experimental animals (Sanders and Whitteridge, 1946) and cases of human nerve injuries (Donoso et al., 1979) suggest almost complete recovery of conduction velocities (to greater than 90 per cent of normal) when regeneration is monitored for very long periods (16 months and greater than 50 months, respectively). These findings are difficult to explain unless it is assumed that internodal length eventually returns to normal, since it is now generally accepted that shortening the normal internodal length reduces conduction velocity (Brill et al., 1977).

BIOCHEMISTRY A very large literature has accumulated concerning the biochemical concomitants of the retrograde reaction to axotomy and subsequent regeneration. A detailed review has been made by Lieberman (1971), and some aspects of the subject have been further updated by Grafstein and McQuarrie (1978). While the morphological changes of the retrograde reaction were initially interpreted as degenerative, the biochemical changes which accompany chromatolysis in fact suggest that the neuron is preparing itself for the metabolic demands of axonal regrowth. The time course of changes in some major constituents of the cell body can be seen in Figure 12–5. The reduction in rough-surfaced endoplasmic reticulum does not indicate a loss of RNA since it results from a dissociation of ribosomes from the outer surfaces of membranous cisternae, with a resultant increase in the proportion of free ribosomes and small polyribosomal aggregates. Although the concentration of total RNA in chromatolytic cells is found to decrease (Gersh and Bodian, 1943; Hyden, 1943; Brattgard et al., 1957; Edstrom, 1959), this is often due to a large increase in neuronal cell volume while the RNA content remains unchanged. After the initial chromatolytic reaction, which in the rabbit hypoglossal neurons corresponds roughly with the period of nerve outgrowth (second to twelfth day), the cellular RNA content increases dramatically. The RNA concentration returns to normal even though cell volume remains large throughout the first 60 days of the maturation period, which is the period of continued axonal enlargement following initial contact with its end-organ (Brattgard et al., 1957; Watson, 1968a). Indeed, the fact that chromatolysis usually involves enlargement of the nucleolus suggests that synthesis of ribosomal RNA may be increasing. Watson (1965) has, in fact, demonstrated autoradiographically that ^{3}H-adenosine incorporation by hypoglossal neurons is increased first in the cell nucleus and then in the cytoplasm. Nucleolar RNA content increases, followed by an increase in cytoplasmic RNA (Watson, 1968a). Actinomycin D, which inhibits the production of DNA-mediated RNA synthesis, causes a more rapid loss of nucleolar RNA after axotomy than in control neurons (Watson, 1968a). Thus, both the rate of synthesis and the rate of turnover of RNA, presumably including ribosomal RNA, is increased following axotomy. In goldfish retinal ganglion cells, as in some other neurons, the increased synthesis of RNA apparently outstrips the increase in cell volume and the cytoplasm becomes intensely hyperchromic rather than pale (Murray and Grafstein, 1969).

Not surprisingly, the result of this increase in RNA production is an increased synthesis of protein, as measured by autoradiography following injection of radio-

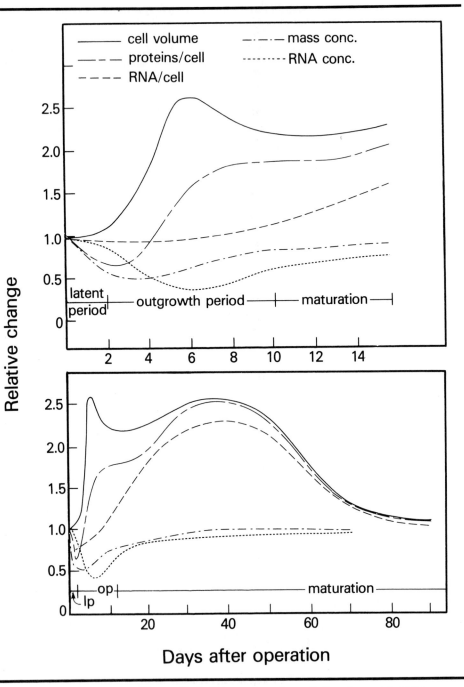

Figure 12-5 Time course of quantitative changes in some nerve cell constituents during regeneration of axotomized rabbit hypoglossal neurons. Upper graph is a time-expanded view of the early changes. (After Brattgard et al., 1957.)

actively labelled amino acid (e.g., Brattgard et al., 1958; see Lieberman, 1971 for review). After a small decrease during the first 4 days, the actual protein content of axotomized rabbit hypoglossal neurons also increases (Brattgard et al., 1957). The increased protein synthesis is clearly not haphazard, since Hall et al. (1977) found that only 10 per cent of the 300 to 400 protein species detectable by two-dimensional acrylamide gel electrophoresis increase following axotomy. A few proteins also decrease. As one would expect of a cell which is synthesizing proteins and other constituents of new axonal processes, some of the increased protein synthesis represents synthesis of glycolytic and respiratory enzymes. During the first few days, when mitochondrial swelling is noted, oxidative metabolism and enzyme levels of the tricarboxylic acid cycle decrease (Watson, 1966a) while glycolysis increases (Watson, 1968b) and glucose-6-phosphate dehydrogenase activity is also increased (Kreutzberg, 1963; Harkonen, 1964), suggesting the possible increased use of the pentose shunt. After the first week, however, oxidative metabolism and the enzyme levels of the tricarboxylic acid cycle increase (Watson, 1966a). This corresponds to the morphological changes of mitochondrial hypertrophy, with an increase in the number and density of cristae seen with electron microscopy (see Lieberman, 1971, for review). The result of increased use of the hexose monophosphate pathway would be to increase cellular levels of NADPH which is required for the synthesis of fatty acids, a major component of lipid membranes. This would be expected for a neuron which must synthesize new axonal membrane. In fact, neuronal lipid content has been found to increase following hypoglossal nerve crush in rabbit (Brattgard et al., 1957). Although glycolysis increases soon after nerve injury, reports conflict as to whether lactic dehydrogenase activity increases. This is not necessarily inconsistent, since lactic dehydrogenase is not a rate-limiting enzyme in glycolysis.

Histochemical studies suggest a great proliferation of lysosomes and lysosomal acid phosphatase following axotomy (Lieberman, 1971). While the significance of this is not clear, it is reasonable to suppose that the increased acid phosphatase activity is required to digest the products of fragmented membranous organelles, such as the cisternae of rough-surfaced endoplasmic reticulum (and Golgi apparatus which, according to some reports, also undergoes dispersion and/or fragmentation following axotomy).

As mentioned earlier, there is evidence for proliferation of the fibrillary components in regenerating axons (Ramón y Cajal, 1928). Although some authors have disagreed, results of most electron microscopic studies suggest a proliferation of both neurofilaments (e.g.,

377

Pannese, 1963; Porter and Bowers, 1963; Prineas, 1969) and neurotubules (Prineas, 1969; Barron et al., 1971). Such a proliferation would be expected in view of the hypothesized role of microtubules in axonal transport, and the enhancement of transport following axotomy (see below). Evidence for increased synthesis of tubulin, the constituent protein of neurofilaments and neurotubules, has been found following axotomy of goldfish retinal ganglion cells (Heacock and Agranoff, 1976) and rat motoneurons (Lasek and Hoffman, 1976).

On the other hand, it is clear that production of certain proteins is unnecessary during axonal regeneration. For example, synthesis of synaptic transmitters would be inappropriate during this time, and axotomy has been shown to result in reduction of transmitter synthetic and degradative enzymes. In cholinergic (motor) neurons, for example, axotomy results in a loss of activity of both choline acetyltransferase (Frizell and Sjostrand, 1974a) and acetylcholinesterase (e.g., Sawyer and Hollinshead, 1945; Gromadzki and Koelle, 1965; Watson, 1966b; Flumerfelt and Lewis, 1975). In noradrenergic neurons there is a decrease in the activities of the synthetic enzymes tyrosine hydroxylase (Cheah and Geffen, 1973; Ross et al., 1975) and dopamine β-hydroxylase (Reis and Ross, 1973; Ross et al., 1975), and of the degradative enzyme monoamine oxidase (Cheah and Geffen, 1973). Similarly, tyrosine hydroxylase activity is reduced following axotomy of dopaminergic neurons (Reis et al., 1978a; Gilad and Reis, 1978). Biochemical and histochemical evidence in these studies suggests a decrease in transmitter levels as well. The sequence of events regarding the activities of enzymes in the monoamine synthetic pathway following axotomy of central catecholaminergic neurons has been reviewed by Reis et al. (1978b). In general, following axotomy, there is a brief (2 to 4-day) period of increased enzyme protein content and activity (peak at 1 to 2 days) which is interpreted as a "pile-up" of enzyme (presumably due to the loss of the distal axon to which the enzyme would ordinarily be transported). As a consequence, transmitter is transiently accumulated in the soma. Thereafter both the activity and actual concentration of enzyme protein are reduced for a period of about 2 to 3 weeks. This decrease is interpreted as a probable reduction of transmitter-related enzyme synthesis (although actual rates of synthesis have not been measured) in favor of production of structural proteins during the phase of axonal regeneration. If the cell does not die, transmitter synthesis then recovers (presumably as synaptic contacts are reformed). Although less complete, there is evidence for similar reversible reductions in transmitter synthetic enzyme contents following axotomy for central serotonergic neurons, peripheral cholinergic neurons, and peripheral noradrenergic neurons. The significance of this sequence of events is that it is the exact inverse of the sequence for RNA and protein synthesis as a whole. This suggests a specificity in the anabolic and catabolic responses of neurons to axotomy for which an adequate mechanism has yet to be discovered.

Specificity of Nerve Regeneration

VERTEBRATE SOMATIC PNS It is clear that the PNS has a great potential for regeneration. However, the functional significance of this depends upon the specificity with which axons can reinnervate their original target tissues. In this regard there is a great difference between fish and amphibians, on the one hand, and mammals on the other. When a mixed motor nerve is cut in a fish or salamander, axonal regeneration is such that coordination of the fin or limb movements is regained perfectly (Sperry, 1950; Weiss, 1936). Despite earlier beliefs that this recovery is due to CNS reorganization, more recent evidence suggests that it is caused by preferential reinnervation of a muscle by its original nerve fibers. The nature of the evidence is rather indirect — that is, by exclusion of the hypothesis of central reorganization, rather than by demonstrating the specific nature of regeneration. Thus, if instead of simple sectioning of a mixed motor nerve the cut ends of nerve branches to opposing muscles are transplanted to the incorrect muscle, in most cases movements remain permanently inappropriate (Mark, 1965; Sperry and Arora, 1965; however, see Sperry, 1950). Specificity of reinnervation in lower vertebrates has also been found in cutaneous innervation. When a skin patch is transplanted from the belly of a tadpole to its back and vice versa, the anomalous wiping responses to tactile stimuli which develop in the frog (Miner, 1956) appear to result from the tendency of nerves to reroute themselves so as to reinnervate their original targets (Sklar and Hunt, 1973; Bloom and Tompkins, 1976; Heidemann, 1977). However, if the cross-grafting is performed after larval stage XV normal reflexes develop (Jacobson and Baker, 1969), suggesting that the degree of regenerative specificity decreases with age.

In contrast with lower vertebrates, section of a mixed motor nerve in mammals does not lead to eventual recovery. The difficulty lies not in an inadequate regenerative response but in the randomness with which motor axons reform connections with target muscles (Weiss and Hoag, 1946; reviewed by Guth, 1956). In addition, as with lower vertebrates, the mammalian CNS is not able to reorganize its connections in order to compensate for inaccurately formed neuromuscular connections (reviewed by Sperry, 1945). Clinical examples of the validity of these tendencies in human nerves are commonly found in the many forms of synkinesias which develop with recovery from lesions of the cranial nerves (Bender, 1936).

379

REGENERATION OF PERIPHERAL NERVE

The reasons for the difference between the selectivity in regeneration of nerves of lower vertebrates and those of mammals are not known. Mark (1969) has postulated that the superior coordination following regeneration of neuromuscular connections in amphibians and fishes is related to the tendency of their muscle fibers to be multiply innervated (Mark et al., 1966). Thus, even though muscle reinnervation may be random, muscle fibers which are innervated by both a correct and incorrect axon can eventually elect to respond only to the correct axon. Experimental evidence for this theory has been found in behavioral, electroneurographic, and morphological studies on cross-innervated antagonistic limb muscles of salamander and extraocular muscles of fish. If one muscle is then reinnervated by the correct nerve, that nerve establishes control of the muscle, provided the density of incorrect neuromuscular junctions is not too great. The incorrect innervation becomes functionless, although morphologically intact neuromuscular junctions remain (Marotte and Mark, 1970a, b; Mark and Marotte, 1972; Mark et al., 1972; Cass et al., 1973). However, when these experiments were repeated by others using intracellular recordings of end-plate potentials, no evidence for functionless neuromuscular junctions or suppression of foreign innervation was found at either extraocular muscles (Scott, 1975) or gill muscles (Frank and Jansen, 1976) of fish. The basis for the remarkable target selectivity in regenerating axons of lower vertebrates is still unclear.

Ironically, when similar experiments were performed on rat limb muscles the correct nerve was able to displace the incorrect nerve (Frank et al., 1975a), accompanied by morphological retraction of foreign neuromuscular junctions. The elimination of neuromuscular synapses from one nerve by a competing nerve depends upon the proximity of the dual innervations along the muscle fiber. When two nerves are implanted close together, competition between them leads to elimination of the synapses of one in a large percentage of cases. However, if they are implanted at opposite poles of the muscle, dual innervation persists (Kuffler et al., 1977). The tendency for regenerating motor axons to displace foreign axon terminals is also seen in partially denervated muscle in which the source of foreign axons is the same nerve. It is well known that when a nerve is partially damaged and some of its target muscle fibers are denervated neighboring intact axons sprout and innervate the denervated muscle fibers, beginning at about 4 or 5 days (reviewed by Edds, 1953). This results in some motor units with greatly expanded territories. In human patients it is manifested by coarse fasciculations on physical examination and giant polyphasic motor unit potentials on electromyography. If the damaged fibers are allowed to regenerate, they will often reinnervate their original muscle fibers (Hoffman, 1951; Guth, 1962). Recent studies using intracellular recording of end-plate potentials in partially denervated mouse muscle have shown that following regeneration of the damaged axons only about 10 per cent of muscle fibers remain doubly innervated. Some of the rest of the initially denervated fibers remain innervated by the foreign sprouts while others are reinnervated by the regenerating axons (Brown and Ironton, 1978). In the latter case it has not yet been shown whether the axon sprouts retract or whether they only become functionally inactive.

It is of interest to note that in many respects the regeneration paradigm mimics normal development of mammalian neuromuscular junctions. Early in their postnatal development muscles are polyneuronally innervated (Redfern, 1970; Bennett and Pettigrew, 1974). During maturation the change to mononeuronal innervation seems to occur by retraction of redundant axon terminals (Korneliussen and Jansen, 1976), and seems to depend upon the distance between competing end-plates. The closer the end-plates the less likely the persistence of multiple innervation (Brown et al., 1976). In lower vertebrates such as amphibians a sizable minority of skeletal muscle fibers remain multiply innervated (Bennett and Pettigrew, 1975; Rotshenker and McMahan, 1976).

The basic mechanisms involved in the competition between axon terminals for innervation of muscle fibers are almost totally unknown. However, when axoplasmic flow is blocked in a salamander nerve by application of colchicine, neighboring nerves sprout and superinnervate the muscle fibers or skin field in the territory of the treated nerve, even though the latter remains morphologically and electrophysiologically intact (Aguilar et al., 1973). Colchicine prevents sprouting in a nerve to which it is applied directly. This suggests that nerve cells may produce a substance which suppresses sprouting in neighboring axons when transported peripherally. When an axon is injured the loss of this transported factor would lead to sprouting in neighboring axons into the territory of the injured one. While such a hypothesis may explain how nerve fibers limit their peripheral fields, it still does not explain how postsynaptic muscle fibers select among competing regenerating axon terminals. Whatever the explanation, the observations described in this section suggest that the failure to achieve accurate reinnervation and recovery of coordination following nerve injury in mammals is not due to a lack of specificity in the recognition of nerve fibers by their proper muscles, nor by the inability of muscle fibers to be temporarily multiply innervated. Rather, they suggest that if several regenerating nerve fibers approach the muscle closely enough the appropriate neuromuscular junctions are

381

formed selectively. It may be, therefore, that the difficulty with mammalian nerve regeneration in comparison with lower vertebrates is that the nerves lack the ability to seek out their correct target muscles when they are separated from those muscles by great distances. Consistent with this notion is the common clinical observation that the prognosis for recovery of function of a denervated muscle or area of skin is greater the more peripheral the nerve injury and subsequent suture (Sunderland, 1947; Seddon, 1948; Kirklin et al., 1949; Shaffer and Cleveland, 1950; Zachary, 1954; Oester and Davis, 1956; Yahr and Beebe, 1956; Omer, 1974; see Sunderland, 1978, for review). On the other hand, the differences in target selectivity between regenerating nerves of small mammals, such as mice, and those of larger amphibians, such as frogs, suggest that the greater recuperative capacity of the latter cannot be accounted for by the differences in the distance of regeneration alone.

Several other observations suggest a great deal of specificity in axon-target organ interaction when regenerating axons, both sensory and motor, are fairly close to their targets. Following sural nerve transection and regeneration, the distributions of peripheral receptor types, nerve conduction velocities, and central projections via dorsal columns are all similar to those in control nerves (Burgess and Horch, 1973; Horch, 1976). From the close correlation among these properties, these authors concluded that a given neuron is likely to have the same receptor function following regeneration as it did before the nerve was cut. Furthermore, when individual patches of skin in the cat are examined before and after femoral cutaneous nerve transection there is a great similarity in the maps of cutaneous dome receptors, suggesting a great specificity in the return of receptors to previous locations on the skin (Burgess et al., 1974). Similarly, regenerating motor axons in both mammals and amphibians show a remarkable tendency to innervate the precise postsynaptic grooves of the muscle end-plate which were occupied previously (Saito and Zacks, 1969; Letinsky et al., 1976). That this precision is related to a property of the postsynaptic end-organ rather than to a specific recognition of that site by its original axon is suggested by the fact that in previously singly innervated muscle fibers the reinnervated grooves may be occupied by more than one axon terminal (Lullman-Rauch, 1971) belonging to more than one axon (Rotshenker and McMahan, 1976). Thus, although the postsynaptic gutters of the muscle end-plate become filled once again with axon terminals, there is variability as to which axons will occupy them. The component of the muscle fiber which attracts the regenerating axon terminals, determines the exact distribution of axonally innervated end-plate membrane, and induces morphological differentiation of presynaptic terminals seems to be the basal lamina of the muscle basement membrane. Sanes et al. (1978) found that when myofibers are damaged and x-irradiated to prevent regeneration the basal laminae remain, and the exact locations of axon terminals on the basal laminae can be identified morphologically. When the muscles are also denervated, regenerating axon terminals reinnervate the basal laminae in the exact locations previously occupied by presynaptic nerve endings. And, once contact is made between a nerve terminal and basal lamina, the nerve terminal develops typical synaptic active zones and vesicle accumulations. Similar factors governing the distribution specificity of cutaneous reinnervation have not yet been described.

AUTONOMIC NERVOUS SYSTEM   Specificity in re-established synaptic connections has also been demonstrated in the mammalian autonomic nervous system. As with skeletal muscle, denervated sympathetic ganglion cells can be reinnervated by a transplanted foreign nerve. The success of the foreign innervation is not as great as that of reinnervation by the normal sympathetic preganglionic nerve (see Purves, 1976, for review). However, unlike skeletal muscle, simultaneous reinnervation by the native presynaptic nerve does not significantly alter the degree to which the foreign nerve synapses with the ganglion cell, and no subsequent displacement of inappropriate synapses seems to occur (Purves, 1976). Paradoxically, when sympathetic preganglionic fibers compete with each other, considerable selectivity is shown in the reinnervation of ganglion cells. For example, the superior cervical ganglion of mammals receives presynaptic innervation from the lower cervical and upper thoracic segments, and different segments innervate ganglion cells with different functions (Langley, 1892). Stimulation of the T1 ventral root of a cat or guinea pig elicits pupillary dilatation and contraction of palpebral smooth musculature, but has little effect upon the vascular smooth muscle of the ear. On the other hand, stimulation of the T4 ventral root causes vasoconstriction and cooling of the ear and piloerection on the face and neck, but has no effects on the eye. Langley (1897) showed that following sectioning of the cervical sympathetic trunk and subsequent regeneration this specificity is re-established when tested after several months. These observations have been confirmed by Guth and Bernstein in cat (1961) and Nja and Purves in guinea pig (1977); analogous observations have been made in the pigeon ciliary ganglion by Landmesser and Pilar (1970). Moreover, regenerating sympathetic preganglionics of the upper three thoracic segments of the cat appear to be able to displace functionally the synaptic terminals of sympathetic preganglionics arising from T4 to T7

383

which had sprouted to innervate the pupillodilator ganglion cells following crush of T1 to T3 ventral roots
(Guth and Bernstein, 1961).

It seems illogical that competitive reinnervation by native sympathetic preganglionics should be able to inac-
tivate or displace synaptic terminals of other sympathetic preganglionics but not those of foreign nerves,
such as the vagus (Purves, 1976). If true, this might
suggest that specificity in re-established synaptic connections occurs if competing regenerating axons with
closely related physical or functional properties at first
distribute their synaptic contacts randomly and subsequently displace one another in accordance with the
functional requirements of the organism. However, this
hypothesis has been rendered implausible by the findings of Nja and Purves (1978b). Using behavioral observations and intracellular recordings of synaptic potentials in superior cervical ganglion cells of guinea pig,
they showed that: (1) the specificity of the end-organ
response is present as soon as any responses are elicitable following a freezing lesion of the cervical sympathetic trunk (15 to 30 days); and (2) from the earliest
times of observable return of synaptic potentials (8 to
19 days) individual ganglion cells tend at first to be
activated by axons of only one spinal segment, and
thereafter by a contiguous subset of spinal segments
(average of 3.0 segments after 6 months), with one
segment being dominant. Consequently, it is unlikely
that specificity in synaptic connections of regenerating
sympathetic preganglionic fibers is superimposed secondarily following an initially random pattern of ganglion cell reinnervation. There is as yet no evidence to
suggest what mechanisms might underlie the specificity in regeneration of autonomic nerves.

The preceding observations on vertebrate PNS may be
summarized as follows. Both mammalian and non-
mammalian vertebrate axons seem able to select appropriate targets at close range. The mechanisms
involved appear to include specific recognition mechanisms between a growing axon and its target organ (muscle, area of skin, or autonomic ganglion cell). In addition,
certain physical or chemical characteristics of the
target tissue may determine the distribution of nerve
terminals on it regardless of which axon innervates
it. In muscle this property seems to reside in the
connective tissue basal membrane. The specificity
of nerve target interaction apparently operates over
longer distances in younger animals than in older.
Thus, cutaneous nerves will seek their original target
skin patch when transplanted from the ventral to
dorsal surface in a tadpole, but not in an adult frog. In
adult mammals regenerating nerves tend to follow the
paths of their degenerating distal stumps but the distribution of axons within branches of these stumps is

384

random. The more proximal the nerve injury the larger the number of branches of the degenerating distal stump, and the greater the likelihood that an axon will not approach its target organ close enough for the mechanisms of selectivity to operate. This hypothesis, applied to the re-establishment of neuromuscular connections, is diagrammed in Figure 12–6. There may well be a degree of randomness and redundancy in initial contacts (Fig. 12–6*B2*) with a subsequent retraction of at least some inappropriate connections (Fig. 12–6*B3*). In the case of regenerating sympathetic preganglionics, specificity seems to be established immediately and step *B2* may not apply.

COMPARISON WITH INVERTEBRATE PNS Several studies have suggested that the axonal response to injury in invertebrates may show some differences in comparison with Wallerian degeneration and subsequent regeneration in vertebrate peripheral nerve. While the majority of invertebrate axons probably undergo Wallerian degeneration, many do not. Instead, regeneration occurs by fusion of the proximal and distal cut ends. Such axons have been described in crustaceans (Hoy et al., 1967; Bittner and Johnson, 1974), the leech (Frank et al., 1975*b*), and the earthworm (Birse and Bittner, 1976). The reasons for this difference are not known, but the axons which have been described thus far as regenerating by fusion are quite large, and may of necessity possess more elaborate biochemical apparatus than vertebrate axons; they may survive longer after being cut off from the soma and thus might still be alive when contacted by their regenerating proximal stumps. However, size of itself cannot be a sufficient explanation, since the giant axons of lamprey spinal cord undergo Wallerian degeneration (Selzer, 1978; Tang and Selzer, 1979).

Even when such mechanisms are not involved, severed invertebrate nerves show a considerable amount of specificity in the reinnervation of target tissues. Some invertebrates are advantageous as models of regeneration since their individual sensory and motor neurons can be identified and impaled with microelectrodes. Their characteristic fields of innervation can be determined by recording responses to skin stimulation or observing muscle responses to intracellular neuronal stimulation. It should therefore be possible to establish the degree of variability in the peripheral fields of individual neurons before and after axotomy and regeneration. This has been done for sensory and motor neurons in the leech (Van Essen and Jansen, 1977). It was found that transected sensory and motor axons usually return to their original target area unless the distal ends of the nerve branches are evulsed. Moreover, once they reach their target area, sensory

385

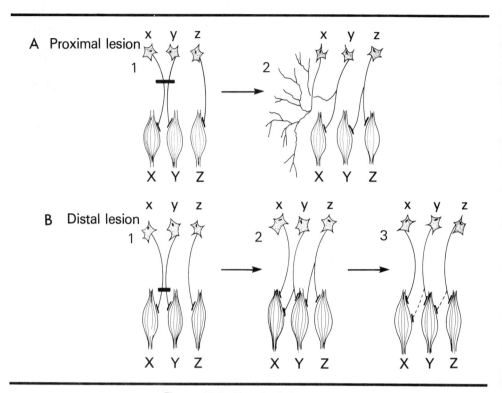

Figure 12–6 Hypothesis based on the experiments described in the text to explain the limited specificity of regeneration of mammalian peripheral nerve fibers. It is assumed that there are at least two types of forces, typified in amphibian PNS, which guide nerve regeneration: long-range forces, which guide fibers into correct nerve branches, and short-range forces, which allow regenerating fibers to select among neighboring muscles supplied by the same nerve. In mammalian PNS the long-range forces seem to be weak or absent. X, Y, and Z are neighboring muscles supplied by motoneurons x, y, and z, respectively. A lesion of x and y far from the muscles *(A1)* results in totally aberrant regeneration of x and the inappropriate reinnervation of X by y *(A2)*. During the prolonged period of denervation, Y is reinnervated by collateral sprouts from neuron z. The result is a loss of coordination among the actions mediated by these muscles. In *B1* the lesion of x and y occurs close to the muscles. Therefore, the choice of paths open to the regenerating axons is limited. Since each regenerating axon sends out several sprouts, even a random pattern of regeneration will result in reinnervation of all the muscle by some sprouts of their original nerve fibers. This results in transient multiple reinnervation of some muscle fibers *(B2)*. However, short-range forces act to bias initial reinnervation toward appropriate nerve-muscle pairs (x-X in *B2*). In addition, perhaps other short-range forces act to eliminate inappropriate connections in muscle fibers which are multiply innervated *(B3)*. The result is a more favorable pattern of reinnervation in distal nerve lesions than in proximal ones.

neurons invariably re-establish their original modality specificity (touch, pressure, or noxious stimuli), and motoneurons always reinnervate the original muscle fiber type (longitudinal, circular, flattener, or annulus erector muscles). Similar specificity has been demonstrated in the regeneration of motor neurons to leg muscles in the cockroach (Pearson and Bradley, 1972), and in the reinnervation of the salivary neuroeffector complex by identified neurons of a mollusc, *Helisoma trivolvis* (Murphy and Kater, 1978). In the case of regenerating motoneurons of the cockroach, knowledge of the normal branching patterns and destinations of identified motor axons has allowed some analysis of the mechanisms of target specificity. Denburg et al. (1977) found that regenerating axons branch profusely, sending processes into both their normal and abnormal nerve branches. Over periods of many weeks, however, incorrect axon branches disappear. It was concluded that target selectivity results from a specific recognition process between an axon and its normal target muscle, and that branches of axons which do not make contact with their correct muscle degenerate. Thus, as with mammalian nerves, invertebrate nerves show a remarkable specificity in re-establishing their original functions. Since distal nerve evulsion prevents accurate regeneration, invertebrate nerves, like those of mammals, seem to require assistance (perhaps in the form of contact guidance by the distal nerve branch) in approaching their original target region. Why larval amphibian nerves seem to require less guidance is not known.

COMPARISON WITH VERTEBRATE CNS A comprehensive review of developments in CNS regeneration is beyond the scope of this chapter. However, the strategies used by the CNS to compensate for or recover lost functions are relevant to the question of whether central reorganization may play a role in establishing functional specificity of peripheral nerve regeneration.

Regeneration (as opposed to collateral sprouting, an important related phenomenon), is generally believed not to occur naturally in mammalian CNS (reviewed by Windle, 1956; Clemente, 1964). This is usually attributed to excessive scar formation blocking the path of regenerating axons. Efforts to induce regeneration in mammalian spinal cord have involved injections of steroids, antimetabolites, or proteolytic enzymes in order to suppress scar formation (Feringa et al., 1974, 1977; see Pettigrew and Windle, 1976, for review). These efforts have resulted in some axonal regeneration but probably not true functional recovery. However, even in the absence of regeneration, a variety of mechanisms are theoretically available to the CNS to compensate for lost anatomical connections. These mechanisms are generally spoken of as "plastic prop-

387

erties'' of the nervous system. They include denervation supersensitivity (Cannon and Rosenblueth, 1949; Stavraki, 1961; Ungerstedt, 1971; Echlin, 1975; Yarbrough and Phillis, 1975; Roper, 1976; Waddington and Cross, 1978), alterations in synaptic efficacy resulting from patterns of use or disuse of neuronal pathways (Kandel and Spencer, 1968; Kandel, 1976, 1977, 1978), and sprouting of nearby axons to occupy a denervated postsynaptic site (Liu and Chambers, 1958; Raisman, 1969; Lynch et al., 1973; Murray and Goldberger, 1974; Goldberger and Murray, 1974; Cotman and Nadler, 1978). Many developments in the study of neuronal plasticity are also reviewed in Rosenzweig and Bennett (1976). Generally, these mechanisms continue to bear only hypothetical relevance to the question of whether CNS reorganization can lead to behavioral recovery. The studies of Goldberger and Murray (1974) address this question more directly. They demonstrated hierarchies of preference in sprouting by neighboring axon bundles in the spinal cord when one of them (pyramidal tract or dorsal root) was cut. The time of sprouting was compared with alterations in spinal reflexes and functional recovery of gait and limb coordination, and it was concluded that in some cases there is a correlation between the time of sprouting and behavioral recovery. What is lacking is evidence as to whether the pattern of sprouting is specific to the behavioral deficit, or whether any behavioral recovery associated with sprouting is a coincidence.

Regeneration in lower vertebrate CNS is more successful, and can be broadly divided into two categories. The first appears to be a point-to-point regeneration of axons to their original targets, as exemplified by the regeneration of the severed optic nerve in amphibians and fish (Fig. 12–7). Results of very long series of experiments involving rotation or other manipulations of the eye or retina, followed by behavioral, electrophysiological, and histological observations on the regenerated visual system, suggest that the axons of the optic nerve grow back to their original locus in the optic tectum, resulting in a predictably anomalous topographic representation of the retina on tectum (Sperry, 1943, 1944, 1948; Gaze, 1959; Gaze and Jacobson, 1963; Jacobson and Gaze, 1965; see Hunt and Jacobson, 1974; Jacobson, 1978 for reviews). This type of regeneration may be seen as similar to that in the PNS, since axons regenerate along a relatively simple nerve matrix and are not hindered or ''distracted'' by contact with other neurons along the way. If point-to-point regeneration does indeed occur, there is no need to postulate a reorganization of other CNS structures in order to explain functional recovery. However, most CNS lesions would involve interruption of at least some long pathways which pass many neurons in their course. Regeneration of these pathways would involve

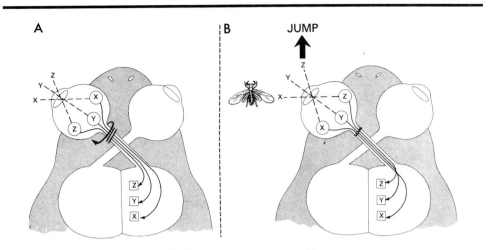

Figure 12–7 Point-to-point regeneration of retinotectal connections of the frog. *A,* Points X, Y, and Z in the visual field of the left eye of a frog normally stimulate ganglion cells X, Y, and Z in the retina. These neurons in turn project to areas X, Y, and Z in the contralateral optic tectum. If the optic nerve is cut, the eye rotated 180°, and the animal allowed to recover, the results are as in *B. B,* The axons of neurons X, Y, and Z have regenerated to their original target areas in the right tectum. The result is that the apparent positions of points X, Y, and Z are reversed. Thus, if an attracting visual stimulus such as a fly is presented at point X, the frog will jump toward point Z.

the possibility of repeated encounters with groups of neurons, some of which have also been partly denervated and are potentially receptive to new synaptic contacts.

A classic example of this type of CNS lesion is spinal cord transection. Even among lower vertebrates the degree of functional recovery from cord section is variable. For example fish, salamanders, and tadpoles all show virtually complete recovery, while adult frogs most often do not (Koppanyi, 1955; Piatt, 1955a,b). Therefore it appears to be true that functional recovery is more complete the younger the animal and the more primitive the species. Yet, even in the most primitive of vertebrates, functional recovery is not accompanied by point-to-point axonal regeneration. The larval sea lamprey, one of the most primitive of all vertebrates, is known to recover swimming coordination following spinal cord transection (Maron, 1959; Hibbard, 1963; Rovainen, 1976; Selzer, 1976). Behavioral studies with surgically manipulated animals have shown that at least part if not all of this recovery is mediated through a regenerative mechanism in the spinal cord (Selzer, 1978). Despite this, studies of the large reticulospinal axons (Müller's and Mauthner's fibers) in serial cross sections suggest that axonal regeneration does not progress beyond a few millimeters across a transection (Rovainen, 1976; Selzer, 1978). Intracellular electrophysiological evidence also supports the notion that behavioral recovery is associated with short distance but not long distance regeneration. In recovered animals neurons caudal to a transection which ordinarily project to the brain (dorsal cells and giant interneurons) can no longer be activated antidromically by stimulating the cord rostral to the transection (Fig. 12–8). However, one of these neuron types, the giant interneuron, which ordinarily is activated monosynaptically by rostral cord stimulation, can be activated only polysynaptically by electrical stimulation of the spinal cord rostral to a transection (Selzer, 1978). From these and other observations it was hypothesized that behavioral recovery does not involve point-to-point regeneration of long axon tracts, but rather short-distance regeneration and synapse formation with neurons in the region of the transection. Information crossing the transection which previously was transmitted centrifugally by direct axonal conduction must now be transmitted by polysynaptic chains. It seems likely, therefore, that after spinal cord transection, unlike the situation in retinotectal regeneration, the CNS must accommodate itself to a new structural arrangement.

Some insight into the reasons for this limited form of regeneration was provided by Bernstein and Bernstein (1967) using goldfish, which ordinarily recover from spinal cord transection by axonal regeneration. When a Teflon shield is inserted into the transection, axonal regeneration and behavioral recovery are prevented. If after 30 days the Teflon is removed, no regeneration follows. The Bernsteins were interested in determining whether the blocking of regeneration under these circumstances is due to the formation of the glial scar. They retransected the spinal cord 1 cm rostral to the original lesion, but this time did not insert a Teflon shield. The result was that descending axons regenerate not only through the new transection but also through the original glial scar. Thus the failure of axon growth after removal of the Teflon shield cannot be ascribed to the mechanical resistance of the scar. Instead the Bernsteins postulated that, when originally deterred from regeneration, the proximal ends of severed axons form synapses with neural elements rostral to the transection, and that this in some way inhibits further regeneration after the Teflon is removed. Retransection eliminates these synapses and allows regeneration. The phenomenon was termed "contact inhibition" because it was felt that contact of axons with postsynaptic neurons inhibits further regeneration. It was later demonstrated by electron microscopy that there is an alteration of the normal pattern of synaptic

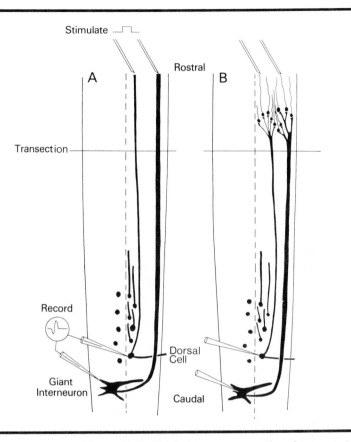

Figure 12–8 Short-distance regeneration of transected lamprey spinal cord. *A,* Two types of rostrally projecting neurons — primary sensory neurons called dorsal cells and secondary sensory neurons called giant interneurons — can normally be activated antidromically by rostral cord stimulation. If the spinal cord is cut and the animal allowed to recover, sensory function returns but these two types of neurons cannot be antidromically activated from the rostral spinal cord. Physiological and histological evidence suggests axonal regeneration in lamprey spinal cord occurs as in *B. B,* Short-distance regeneration is postulated for primary and second order sensory cells. Sensory function would have to be reestablished through synapse formation (not yet proved) with interneurons in the region of the transection. (From Selzer, 1978.)

organization in the spinal cord just rostral to the Teflon shield, suggesting that the cut axons have formed axo-axonal and axodendritic synapses in the area (Bernstein and Bernstein, 1969). If this hypothesis is accepted the point-to-point regeneration of retinotectal connections in amphibia may still be explained on the basis of the short distance which axons must travel through neuron groups that have been denervated before reaching their appropriate target neurons.

ANALOGY BETWEEN SPINAL CORD REGENERATION IN LOWER VERTEBRATES AND SPROUTING IN PNS

If the point-to-point regeneration in the retinotectal system can be likened to regeneration of cut peripheral nerves, the short-distance regeneration seen in spinal axons of lower vertebrates can be compared for instructional purposes with collateral sprouting. Several types of experimental and natural circumstances lead to sprouting of axons in the absence of physical injury. In addition to denervation of neighboring muscles, skin, or neurons, sprouting can also result from local injection of botulinum toxin (Watson, 1969). This toxin blocks transmitter release at the neuromuscular junction (Guyton and MacDonald, 1947; Ambache, 1949; Burgen et al., 1949; Brooks, 1954), and thus produces a functional denervation (see below). Blockage of nerve action potentials by tetrodotoxin also induces sprouting (Brown and Ironton, 1977), presumably by a similar mechanism. There is no reason to distinguish between regeneration and sprouting in regard to their anatomical appearance or basic mechanisms. Both involve outgrowth from the region of the nerve terminal or from the distalmost nodes of Ranvier. The elongation seems to involve deposition of membranous material in the region of the growth cone rather than along the axon shaft or initial segment (Bray, 1973; Bunge, 1973). While some differences have been described between sprouting and regeneration with regard to the details of concomitant biochemical and morphological changes in the cell body, these may well relate to the circumstances of the new axonal growth rather than to differences in the mechanism of elongation. The fundamental difference between the two processes is that sprouting occurs close to the target tissue and thus may be more likely to reflect trophic influences of that target tissue than axonal regeneration. The short-distance regeneration of lower vertebrate spinal axons is analogous with sprouting — i.e., the distribution of regenerating synaptic terminals is probably affected most by the short range forces underlying selectivity and competition for postsynaptic sites already discussed in relation to peripheral nerve. Clearly this analogy and the various hypotheses which will be discussed to mediate the analogy are very speculative. They are raised here only because the various experimental results relating to the control of sprouting and short-distance CNS regeneration are so disparate, and often seem so contradictory, that it is useful to see whether it is at all possible to resolve them.

The concept of contact inhibition in CNS would seem to imply either that axons are preprogrammed to form a specific maximum number of synaptic boutons, or that some or any postsynaptic neuron transfers to the presynaptic axon an inhibitory substance or factor (e.g., electric) which suppresses further sprouting or axon elongation. In either case, while the principle has not been tested directly, some observations on sprouting of motor axons would tend to contradict it. The fact that motor axons can sprout and increase the number of synaptic contacts they make when neighboring muscle fibers are denervated shows that the natural number of synaptic contacts made by motor axons is not limited by a property intrinsic to the neuron. Similarly, since axons with their full complement of synaptic connections can sprout to neighboring denervated muscle fibers, it is unlikely that the postsynaptic muscle end-plate is supplying an inhibitory substance which limits its own axon's growth. On the contrary Pestronk and Drachman (1978) have adduced evidence which suggests that muscle fibers may exert a positive influence upon sprouting through their extrajunctional acetylcholine receptors. Sprouting in nerve fibers was induced by chronically blocking release of acetylcholine with botulinum toxin or by producing disuse of muscle fibers with repeated local injections of tetrodotoxin. It was found that the degree of sprouting is correlated with the levels of extrajunctional acetylcholine receptors, and that the sprouting is inhibited by blocking the receptors with α-bungarotoxin. On the other hand, we have seen that axons compete with each other for postsynaptic sites, and that interruption of axonal transport in salamander axons by focal application of colchicine can induce sprouting in nearby fibers. This suggests the possibility that synapse density in a region may be regulated by an axonally transported substance which inhibits axon growth or sprouting when released into the extracellular space by the nerve terminal (Aguilar et al., 1973).

Some researchers have proposed that nerve injury or muscle denervation causes the local release of a sprout-inducing substance (Van Harreveld, 1947; Hoffman and Springell, 1951; Edds, 1953; Rotshenker, 1978). Denervation of one cutaneous-pectoris muscle in the frog can result in sprouting (measured as the percentage of multiply innervated muscle fibers) in the nerve to the same muscle on the opposite side (Rotshenker and McMahan, 1976). The sprouting occurs even when the denervated muscle and its distal cut nerve are removed (Rotshenker, 1978). Thus, if a sprout-inducing substance is being released, it is coming neither from denervated muscle nor from degenerating axon. Rotshenker suggests that it comes from the damaged neurons and is released in the spinal cord. However, these results could also be explained by the loss of production or release by damaged neurons of a sprout-inhibiting factor, especially if that factor were ordinarily released within the spinal cord where the contralateral motoneurons could be preferentially affected. Rotshenker's (1978) findings can be reconciled with those of Aguilar et al, (1973) regarding the sprout-inducing effects of colchicine if it is assumed either that colchicine is acting as a nonspecific injury to the axon or that a sprout-inhibiting substance is supplied by a given muscle fiber to its presynaptic axon terminal. In the latter case, the substance would be carried to the soma by retrograde transport. In the spinal cord the substance might be released into the extracellular space, where it would affect those neurons closest to it, which would primarily include neurons innervating the same muscle. If a large number of motoneurons are simultaneously injured the effect might be reflected in other nearby motoneuron pools, including the homologous contralateral motor nucleus. Such a mechanism would be compatible with both the notion of contact inhibition and the ability of nerve fibers to sprout even when their own neuromuscular connections remain intact.

Regardless of whether sprouting is induced by release of an inducing factor or loss of an inhibiting factor, the above observations suggest that axon competition may operate in CNS as it does on neuromuscular innervation to limit the territories of synaptic distribution of regenerating severed axons. This competition might or might not be accompanied by a form of contact inhibition. It may be imagined that when the spinal cord is transected descending axons undergo Wallerian degeneration caudal to the cut. Many neurons would lose part of their complement of synaptic input, and the total synaptic density would decrease. At this point sprouting might be induced in nearby axons, and a competition would be set up between regenerating severed axons and sprouts of intact nearby axons in the formation of synaptic boutons in the region. Assuming that regenerating axon tips are similarly affected by the factors which limit the sprouting of intact axons (not at all established yet), the postsynaptic territory of a regenerating axon would be governed by the relative magnitudes of the initial delays and growth rates of the local sprouts and regenerating axon branches, as well as by the transsynaptic accumulation of a sprout-inhibiting factor as more and more synapses are formed. Axons might well regenerate more slowly through a dense neuropil than within a nerve sheath. This might explain the relative success of point-to-point regeneration in retinotectal connections since the retinal ganglion cell axons regenerate along the optic nerve, and not through neuron groups, until they reach the optic tectum. Thus, they might be in a relatively favorable position when competing with potential sprouting axons for contact with denervated postsynaptic sites. Moreover, if sprouting is induced by release of a sprout-inducing substance or loss of an inhibitory substance ordinarily released by neuron somata, then the absence of a large population of axotomized neurons within the tectum would mean that little stimulus for sprouting exists in nearby intact axons.

SPECIFICITY OF REGENERATION IN INVERTEBRATE CENTRAL GANGLIA

Among invertebrates, the leech has demonstrated some degree of specificity in the regeneration of synaptic linkages between identified neurons of different ganglia following transection of the connective nerves (Baylor and Nicholls, 1971; Jansen and Nicholls, 1972). However, it is not clear whether the regenerated contacts described in these studies are monosynaptic, as they are in the nontransected animal. If they are not monosynaptic, then the leech connectives may behave similarly to the spinal cord of lamprey larvae in regard to the mechanisms underlying recovery of function following disconnection of different levels of CNS.

CAN CNS REMODELLING CONTRIBUTE TO BEHAVIORAL RECOVERY?

It should now be apparent that models of CNS regeneration are of interest in the consideration of mechanisms of specificity in peripheral nerve-target organ recognition for two important reasons:

1. By allowing comparison of peripheral nerve with various degrees of increased complexity in the path and targets of regeneration, these models serve as natural controls for experiments on peripheral nerve regeneration and sprouting.
2. The model of functional recovery following spinal cord transection in lower vertebrates shows that exact point-to-point regeneration is not necessary for such recovery, and that "remodelling" of central connections may, under some circumstances, underlie successful responses to injury.

If this is true for CNS regeneration, then there is still a possibility that such plastic responses of CNS, either structural or physiological, may be involved in the recovery of function following less than exact regeneration of peripheral nerves to their target tissues.

We have seen that the behavioral studies of Sperry and others on cross-innervation of antagonistic muscles fail to provide evidence for recovery of normal muscle coordination (as opposed to learned compensation for the loss of some muscles by use of others) in mammals and, in most instances, in lower vertebrates also. It should also be emphasized that intracellular neurophysiological studies on the distribution of Ia afferent input to motoneurons of cross-innervated muscles in cats fail to demonstrate consistent evidence for what Sperry (1950) called "myotypic respecification" of motoneuronal function. This theory, proposed by Weiss (1936) and others in one form or another since before the turn of the century, suggests that the central connections of motoneurons can be modulated or altered either morphologically or physiologically, according to the function of the muscles they reinnervate when their axons are transplanted into foreign muscles (see Sperry, 1945, for a critical review). Ia afferents from one muscle ordinarily activate most strongly the motoneurons to the same muscle; they activate motoneurons to synergists less strongly, and inhibit motoneurons to antagonists. Despite occasional small shifts in EPSP size (Eccles et al., 1960, 1962) in the direction predicted by the theory of myotypic modulation (but which could also be explained without invoking myotypic modulation), these relationships are qualitatively unchanged by cross-innvervation of agonistic or antagonistic muscles (Eccles et al., 1962), and do not involve changes in the percentages of motoneurons in different motor nuclei which receive monosynaptic excitation from individual Ia afferents (Mendell and Scott, 1975). However, these studies were on mammals, which show relatively poor specificity in recovery from transection of mixed motor nerves. Similar studies have not been performed on those species, such as salamander, which show good recovery following mixed motor nerve injury. Although Sperry rejected the theory of myotypic modulation for adult mammals, he left open the possibility of its operating in more primitive vertebrates (Sperry, 1941, 1950); thus, it might be an influence on the development of the embryonic nervous system in mammals. Only a few tests of the notion that plastic changes in CNS organization can compensate for inaccurate peripheral nerve regeneration have been done thus far using intracellular recording techniques. It would seem that this theory cannot yet be rejected, even in adult mammals.

Factors Which Affect Nerve Regeneration

AXOPLASMIC TRANSPORT The characteristics of axoplasmic transport are described in detail in this volume by Pleasure (Chapter 6). In brief, substances are transported from the cell body by one of at least two transport systems: (1) fast axoplasmic transport, which in mammals has a rate of about 410 mm/day; and (2) a slower component, which carries substances having a very wide range of rates, in some instances as low as 1 mm/day. It is postulated that substances are transported along the neurofilament system, since drugs such as colchicine which block axonal transport also bind to tubulin and, at high concentrations, induce disassembly of microtubules and filaments. Ochs (1975) and Ochs and Worth (1978) have suggested a unitary theory of axonal transport based upon the concept that transported substances bind to neurofilaments which are pushed along by making and breaking of cross-bridges with the stationary microtubules, analogous with the sliding filament hypothesis of muscle contraction. According to this hypothesis the slow transport system could arise from the tendencies of some substances to be loosely bound to the sliding filaments, and thus continually make and break contact with different filaments on their way along the axon. Whether or not this is true, many studies have claimed to show differential effects upon the rates of fast and slow transport by various physical and chemical agents. Several hypotheses concerning mechanisms of transport are still being considered including the theory, based upon the original findings of Weiss and Hiscoe (1948), that slow transport represents a peristaltic movement of axoplasm (see Grafstein, 1977). Thus, the two transport rates are conveniently envisioned as comprising separate systems.

Among the substances transported by fast axoplasmic transport are secretion products, such as the dense core vesicles containing norepinephrine and dopamine-β-hydroxylase in sympathetic neurons, transmitter-related enzymes, such as acetylcholinesterase, other proteins and polypeptides of varying sizes, especially structural proteins such as mucopolysaccharide proteins, glycoproteins, and other constituents of membrane such as cholesterol, glycolipids, and phospholipids. Other proteins, such as tubulin itself, many cytoplasmic proteins, many small molecules of various types, and some particulate structures, such as mitochondria, have a net outward transport at rates in the slow transport range. A general correlation has been made between substances produced by rough-surfaced endoplasmic reticulum and those which are transported by fast transport, while products of free polyribosomes generally seem to travel via the slow transport system (Price and Porter, 1972). Substances are also transported in a retrograde fashion, from nerve terminals to the soma. Maximum rates for this process are estimated at about half those of fast anterograde transport.

Strong a priori arguments can be made for involvement of both anterograde and retrograde transport in regeneration. It is obvious from the fact that distal segments of cut axons undergo irreversible degeneration that axons (at least in vertebrates) do not possess the necessary machinery for synthesis of those substances necessary for their own maintenance. Thus, clearly anterograde transport is necessary to the survival of regenerating axons, as it is to axons in general. But, in addition, the absence of rough-surfaced endoplasmic reticulum and free polyribosomes in axons means that the protein components of newly formed membrane, axoplasmic matrix, and microtubule and microfilament systems must generally be manufactured in the soma and trans-

397

ported to the periphery. Teleologically one might expect, therefore, that axonal regeneration would be accompanied by an increase in the rate and volume of axonal transport. This is indeed the case in goldfish optic nerve, where the rates of both slow and fast transport are markedly increased following nerve section (Grafstein and Murray, 1969; McQuarrie, 1977). However, in mammalian nerve, the rate of fast transport seems unchanged by axotomy (Ochs, 1976; Bisby, 1978), and there is still considerable disagreement as to whether regeneration is accompanied by significant changes in the volume of fast transport (Kreutzberg and Schubert, 1971; Frizell and Sjostrand, 1974a; Ochs, 1976; Griffin et al., 1976; Bisby, 1978).

The situation regarding the rate and volume of slow transport is equally unclear (Frizell and Sjostrand, 1974b; Kreutzberg and Schubert, 1971; Lasek and Hoffman, 1976). O'Brien (1978) found an increase in the accumulation of acetylcholine but a decrease in accumulation of choline acetyltransferase and cholinesterase behind a crush in regenerating peripheral nerve. However, these findings do not distinguish transport rate from synthesis rate or transport volume. Indirect evidence for a role of the soma in regeneration of the axon has been found by McQuarrie (1977), who showed that cycloheximide-induced inhibition of protein synthesis in the cell body causes a reduction in the rate of axonal growth following optic nerve crush in goldfish. In addition, Griffin et al. (1976) showed a preferential incorporation of fast transported protein into the regenerating portion of transected motor axons. Nevertheless, a critical experiment has not yet been performed to demonstrate whether selective blocking of axonal transport proximally (with focally applied colchicine, for example) will prevent axonal regeneration. While colchicine does seem to inhibit axonal outgrowth when applied to the cut axon tip (Pinner-Poole and Campbell, 1969), it is not clear if this effect is related to an effect on axonal transport (Grafstein, 1971; Grafstein et al., 1970). Colchicine applied to nerves in salamander does inhibit collateral sprouting in response to injury of a neighboring nerve (Aguilar et al., 1973).

Circumstantial evidence suggests that retrograde transport may be important in providing a signal from the injured axon to the cell body to initiate the axon reaction. Injured axons are known to take up proteins such as horseradish peroxidase and to transport them to the soma in advance of the chromatolytic reaction (Kristensson and Olsson, 1974). Colchicine, which also blocks retrograde axonal transport, can induce many of the perikaryal changes associated with axotomy when applied onto nerves focally (Pilar and Landmesser, 1972). It is conceivable that a substance ordinarily not present in the axon could be picked up at the site of a lesion and transported to the soma, where it might trigger some part of the axon reaction. Alternatively, substances might ordinarily be supplied to intact axon terminals by some element in their natural environment, such as the postsynaptic membrane or end-organ, which when transported to the soma suppresses chromatolysis or other aspects of the axon reaction. Axotomy might then eliminate a tonic suppression of the axon reaction. The latter hypothesis would seem to be contradicted by the observations of Watson (1968a), who found that following hypoglossal axotomy the increase in nucleolar nucleic acid, which reaches a peak at between 5 and 10 days, declines in the usual way regardless of whether or not the nerve is allowed to reinnervate the tongue. In fact, the same retrograde axon reaction is elicitable again in nerves which have been previously cut and forced to form a neuroma. Moreover, the time course of the changes in nucleic acid concentration, including the late decline, is delayed longer the further the cut is from the soma. This is the opposite of what one would expect if the end-organ were supplying a chromatolysis-suppressing substance, since the more peripheral the lesion the shorter the regenerating path and the sooner contact with the end-organ is re-established. As with anterograde transport, following nerve injury the volume of retrogradely transported proteins is increased in goldfish optic nerves (Grafstein and McQuarrie, 1978), although whether the rate of transport is increased is not clear. Again, in other animals the effects of nerve injury on retrograde transport appear to vary (Halperin and La-Vail, 1975; Frizell et al., 1976).

Cragg (1970) has considered in detail several hypothetical mechanisms for the signalling of axon injury in initiating the cell body response. Based upon Watson's (1968a) data in rabbit hypoglossal neurons for the latency of the increase in nucleolar RNA as a function of distance of the transection from the soma, Cragg calculated a rate for the travelling of a hypothetical "signal" for the cell body reaction of 4 to 5 mm per day. This rate is considerably slower than the rates of retrograde transport described thus far for various types of substances in mammalian nerve. However, analogous morphological observations on the latency of chromatolysis in rat dorsal root ganglion cells suggest a rate for the "signal" which is of the same order of magnitude as the rate of retrograde transport (Kristensson and Olsson, 1975). In any case, there is no strong reason to believe that some substances may not be transported retrogradely at much slower rates than those established for the few proteins which have been examined thus far. In addition, as Grafstein and McQuarrie (1978) pointed out, it may be that different signals exist for different aspects of the retrograde reaction. If this is true, then it might be that some signals involve retrograde transport and others do not. The possibility that retrograde transport of promoting or inhibiting substances may play a role in the maintenance of the peripheral territories of axons and in collateral sprouting has already been discussed.

NERVE GROWTH FACTOR This name is given to an extract of certain mouse sarcomas which are found to promote the enlargement of sensory and sympathetic ganglia (Levi-Montalcini and Hamberger, 1951, 1953; Levi-Montalcini, 1952). The substance also promotes the outgrowth of axons from ganglia in tissue culture (Levi-Montalcini et al., 1954), thus encouraging the hope that trophic substances may aid in the process of nerve regeneration. Nerve growth factor (NGF) has been found in many nontumor tissues, particularly the submaxillary gland of the male mouse but in lower quantities in almost all tissues, including brain (Levi-Montalcini and Angeletti, 1968). Mouse submaxillary gland NGF has been purified and found to be a protein consisting of three subunits; the beta subunit, a dimer of a peptide of approximately 14,000 molecular weight is the active portion (Angeletti et al., 1971). Its amino acid sequence has been determined (Angeletti and Bradshaw, 1971; Angeletti et al., 1973), and antiserum to the purified NGF has been prepared (Cohen, 1960). When injected into young animals anti-NGF produces destruction of the sympathetic nervous system (immunosympathectomy). However its action, like that of NGF itself, seems to be limited mostly to sympathetic neurons at all stages of development and to embryonic sensory ganglion cells. A role for NGF in the growth of most nerves therefore appears unlikely. Nevertheless, NGF has been shown to enhance regeneration in amphibian optic nerve (Turner and Glaze, 1977). In addition, several growth-promoting factors have been found to affect nonneural tissues (Gospodarovicz and Moran, 1976), and evidence has been found for the existence of a high molecular weight substance produced by rat muscle, lung, and cultured fibroblasts which, unlike NGF, enhances neurite outgrowth from spinal cord slices (Dribin and Barrett, 1978). It seems likely that a knowledge of the mechanisms of action of NGF will prove useful to understanding the regulation of nerve regeneration. One of the most dramatic effects of NGF is the induction of microtubule production (Levi-Montalcini et al., 1968). Considering the probable role of microtubules in axoplasmic transport, and the likely importance of axoplasmic transport in sustaining nerve growth, this action of NGF would seem to be quite relevant to its role in promoting axon outgrowth.

NGF obviously plays an important role in maintaining sympathetic neurons, but its role is not limited to induction of neurite outgrowth. NGF has also been shown to induce an increase in the activities of some enzymes in the catecholamine synthetic pathway: tyrosine hydroxylase, dopamine β-hydroxylase (Thoenen et al., 1971), and phenylethanolamine-N-methyltransferase (Liuzzi et al., 1977). There is even a suggestion that NGF may affect the development of electrophysiological properties of sympathetic neurons. In a rat pheochromocytoma cell line, NGF can induce the ability to generate action potentials and sensitivity to acetylcholine (Dichter et al., 1977), as well as trigger neurite outgrowth.

Even when NGF does not induce changes in physiological or morphological properties it may prevent the changes produced by axotomy. Nja and Purves (1978a) found little effect upon either the potency or number of synaptic contacts onto superior cervical ganglion cells of adult guinea pigs when exogenous NGF was applied to the ganglia in vivo. However, NGF reduced the depression of synaptic transmission and loss of synaptic contacts onto the ganglion cells which ordinarily follows postganglionic axotomy by 50 per cent. In addition to this effect NGF also prevented chromatolysis and other morphological changes associated with the retrograde axon reaction. It was postulated (Nja and Purves, 1978a) that axotomy causes a reduction in the amount of NGF which is ordinarily supplied by the target issue to the soma by retrograde transport; NGF would be necessary to maintain the normal physiological and morphological characteristics of the ganglion cells. (Similar conclusions were drawn by Hendry, 1975, regarding the ability of NGF to prevent death of axotomized sympathetic neurons in young rats.) If one of these characteristics is the production of a second trophic substance analogous to NGF, the loss of production of such a factor might result in a loss of transsynaptic trophic effect on presynaptic terminals, resulting in bouton retraction. Such a hypothesis is attractive because it encourages the belief in multiple neurotrophic factors, and the expectation that the actions of NGF can be used as models for more general neurotrophic principles.

The site of action of NGF is far from clear. It is known that NGF is selectively transported retrogradely by axons of sympathetic neurons (Hendry et al, 1974) and dorsal root ganglion cells (Stockel et al., 1975), but not by motor neurons (Stockel and Thoenen, 1975). Many of the effects of NGF are presumably mediated by this selective, high affinity retrograde transport system and subsequent intracellular actions. For example Paravicini et al. (1975) showed that NGF injected into the anterior chamber of the rat eye results in increased activity of tyrosine hydroxylase only in the ipsilateral superior cervical ganglion. No increased enzyme activity results if NGF is administered systemically. Moreover,the increase in enzyme activity induced by intraocular injection can be blocked by injection of colchicine into the superior cervical ganglion or by axotomy. Thus, it seems clear that the retrograde transport of NGF is biologically important to its action upon tyrosine hydroxylase activity.

Conversely, the immediate effect of NGF on neurite outgrowth is apparently mediated by a surface membrane effect. Frazier et al. (1973) showed that neurite outgrowth, and even protection from cell necrosis, can be imparted by culturing sympathetic and sensory ganglion cells in the presence of NGF which is tightly bound to sepharose beads. No NGF disassociates from the beads, and the beads are too large to enter the neurons. Presumably, therefore, some actions of NGF are mediated by binding to a surface membrane receptor. Similarly, Campenot (1977) found that when sympathetic neurons are grown in a special chamber in which distal dendrites are separated from the soma by a fluid-impermeable barrier, neurite outgrowth is related to the presence of NGF in the vicinity of the distal neurites but not in that part of the chamber containing the soma and proximal neurites. An analogy has been made between NGF and insulin, both with regard to structure and site of action (Bradshaw et al., 1974). A surface receptor mechanism for NGF action suggests the possibility of involvement of a "second messenger," such as a cyclic nucleotide. However the literature is conflicting as to whether either adenosine 3', 5' cyclic monophosphate (cAMP) or guanosine 3', 5' cyclic monophosphate (cGMP) is involved in the actions of NGF on neurite outgrowth and enzyme induction (Frazier et al., 1973; Hier et al., 1973; Bradshaw et al., 1974; Nikodijevic et al., 1975; Otten et al., 1978).

ROLE OF SCHWANN CELLS Since the early light microscopic observations of Ramón y Cajal it has been a common belief that axonal regeneration is facilitated by Schwann cells (cf. Holmes and Young, 1942). We have noted that following nerve section and Wallerian degeneration Schwann cells proliferate and form orderly arrays called bands of Büngner along the endoneurial margin. The work of Weiss et al. (1941, 1944) emphasized the fact that physical features in the environment of regenerating axons influence the path of regeneration through tensional lines of stress and contact guidance. Weddell (1942), using the methylene blue staining technique, showed that in the region of the transection gap regenerating sprouts invariably follow a course along a band of Schwann cells. The phenomenon is so striking that it has been generally believed that one of the reasons for the comparative inefficiency of central nervous system regeneration is the absence of an exclusive relationship between the myelin-forming cells (oligodendroglia) and single axons, so that bands similar to the bands of Büngner of peripheral nerve degeneration are not formed. It is unlikely that this is true since unmyelinated nerves seem equally capable of regeneration, despite the fact that a single Schwann cell normally surrounds more than one axon, and the number of axons per Schwann cell actually increases with regeneration because of axon sprouting (Bray et al., 1972; Dyck and Hopkins, 1972; Aguayo et al., 1973). Moreover, as discussed above, the optic nerves of amphibia and fish regenerate well despite the fact that they are myelinated in typical CNS fashion by oligodendroglia.

Nevertheless, a regeneration-promoting function of Schwann cells is certainly possible. Although the possible supporting role of these cells for their axons has not been well studied, several observations suggest that Schwann cells may be important in specifying the diameters of regenerating axons. When a distal nerve stump of an animal is grafted onto a proximal stump of the same or another animal, the grafted stump undergoes Wallerian degeneration and regenerating axons from the proximal stump become ensheathed and myelinated by the Schwann cells of the graft (Weinberg and Spencer, 1975, 1976; Aguayo et al., 1976a, b). When a length of nerve from a Trembler mutant mouse is grafted onto the sciatic nerve of a normal mouse, the normal axons regenerating into the graft develop the reduced diameter and thin myelin sheaths characteristic of the Trembler mouse. Conversely, abnormal axons in a Trembler mouse develop larger diameters and normal myelin thickness when regenerating into a graft of normal nerve (Aguayo et al., 1977a). Similar observations have been made for the neuropathy of quaking mice (Aguayo et al., 1977c). This line of research has been extended to xenografts of human normal and abnormal nerves transplanted into mouse, with the exciting result that the accumulation of metachromatic granules and the demyelination of metachromatic leukodystrophy is shown to be an intrinsic abnormality of the Schwann cell, and not dependent upon the axon (Aguayo et al., 1977b). In a variety of circumstances in which CNS demyelination occurs in both humans and experimental animals, Schwann cells have been observed to invade the demyelinated area and remyelinate the CNS axons. However, the myelin which is formed is typical of peripheral nerve myelin, with such features as its one-to-one relationship between supporting cell and axon, doubled intraperiod lines, outer collar of cytoplasm, and basement membrane (Ghatak et al., 1973; Blakemore, 1975, 1977; Snyder et al., 1975; Raine, 1976). On the other hand, ectopic oligodendrocytes can form CNS-type myelin around the denuded axons found in spinal roots of dystrophic mice (Weinberg et al., 1975). Weinberg and Spencer (1979) also reported that oligodendrocytes from a graft of optic nerve produce central myelin around regenerating peripheral axons. Thus, in many cases, the myelin-forming cells can specify the nature of the myelin to be formed regardless of the location or origin of the axon.

Results of other studies, however, suggest that the myelin-forming behavior of a Schwann cell may be influenced by its axon. With very few exceptions, in both CNS and PNS, myelin is associated only with axons, and Schwann cells will not form myelin around nonaxonal structures in tissue culture (see Spencer and Weinberg, 1978). However, the presence of axons will induce Schwann cell multiplication and myelination in vitro (Wood and Bunge, 1975). Particularly convincing evidence regarding the regulatory role of axons in myelination includes observations on the behavior of Schwann cells of cross-anastomosed myelinated and unmyelinated nerves (Fig. 12–9). When the proximal stump of a myelinated nerve is anastomosed to the distal stump of an unmyelinated nerve, the axons regenerating into the distal stump become normally myelinated (Weinberg and Spencer, 1975; Aguayo et al., 1976b). The reverse is true when an unmyelinated nerve regenerates into a myelinated nerve distal stump (Aguayo et al., 1976b; Weinberg and Spencer, 1976). Experiments using autoradiographic labelling of Schwann cells to distinguish donor cells from host cells in nerve graft experiments show that the Schwann cells within the graft (or distal stump in cross-anastomosis experiments) do in fact originate from the degenerated donor axons (Aguayo et al., 1976a, b; Weinberg and Spencer, 1976). For example, Aguayo et al. (1976a) injected 1-month-old inbred mice with tritiated thymidine, thus labelling the Schwann cells which were still multiplying. One month later lengths of cervical sympathetic trunk, an unmyelinated nerve, were grafted from injected donors into sural nerves (which normally contain myelinated fibers) of uninjected recipient mice (Fig. 12–10A). The regenerating sural axons are myelinated by labelled Schwann cells within the graft (Fig. 12–10B). Thus the Schwann cells within the grafts originate in the grafts and do not migrate from the proximal or distal ends of the host nerves. This conclusion is further supported by radioautographic studies of crushed unmyelinated nerves (mouse cervical sympathetic trunk) showing that Schwann cells, which proliferate mostly at the site of the crush (Romine et al., 1976), do not migrate into the distal stump during axon regeneration (Romine et al., 1975).

The conclusion to be drawn from all these studies is that Schwann cells are multipotential and that whether or not they form myelin depends upon the axon with which they become associated. Growing tips of myelin-

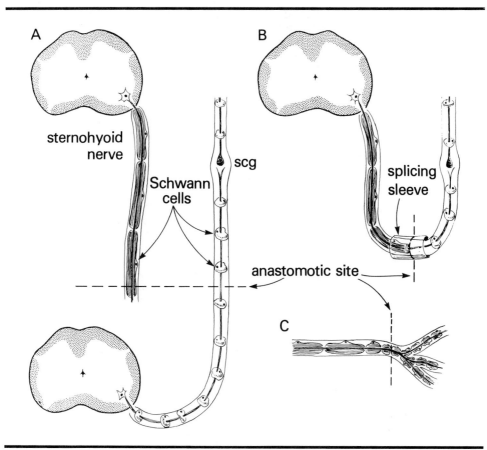

Figure 12–9 Induction of myelin-forming activity in Schwann cells of an unmyelinated nerve of a rat by cross-anastomosis with the proximal stump of a myelinated nerve. *A,* Diagram illustrating origin and direction of fiber pathways of the predominantly myelinated sternohyoid nerve *(left)* and the largely unmyelinated cervical sympathetic trunk *(right);* scg, superior cervical ganglion. *B,* The proximal stump of the sternohyoid nerve is anastomosed to the distal stump of the cervical sympathetic trunk. The result will be Wallerian degeneration of the axons in the distal stump, leaving the Schwann cells to make contact with regenerating axons of the proximal stump of sternohyoid. *C,* As the sternohyoid axons grow into the distal stump they are myelinated by Schwann cells of the generated sympathetic trunk. Evidence for the origin of these Schwann cells is shown in Fig. 12–10. (Adapted from Weinberg and Spencer, 1975. By permission of Chapman and Hall, Ltd., Publishers.)

ated axons will induce myelination, whereas growing tips of unmyelinated axons will not. The mechanisms involved in this axonal regulation of Schwann cell function are not known; several hypotheses are examined in a review by Spencer and Weinberg (1978).

405

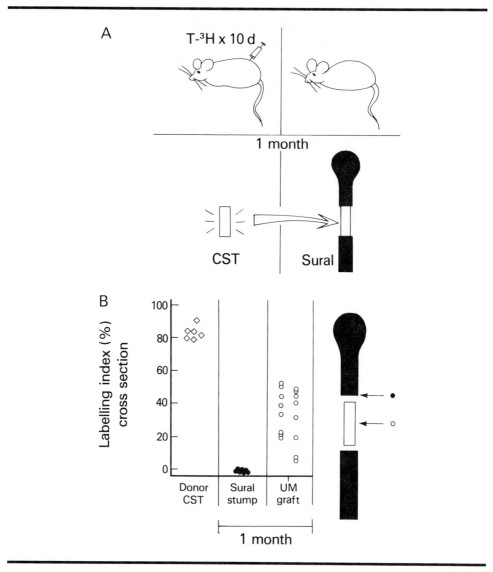

Figure 12–10 Demonstration that axons regenerating into a graft of unmyelinated nerve are myelinated by the Schwann cells of the graft (i.e., Schwann cells which originally did not form myelin). *A,* In 1-month-old inbred mice, labelled cervical sympathetic trunks (CSTs) from animals injected neonatally with tritiated thymidine (T-³H) for 10 days (donor CSTs) were grafted to unlabelled sural nerves of litter mates (hosts). These mice were sacrificed 1 month later. *B,* Labelling indices in cross sections of the unmyelinated fibers of donor CSTs (diamonds) averaged 83.5 ± 1.8 (mean $\pm$ S.E.M.). 1 month later, when grafts contain large numbers of myelinated fibers, Schwann cells in the proximal sural stump *(filled circles)* are unlabelled. In the grafts indices for unmyelinated fibers (V) averaged 36.1 ± 4.7, and for myelinated fibers (M) 31.7 ± 6.3. On the right side of the figure a schematic representation of the experimental model is depicted; sural nerves are represented in black, and CSTs in white. (Adapted from Aguayo et al., 1976 *a.* By permission of Chapman and Hall, Ltd., Publishers.)

SURGICAL REPAIR A great deal has been written about the various factors which affect the success of peripheral nerve regeneration and its promotion by surgical repair. Unfortunately, very little of this literature is based upon controlled studies, and one gets the impression that the actual technique employed is less important than either the natural healing process or the skill and carefulness of the surgeon. The fundamental principles involved have been recognized since the early work of Ramón y Cajal:

1. The quality and speed of regeneration of a severed nerve depend upon the width of the gap between the proximal and distal cut ends.
2. The success of regeneration is greatly enhanced by the ability of regenerating nerve fibers to find their way into the vacated endoneurial tubes of the distal stump, which act as mechanical guides for axon elongation, and perhaps have other beneficial effects.
3. The scar tissue developed at the site of a transection acts as a physical barrier to nerve growth, contributes to the disorientation of growing axon tips and, therefore, perhaps promotes neuroma formation, all of which makes it less likely that regenerating axons will find their way to receptive endoneurial sheaths.

Most modifications of surgical technique have been made in order to minimize one or more of these factors. The most informative reference on the subject remains Sunderland's (1978) encyclopedic monograph. Useful technical information may also be found in Rand's (1978) monograph on microneurosurgery, in the proceedings of a symposium on operative nerve injuries edited by Simeone (1972), and in Seddon's (1975) volume concerning operative nerve lesions.

Even when new methods are based upon animal experiments they often do not prove to be more advantageous than standard techniques. For example, the usual method of nerve repair since before the turn of the century has been to approximate the cut ends by suture, in order to minimize the regeneration gap. Based upon experiments with over 700 nerve transections in a variety of experimental animals, Weiss (1944) concluded that superior results could be obtained by ensheathing the cut nerve ends in an arterial splice and filling the gap with a plasma clot. The clot establishes lines of tension between the proximal and distal nerve ends and regenerating fibers orient themselves along these lines of tension. Weiss's objection to the standard suturing technique was that it did not establish lines of tension for fibers to grow along. Despite this experimental work in the laboratory of one of the most eminent scientists in the field of regeneration since Ramón y Cajal arterial sleeve splicing, including several technical modifica-

407

tions, has largely been abandoned. Similar fates have befallen techniques for bridging transection gaps with such materials as millipore filters, decalcified bone, veins, nerve heterografts, and nerve homografts from cadavers (see Sunderland, 1978, for review).

The only method which appears to rival end-to-end suture in effectiveness is the use of autogenous nerve grafts (Seddon, 1947; Bjorkesten, 1948). These can be used in the repair of nerve injuries where the distance between proximal and distal cut ends is too great for end-to-end suture. The graft must come from a relatively dispensable nerve. Therefore the sural, superficial radial or other small sensory nerves are used, all of which are relatively dispensable because they innervate skin and not muscle. Therefore, the technique is limited to the repair of relatively small nerves, such as digital or facial nerves. When gaps in larger nerves must be bridged cable grafts of several lengths of sural nerve in parallel are formed, requiring a longer length of graft nerve. Surgeons have also resorted to homografts prepared from cadavers to repair large nerves. The major difficulty with this technique is immunological graft rejection. To reduce immunogenecity frozen stored homografts have been treated with ionizing radiation before implantation (Campbell et al., 1963; Marmor, 1963, 1967). Additional protection from graft rejection has been sought by immunosuppressive therapy, but without beneficial results (Marmor, 1972). Thus far nerve homografting has proved disappointing, despite occasional therapeutic successes.

One final aspect of the influence of surgical manipulation on nerve regeneration warrants comment. It has been mentioned that, even in mammals, competition among regenerating fibers favors innervation of muscle by the appropriate axons. Thus, if it were possible to improve the routing of regenerating fibers in a mixed nerve, one would expect appropriate neuromuscular connections to be formed as axons approach the muscle. The advent of the surgical microscope has encouraged the use of internal neurolysis (the clearing of scar tissue within the epineurium) and apposition by suture of individual funiculi within the severed nerve under microscopic control (e.g., Khodadad, 1972; Rand, 1978). This method has two serious limitations which are highlighted by the studies of Sunderland in the 1940's on the longitudinal variation in funicular organization of various peripheral nerves (reviewed by Sunderland, 1978). First, individual funiculi migrate very precipitously within the epineurium, so their patterns will be very different in the proximal and distal cut edges if there has been any appreciable loss of nerve tissue in between. Second, there is a great amount of crossing over of nerve fibers between various funiculi so that the funiculi are constantly being resorted, and even their numbers in cross section vary greatly within the space of a few centimeters (Fig. 12–11). Therefore, even if

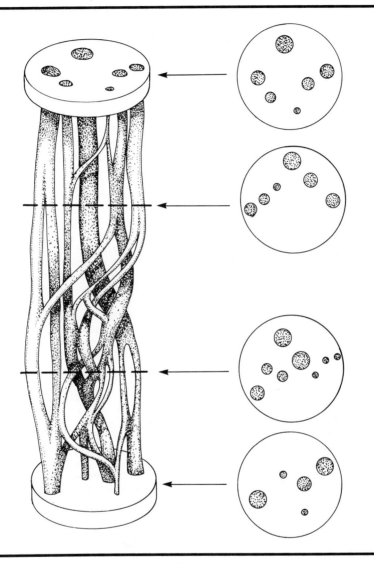

Figure 12–11 Funicular plexus formations in a 3-cm segment of a specimen of the musculocutaneous nerve of the arm. The circles to the right represent approximate cross sections at different levels of the plexus drawing on the left. Note that both the number of fascicles and their positions within the nerve vary from one level to another. (Modified from Sunderland, 1978.)

a regenerating fiber finds its native funiculus, it will not necessarily be directed to its native muscle. Sunderland (1978) concluded that the technique has limited value unless specific knowledge of the funicular structure of the nerve involved at and below the level of injury suggests that these limitations will not be significant.

409

In general, therefore, surgical repair seems to have improved little over the years. The best technique still seems to be simple end-to-end suture of the nerve, where possible, and nerve autografting when a long gap is present. I suspect that funicular repair may in some cases yield better results mainly by forcing the surgeon to be more careful in handling the nerve, and because only surgeons who are skillful can attempt it. It has not yet been possible to influence the course of regenerating fibers within a nerve enough to take advantage of what appears to be a tendency toward specificity in axon muscle fiber recognition at close range.

SUMMARY AND CONCLUSIONS

Following injury to a peripheral nerve a series of degenerative changes occur in the distal trunk (Wallerian degeneration), which leaves a receptive lattice of endoneurial sheaths lined with rows of Schwann cells. Simultaneous changes occur in the proximal axon and cell body which have often been described as degenerative, but many of these represent metabolic alterations in preparation for the demands of axonal regeneration. These changes, collectively called the retrograde axon reaction, include dispersion of rough-surfaced endoplasmic reticulum, an increase in free ribosomes and polysomes, an increase in total cellular, nuclear and nucleolar RNA and total cellular protein, a shift in the types of proteins synthesized, probable increases in the rates of various components of axoplasmic transport (in some cases), and retraction of presynaptic boutons from the axotomized neuron. Even this last change could be helpful in functional recovery since it leaves open possibilities for alterations, either qualitative or quantitative, in the afferent connections of motoneurons to compensate for imprecisions in regeneration of neuromuscular connections. To consider these possibilities is to resurrect a theory originally proposed by Weiss, and rephrased by Sperry, that when nerves innervate muscles, either during embryonic development or after regeneration, those muscles can affect the central connections of the neurons that innervate them (the theory of myotypic specification of motoneurons). Thus, if the reinnervating neuron is different from the original, shifts in central connections can respecify the motoneuron so that its behavior is appropriate to its new target. A great deal of research by Sperry, Mark, Eccles, and others has tended not to support this notion when applied to cross-union of nerves to antagonistic muscles in mammals and most lower vertebrates. However, more subtle shifts in the potency of afferent interconnections among agonistic motoneurons and alterations in descending inputs to motoneurons have not been ruled out. Indeed, given the great degree of plasticity already discovered in synaptic connections of nonlesioned animals, and the potential for functional recovery in lower vertebrates using aberrant regeneration patterns after spinal cord transection, it seems most likely that some CNS remodelling may act over long periods in promoting functional recovery.

Nevertheless, it remains true that return of function following nerve injury is more likely the more primitive the animal and the younger the animal. Despite morphological and physiological regeneration mammals generally do not recover proper limb coordination following mixed nerve or spinal root transection. Only part of the problem lies in directing nerve regrowth into the distal stump and avoiding neuroma formation. Perhaps an even greater problem is the lack of specificity in the routing of fibers within the distal stump toward the correct funiculi and terminal nerve branches. If this could be accomplished, even partially, experimental evidence suggests that short-range trophic influences would effect accurate sorting of nerve terminals and target muscle fibers. Neurosurgical approaches, including funicular suture, have not yet achieved this goal. Research into the nature of trophic interactions which determine nerve-target organ specificity may ultimately provide answers to the question of why nerves of more primitive vertebrates seem better able to achieve initial orientation, as though trophic influences were acting at longer range. Similarly, research into possible compensatory mechanisms in CNS may provide clues to the abilities of primitive vertebrates to achieve functional recovery in the face of aberrant regeneration of central axons, such as after spinal cord transection. If such mechanisms could be enhanced in mammals they might allow remodelling of central connections to compensate for imprecisions in peripheral nerve regeneration.

References Abercrombie, M., Evans, D. H. L., and Murray, J. G.: Nuclear multiplication and cell migration in degenerating unmyelinated nerves. J. Anat., *93*:9, 1959.

Aguayo, A. J., Attiwell, M., Trecarten, J., Perkins, S., and Bray, G. M.: Abnormal myelination in transplanted Trembler mouse Schwann cells. Nature, *265*:73, 1977a.

Aguayo, A. J., Charron, L., and Bray, G. M.: Potential of Schwann cells from unmyelinated nerves to produce myelin: A quantitative ultrastructural and radiographic study. J. Neurocytol., *5*:565, 1976*a*.

Aguayo, A. J., Epps, J., Charron L., and Bray, G. M.: Multipotentiality of Schwann cells in cross-anastomosed and grafted myelinated and unmyelinated nerves: quantitative microscopy and radioautography. Brain Res., *104*:1, 1976*b*.

Aguayo, A. J., Kasarjian, J., Samene, E., Kongshavn, P., and Bray, G. M.: Myelination of mouse axons by Schwann cells transplanted from normal and abnormal human nerves. Nature, *268*:753, 1977*b*.

Aguayo, A. J., Mizuno, K., and Bray, G. M.: Schwann cell transplantation: Evidence for a primary sheath cell disorder causing hypomyelination in quaking mice. J. Neuropathol. Exp. Neurol., *36*:595, 1977*c*.

411

REGENERATION OF PERIPHERAL NERVE

Aguayo, A. J., Peyronnard, J. M., and Bray, G. M.: A quantitative ultrastructural study of regeneration from isolated proximal stumps of transected unmyelinated nerves. J. Neuropathol. Exp. Neurol., 32:256, 1973.

Aguilar, C. E., Bisby, M. A., Cooper, E., and Diamond, J.: Evidence that axoplasmic transport of trophic factors is involved in the regulation of peripheral nerve fields in salamanders. J. Physiol. (Lond.), 234:449, 1973.

Allt, G.: Pathology of the peripheral nerve. In Landon, D. N. (ed.): The Peripheral Nerve. London, Chapman and Hall, 1976, pp. 666–739.

Ambache, N.: Peripheral action of Cl. botulinum toxin. J. Physiol. (Lond.), 108:127, 1949.

Angeletti, R. H., and Bradshaw, R. A.: Nerve growth factor from mouse submaxillary gland: Amino acid sequence. Proc. Natl. Acad. Sci. U.S.A., 68:2417, 1971.

Angeletti, R. H., Bradshaw, R. A., and Wade, R. D.: Subunit structure and amino acid composition of mouse submaxillary gland nerve growth factor. Biochemistry, 10:463, 1971.

Angeletti, R. H., Hermodsen, M. A., and Bradshaw, R. A.: Amino acid sequences of mouse 2.5 S nerve growth factor. II. Isolation and characterization of the thermolytic and peptic peptides and complete covalent structure. Biochemistry, 12:100, 1973.

Barr, M. L., and Hamilton, J. D.: A quantitative study of certain morphological changes in spinal motor neurons during axon reaction. J. Comp. Neurol., 89:93, 1948.

Barron, K. D., Chiang, T. Y., Daniels, A. C., and Doolin, P. F.: Subcellular accompaniments of axon reaction in cervical motoneurons of the cat. In Zimmerman, H. M. (ed.): Progress in Neuropathology, Vol. 1. New York, Grune and Stratton, 1971, pp. 255–277.

Baylor, D. A., and Nicholls, J. G.: Patterns of regeneration between individual nerve cells in the central nervous system of the leech. Nature, 232:268, 1971.

Bender, M. B.: The nerve supply to the orbicularis muscle and the physiology of movements of the upper eyelid, with particular reference to the pseudo-Graefe phenomenon. Arch. Ophthalmol., 15:21, 1936.

Bennett, M. R., and Pettigrew, A. G.: The formation of synapses in striated muscle during development. J. Physiol. (Lond.), 241:515, 1974.

Bennett, M. R., and Pettigrew, A. G.: The formation of synapses in amphibian striated muscle during development. J. Physiol. (Lond.), 252:203, 1975.

Bernstein, J. J., and Bernstein, M. E.: Effect of glial-ependymal scar and Teflon arrest on the regenerative capacity of goldfish spinal cord. Exp. Neurol., 19:25, 1967.

Bernstein, J. J., and Bernstein, M. E.: Ultrastructure of normal regeneration and loss of regenerative capacity following Teflon blockage in goldfish spinal cord. Exp. Neurol., 24:538, 1969.

Berry, C. M., Grundfest, H., and Hinsey, J. C.: The electrical activity of regenerating nerves in the cat. J. Neurophysiol., 7:103, 1944.

Birse, S. C., and Bittner, G. D.: Regeneration of giant axons in earthworms. Brain Res., *113*:575, 1976.

Bisby, M. A.: Fast axonal transport of labeled protein in sensory axons during regeneration. Exp. Neurol., *61*:281, 1978.

Bittner, G. D., and Johnson, A. L.: Degeneration and regeneration in crustacean peripheral nerves. J. Comp. Physiol., *89*:1, 1974.

Bjorkesten, G.: Clinical experience with nerve grafting. J. Neurosurg., *5*:450, 1948.

Black, M. M., and Lasek, R. J.: Slowing of the rate of axonal regeneration during growth and maturation. Exp. Neurol., *63*:108, 1979.

Blackwood, W., and Corsellis, J. A. N.: Greenfield's Neuropathology, 3rd ed. London, Edward Arnold, 1976.

Blakemore, W. F.: Remyelination by Schwann cells of axons demyelinated by intraspinal injection of 6-aminonicotinamide in the rat. J. Neurocytol., *4*:75, 1975.

Blakemore, W. F.: Remyelination of CNS axons by Schwann cells transplanted from the sciatic nerve. Nature, *266*:68, 1977.

Blinzinger, K., and Kreutzberg, G.: Displacement of synaptic terminals from regenerating motoneurons by microglial cells. Z. Zellforsch. Mikrosk. Anat., *85*:145, 1968.

Bloom, E. M., and R. Tompkins: Selective reinnervation in skin rotation grafts in *Rana pipiens*. J. Exp. Zool., *195*:236, 1976.

Bodian, D.: Nucleic acid in nerve-cell regeneration. Symp. Soc. Exp. Biol., *1*:163, 1947.

Bradley, W. G., and Asbury, A. K.: Duration of synthesis phase in neurilemma cells in mouse sciatic nerve during degeneration. Exp. Neurol., *26*:275, 1970.

Bradshaw, R. A., Hogue-Angeletti, R. H., and Frazier, W. A.: Nerve growth factor and insulin: Evidence of similarities in structure, function, and mechanism of action. Recent Prog. Horm. Res., *38*:575, 1974.

Brattgard, S. O., Edstrom, J. E., and Hyden, H.: The chemical changes in regenerating neurons. J. Neurochem., *1*:316, 1957.

Brattgard, S. O., Hyden, H., and Sjostrand, J.: Incorporation of ortic acid-^{14}C and lycine-^{14}C in regenerating single nerve cells. Nature, *182*:801, 1958.

Bray, D.: Model for membrane movements in the neural growth cone. Nature, *244*:93, 1973.

Bray, G. M., and Aguayo, A. J.: Regeneration of peripheral unmyelinated nerves. Fate of the axonal sprouts which develop after injury. J. Anat., *117*:517, 1974.

Bray, G. M., Aguayo, A. J., and Martin, J. B.: Immunosympathectomy: Late effects on composition of rat cervical sympathetic trunks and influence on axonal regeneration after crush. Acta. Neuropathol., *26*:345, 1973.

Bray, G. M., Peyronnard, J. M., and Aguayo, A. J.: Reactions of unmyelinated nerve fibers to injury. An ultrastructural study. Brain Res., *42*:297, 1972.

Brill, M. H., Waxman, S. G., Moree, J. W., Joyner, R. W.: Conduction velocity in myelinated fibers: Computed dependence on internode distance. J. Neurol. Neurosurg. Psychiatry, *40*:769, 1977.

413

REGENERATION OF PERIPHERAL NERVE

Brooks, V. B.: The action of botulinum toxin on motor-nerve filaments. J. Physiol. (Lond.), *123*:501, 1954.

Brown, M. C., and Ironton, R.: Motor neurone sprouting induced by prolonged tetrodotoxin block of nerve action potentials. Nature, *265*:459, 1977.

Brown, M. C., and Ironton, R.: Sprouting and regeneration of neuromuscular synapses in partially denervated mammalian muscles. J. Physiol. (Lond.), *278*:325, 1978.

Brown, M. D., Jansen, J. K. S., and Van Essen, D.: Polyneuronal innervation of skeletal muscle in newborn rats and its elimination during maturation. J. Physiol., (Lond.), *261*:387, 1976.

Bunge, M. B.: Fine structure of nerve fibers and growth cones of isolated sympathetic neurons in culture. J. Cell Biol., *56*:713, 1973.

Burgen, A. S. V., Dicken, F., and Zatman, L. J. Action of botulinum toxin on neuromuscular junction. J. Physiol. (Lond.), *109*:10, 1949.

Burgess, P. R., English, K. B., Horch, K. W., and Stensaas, L. J.: Patterning in the regeneration of type I cutaneous receptors. J. Physiol. (Lond.), *236*:57, 1974.

Burgess, P. R., and Horch, K. W.: Specific regeneration of cutaneous fibers in the cat. J. Neurophysiol., *36*:101, 1973.

Campbell, B.: The effects of retrograde degeneration upon reflex activity of ventral horn neurones. Anat. Rec., *88*:25, 1944.

Campbell, J. B., Bassett, C. A. L., and Bohler, J.: Frozen irradiated homografts shielded with microfilter sheaths in peripheral nerve surgery. J. Trauma, *3*:303, 1963.

Campenot, R. B.: Local control of neurite development by nerve growth factor. Proc. Natl. Acad. Sci. U.S.A., *74*:4516, 1977.

Cannon, W. B., and Rosenblueth, A.: The Supersensitivity of Denervated Structures. New York, Macmillan, 1949.

Cass, D. T., Sutton, T. U., and Mark, R. F.: Competition between nerves for functional connections with axolotl muscles. Nature, *243*:201, 1973.

Cheah, T. B., and Geffen, L. B.: Effects of axonal injury on norepinephrine, tyrosine hydroxylase and monoamine oxidase levels in sympathetic ganglia. J. Neurobiol., *4*:443, 1973.

Clemente, C. D.: Regeneration in the vertebrate central nervous system. Int. Rev. Neurobiol., *6*:257, 1964.

Cohen, S.: Purification of a nerve growth promoting protein from the mouse salivary gland and its neurocytotoxic antiserum. Proc. Natl. Acad. Sci. U.S.A., *46*:302, 1960.

Cook, W. H., Walker, J. H., and Barr, M. L.: A cytological study of transneuronal atrophy in the cat and rabbit. J. Comp. Neurol., *94*:267, 1951.

Cotman, C. W., and Nadler, J. V.: Reactive synaptogenesis in the hippocampus. *In* Cotman, C. W. (ed.): Neuronal Plasticity. New York, Raven Press, 1978, pp. 227–271.

Cragg, B. G.: What is the signal for chromatolysis? Brain Res., *23*:1, 1970.

REGENERATION OF PERIPHERAL NERVE

Cragg, B. G., and Thomas, P. K.: Changes in conduction velocity and fiber size proximal to peripheral nerve lesions. J. Physiol. (Lond.), *157*:315, 1961.

Cragg, B. G., and Thomas, P. K.: The conduction velocity of regenerated peripheral nerve fibers. J. Physiol., (Lond.). *171*:164, 1964.

Cull, R. E.: Role of nerve-muscle contact in maintaining synaptic connections. Exp. Brain Res., *20*:307, 1974.

Denburg, J. L., Seecof, R. L., and Horridge, G. A.: The path and rate of growth of regenerating motor neurons in the cockroach. Brain Res., *125*:213, 1977.

Denny-Brown, D., and Brenner, C.: The effect of percussion of nerve. J. Neurol. Neurosurg. Psychiatry, *7*:76, 1944.

Dichter, M. A., Tischler, A. S., and Greene, L. A.: Nerve growth factor-induced increase in electrical excitability and acetylcholine sensitivity of a rat pheochromocytoma cell line. Nature, *268*:501, 1977.

Donat, J. R., and Wisniewski, H. M.: The spatio-temporal pattern of Wallerian degeneration in mammalian peripheral nerves. Brain Res., *53*:41, 1973.

Donoso, R. S., Ballantyne, J. P., and Hansen, S.: Regeneration of sutured human peripheral nerves: An electrophysiological study. J. Neurol. Neurosurg. Psychiatry, *42*:97, 1979.

Downman, C. B. B., Eccles, J. C., and McIntyre, A. K.: Functional changes in chromatolyzed motoneurones. J. Comp. Neurol., *98*:9, 1953.

Dribin, L. B., and Barrett, J. N.: Enhancement of axonal outgrowth from spinal cord explants by conditioned medium. Neurosci. Abstr., *4*:602, 1978.

Droz, B.: Synthetic machinery and axoplasmic transport: Maintenance of neuronal connectivity. *In* Tower, D. B. (ed.): The Nervous System, Vol. 1: The Basic Neurosciences. New York, Raven Press, 1975, pp. 111–127.

Duce, I. R., Reeves, J. F., and Keen, P.: Scanning electron microscope study of the development of free axonal sprouts at the cut ends of dorsal spinal nerve roots in the rat. Cell Tissue. Res., *170*:507, 1976.

Dyck, P. J., and Hopkins, A. P.: Electron microscopic observations on degeneration and regeneration of unmyelinated nerves. Brain, *95*:233, 1972.

Ebeling, P., Gilliatt, R. W., and Thomas, P. K.: A clinical and electrical study of ulnar nerve lesions in the hand. J. Neurol. Neurosurg. Psychiatry, *23*:1, 1960.

Eccles, J. C., Eccles, R. M., and Magni, F.: Monosynaptic excitatory action of motoneurons regenerated to antagonistic muscles. J. Physiol. (Lond.), *154*:68, 1960.

Eccles, J. C., Eccles, R. M., Shealy, C. N., and Willis, E. F.: Experiments utilizing monosynaptic excitatory action on motoneurons for testing hypotheses relating to specificity of neuronal connection. J. Neurophysiol., *25*:559, 1962.

Eccles, J. C., Krnjevic, K. and Miledi, R.: Delayed effects of peripheral severance of afferent nerve fibres on the efficiency of their central synapsis. J. Physiol. (Lond.), *145*:204, 1959.

415

Eccles, J. C., Libet, B., and Young, R. R.: The behavior of chromatolyzed motoneurons studied by intracellular recording. J. Physiol. (Lond.), *143*:11, 1958.

Echlin, F.: Time course of development of supersensitivity to topical acetylcholine in partially isolated cortex. Electroencephalogr. Clin. Neurophysiol., *38*:225, 1975.

Edds, M. V., Jr.: Collateral nerve regeneration. Q. Rev. Biol., *28*:260, 1953.

Edstrom, J. E.: RNA changes in the motoneurons of the frog during axonal regeneration. J. Neurochem., *5*:43, 1959.

Erlanger, J., and Schoepfle, G. M.: A study of nerve degeneration and regeneration. Am. J. Physiol., *147*:550, 1946.

Estable, C., Acosta-Ferreira, W., and Sotelo, J. R.: An electron microscope study of the regenerating nerve fibers. Z. Zellforsch. Mikrosk. Anat., *46*:387, 1957.

Evans, D. H. L., and Murray, J. G.: Regeneration of non-medullated nerve fibers. J. Anat., *88*:465, 1954.

Feringa, E. R., Shuer, L. M., Vahlsing, H. L., and Davis, S. W.: Regeneration of corticospinal axons in the rat. Ann. Neurol., *2*:315, 1977.

Feringa, E. R., Wendt, J. S., and Johnson, R. D.: Immunosuppressive treatment to enhance spinal cord regeneration in rats. Neurology, *24*:287, 1974.

Flumerfelt, B. A., and Lewis, P. R.: Cholinesterase activity in the hypoglossal nucleus of the rat and the changes produced by axotomy: A light and electron microscopic study. J. Anat., *119*:309, 1975.

Forman, D. S., and Berenberg, R. A.: Regeneration of motor axons in the rat sciatic nerve studied by labeling with axonally transported radioactive proteins. Brain Res., *156*:213, 1978.

Frank, E., and Jansen, J. K. S.: Interaction between foreign and original nerves innervating gill muscles in fish. J. Neurophysiol., *39*:84, 1976.

Frank, E., Jansen, J. K. S., Lomo, T., and Westergaard, R. H.: The interaction between foreign and original motor nerves innervating the soleus muscle of rats. J. Physiol., (Lond.), *247*:725, 1975*a*.

Frank, E., Jansen, J. K. S., and Rinvik, E.: A multisomatic axon in the central nervous system of the leech. J. Comp. Neurol., *159*:1, 1975*b*.

Frazier, W. A., Ohlendorf, C. E., Boyd, L. F., Aloe, L., Johnson, E. M., Ferrendelli, J. A., and Bradshaw, R. A.: Mechanism of action of nerve growth factor and cyclic AMP on neurite outgrowth in embryonic chick sensory ganglia: Demonstration of independent pathways of stimulation. Proc. Natl. Acad. Sci. U.S.A., *70*:2448, 1973.

Frizell, M., McLean, W. G., and Sjostrand, J.: Retrograde axonal transport of rapidly migrating labelled proteins and glycoproteins in regenerating peripheral nerves. J. Neurochem., *27*:191, 1976.

Frizell, M., and Sjostrand, J.: Transport of proteins, glycoproteins, and cholinergic enzymes in regenerating hypoglossal neurons. J. Neurochem., *23*:651, 1974*a*.

Frizell, M., and Sjostrand, J.: The axonal transport of slowly migrating ^{3}H-leucine-labelled proteins and the regeneration rate in regenerating hypoglossal and vagus nerves of the rabbit. Brain Res., *81*:267, 1974*b*.

Fukami, Y., and Ridge, R. M. A. P.: Electrophysiological and morphological changes at extrafusal end-plates in the snake following chronic denervation. Brain Res., *29*:139, 1971.

Gaze, R. M.: Regeneration of the optic nerve of *Xenopus laevis*. Q. J. Exp. Physiol., *44*:209, 1959.

Gaze, R. M., and Jacobson, M.: A study of the retino-tectal projection during regeneration of the optic nerve in the frog. Proc. R. Soc. Lond. [Biol.], *157*:420, 1963.

Geist, F. D.: Chromatolysis of efferent neurons. Arch. Neurol. Psychiatry, *29*:88, 1933.

Gersh, I., and Bodian, D.: Some chemical mechanisms in chromatolysis. J. Cell. Comp. Physiol., *21*:253, 1943.

Ghatak, N., Hirano, A., Doron, Y., and Zimmerman, H. M.: Remyelination in MS with peripheral type myelin. Arch. Neurol., *29*:262, 1973.

Gilad, G., and Reis, D. J.: Reversible reduction of tyrosine hydroxylase enzyme protein during the retrograde reaction in mesolimbic dopaminergic neurons. Brain Res., *149*:141, 1978.

Gilliat, R. W.: Nerve conduction: Motor and sensory. *In* Licht, S. (ed.): Electrodiagnosis and Electromyography, 2nd ed. Baltimore, Waverly Press, 1961, pp. 385–411.

Gilliat, R. W., and Hjorth R. J.: Nerve conduction during Wallerian degeneration in the baboon. J. Neurol. Neurosurg. Psychiatry, *35*:335, 1972.

Glees, P.: Observations on the structure of the connective tissue sheaths of cutaneous nerves. J. Anat., *77*:153, 1943.

Goldberger, M. E., and Murray, M.: Restitution of function and collateral sprouting in the cat spinal cord: The deafferented animal. J. Comp. Neurol., *158*:37, 1974.

Gospodarovicz, D., and Moran, J. S.: Growth factors in mammalian cell culture. Ann. Rev. Biochem. *45*:531, 1976.

Grafstein, B.: Role of slow axonal transport in nerve regeneration. Acta Neuropathol. [Suppl.] (Berl.) 5:144, 1971.

Grafstein, B.: Axonal transport: The intracellular traffic of the neuron. *In* Kandel, E. R. (ed.): Handbook of Physiology. Section I: The Nervous System, Vol. I. Cellular Biology of Neurons, Part I. Bethesda, American Physiological Society, 1977, pp. 691–717.

Grafstein, B., McEwen, B. S., and Shelanski, M. L.: Axonal transport of neurotubule protein. Nature, *227*:289, 1970.

Grafstein, B., and McQuarrie, I. G.: Role of the nerve cell body in axonal regeneration. *In* Cotman, C. W. (ed.): Neuronal Plasticity. New York, Raven Press, 1978, pp. 155–195.

Grafstein, B., and Murray, M.: Transport of protein in goldfish optic nerve during regeneration. Exp. Neurol., *25*:494, 1969.

Griffin, J. W., Drachman, D. B., and Price, D. L.: Rapid axonal transport in motor nerve regeneration. J. Neurobiol., *7*:355, 1976.

Grinnell, A. D.: Specificity of neurons and their interconnections. *In* Kandel, E. R. (ed.): Handbook of Physiology. Section I: The Nervous System, Vol. I. Cellular Biology of Neurons,

417

Part 2. Bethesda, American Physiological Society, 1977, pp. 803–853.

Gromadzki, C. G., and Koelle, G. B.: The effect of axotomy on the acetyl-cholinesterase of the superior cervical ganglion of the cat. Biochem. Pharmacol., *14*:1745, 1965.

Guth, L.: Regeneration in the mammalian peripheral nervous system. Physiol. Rev., *36*:441, 1956.

Guth, L.: Neuromuscular function after regeneration of interrupted nerve fibers into partially denervated muscle. Exp. Neurol., *6*:129, 1962.

Guth, L., and Bernstein, J. J.: Selectivity in the reestablishment of synapses in the superior cervical sympathetic ganglion of the cat. Exp. Neurol., *4*:59, 1961.

Gutmann, E., Guttmann, L., Medawar, P. B., and Young, J. Z.: The rate of regeneration of nerve. J. Exp. Biol., *19*:14, 1942.

Gutmann, E., and Sanders, F. K.: Recovery of fibre numbers and diameters in the regeneration of peripheral nerves. J. Physiol. (Lond.), *101*:489, 1943.

Guyton, A. C., and MacDonald, M. A.: Physiology of botulinus toxin. Arch. Neurol. Psychiatry, *57*:578, 1947.

Hall, M. E., Wilson, D. L., and Stone, G. C.: Changes in protein metabolism following axotomy: A two-dimensional analysis. Neurosci. Abstr., *3*:426, 1977.

Halperin, J. J., and LaVail, J. H.: A study of the dynamics of retrograde transport and accumulation of horseradish peroxidase in injured neurons. Brain Res., *100*:253, 1975.

Hamberger, A., Hansson, H. and Sjostrand, J.: Surface structure of isolated neurones. J. Cell Biol., *47*:319, 1970.

Hamberger, C. A., and Hyden, H.: Transneuronal chemical changes in Deiter's nucleus. Acta Otolaryngol. [Suppl.] (Stockh.), *75*:82, 1949.

Harkonen, M.: Carboxylic esterases, oxidative enzymes and catecholamines in the superior cervical ganglion of the rat and the effect of pre- and post-ganglionic nerve division. Acta Physiol. Scand. *63*[Suppl. 237]:1, 1964.

Heacock, A. M., and Agranoff, B. W.: Enhanced labeling of a retinal protein during regeneration of optic nerve in goldfish. Proc. Natl. Acad. Sci. U.S.A., *73*:828, 1976.

Heidemann, M. K.: Neurophysiological and behavioral evidence for selective reinnervation in skin-grafted *Rana pipiens*. Proc. Natl. Acad. Sci. U.S.A., *74*:5749, 1977.

Hendry, I. A.: The response of adrenergic neurons to axotomy and nerve growth factor. Brain Res., *94*:87, 1975.

Heuser, J., and Reese, T. S.: Stimulation-induced uptake and release of peroxidase from synaptic vesicles in frog neuromuscular junctions. Anat. Rec., *172*:329, 1972.

Hibbard, E.: Regeneration in the severed spinal cord of chordate larvae of *Petromyzon marinus*. Exp. Neurol., *7*:175, 1963.

Hier, D. B., Arnason, B. G., and Young, M.: Nerve growth factor: Relationship to the cyclic AMP system of sensory ganglia. Science, *182*:79, 1973.

Hiscoe, H. B.: The distribution of nodes and incisures in normal and regenerated nerve fibers. Anat. Rec., *99*:447, 1947.

Hodes, R. M. G., Larrabee, M. G., and German, W.: The human

electromyogram in response to nerve stimulation and the conduction velocity of motor axons. Arch. Neurol., Psychiatry, 60:340, 1948.

Hoffman, H.: Fate of interrupted nerve fibers regenerating into partially denervated muscle. Aust. J. Exp. Biol. Med. Sci., 29:211, 1951.

Hoffman, H., and Springell, P. H.: An attempt at the chemical identification of neurocletin (the substance evoking axon sprouting). Aust. J. Exp. Biol. Med. Sci., 29:417, 1951.

Holmes, W., and Young, J. Z.: Nerve regeneration after immediate and delayed suture. J. Anat., 77:63, 1942.

Holtzman, E., and Novikoff, A. B.: Lysosomes in the rat sciatic nerve following crush. J. Cell Biol., 27:651, 1965.

Honjin, R., Nakamura, T., and Imura, M.: Electron microscopy of peripheral nerve fibres. IV. On the axoplasmic changes during Wallerian degeneration. Okajimas Folia Anat. Jpn., 33:131, 1959.

Hopkins, A. P., and Lambert, E. H.: Conduction in regenerating unmyelinated fibres. Brain, 95:213, 1972.

Horch, K. W.: Ascending collaterals of cutaneous neurons in the fasciculus gracilis of the cat during peripheral nerve regeneration. Brain Res., 117:19, 1976.

Hoy, R. R., Bittner, G. D., and Kennedy, D.: Regeneration in crustacean motor neurons: Evidence for axonal fusion. Science, 156:251, 1967.

Huizar, P., Kuno, M., Kudo, N., and Miyata, Y.: Reaction of intact spinal motoneurones to partial denervation of the muscle. J. Physiol., 265:175, 1977.

Hunt, R. K., and Jacobson, J.: Neuronal specificity revisited. Curr. Top. Dev. Biol., 8:203, 1974.

Hyden, H.: Protein metabolism in the nerve cell during growth and function. Acta. Physiol. Scand. 6 [Suppl. 17]:1, 1943.

Jacobson, M.: Developmental Neurobiology, 2nd ed. New York, Plenum Press, 1978.

Jacobson, M., and Baker, R. E.: Development of neuronal connections with skin grafts in frogs: Behavioral and electrophysiological studies. J. Comp. Neurol., 137:121, 1969.

Jacobson, M., and Gaze, R. M.: Selection of appropriate tectal connections by regenerating optic nerve fibers in adult goldfish. Exp. Neurol., 13:418, 1965.

Jacobson, S., and Guth, L.: An electrophysiological study of the early stages of peripheral nerve regeneration. Exp. Neurol., 11:48, 1965.

Jansen, J. K. S., and Nicholls, J. G.: Regeneration and changes in synaptic connections between individual nerve cells in the central nervous system of the leech. Proc. Natl. Acad. Sci. U.S.A., 69:636, 1972.

Joseph, J.: Absence of cell multiplication during degeneration of non-myelinated nerves. J. Anat., 81:135, 1947.

Kandel, E. R.: Cellular Basis of Behavior. San Francisco, W. H. Freeman, 1976, pp. 1288–1351.

Kandel, E. R.: Neuronal plasticity and the modification of behavior. In Kandel, E. R. (ed.): Handbook of Physiology. Section

419

I: The Nervous System, Vol. I. Cellular Biology of Neurons, Part 2. Bethesda, American Physiological Society, 1977, pp. 1137–1182.

Kandel, E. R., and Spencer, W. A.: Cellular neurophysiological approaches in the study of learning. Physiol. Rev., *48*:65, 1968.

Kerns, J. M., and Hinsman, E. J.: Neuroglial response to sciatic neurectomy. II. Electron microscopy. J. Comp. Neurol., *151*:255, 1973.

Khodadad, G.: Microsurgical techniques in repair of peripheral nerves. Surg. Clin. North Am., *52*:1157, 1972.

Kiernan, J. A.: Estimation of lengths of regenerated axons in nerves. Exp. Neurol., *56*:431, 1977.

King, R. H. M., and Thomas, P. K.: Electron microscope observations on aberrant regeneration of unmyelinated axons in the vagus nerve of the rabbit. Acta Neuropathol. (Berl.), *18*:150, 1971.

Kiraly, J. K., and Krnjevic, K.: Some retrograde changes in function of nerves after peripheral section. Q. J. Exp. Physiol., *44*:244, 1959.

Kirklin, J. W., Murphy, F., and Berkson, J.: Suture of peripheral nerves: Factors affecting prognosis. Surg. Gynecol. Obstet., *88*:719, 1949.

Koppanyi, T.: Regeneration in the central nervous system of fishes. *In* Windle, W. F. (ed.): Regeneration in the Central Nervous System. Springfield: Charles C Thomas, 1955, pp. 3–19.

Korneliussen, H., and Jansen, J. K. S.: Morphological aspects of the elimination of polyneuronal innervation of skeletal muscle fibres in newborn rats. J. Neurocytol., *5*:591, 1976.

Kreutzberg, G. W.: Changes of Coenzyme (TPN) diaphorase and TPN-linked dehydrogenase during axonal reaction of the nerve cell. Nature, *199*:393, 1963.

Kreutzberg, G. W., and Schubert, P.: Changes in axonal flow during regeneration of mammalian motor nerves. Acta Neuropathol. [Suppl.], (Berl.) *5*:70, 1971.

Kristensson, K., and Olsson, Y.: Retrograde transport of horseradish peroxidase in transected axons. I. Time relationships between transport and induction of chromatolysis. Brain Res., *79*:101, 1974.

Kristensson, K., and Olsson, Y.: Retrograde transport of horseradish perioxidase in transected axons. II. Relations between rate of transfer from the site of injury to the perikaryon and the onset of chromatolysis, J. Neurocytol., *4*:653, 1975.

Kuffler, D., Thompson, W., and Jansen, J. K. S.: The elimination of synapses in multiply innervated skeletal muscle fibres of the rat: Dependence on distance between end-plates. Brain Res., *138*:353, 1977.

Kugelberg, E., Edstrom, L. and Abbruzzese, M.: Mapping of motor units in experimentally reinnervated rat muscle. J. Neurol. Neurosurg. Psychiatry, *33*:319, 1970.

Kuno, M.: Response of spinal motoneurones to section and restoration of peripheral motor connections. Cold Spring Harbor Symp. Quant. Biol., *40*:456, 1976.

Kuno, M., and Llinas, R.: Enhancement of synaptic transmission by dendritic potentials in chromatolyzed motoneurones of the cat. J. Physiol., *210*:807, 1970a.

Kuno, M., and Llinas, R.: Alteration of synaptic action in chromatolysed motoneurones of the cat. J. Physiol., *210*:823, 1970*b*.

Kuno, M., Miyata, Y., and Muñoz-Martinez, E. J.: Differential reaction of fast and slow alpha motoneurones to axotomy. J. Physiol., (Lond.) *240*:725, 1974*a*.

Kuno, M., Miyata, Y., and Muñoz-Martinez, E. J.: Properties of fast and slow alpha motoneurones following motor reinnervation. J. Physiol., (Lond.) *242*:273, 1974*b*.

Lampert, P. W.: A comparative study of reactive, degenerating, regenerating and dystrophic axons. J. Neuropathol. Exp. Neurol., *26*:345, 1967.

Landis, S. C.: Growth cones of cultured sympathetic neurons containing adrenergic vesicles. J. Cell Biol., *78*:R8, 1978.

Landmesser, L., and Pilar, G.: Selective re-innervation of two cell populations in the adult pigeon ciliary ganglia. J. Physiol., (Lond.), *211*:203, 1970.

Landley, J. N.: On the origin from the spinal cord of the cervical and upper thoracic sympathetic fibres, with some observations on white and grey rami communicantes. Philos. Trans. R. Soc. Lond. [Biol.], *183*:85, 1892.

Langley, J. N.: On the regeneration of pre-ganglionic and of post-ganglionic visceral nerve fibres. J. Physiol. (Lond.), *22*:215, 1897.

Lasek, R. J., and Hoffman, P. N.: The neuronal cytoskeleton, axonal transport, and axonal growth. *In* Goldman, R., Pollard, T., and Rosenbaum, J. (eds.): Cell Motility, Book C., Microtubules and Related Proteins. Cold Spring Harbor, N.Y., Cold Spring Harbor Laboratory, 1976, pp. 1021–1051.

Lee, J. C.-Y.: Electron microscopy of Wallerian degeneration. J. Comp. Neurol., *120*:65, 1963.

Lentz, T. L.: Fine structure of nerves in the regenerating limb of the newt *Triturus*. Am. J. Anat. *121*:647, 1967.

Letinsky, M. S., Fischbeck, K. H., and McMahan, V. J.: Precision of reinnervation of original postsynaptic sites in frog muscle after a nerve crush. J. Neurocytol., *5*:691, 1976.

Levi-Montalcini, R.: Effects of mouse tumor transplantation on the nervous system. Ann. N.Y. Acad. Sci., *55*:330, 1952.

Levi-Montalcini, R., and Angeletti, P. V.: Nerve growth factor. Physiol. Rev., *48*:534, 1968.

Levi-Montalcini, R., Caramia, F., Luse, S. A., and Angeletti, P. V.: In vitro effects of the nerve growth factor on the fine structure of the sensory nerve cells. Brain Res., *8*:347, 1968.

Levi-Montalcini, R., and Hamberger V.: Selective growth-stimulating effects of mouse sarcoma on the sensory and sympathetic nervous system of the chick embryo. J. Exp. Zool., *116*:321, 1951.

Levi-Montalcini, R., and Hamberger, V.: A diffusible agent of mouse sarcoma, producing hyperplasia of sympathetic ganglia and hyperneurotization of the chick embryo. J. Exp. Zool. *123*:233, 1953.

Levi-Montalcini, R., Meyer, H., and Hamberger, V.: In vitro experimentation on the effects of mouse sarcoma 180 and 37 on the spinal and sympathetic ganglia of the chick embryo. Cancer Res., *14*:49, 1954.

421

Lieberman, A. R.: The axon reaction: A review of the principal features of perikarial responses to axon injury. Int. Rev. Neurobiol., *14*:49, 1971.

Lieberman, A. R.: Some factors affecting retrograde neuronal responses to axonal lesions. *In* Bellairs, R., and Gray, E. G. (eds.): Essays on the Nervous System. Oxford, Clarendon Press, 1974, pp. 71–105.

Liu, C. N., and Chambers, W. W.: Intraspinal sprouting of dorsal root axons. Arch. Neurol. Psychiatry, *79*:46, 1958.

Liuzzi, A., Foppen, F. H., and Kopin, I. J.: Stimulation and maintenance by nerve growth factor phenylethanolamine-N-methyltransferase in superior cervical ganglia of adult rats. Brain Res., *138*:309, 1977.

Lullman-Rauch, R.: The regeneration of neuromuscular junctions during spontaneous reinnervation of the rat diaphragm. Z. Zellforsch. Mikrosk. Anat., *121*:593, 1971.

Lynch, G., Deadwyler, S., and Cotman, C.: Postlesion axonal growth produces permanent functional connections. Science, *180*:1364, 1973.

Marinesco, G.: La Cellule Nerveuse. Paris, Doin, 1909.

Mark, R. F.: Fin movement after regeneration of neuromuscular connections: An investigation of myotypic specificity. Exp. Neurol., *12*:292, 1965.

Mark, R. F.: Matching muscles and motoneurones. A review of some experiments on motor nerve regeneration. Brain Res., *14*:245, 1969.

Mark, R. F., and Marotte, L. R.: The mechanism of selective reinnervation of fish eye muscles. III. Functional, electrophysiological and anatomical analysis of recovery from section of the third and fourth nerves. Brain Res., *46*:131, 1972.

Mark, R. F., Marotte, L. R., and Mart, P. E.: The mechanism of selective reinnervation of fish eye muscles. IV. Identification of repressed synapses. Brain Res., *46*:149, 1972.

Mark, F. R., von Campenhausen, A., and Lischinski, D. J.: Nerve muscle relations in the salamander: Possible relevance to nerve regeneration and muscle specificity. Exp. Neurol., *16*:438, 1966.

Marmor, L.: Regeneration of peripheral nerve defects by irradiated homografts. Lancet, *1*:1191, 1963.

Marmor, L.: Peripheral Nerve Regeneration Using Nerve Grafts. Springfield, Ill., Charles C Thomas, 1967.

Marmor, L.: Nerve grafting in peripheral nerve repair. Surg. Clin. North Am., *52*:1177, 1972.

Maron, K.: Regeneration capacity of the spinal cord in *Lampetra fluviatilis* larvae. Folia Biol. (Warsaw), *7*:179, 1959.

Marotte, L. R., and Mark, R. F.: The mechanism of selective reinnervation of fish eye muscle. I. Evidence from muscle function during recovery. Brain Res., *19*:41, 1970*a*.

Marotte, L. R., and Mark, R. F.: The mechanism of selective reinnervation of fish eye muscle. II. Evidence from electron microscopy of nerve endings. Brain Res., *19*:53, 1970*b*.

Matthews, M. R., Cowen, W. M., and Powell, T. S. P.: Transneuronal cell degeneration in the lateral geniculate nucleus of the macaque monkey. J. Anat., *94*:145, 1960.

Matthews, M. R., and Nelson, V. H.: Detachment of structurally intact nerve endings from chromatolytic neurones of rat superior cervical ganglion during depression of synaptic transmission induced by postganglionic axotomy. J. Physiol. (Lond.), *245*:91, 1975.

McIntyre, A. K., Bradley, K., and Brock, L. G.: Responses of motoneurones undergoing chromatolysis. J. Gen. Physiol., *42*:931, 1959.

McQuarrie, I. G.: Axonal regeneration in the goldfish optic system: The role of the nerve cell body. Ph.D. Thesis, Cornell University Graduate School of Medical Sciences, 1977. (Cited in Grafstein and McQuarrie, 1978.)

Mendell, L. M., Munson, J. B., and Scott, J. G.: Alterations of synapses on axotomized motoneurones. J. Physiol. (Lond.), *255*:67, 1976.

Mendell, L. M., and Scott, J. G.: The effect of peripheral nerve cross-union on connections of single Ia fibers to motoneurones. Exp. Brain Res., *22*:221, 1975.

Miner, N.: Integumental specification of sensory fibers in the development of cutaneous local sign. J. Comp. Neurol., *105*:161, 1956.

Morris, J. H., Hudson, A. F., and Weddell, G. A study of degeneration and regeneration in the divided rat sciatic nerve based on electron microscopy. II. The development of the "Regenerating Unit." Z. Zellforsch., *124*:103, 1972.

Murphy, A. D., and Kater, S. B.: Specific reinnervation of a target organ by a pair of identified molluscan neurons. Brain Res., *156*:322, 1978.

Murray, M., and Goldberger, M. E.: Restitution of function and collateral sprouting in the cat spinal cord: The partially hemisected animal. J. Comp. Neurol., *158*:19, 1974.

Murray, M., and Grafstein, B.: Changes in the morphology and amino acid incorporation of regenerating goldfish optic neurons. Exp. Neurol., *23*:544, 1969.

Napier, J. R.: The significance of Tinel's sign in peripheral nerve injuries. Brain, *72*:63, 1949.

Nathaniel, E. J. H., and Pease, D. C.: Regenerative changes in rat dorsal roots following Wallerian degeneration. J. Ultrastruct. Res., *9*:533, 1963.

Nikodijevic, B., Nikodijevic, O., Wong Yu, M. Y., Pollard, H., and Guroff, G.: The effect of nerve growth factor on cyclic AMP levels in superior cervical ganglia of the rat. Proc. Natl. Acad. Sci. U.S.A., *72*:4769, 1975.

Nissl, F.: Über die Veranderungen der Ganglienzellen am Facialiskern des kaninchens nach Ausreissung der Nerven. All. Z. Psychiat., *48*:197, 1892.

Nja, A., and Purves, D.: Reinnervation of guinea-pig superior cervical ganglion cells by preganglionic fibers arising from different levels of the spinal cord. J. Physiol., *272*:633, 1977.

Nja, A., and Purves, D.: The effects of nerve growth factor and its antiserum on synapses in the superior cervical ganglion of the guinea-pig. J. Physiol., *277*:53, 1978*a*.

Nja, A., and Purves, D.: Specificity of initial synaptic contacts made on guinea-pig superior cervical ganglion cells during re-

423

generation of the cervical sympathetic trunk. J. Physiol., *281*:45, 1978*b*.

O'Brien, R. A. D.: Axonal transport of acetylcholine, choline acetyltransferase and cholinesterase in regenerating peripheral nerve. J. Physiol. (Lond.), *282*:91, 1978.

Ochs, S.: A unitary concept of axoplasmic transport based on the transport filament hypothesis. *In* Bradley, W. G., Gardner-Medwin, D., and Walton, J. N. (eds.): Third International Congress on Muscle Diseases. Amsterdam, Excerpta Medica, Vol. 360, 1975, pp. 189–194.

Ochs, S.: Fast axoplasmic transport in the fibres of chromatolyzed neurones. J. Physiol. (Lond.), *255*:249, 1976.

Ochs, S., and Worth, R. M.: Axoplasmic transport in normal and pathological systems. *In* Waxman, S. G. (ed.): Physiology and Pathobiology of Axons. New York, Raven Press, 1978, pp. 251–264.

Oester, Y. T., and Davis, L.: Recovery of sensory function. *In* Woodhall, B., and Beebe, G. W., (eds.): Peripheral Nerve Regeneration — A Follow-up Study of 3,656 World War II Injuries. Washington, U.S. Government Printing Office, 1956, V.A. Medical Monograph. Chapter 5.

Omer, G. E.: Injury to nerves of the upper extremity. J. Bone Joint Surg. [Am.], *56-A*:1615, 1974.

Otten, V., Hatanaka, H., and Thoenen, H.: Role of cyclic nucleotides in NGF-mediated induction of tyrosine hydroxylase in rat sympathetic ganglia and adrenal medulla. Brain Res., *140*:385, 1978.

Pannese, E.: Investigations on the ultrastructural changes of the spinal ganglion neurons in the course of axon regeneration and cell hypertrophy. I. Changes during axon regeneration. Z. Zellforsch., *60*:711, 1963.

Paravicini, U., Stockel, K., and Thoenen, H.: Biological importance of retrograde axonal transport of nerve growth factor in adrenergic neurons. Brain Res., *84*:279, 1975.

Pearson, K. G., and Bradley, A. B.: Specific regeneration of excitatory motor neurons to leg muscles in the cockroach. Brain Res., *47*:492, 1972.

Pestronk, A., and Drachman, D. B.: Motor nerve sprouting and acetyl-choline receptors. Science, *199*:1223, 1978.

Pettigrew, R. K., and Windle, W. F.: Factors in recovery from spinal cord Injury. Exp. Neurol., *53*:815, 1976.

Piatt, J.: Regeneration in the spinal cord of amphibia. *In* Windle, W. F. (ed.): Regeneration in the Central Nervous System. Springfield, Ill., Charles C Thomas, 1955*a*, pp. 20–46.

Piatt, J.: Regeneration of the spinal cord in the salamander. J. Exp. Zool., *129*:177, 1955*b*.

Pilar, G., and Landmesser, L.: Axotomy mimicked by localized colchicine application. Science, *177*:1116, 1972.

Pinner-Poole, B., and Campbell, J. B.: Effects of low temperature and colchicine on regenerating sciatic nerve. Exp. Neurol., *25*:603, 1969.

Porter, K. R., and Bowers, M. B.: A study of chromatolysis in motor neurons of the frog *Rana pipiens*. J. Cell Biol., *19*:56, 1963.

Price, D. L., and Porter, K. R.: The response of ventral horn neurons to axonal transection. J. Cell Biol., *53*:24, 1972.

Prineas, J.: The pathogenesis of dying-back polyneuropathies. I. An ultrastructural study of experimental triortho-cresyl phosphate intoxication in the cat. J. Neuropathol. Exp. Neurol., *28*:571, 1969.

Purves, D.: Functional and structural changes in mammalian sympathetic neurones following interruption of their axons. J. Physiol. (Lond.), *252*:429, 1975.

Purves, D.: Competitive and non-competitive reinnervation of mammalian sympathetic neurones by native and foreign fibres. J. Physiol. (Lond.), *261*:453, 1976.

Raine, C. S.: On the occurrence of Schwann cells in the normal central nervous system. J. Neurocytol., *5*:371, 1976.

Raisman, G.: Neuronal plasticity in the septal nuclei of the adult rat. Brain Res., *14*:25, 1969.

Ramón y Cajal, S.: Degeneración y Regeneración del Sistema Nervioso. Madrid, Nicolas Moya, 1914.

Ramón y Cajal, S.: Degeneration and Regeneration of the Nervous System. London, Oxford University Press, 1928. (Translated and edited by R. M. May.)

Rand, R. W.: Microneurosurgery, 2nd ed. St. Louis, C. V. Mosby, 1978.

Redfern, P. A.: Neuromuscular transmission in newborn rats. J. Physiol (Lond.), *209*:701, 1970.

Rees, R. P., Bunge, M. B., and Bunge, R. P.: Morphological changes in the neuritic growth cone and target neuron during synaptic junction development in culture. J. Cell Biol., *68*:240, 1976.

Reis, D. J., and Ross, R. A.: Dynamic changes in brain dopamine β-hydroxylase activity during anterograde and retrograde reactions to injury of central noradrenergic neurons. Brain Res., *57*:307, 1973.

Reis, D. J., Gilad, G., Pickel, V. M., and Joh, T. H.: Reversible changes in the activities and amounts of tyrosine hydroxylase in dopamine neurons of the substantia nigra in response to axonal injury as studied by immunochemical and immunocytochemical methods. Brain Res., *144*:325, 1978*a*.

Reis, D. J., Ross, R. A., Gilad, G., and Joh, T. H.: Reaction of central catacholaminergic neurons to injury: Model systems for studying neurobiology of central regeneration and sprouting. *In* Cotman, C. W. (ed.): Neuronal Plasticity. New York, Raven Press, 1978*b*, pp. 197–226.

Romine, J. S., Aguayo, A. J., and Bray, G. M.: Absence of Schwann cell migration along regenerating unmyelinated nerve. Brain Res., *98*:601, 1975.

Romine J. S., Bray, G. M., and Aguayo, A. J.: Schwann cell multiplication after crush injury of unmyelinated fibers. Arch. Neurol., *33*:49, 1976.

Roper, S.: The acetylcholine sensitivity of the surface membrane of multiply-innervated parasympathetic ganglion cells in the mudpuppy before and after partial denervation. J. Physiol. (Lond.), *254*:455, 1976.

Rosenzweig, M. R., and Bennett, E. L.: Neural Mechanisms of Learning and Memory. Cambridge, Massachusetts, M.I.T. Press, 1976.

Ross, R. A., Joh, T. H., and Reis, D. J.: Reversible changes in the accumulation and activities of tyrosine hydroxylase and dopamine β-hydroxylase in neurons of nucleus locus ceruleus during the retrograde reaction. Brain Res., 92:57, 1975.

Rotshenker, S.: Sprouting of intact motor neurons induced by neuronal lesion in the absence of denervated muscle fibers and degenerating axons. Brain Res., 155:354, 1978.

Rotshenker, S., and McMahan, U. G.: Altered patterns of innervation in frog muscle after denervation. J. Neurocytol., 5:719, 1976.

Rotter, A., Birdsall, N. J. M., Burgen, A. S. V., Field, P. M., and Raisman, G.: Axotomy causes loss of muscarinic receptors and loss of synaptic contacts in the hypoglossal nucleus. Nature, 266:734, 1977.

Rovainen, C. M.: Regeneration of Müller and Mauthner axons after spinal transection in larval lampreys. J. Comp. Neurol., 168:545, 1976.

Saito, A., and Zacks, S. I.: Fine structure observations of denervation and reinnervation of neuromuscular junctions in mouse foot muscle. J. Bone Joint Surg. [Am.], 51-A:1163, 1969.

Sanders, F. K., and Whitteridge, D.: Conduction velocity and myelin thickness in regenerating nerve fibres. J. Physiol. (Lond.), 105:152, 1946.

Sanes, J. R., Marshall, L. M., and McMahan, V. J.: Reinnervation of muscle fiber basal lamina after removal of myofibers: Differentiation of regenerating axons at original synaptic sites. J. Cell Biol., 78:176, 1978.

Sawyer, C. H., and Hollinshead, W. H.: Cholinesterases in sympathetic fibers and ganglia. J. Neurophysiol., 8:135, 1945.

Schlaepfer, W. W.: Calcium-induced degeneration of axoplasm in isolated segments of rat peripheral nerve. Brain Res., 69:203, 1974.

Schlaepfer, W. W., and Bunge, R. P.: Effects of calcium ion concentration on the degradation of amputated axons in tissue culture. J. Cell Biol., 59:456, 1973.

Schröder, J. M.: Degeneration and regeneration of myelinated nerve fibers in experimental neuropathies. In Dyck, P. J., Thomas, P. K., and Lambert, E. H., (eds.): Peripheral Neuropathy. Philadelphia, W. B. Saunders, 1975, pp. 337–362.

Scott, S. A.: Persistence of foreign innervation on reinnervated goldfish extraocular muscles. Science, 189:644, 1975.

Seddon, H. J.: Three types of nerve injury. Brain, 66:237, 1943.

Seddon, H. J.: The use of autogenous grafts for the repair of large gaps in peripheral nerves. Br. J. Surg., 35:151, 1947.

Seddon, H. J.: War injuries of peripheral nerves. Br. J. Surg., War Suppl. No. 2, Wounds of the Extremities:325, 1948.

Seddon, H. J.: Surgical Disorders of Peripheral Nerves, 2nd ed. Edinburgh, Churchill Livingstone, 1975.

Seddon, H. J., Medawar, P. B., and Smith, H.: Rate of regeneration of peripheral nerves in man. J. Physiol. (Lond.), 102:191, 1943.

Selzer, M. E.: Regeneration of transected lamprey spinal cord. J. Neuropathol. Exp. Neurol., 35:349, 1976.

Selzer, M. E.: Mechanisms of functional recovery and regeneration after spinal cord transection in larval sea lamprey. J. Physiol. (Lond.), 277:395, 1978.

Shaffer, J. M., and Cleveland, F.: Delayed suture of sensory nerves of the hand. Ann. Surg., 131:556, 1950.

Simeone, F., ed.: Symposium on Operative Nerve Injuries. Surg. Clin. North. Am., 52:1972.

Sklar, J. H., and Hunt, R. K.: The acquisition of specificity in cutaneous sensory neurons: A reconsideration of the integumental specification hypothesis. Proc. Natl. Acad. Sci. U.S.A., 70:3684, 1973.

Snyder, D. H., Valsamis, M. P., Stone, S. H., and Raine, C. S.: Progressive and reparatory events in chronic experimental allergic encephalomyelitis. J. Neuropathol. Exp. Neurol., 34:209, 1975.

Spencer, P. S., and Weinberg, H. J.: Axonal specification of Schwann cell expression and myelination. In Waxman, S. G. (ed.): Physiology and Pathobiology of Axons. New York, Raven Press, 1978, pp. 389–405.

Sperry, R. W.: The effect of crossing nerves to antagonistic limb muscles in the hind limb of the rat. J. Comp. Neurol., 75:1, 1941.

Sperry, R. W.: Visuomotor coordination in the newt (Triturus viridescens) after regeneration of the optic nerves. J. Comp. Neurol., 79:33, 1943.

Sperry, R. W.: Optic nerve regeneration with return of vision in anurans. J. Neurophysiol., 7:57, 1944.

Sperry, R. W.: The problem of central nervous reorganization after nerve regeneration, and muscle transposition. Q. Rev. Biol., 20:311, 1945.

Sperry, R. W.: Orderly patterning of synaptic associations in regeneration of intracentral fiber tracts mediating visuomotor coordination. Anat. Rec., 102:63, 1948.

Sperry, R. W.: Myotypic specificity in teleost motoneurones. J. Comp. Neurol., 93:277, 1950.

Sperry, R. W., and Arora, H. L.: Selectivity in regeneration of the oculomotor nerve in the cichlid fish Astronotus ocellatus. J. Embryol. Exp. Morphol., 14:307, 1965.

Stavraki, G. W.: Supersensitivity Following Lesions of the Nervous System. Toronto, University of Toronto Press, 1961.

Stockel, K., Schwab, M., and Thoenen, H.: Specificity of retrograde transport of nerve growth factor (NGF) in sensory neurons: A biochemical and morphological study. Brain Res., 89:1, 1975.

Stockel, K., and Thoenen, H.: Retrograde axonal transport of nerve growth factor: Specificity and biological importance. Brain Res., 85:337, 1975.

Sumner, A.: Physiology of dying-back neuropathies. In Waxman, S. G. (ed.): Physiology and Pathobiology of Axons. New York, Raven Press, 1978, pp. 349–359.

Sumner, B. E. H.: A quantitative analysis of the response of presynaptic boutons to postsynaptic motor neuron axotomy. Exp. Neurol., 46:605, 1975.

Sumner, B. E. H.: Quantitative ultrastructural observations on the inhibited recovery of the hypoglossal nucleus from the axotomy response when regeneration of the hypoglossal nerve is prevented. Exp. Brain Res., 26:141, 1976.

Sumner, B. E. H., and Sutherland, F. I.: Quantitative electron microscopy of the injured hypoglossal nucleus of the rat. J. Neurocytol., 2:315, 1973.

Sunderland, S.: Course and rate of regeneration of motor fibers following lesions of the radial nerve. Arch. Neurol. Psychiatry, 56:133, 1946.

Sunderland, S.: Rate of regeneration in human peripheral nerves. Arch. Neurol. Psychiatry, 58:251, 1947.

Sunderland, S.: Nerves and Nerve Injuries, 2nd edition. London, Churchill Livingstone, 1978.

Sunderland, S., and Bradley, K. C.: Endoneurial tube shrinkage in the distal segment of a severed nerve. J. Comp. Neurol., 93:411, 1950.

Sunderland, S., and Bradley, K. C.: Rate of advance of Hoffmann-Tinel sign in regenerating nerves. Arch. Neurol. Psychiatry, 67:650, 1952.

Tang, D., and Selzer, M. E.: Projections of lamprey spinal neurons determined by the retrograde axonal transport of horseradish peroxidase. J. Comp. Neurol., 188:629, 1979.

Tennyson, V. M.: The fine structure of the axon and growth cone of the dorsal root neuroblast of the rabbit embryo. J. Cell Biol., 44:62, 1970.

Terry, R. D., and Harkin, J. C.: Regenerating peripheral nerve sheaths following Wallerian degeneration. Exp. Cell. Res., 13:193, 1957.

Thoenen, H., Angeletti, P. V., Levi-Montalcini, R., and Kettler, R.: Selective induction by nerve growth factor of tyrosine hydroxylase and dopamine beta-hydroxylase in the rat superior cervical ganglia. Proc. Natl. Acad. Sci. U.S.A., 68:1598, 1971.

Thomas, P. K.: Motor nerve conduction in the carpal tunnel syndrome. Neurology, 10:1045, 1960.

Thomas, P. K.: Changes in the endoneurial sheaths of peripheral myelinated nerve fibers during Wallerian degeneration. J. Anal, 98:175, 1964a.

Thomas, P. K.: The deposition of collagen in relation to Schwann cell basement membrane during peripheral nerve regeneration. J. Cell Biol., 23:375, 1964b.

Thulin, C. A.: Electrophysiological study of consecutive changes of feline ventral root reflexes during degeneration and regeneration following peripheral nerve section. Exp. Neurol., 4:531, 1961.

Tinel, J.: Le signe du fourmillement dans le lesions des nerfs peripheriques. Presse Med., 23:388, 1915.

Torvik, A.: Transneuronal changes in the inferior olive and pontine nuclei in kittens. J. Neuropathol. Exp. Neurol., 15:119, 1956.

Torvik, A., and Heding, A.: Histological studies on the effect of actinomycin D on retrograde nerve cell reaction in the facial nucleus of mice. Acta Neuropathol. (Berl.), 9:146, 1967.

Torvik, A., and Heding, A.: Effects of actinomycin D on retrograde nerve cell reaction. Further observations. Acta Neuropathol. (Berl.), 14:62, 1969.

Turner, J. E., and Glaze, K. A.: Regenerative repair in the severed optic nerve of the newt (Triturus viridescens): Effect of nerve growth factor. Exp. Neurol., 57:687, 1977.

Ungerstedt, U.: Postsynaptic supersensitivity after 6-hydroxydopamine-induced degeneration of the nigro-striatal dopamine system. Acta Physiol. Scand. Suppl., 367:69, 1971.

Van Essen, D. C., and Jansen, J. K. S.: The specificity of reinnervation by identified sensory and motor neurones in the leech. J. Comp. Neurol., 171:433, 1977.

Van Harreveld, A.: On the mechanisms of spontaneous reinnervation in paretic muscles. Am. J. Physiol., 130:670, 1947.

Vial, J. D.: The early changes in the axoplasm during Wallerian degeneration. J. Biophys. Biochem. Cytol., 4:551, 1958.

Vizoso, A. D., and Young, J. Z.: Internode length and fiber diameter in developing and regenerating nerves. J. Anat., 82:110, 1948.

Waddington, J. L., and Cross, A. J.: Denervation supersensitivity in the striatonigral GABA pathway. Nature, 276:618, 1978.

Waller, A. V.: Experiments on the section of the glossopharyngeal and hypoglossal nerves of the frog, and observation on the alterations produced thereby in the structure of their primitive-fibres. Philos. Trans. R. Soc. Lond. [Biol.], 140:423, 1850.

Watson, W. E.: An autoradiographic study of the incorporation of nucleic acid precursors by neurones and glia during nerve regeneration. J. Physiol. (Lond.), 180:741, 1965.

Watson, W. E.: Some quantitative observations upon the oxidation of substrates of the tricarboxylic acid cycle in injured neurons. J. Neurochem., 13:849, 1966a.

Watson, W. E.: Quantitative observations upon acetylcholine hydrolase activity of nerve cells after axotomy. J. Neurochem., 13:1549, 1966b.

Watson, W. E.: Observations on the nucleolar and total cell body nucleic acid of injured nerve cells. J. Physiol (Lond.), 196:655, 1968a.

Watson, W. E.: Anaerobic glycolytic capacity of nerve cells after axotomy. J. Physiol. (Lond.), 198:77, 1968b.

Watson, W. E.: The response of motor neurones to intramuscular injection of botulinum toxin. J. Physiol. (Lond.), 202:611, 1969.

Watson, W. E.: Cellular responses to axotomy and to related procedures. Br. Med. Bull., 30:112, 1974.

Webster, H. de F.: The relationship between Schmidt-Lantermann incisures and myelin segmentation during Wallerian degeneration. Ann. N.Y. Acad. Sci., 122:29, 1965.

Weddell, G.: Axonal regeneration in cutaneous nerve plexuses. J. Anat., 77:49, 1942.

Weddell, G., and Glees, P.: The early stages in the degeneration of cutaneous nerve fibres. J. Anat., 76:65, 1941.

429

Weinberg, E. L., and Spencer, P. S.: Studies on the control of myelinogenesis. III. Signalling of oligodendrocyte myelination by regenerating peripheral axons. Brain Res., *162*:273, 1979.

Weinberg, H. J., and Spencer, P. S.: Studies on the control of myelinogenesis. I. Myelination of regenerating axons after entry into a foreign unmyelinated nerve. J. Neurocytol., *4*:395, 1975.

Weinberg, H. J., and Spencer, P. S.: Studies on the control of myelination. II. Evidence for neuronal regulation of myelination. Brain Res., *113*:363, 1976.

Weinberg, H. J., Spencer, P. S., and Raine, C. S.: Aberrant PNS development in dystrophic mice. Brain Res., *88*:532, 1975.

Weiss, P.: Selectivity controlling the central-peripheral relations in the nervous system. Biol. Rev., *11*:494, 1936.

Weiss, P.: Nerve patterns: The mechanics of nerve growth. Growth, *5* (Suppl.):163, 1941.

Weiss, P.: The technology of nerve regeneration: A review. Sutureless tubulation and related methods of nerve repair. J. Neurosurg., *1*:400, 1944.

Weiss, P., and Hiscoe, H. B.: Experiments on the mechanism of nerve growth. J. Exp. Zool., *107*:315, 1948.

Weiss, P., and Hoag, A.: Competitive reinnervation of rat muscles by their own and foreign nerves. J. Neurophysiol., *9*:413, 1946.

West, J. R.: Early history of mammalian nerve regeneration. Neurosci. Behav. Rev., *2*:27, 1978.

Wettstein, R., and Sotelo, J. R.: Eelectron microscope study on the regenerative process of peripheral nerves of mice. Z. Zellforsch. Mikrosk. Anta., *59*:708, 1963.

Williams, P. L., and Hall, S. M.: Prolonged in vivo observations of normal peripheral nerve fibers and their acute reactions to crush and deliberate trauma. J. Anat., *108*:397, 1971*a*.

Williams, P. L., and Hall, S. M.: Chronic Wallerian degeneration — an in vivo and ultrastructural study. J. Anat., *109*:487, 1971*b*.

Windle, W. F.: Regeneration of axons in the vertebrate central nervous system. Physiol. Rev., *36*:427, 1956.

Wood, P. M., and Bunge, R. P.: Evidence that sensory axons are mitogenic for Schwann cells. Nature, *256*:662, 1975.

Yahr, M. D., and Beebe, G. W.: Recovery of motor function. *In* Woodhall, B., and Beebe, G. W. (eds.): Peripheral Nerve Regeneration — A Follow-up Study of 3,656 World War II Injuries. Washington, U.S. Government Printing Office, 1956. V.A. Medical Monograph, Chapter 3.

Yamada, K. M., Spooner, B. S., and Nessels, N. K.: Ultrastructure and function of growth cones and axons of cultured nerve cells. J. Cell Biol., *49*:614, 1971.

Yarbrough, G. G., and Phillis, J. W.: Supersensitivity of central neurons — a brief review of an emerging concept. Can. J. Neurol. Sci., *2*:147, 1975.

Young, J. Z.: The functional repair of nervous tissue. Physiol. Rev., *22*:318, 1942.

REGENERATION OF PERIPHERAL NERVE

Zachary, R. B.: Results of nerve suture. *In* Seddon, H. J. (ed.): Peripheral Nerve Injuries. London, Her Majesty's Stationary Office, 1954, p. 354; Medical Research Council Special Report Series, No. 282.

Zelena J., Lubinska, L., and Gutmann, E.: Accumulation of organelles at the ends of interrupted axons. Z. Zellforsch. Microsk. Anat., *91*:200, 1968.

Autonomic Nervous System

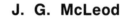

13

J. G. McLeod

ANATOMY The anatomy of the autonomic nervous system will be only briefly reviewed; more detailed accounts are available elsewhere (Mitchell, 1953; Kuntz, 1953; Pick, 1970; Johnson and Spalding, 1974; Appenzeller, 1976; Gabella, 1976). The autonomic nervous system consists of two major divisions — the sympathetic (thoracolumbar division) and the parasympathetic (craniosacral outflow).

Sympathetic Nervous System The central connections of the sympathetic nervous system are not known precisely. The main center for control lies in the hypothalamus, but autonomic effects can be produced by stimulation of the fronto-orbital cortex, temporal cortex, piriform lobe, and parts of the amygdala (Korner, 1971).

Descending pathways from the hypothalamus synapse with the cells of the preganglionic sympathetic efferents in the intermediolateral cell column of the spinal cord, which extends from T1 to L2. The axons emerge from the spinal cord through the anterior roots and join the sympathetic chain through the white rami (Fig. 13–1). The sympathetic chain consists of a series of ganglia and nerve fibers which extends from the base of the skull to the coccyx. There are three cervical ganglia, the upper, middle, and lower (stellate) ganglia, ten to twelve thoracic ganglia, four lumbar ganglia, and four to five sacral ganglia. The preganglionic fibers which enter the chain through the white rami may synapse in the nearest ganglion, pass up or down in the sympathetic chain before making their synapse, or pass through the chain to synapse at more peripheral ganglia such as the celiac and other mesenteric ganglia (Fig. 13–1). Peripheral ganglia, such as the inferior mesenteric ganglion, are not simply relay stations but receive an afferent input from the structure that they innervate, and integrate information from several sources (Szurszewski and Weems,

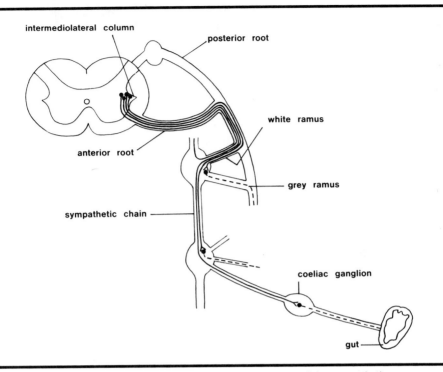

Figure 13–1 Schematic diagram of the sympathetic nervous system. Preganglionic myelinated fibers are represented by continuous lines (———) and postganglionic fibers by interrupted lines (- - - -).

1976). Postganglionic sympathetic fibers are unmyelinated, and those arising from the ganglia of the sympathetic chain join the main nerve trunks by way of the grey rami communicantes and are distributed to the skin and blood vessels (Fig. 13–1). The sympathetic innervation of the different body structures has been studied in detail (Bonica, 1968). In brief, the segmental innervation of the eye is from T1; heart, T1-4; upper limb, T2-8; abdominal viscera via splanchnic nerve, T6-L2; lower limbs, T10-L2; and pelvic viscera and genitourinary system, T6-L1.

The preganglionic sympathetic efferent fibers are myelinated B fibers (Gasser and Erlanger, 1927) that range in diameter from 1 to 3 μm and conduct with a velocity of 10 to 12 meters per second. The postganglionic unmyelinated C fibers conduct at velocities of 1 to 2 meters per second.

The preganglionic fibers in the sympathetic nervous system are cholinergic. Postganglionic fibers are noradrenergic, except those innervating sweat glands, the adrenal medulla, and some vasodilator fibers to muscles.

433

Afferent fibers also travel in the sympathetic nervous system. There are large and small diameter myelinated fibers and unmyelinated C fibers. The smaller fibers convey the sensations of visceral pain and converge with somatic afferent fibers onto single cells in the thalamus and elsewhere in the central nervous system, thus providing the physiological and anatomical substrate for the phenomenon of referred pain (McLeod, 1958, 1961).

Parasympathetic Nervous System

The hypothalamus and other suprabulbar centers maintain central control over the divisions of the parasympathetic nervous system. Parasympathetic fibers leave the brain stem in the third, seventh, ninth, and tenth cranial nerves and the sacral cord in the second, third, and fourth sacral nerves. The parasympathetic fibers in the third cranial nerves supply the pupillary and ciliary muscles, those in the seventh cranial nerves supply the lacrimal, submandibular, and sublingual salivary glands, the parotid gland is supplied by parasympathetic fibers in the ninth cranial nerve, the vagus nerve innervates the thoracic and abdominal viscera, and the sacral outflow supplies the genitourinary system and large bowel. The ganglia lie close to the innervated structures, and the postganglionic fibers are short in length. Both pre- and postganglionic fibers in the sympathetic nervous system are cholinergic.

HISTOLOGICAL AND ELECTROPHYSIO-LOGICAL PROPERTIES OF THE AUTONOMIC NERVOUS SYSTEM

The histological structure of the white rami, sympathetic trunk, and splanchnic nerve of the cat was studied in detail by Ranson and Billingsley (1918a, b). They consist mainly of small myelinated fibers in the 1- to 3-μm range but there are also larger fibers in the 8- to 13-μm range. The larger diameter fibers are mainly afferent fibers and the small myelinated fibers are mainly preganglionic sympathetic efferent fibers. Other studies of the splanchnic nerve of the cat have confirmed the earlier studies and shown that there are two major peaks in the histogram of fiber diameter distribution at 2 to 3 μm and 9 to 10 μm (McLeod, 1958; Post, 1976; Post and McLeod, 1977a).

Sympathetic Nervous System

The histological structure of the sympathetic chain, white rami, and splanchnic nerve has also been studied in man (Pick and Sheehan, 1946; Takahashi, 1966; Walsh, 1971; Appenzeller and Ogin, 1973; Low et al., 1975a, b). The fiber diameter distribution of myelinated fibers is similar in all three nerves (Walsh, 1971) (Fig. 13–2). Most of the fibers are in the range of 2 to 6 μm, but there is another distinct group of larger fibers with a peak at about 12 μm; the large myelinated fibers, and some of the small myelinated fibers, are afferent. Internodal lengths in the sympathetic chain and in the white rami are shorter in relation to fiber diameter than those in the peripheral nervous system (Fig. 13–3). A recent morpho-

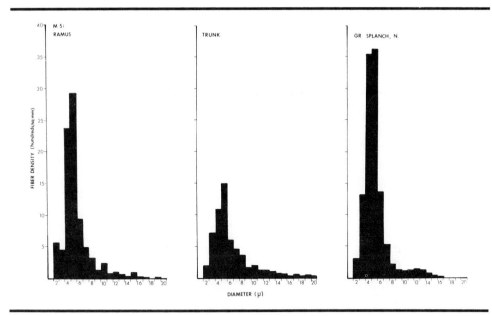

Figure 13–2 Control human subject. Diameter distribution of myelinated fiber in white ramus, sympathetic trunk, and greater splanchnic nerve. (From Walsh, 1971.)

metric analysis of the preganglionic neurons in the spinal cord of man and of the sympathetic preganglionic fibers in the ventral root has shown that the preganglionic fibers range in diameter from 1.5 to 4.7 μm, with a peak at 2.5 μ. There is a progressive reduction with age of both cells and fibers (Low et al., 1977; Low and Dyck, 1977).

The compound action potential recorded from the greater splanchnic nerve of the cat on stimulating the sympathetic trunk consists of an Aβ wave, which represents activity in the largest myelinated fibers and has a maximum conduction velocity of 70 to 75 m/sec, a smaller A$\gamma\delta$ wave with a maximum conduction velocity of 30 to 35 m/sec, a large B wave which represents conduction in the preganglionic myelinated efferent fibers and has a maximum conduction velocity of 10 to 12 m/sec, and a C wave representing conduction in the unmyelinated fibers with a maximum conduction velocity of 1 to 2 m/sec (Amassian, 1951; Widen, 1955; McLeod, 1958; Post and McLeod, 1977a) (Fig. 13–4). Although Gasser and Erlanger (1927) believed that the B fibers had distinct physiological properties, it is now considered that they do not differ from other myelinated fibers of the same diameter (Paintal, 1973a).

There is both convergence and divergence of preganglionic fibers onto sympathetic ganglion cells, and interneurons are also present in the sympathetic ganglia

435

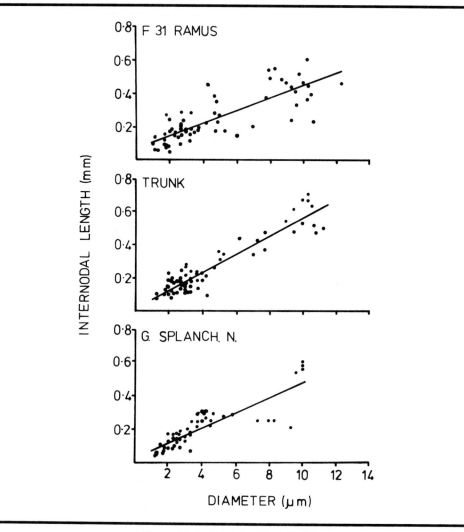

Figure 13–3 Control subject. Relationship between internodal length and diameter of myelinated fibers in human white ramus (*top*), sympathetic trunk (*middle*), and splanchnic nerve (*bottom*).

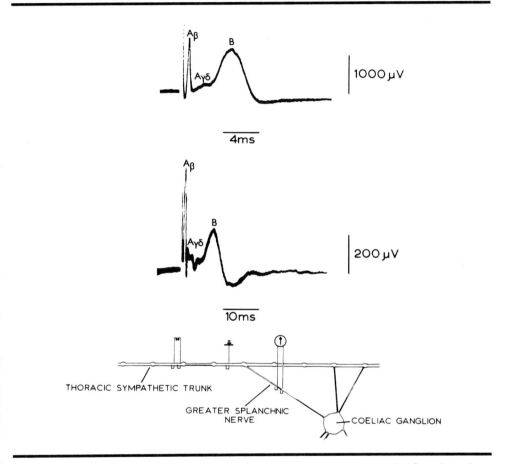

Figure 13–4 Compound action potential recorded from the cat's greater splanchnic nerve and sympathetic trunk. The upper trace is from a control cat, while the lower trace is from a cat severely poisoned with acrylamide. The experimental arrangement is shown below, with stimulating electrodes on the sympathetic trunk and recording electrodes on the greater splanchnic nerve.

(Gabella, 1976; Njå and Purves, 1977). Postsynaptic excitatory and postsynaptic inhibitory synaptic potentials may be recorded from ganglion cells following a preganglionic volley.

Vagus Nerve The histological structure of the vagus nerve has been studied in the cat (Foley and Dubois, 1937; Agostoni et al., 1957; Post, 1976; Post and McLeod, 1977a) and in the rabbit (Evans and Murray, 1954). In the cat only about 16 per cent of the fibers of the cervical vagus are myelinated and they have a unimodal fiber diameter distribution, with a peak at about 4 μm and a range of fibers from 2 to 16 μm. Most of the efferent fibers to the heart are unmyelinated or are small diameter myelinated fibers (Agostoni et al., 1957). The morphometry of the vagus nerve has also been studied in man (Schnitzlein et al., 1958; Hoffman and Schnitzlein, 1961) in whom nearly 80 per cent of the fibers in the cervical vagus are unmyelinated. The compound action potential of the vagus nerve of cats and guinea pigs shows a large Aβ, an A$\gamma\delta$, and a very large C wave (Li et al., 1977; Tuck, 1978) (Figs. 13–5 and 13–6).

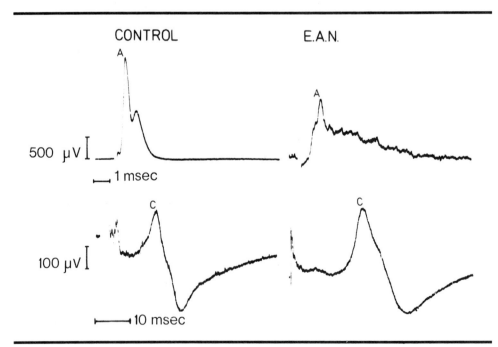

Figure 13–5 Compound action potentials recorded from the cervical vagus nerve of a control guinea pig (*left*) and a guinea pig with E.A.N. (*right*). Note the dispersion of the A wave and the normal C wave in E.A.N. Conduction distance 19.2 mm.

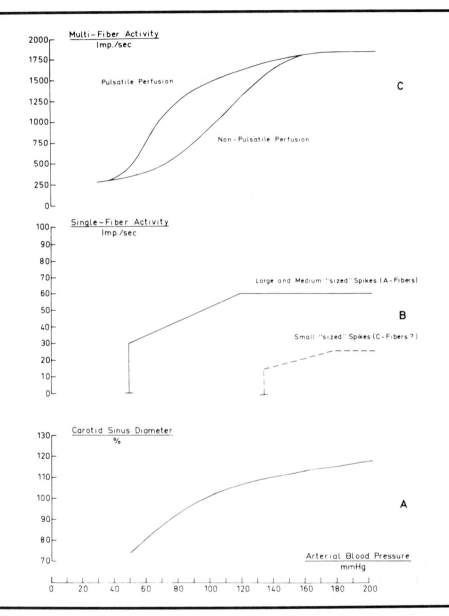

Figure 13–6 Schematic representation of carotid sinus barore-ceptor activity related to pressure-diameter relationship of carotid sinus. *A*, Pressure-diameter relationship. *B*, Typical status stimulus response curves of two "functional subgroups" of baroreceptor afferents (single fiber recordings). *C*, Multifiber activity observed when pulsatile or nonpulsatile perfusion of isolated carotid sinus is performed. (From Kirchheim, 1976.)

PHYSIOLOGY

Vasomotor Tone

Vasomotor tone determines peripheral resistance and is controlled almost entirely by the sympathetic nervous system. Postganglionic sympathetic unmyelinated fibers course mainly by way of somatic nerves to innervate the small peripheral blood vessels in skin and muscles. In the case of mesenteric blood vessels, preganglionic fibers synapse in the celiac and other abdominal ganglia from which unmyelinated fibers pass directly to the splanchnic vascular bed. Adrenergic fibers are chiefly responsible for maintaining constrictor tone in muscle resistance beds, and vasodilatation results from inhibition of the tonic vasoconstrictor fiber activity (Roddie et al., 1957). Some muscle blood vessels are innervated by sympathetic cholinergic vasodilator fibers.

Microelectrode studies of sympathetic activity in human muscle and skin nerves have greatly advanced our understanding of the functions of the sympathetic nervous system in man. Sympathetic activity in muscle nerves is increased by maneuvers accompanied by vasoconstriction and increased peripheral resistance, such as Valsalva's maneuver and body tilting (Hagbarth and Vallbo, 1968; Delius et al., 1972a, b). Body cooling does not significantly influence sympathetic activity in muscle nerves (Delius et al., 1972b). The influence of the baroreceptors on sympathetic muscle nerve activity is discussed below.

Sympathetic activity in human skin nerves is increased by mental stress and emotional stimuli but is not significantly changed by alteration of body posture or the Valsalva maneuver. Skin nerve activity is increased by cooling and reduced by warming (Hagbarth et al., 1972; Delius et al., 1972c; Hallin and Torebjork, 1974).

The veins are also innervated by the sympathetic nervous system, stimulation of which causes venoconstriction (Holman and McLean, 1967). Reflex venomotor activity occurs in response to body tilting, the Valsalva maneuver, cooling, and other stimuli, and may play a part in the redistribution of the blood volume (Page et al., 1955).

Control of Blood Pressure and Heart Rate

There have been a number of reviews of the neural control of the cardiovascular system (Korner, 1971; Kirchheim, 1976; Oberg, 1976). The main reflexes are those whose afferent limbs arise from the arterial baroreceptors, pulmonary arterial receptors, and cardiac mechanoreceptors. Of these, the arterial baroreceptors are the most important in controlling heart rate and blood pressure and are the only ones which will be considered in this review, since their reflex arcs are affected by disease of the peripheral nervous system and they can be tested clinically.

440

ARTERIAL BARORECEPTORS The major systemic arterial baroreceptors are in the carotid sinus and aortic arch; less important baroreceptors exist in the common carotid and subclavian arteries. The *carotid sinus* is supplied by the sinus nerve, a branch of the glossopharyngeal nerve. Anatomically the carotid sinus has a thinner media, significantly less smooth muscle, and higher elastin content than the adjacent internal, external, and common carotid arteries (Kirchheim, 1976). Two distinct types of receptor endings, types 1 and 2, are recognized. They are located only in the adventitia, mainly at the medial-adventitial border and are stimulated by mechanical deformation of the arterial wall.

The carotid sinus nerve of the different animal species studied, including man, contains myelinated fibers which range in diameter from 2 to 12 μm, and most of these are in the 2- to 5-μm diameter range; it also contains some unmyelinated fibers (Gerard and Billingsley, 1923; Eyzaguirre and Uchizono, 1961; Kirchheim, 1976). Sympathetic nerve endings of the adrenergic type in the carotid sinus may have an efferent influence on the sensitivity or set-point of baroreceptors (Kirchheim, 1976). The *aortic arch* is supplied by branches of the vagus nerve. The baroreceptor endings are situated mainly in aortic arch areas that are free of smooth muscle, and the receptors are very similar to the type 2 receptors of the carotid sinus (Kirchheim, 1976). The majority of fibers to the aortic arch receptors are myelinated and in the cat range in diameter from 2 to 10 μm, although most are in the 2- to 6-μm range. Conduction velocities in these fibers range from 12 to 53 m/sec (Paintal, 1973*b*). Unmyelinated baroreceptor afferent fibers are present in some species (Paintal, 1973*b*; Thorén et al., 1977).

Both the aortic and carotid baroreceptors are slowly adapting mechanoreceptors that respond to circumferential stretch due to transmural pressure and to longitudinal stretches (Kirchheim, 1976). Neurophysiological recordings from afferent fibers have demonstrated spike activity in both myelinated A fibers and in unmyelinated C fibers (Paintal, 1973*b*; Kirchheim, 1976; Thorén et al., 1977). The types of electrical activity which may be recorded in single fiber or multifiber preparations of baroreceptor reflex afferents have been reviewed (Paintal, 1973*b*; Kirchheim, 1976). Both carotid and aortic baroreceptor afferents behave in a qualitatively similar manner. Afferent fibers have different thresholds and firing characteristics according to their diameter and receptor endings but, in general, there is a linear relationship between the intra-arterial pressure and impulse frequency in the range between the threshold and maximum firing rate. Pulsatile pressures produce a higher frequency of discharge than static pressures, but the total number of impulses per second is the same in both cases (Paintal, 1973b). In multifiber preparations the stimulus-response curves tend to be more sigmoid than those obtained from single fiber preparations, and the most sensitive part of the curve is close to the mean pressure level in a normal animal (Kirchheim, 1976) (Fig. 13–6). In single fiber recordings from normal carotid sinus or aortic nerves at normal blood pressure (i.e., about 100 mm Hg) the firing occurs in bursts, with most activity during systole and very little during diastole. Only at higher pressures (130 to 150 mm Hg) does firing become continuous throughout the greater part of the cycle. It is mainly the large spike fibers that show this behavior, whereas the firing of the units yielding small spikes is usually more or less continuous.

Korner (1971) has emphasized the importance in cardiovascular control of the integration within the central nervous system of all the afferent inputs concerned with autonomic activity. The major input to the central nervous system is from the carotid sinus and aortic baroreceptors, whose afferents enter the medulla through the ninth and tenth cranial nerves and pass to the nucleus of the tractus solitarius. There are bilateral projections to the medial reticular formation, hypothalamus, basal ganglia, fronto-orbital cortex, temporal cortex, cingulate gyrus, and connected rhinencephalic regions.

INFLUENCE OF BARORECEPTOR AFFERENTS ON CARDIOVASCULAR EFFECTOR ORGANS In studies of open loop reflexes the static stimulus-response curve relating the fall in mean systemic blood pressure to the rise in the carotid sinus or aortic arch pressure is a sigmoid curve. The reflex control of the systemic vascular resistance by the carotid sinus baroreceptors is determined by both the local mean pressure and the pulse pressure in the carotid sinus. In contrast, the aortic arch baroreceptors are influenced mainly by mean pressure (Angell-James and Daly, 1970). The aortic arch baroreceptors have a higher threshold than those of the carotid sinuses, and the sigmoid stimulus-response curve for the aortic arch baroreflex is displaced to the right in the dog (Donald and Edis, 1971) (Fig. 13–7). These findings suggest that the aortic arch is more involved in the control of high blood pressure than is the carotid sinus, but their relative contributions to systemic blood pressure control in intact animals remains uncertain.

Direct recording from sympathetic efferent fibers in man and animals has provided further information about the mechanisms of blood pressure and heart rate control. In vasomotor fibers there are pulse-

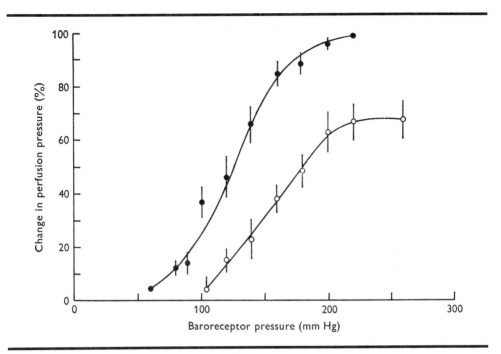

Figure 13–7 Stimulus-response curves for the carotid (●) and aotic arch (○) baroreflexes in 11 dogs. Response in perfusion pressure is expressed as the percentage of maximal change evoked by carotid distention (mean ± S.E.). The aortic arch curve is displaced to the right and its maximal slope and height are less than those for the carotid sinus curve. (From Donald and Edis, 1971.)

synchronous, rhythmic bursts of impulses which are also related to the respiratory cycle (Adrian et al., 1932; Hagbarth and Vallbo, 1968; Kirchheim, 1976). The rhythm is dependent upon the input from baroreceptor afferents. Elevation of arterial blood pressure in the carotid sinus and aortic arch causes reflex inhibition of the sympathetic efferent activity, but there are differences in response to baroreceptor stimulation in nerves to different organs (Ninomiya et al., 1971; Ninomiya and Irisawa, 1975; Delius et al., 1972a, b, c; Kendrick et al., 1972a, b; Wallin et al., 1975; Oberg, 1976). For example, stimulation of the carotid sinus nerve in man causes a reduction in muscle nerve sympathetic activity but no reproducible effect on skin nerve activity (Wallin et al., 1975).

Increased blood pressure causes reflex slowing of the heart through a baroreceptor reflex, the efferent limb of which is in the vagus (Eckberg et al., 1972; Pickering et al., 1972b, c). Tachycardia in response to lowering of blood pressure results from inhibition of vagal activity and increased sympathetic activity; the vagal effects are im-

443

mediate but the sympathetic effects are delayed until several seconds after the change in blood pressure has occurred (Korner, 1971; Kirchheim, 1976). There is indirect evidence that aortic baroreceptors influence heart rate more and vascular beds less than do carotid baroreceptors (Eckberg et al., 1972; Oberg, 1976).

EFFECT OF POSTURE ON HEART RATE AND BLOOD PRESSURE On standing up, about 700 ml of blood leave the chest and are pooled in the abdomen and legs (Sjostrand, 1953). There may be a slight fall in systolic blood pressure but usually the diastolic pressure remains unaltered or increases (Currens, 1948). Reduced blood pressure in arterial baroreceptors produces marked vasoconstriction in skeletal muscle resistance vessels, and there is an increase in the rate and force of cardiac contraction (Brigden et al., 1950; and see Kirchheim, 1976). It has been shown by intraneural recording from muscle nerves in man that head uptilting and the Valsalva maneuver cause an increase in sympathetic muscle nerve activity (Delius et al., 1972*b*). No significant change occurs in sympathetic activity in skin nerves (Delius et al., 1972*c*). Using a similar technique, Burke et al. (1977) have shown that there is an increase in sympathetic activity in muscle nerves changing from lying to sitting and from sitting to standing positions. The increase in sympathetic activity is accompanied by an increase in heart rate. These findings emphasize the importance of heart rate in maintaining blood pressure during the upright posture, as well as that of vasoconstrictor mechanisms.

The splanchnic vascular bed plays an important part in human blood pressure regulation. There is a decrease in hepatic blood flow upon assuming the upright posture, and this is abolished by splanchnicectomy (Culbertson et al., 1951; Wilkins et al., 1951). Other studies in which lower body negative pressure has been applied to normal subjects have confirmed the importance of the splanchnic vascular bed in human blood pressure control, and have indicated that decreased splanchnic conductance accounts for approximately one third of the reduction in total vascular conductance during the procedure (Rowell et al., 1972). Low pressure baroreceptors in the cardiopulmonary region may be responsible for initiating splanchnic and forearm vasoconstriction (Johnson et al., 1974). Further evidence of the importance of the mesenteric vascular bed is that sympathectomy has little influence on blood pressure control until the splanchnic nerves are sectioned (White and Smithwick, 1944; Wilkins et al., 1951); also, patients with spinal cord lesions do not develop significant postural hypotension unless the lesion lies above the level of the splanchnic outflow at T6 (Guttmann and Whitteridge, 1947). Constriction of venous capacitance beds may cause a redistribution of blood during postural changes (Page et al., 1955), but it does not appear to be an essential part of the compensatory vascular response for maintenance of systemic arterial blood pressure in the upright position (Samueloff et al., 1966). The renin-angiotensin system may also play a role in adjustment of blood pressure with alteration of posture (Cowley and Guyton, 1972; and see Oberg, 1976).

Control of Sweating

The eccrine sweat glands occur over most of the body and are innervated by postganglionic sympathetic nerve fibers in which acetylcholine is the neurotransmitter. Sweating is initiated by a rise in the central temperature acting upon the hypothalamus, and also probably reflexly from skin receptors (Kerslake, 1955). In certain areas (e.g., face, hands, feet, and axillae) the eccrine glands also respond to emotion. They can be stimulated chemically, even when denervated, by pilocarpine 5 to 15 mg administered I.M. There is a segmental innervation of the eccrine glands which is related approximately to the sensory dermatomes (List and Peet, 1938; Randall et al., 1952; Richter and Otenasek, 1946).

The apocrine glands in the axillae, nipples, and anogenital region respond to emotional stimuli and are stimulated by circulating adrenaline. They are probably not under the control of the autonomic nervous system (Evans, 1957).

Control of Pupillary Responses

The pupil is innervated by sympathetic and parasympathetic fibers. The adrenergic sympathetic postganglionic fibers arise from the superior cervical ganglion and ascend around the internal carotid artery to join the first division of the trigeminal nerve. They supply the dilator muscle of the pupil and some fibers innervate blood vessels in the orbit.

Parasympathetic fibers to the pupil course in the third nerve. Constrictor fibers to the pupil synapse in the ciliary ganglion, and cholinergic postganglionic fibers run in the short ciliary nerves to the sphincter pupillae muscle (Gabella, 1976).

Control of the Urinary Bladder

The smooth muscle of the bladder is innervated by sympathetic and parasympathetic fibers, while the external sphincter receives only somatic innervation.

Parasympathetic preganglionic fibers originate from the grey matter of sacral cord segments S2-4, emerge through the ventral roots, and travel in the pelvic nerves to form a diffuse subserosal network on the bladder surface. They synapse with postganglionic cells which

445

innervate the smooth muscle, causing the detrusor muscle to contract and the bladder neck to shorten and thus allow the passage of urine. Afferent fibers responsible for reflex bladder contraction run with the parasympathetic nerves to enter the spinal cord through the S2-4 dorsal roots.

Sympathetic preganglionic efferent fibers arise from the intermediolateral column of the spinal grey matter in T1-L2 segments. They run through the sympathetic ganglia and splanchnic nerves to the hypogastric plexus. Postganglionic fibers arise from cells in the hypogastric or vesical plexus and innervate the bladder musculature. Evidence concerning the function of the sympathetic efferents is conflicting, but they appear to play little part in the act of micturition (Kuru, 1965; Nyberg-Hansen, 1966; Plum, 1962). Sympathetic afferent fibers play no part in the micturition reflex.

TESTS OF AUTONOMIC FUNCTION

Tests of Sudomotor Function

The method of performing sweat tests has been described by Guttmann (1941), who defined the areas in which sweating occurs by covering the patient with a blue powder, quinizarin, that turns red when wet. Starch powder and iodine may also be used or alazarin red, which turns a deep violet when sweating occurs (Low et al., 1975a). The patient is warmed by raising the ambient temperature with a heat cradle until either the sublingual temperature has risen by 1° C or brisk sweating occurs over the forehead. Aspirin may also be given by mouth to stimulate sweating. Quantitative methods of measuring sweat production have been described (Young et al., 1975). Sweating may also be measured indirectly by recording changes in skin resistance (Richter, 1946; Ratcliffe and Jepson, 1950).

In peripheral nerve lesions anhidrosis usually occurs in the area of sensory loss because postganglionic sympathetic fibers are present in the peripheral nerve trunks. Guttmann (1940) demonstrated that the sweat test may be useful in the assessment of patients with peripheral nerve lesions. In acute and chronic polyneuropathies of different types sweating is usually impaired predominantly over the distal parts of the extremities, but also on the trunk.

Local hyperhidrosis may be seen in partial nerve injuries such as causalgia, and when there is pressure on nerve roots such as occurs in malignancy (Pool, 1956; Walsh et al., 1976) (Fig. 13–8) or on the lower brachial plexus by a cervical rib (Telford, 1942). Excess sweating may also occur in tetanus due to sympathetic overactivity (Kerr et al., 1968).

446

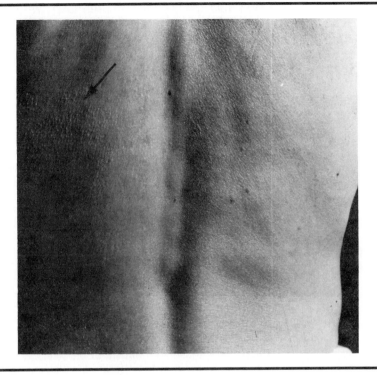

Figure 13–8 Spontaneous piloerection (*arrow*) in area of hidrosis on left side of thorax in a patient with underlying carcinoma of the lung.

Tests of Peripheral Vasomotor Control Peripheral blood flow is usually measured in the hand, forearm, foot, or leg by a variety of techniques, including venous occlusion plethysmograpy, mercury-in-rubber strain gauge plethysmography, measurement of skin temperature, and measurement of heat exchange using the heat flow discs on the skin. Alterations in finger blood flow reflect changes in the skin circulation, whereas forearm blood flow is mainly a manifestation of circulation through muscles. Vasodilatation is achieved by release of vasoconstrictor tone (Roddie et al., 1957).

RADIANT HEATING OF TRUNK The change in blood flow to the hand following application of radiant heat to the trunk was measured by Kerslake and Cooper (1950) and Cooper and Kerslake (1954). A rapid increase in the blood flow normally results from vasodilatation, which seems to be effected through a reflex mechanism and not by a rise in central temperature. The pathways are above C5 and are probably through the brain stem (Appenzeller and Schnieden, 1963).

447

APPLICATION OF ICE TO FOREHEAD AND NECK

Application of ice to the forehead and neck induces reflex vasoconstriction in the hand. The technique has a reproducible and detectable effect in normal individuals (De la Lande et al., 1960; Jamieson et al., 1971).

IMMERSION OF HAND IN HOT WATER Immersing one hand in hot water causes vasodilatation in the opposite hand and a concomitant increase in blood flow. This reflex is thought to be due to elevation in central temperature (Pickering, 1932).

MENTAL ARITHMETIC, NOISE, PAIN, AND EMOTIONAL STIMULI Emotional stress applied in various ways, such as performing mental arithmetic, causes an increase in heart rate and mean arterial blood pressure but has a variable effect on skin blood flow, which depends upon the initial environmental temperature (Ludbrook and Vincent, 1974; Ludbrook et al., 1975). Mental arithmetic causes an increase in sympathetic activity to skin vessels and a reduction in sympathetic activity to muscle vessels, the latter probably being mediated by inhibition of baroreceptors (Delius et al., 1972a, b, c). Since not all normal subjects have a rise in blood pressure in response to cold, loud noise, and mental arithmetic, the absence of reflex rise in blood pressure to these stimuli cannot be taken as firm evidence of a lesion in the efferent sympathetic pathways (Johnson and Spalding, 1974).

HAND GRIP Sustained hand grip for up to 5 minutes results in an increase in heart rate and in systolic and diastolic blood pressures. The blood pressure rise is partly due to increased output and partly to peripheral vasoconstriction. The response is impaired in diseases affecting the autonomic reflexes, such as diabetes and uremia. It is a useful screening test for autonomic dysfunction (Ewing et al., 1974; Ewing and Winney, 1975).

INSPIRATORY GASP A sudden inspiratory gasp causes a reduction of blood flow through the hand. The reflex is present in patients with cervical cord lesions above the sympathetic outflow to the hand and, hence, the pathway passes mainly through the spinal cord (Gilliatt, 1948; Gilliatt et al., 1948).

Tests of Baroreceptor Function

VALSALVA MANEUVER The subject is asked to maintain a column of mercury at 40 mm pressure for 10 to 15 seconds while in a semirecumbent posture. The blood pressure is recorded continuously through an intra-arterial catheter and the electrocardiogram (ECG) is monitored continuously. The patient should be given two or three practice attempts before a final recording is made.

There are four main phases in the response of arterial blood pressure to the Valsalva maneuver (Sharpey-Schafer and Taylor, 1960; Johnson and Spalding, 1974; Bannister et al., 1977) (Fig. 13–9).

Phase I There is a rise in arterial blood pressure due to the increased intrathoracic pressure being transmitted to the aorta.

Phase II There is a gradual reduction in the systolic, diastolic, and mean arterial blood pressures for several seconds, after which they plateau and may begin to rise. This is attributed to a reduction in venous return and cardiac output, followed by reflex vasoconstriction. There is also an increase in heart rate during phase II. The effectiveness of blowing may be assessed by the ratio of the fall in pulse pressure during phase II to the resting pulse pressure, and it is normally greater than 60 per cent (Bannister et al., 1977).

Phase III For about 2 seconds after the release of blowing pressure there is a sudden drop in intrathoracic pressure, resulting in an abrupt drop in the mean arterial blood pressure.

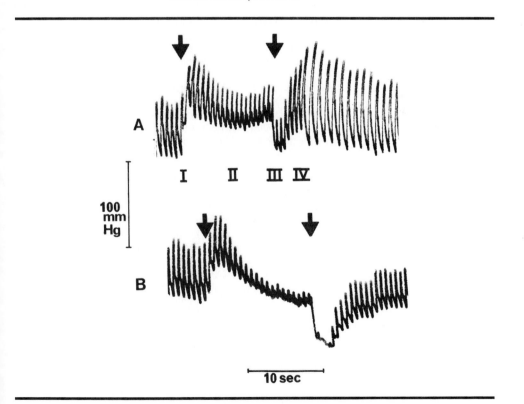

Figure 13–9 Normal Valsalva response in control subject (A) and blocked response in a patient with amyloid disease (B).

Phase IV The systolic and mean arterial blood pressures rise above the resting level. The pulse pressure increases above that in phase II, and the diastolic pressure usually rises but occasionally does not. The blood pressure returns to resting levels after a period of about 90 seconds. The overshoot in phase IV is usually attributed to reflex vasoconstriction (Sharpey-Schafer, 1953; Sarnoff et al., 1948), but increased cardiac output may be an important factor (Stone et al., 1965). The overshoot may be quantitated by relating the percentage change in pulse pressure during phase II to the percentage change in diastolic pressure during phase IV (Sharpey-Schafer, 1955; Sharpey-Schafer and Taylor, 1960).

Clear evidence of an abnormal Valsalva response due to impaired circulatory reflexes (Johnson and Spalding, 1974) is: (1) absence of systolic blood pressure overshoot in phase IV; (2) lower heart rate in phase II than in phase IV; (3) fall in mean arterial blood pressure in phase II below 50 per cent of the previous resting mean arterial pressure. An impaired or blocked Valsalva response may occur as a result of a wide range of conditions, which include: (1) heart disease and heart failure (Sharpey-Schafer, 1955; Gorlin et al., 1957); (2) asthma, emphysema (Barraclough and Sharpey-Schafer, 1963); (3) idiopathic orthostatic hypotension (Johnson et al., 1966); (4) cerebrovascular disease (Appenzeller and Descarries, 1964; (5) cervical cord lesions (Johnson et al., 1969); (6) drugs (Barraclough and Sharpey-Schafer, 1963; (7) tabes dorsalis (Sharpey-Schafer, 1956); (8) Holmes-Adie syndrome (Johnson et al., 1971); and (9) acute and chronic polyneuropathies (Scharpey-Schafer and Taylor, 1960; Watson, 1962). In neurological diseases a blocked Valsalva response may be a result of a lesion in the afferent or efferent limb of the reflex arc, or both.

VALSALVA RATIO The Valsalva ratio is a simple quantitative assessment of baroreceptor function which obviates the need for arterial catheterization. The patient performs the Valsalva maneuver while the ECG is monitored continuously. The Valsalva ratio is the ratio of the longest pulse interval to the shortest pulse interval during the maneuver (Levin, 1966). In over 96 per cent of controls the Valsalva ratio is greater than 1.5 (Levin, 1966; Low et al., 1975a). Although the Valsalva ratio is a useful screening test, it is a less sensitive measure of baroreceptor function than a full evaluation of the hemodynamic events which occur throughout the Valsalva maneuver, and it may be normal in patients who fail to show overshoot of the blood pressure in phase IV of the response (Low et al., 1975a).

CHANGE OF POSTURE The alteration in blood pressure and pulse rate with change in posture may be measured with the patient on a tilt table (Brigden et al., 1950). The blood pressure and pulse rate are monitored continuously with the patient lying supine until a steady state is achieved for about 10 minutes. The patient is then tilted 60°, or allowed to stand, while the blood pressure and pulse rate are monitored continuously. In normal subjects there is little or no fall in systolic or diastolic blood pressure (Currens, 1948). In patients with postural hypotension, there may be a marked drop in blood pressure which can lead to syncope.

SUBATMOSPHERIC PRESSURE TO THE LOWER PART OF THE BODY Instead of using a tilt table the pressure may be reduced in the legs and lower part of the body by enclosing the lower limbs and pelvis in an airtight metal box and reducing the pressure inside by means of a domestic vacuum cleaner. The pressure can be adjusted to levels 70 mm Hg below atmospheric pressure (Brown et al., 1964; Bannister et al., 1967).

NECK CHAMBER Carotid sinus transmural pressure may be altered by applying positive and negative pressures to a sealed chamber placed around the neck of conscious subjects (Eckberg et al., 1975; Ludbrook et al., 1977).

STIMULUS-RESPONSE CURVES The baroreceptor function may be assessed more precisely than with the Valsalva maneuver by measuring the heart rate response to alterations of blood pressure, whether spontaneous or induced (Martin et al., 1968; Bannister and Oppenheimer, 1972; Low et al., 1975a, b). The blood pressure may be reduced by tilting, lower body suction, or administration of intravenous glyceryl trinitrate, which causes peripheral vasodilatation. The blood pressure may be elevated with phenylephrine, a directly acting alpha-adrenergic agent which produces little or no cardiac effect in doses used to produce vasoconstriction (Varma et al., 1960; Loggie and Van Maanen, 1972), and which has been used to assess baroreceptor function in man (Robinson et al., 1966; Smyth et al., 1969; Korner et al., 1974). Pickering et al. (1967) plotted the systolic blood pressure of each successive pulse against the R-R interval of the next beat. Korner et al. (1972, 1974) studied the steady state properties of baroreceptor function in man and animals by plotting the stimulus-response curve over a wide range of arterial pressures, following injections of phenylephrine and glyceryl trinitrate. From their studies the authors derived various parameters, including heart period range (the difference between maximum and minimum heart period in response to induced blood pressure alterations) and mean gain (the slope of the curve of the pooled data between one standard deviation above and one standard deviation below the estimated blood

451

pressure at the middle of the heart period range — i.e., the mean heart period). These measurements help to define the range of the heart rate response as well as the maximum rate of response to alterations in mean arterial pressure. That is, one is able to quantitate not only the upper limits of the subject's heart rate response to major alterations in blood pressure but also the rate of change of the heart rate to minor alterations in blood pressure. The baroreceptor response curves may be abnormal even when the Valsalva response is normal (Low et al., 1975a), and are a more sensitive index of baroreceptor function than the Valsalva maneuver. The heart period-mean blood pressure curve is sigmoid (Fig. 13–10). The portion of the curve above the resting point tends to be a measure of vagal tone of the heart in response to mean arterial pressure elevation produced by phenylephrine, and the curve below the resting point tends to be a measure of the sympathetic tone in response to mean arterial pressure fall produced by glyceryl trinitrate.

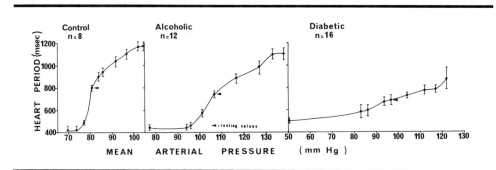

Figure 13–10 Stimulus-response curves relating heart period to mean arterial pressure in control subjects and patients with diabetic and alcoholic peripheral neuropathy.

Denervation Supersensitivity

Denervation supersensitivity may result from degeneration of postganglionic sympathetic nerve fibers. It is manifested by an abnormal pressor response to graded doses of intravenous phenylephrine, noradrenaline, or adrenaline (Smith and Dancis, 1964; Moorhouse et al., 1966; Martin et al., 1968; Low et al., 1975a, b) (Fig. 13–11).

Axon Reflex

Intradermal injection of acetylcholine (5 to 10 mg) stimulates an axon reflex in postganglionic sympathetic fibers, causing local piloerection and sweating. The axon reflex may be used to test the integrity of the postganglionic sympathetic pathways for sweating and piloerection

(Barany and Cooper, 1956). Acetylcholine may also be electrophoresed through the skin (MacMillan and Spalding, 1969). When postganglionic sympathetic fibers have degenerated, such as occurs with ganglionic and postganglionic lesions, the axon reflex may be abolished.

Tests of Cardiac Innervation

The sympathetic and vagal innervation of the heart may be tested by measuring the heart rate response to induced changes in blood pressure (see above). Impairment of vagal innervation may also be demonstrated by a reduction in the normal increase in heart rate to sustained hand grip (Ewing et al., 1974), the loss of beat-to-beat variation in heart rate with respiration (Wheeler and Watkins, 1973), or the absence of increase in heart rate after atropine.

Tests of Pupillary Innervation

Methacholine (Mecholyl) 2.5 per cent does not affect the size of the normal pupil but causes pupillary constriction in lesions of the parasympathetic innervation as a result of denervation supersensitivity. Homatropine 5 per cent causes dilatation of the normal pupil by blocking the action of acetylcholine but has a less pronounced effect when there is a lesion of the sympathetic innervation. Cocaine 4 per cent is a sympathomimetic agent which causes dilatation of the normal pupil. If there has been interruption of the sympathetic innervation outside the central nervous system, pupillary dilatation does not occur.

Tests of Bladder Function

The cystometrogram records the relationship of bladder volume to intravesical pressure. As the bladder is filled, the pressure rises gradually with each filling increment. Low level rhythmic contractions associated with a transient sensation of urgency usually develop at volumes of about 150 to 200 ml, and a sense of fullness at about 150 to 300 ml. Reflex micturition then starts with rhythmic waves of increasing amplitude, developing into a sustained contraction of the detrusor muscle. Bladder tone — i.e., the slope of the pressure-volume curve — is a function of the intrinsic properties of the smooth muscle of the bladder wall and is not affected directly by denervation or spinal cord section (Plum, 1962). However, loss of bladder tone may result from overdistention of the bladder, whether the initial cause is a lesion of the corticospinal connections, the sacral reflex arc, or simply psychogenic inhibition of the desire to void. A hypertonic bladder indicates a small contracted bladder, usually the result of chronic cystitis whether or not an upper motor neuron lesion is present. Rhythmic contractions of the bladder, like its tone, are an inherent property of the smooth muscle and are not related to its innervation.

453

Summary of Tests of Autonomic Function

The total baroreflex arc is tested by the Valsalva maneuver and by measurement of heart rate response to induced change of blood pressure. With the latter test it may be possible to recognize disorders affecting predominantly vagal or sympathetic innervation of the heart. The sympathetic efferent pathway is assessed by a number of tests, including the sweat test, measurement of the vasoconstrictor response to ice, noise, inspiratory gasp, hand grip, or the vasodilator response to radiant heat. Postganglionic sympathetic efferent lesions may be detected by impairment of the acetylcholine axon reflex or by the presence of denervation supersensitivity. There are no direct tests of the afferent limb of the baroreflex arc alone.

Relatively simple screening tests for autonomic dysfunction are the sweat test, tests for postural hypotension, measurement of the Valsalva ratio, measurement of heart rate and blood pressure response to hand grip, and the presence or absence of respiratory arrhythmia.

Innervation of the pupil and bladder may be tested separately.

AUTONOMIC DYSFUNCTION IN PERIPHERAL NEUROPATHY

Diabetes

Rundles (1945) wrote the first comprehensive account of the autonomic complications of diabetes, which include diarrhea, sphincter disturbances, impotence, and postural hypotension. Postural hypotension has been observed in diabetics by a number of workers (Rundles, 1945; Berner, 1952; Odel et al., 1955; Malins and French, 1957; Sharpey-Schafer and Taylor, 1960; Low et al., 1975a; Ewing et al., 1976a). The mechanism of postural hypotension is complex and has been discussed above. It is probably due to a combination of impairment of baroreflex activity and of peripheral and splanchnic vasoconstriction due to segmental demyelination and degeneration of small myelinated and unmyelinated fibers.

An abnormal Valsalva maneuver was reported in some patients with diabetic neuropathy by Sharpey-Schafer and Taylor (1960), and many other workers have subsequently confirmed their findings. Sharpey-Schafer and Taylor (1960) concluded that the abnormalities of the Valsalva maneuver were due to an afferent rather than an efferent limb lesion, but Bennett et al. (1976) reached the opposite conclusion. Postural hypotension cannot be correlated directly with the impairment of the Valsalva response because, in some patients with postural hypotension, the Valsalva is normal (Low et al., 1975a) and in other patients with an abnormal Valsalva response there is no postural hypotension (Bennett et al., 1976; Fraser et al., 1977).

There is other evidence of cardiac denervation in diabetes. There is impairment of the beat-to-beat variation in heart rate (Wheeler and Watkins, 1973; Lloyd-Mostyn and Watkins, 1975) which indicates vagal involvement. The absence of respiratory arrhythmia may occur early in the disease and in the absence of clinical peripheral neuropathy (Fekete et al, 1976; Neubauer and Gundersen, 1976; Gundersen and Neubauer, 1977). Persistent tachycardia may also occur in diabetics (Wheeler and Watkins, 1973; Low et al., 1975a), indicating a vagal efferent lesion. There is impairment of baroreceptor reflex responses and, in some patients, the heart appears to be completely denervated (Low et al., 1975a; Bennett et al., 1976; Lloyd-Mostyn and Watkins, 1976). The studies of baroreflex responses to changes in blood pressure indicate that both the sympathetic and vagal efferent innervation of the heart may be impaired in patients with diabetic neuropathy.

Denervation supersensitivity (Moorhouse et al., 1966; Frank et al., 1972; Low et al., 1975a) may be present, indicating involvement of sympathetic efferent pathways (Fig. 13–11). Pathological involvement of the unmyelinated fibers and small myelinated fibers may be an early feature of diabetic neuropathy, and is consistent with the finding of denervation hypersensitivity (Martin, 1953; Brown et al., 1976; Low et al., 1975a).

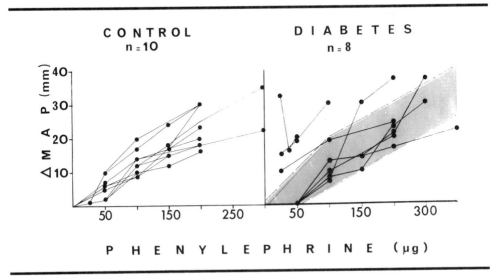

Figure 13–11 Denervation supersensitivity in diabetes. The changes in mean arterial pressure (Δ MAP, mm Hg) with graded doses of intravenous phenylephrine are shown in control and in diabetic subjects. Shaded area indicates control range.

455

Disturbances of reflex vasomotor response to body heating and cooling and to local heating and cooling have been demonstrated in diabetics (Martin, 1953; Moorhouse et al., 1966). Abnormal vasoconstrictor responses to ice and noise indicate lesions in the sympathetic efferent pathways (Frank et al., 1972).

Impotence is a well recognized complication of diabetes (Rundles, 1945; Martin, 1953; Buck et al., 1974), and may be due to the degeneration of the parasympathetic nerve endings in the corpora cavernosa that has been demonstrated pathologically (Faerman et al., 1974).

Diabetic diarrhea (Rundles, 1945; Martin, 1953; Malins and French, 1957; Whalen et al., 1969) is well recognized, and abnormal esophageal motility also occurs (Vela and Balart, 1970). In this context abnormalities demonstrated pathologically in the extrinsic and intrinsic parasympathetic fibers to the esophagus are of considerable importance (Smith, 1974).

Bladder dysfunction with incontinence or retention may also occur (Rundles, 1945). Decreased bladder sensation and increased bladder capacity may be demonstrated on cystometry (Buck et al., 1974). Decreased sweating (Martin, 1953; Low et al., 1975a) over the extremities is common, and increased facial sweating after food may also occur (Watkins, 1973).

Ewing et al. (1976a) have demonstrated that the abnormalities in autonomic function studies correlate with abnormalities of motor conduction velocity in the peripheral nerves. The prognosis in patients with diabetic autonomic neuropathy is poor (Ewing et al., 1976b).

Pathological studies of the autonomic nervous system in diabetic neuropathy are limited. Giant neurons in the sympathetic ganglia have been noted (Appenzeller and Richardson, 1966). Low et al. (1975a) made an autopsy study of the splanchnic nerves in patients with diabetic neuropathy and found that there was a significant loss of myelinated fibers and evidence of segmental demyelination in teased nerve fibers (Figs. 13–12 and 13–13). In another study, Appenzeller and Ogin (1974) found an increased fiber density in the white rami and abnormally short internodes, suggesting degeneration and regeneration.

Alcohol Although postural hypotension is common in Wernicke's encephalopathy, where it is probably the result of impaired sympathetic outflow at central or peripheral levels (Gravellese and Victor, 1957; Birchfield, 1964; Victor et al., 1971), it is not a common feature of uncomplicated alcoholic neuropathy (Low et al., 1975b).

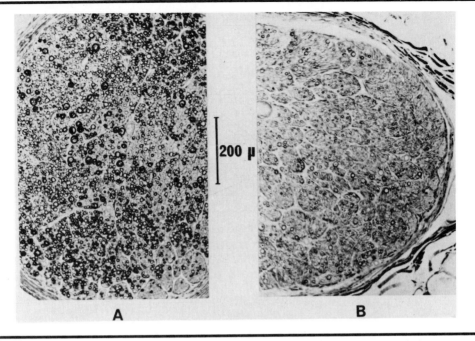

200 μ

A   B

Figure 13–12 Transverse sections of greater splanchnic nerve from a control subject (A) and a patient with diabetic neuropathy (B). There is a reduction in myelinated fibers in (B).

Of the seven patients with alcoholic peripheral neuritis studied by Barraclough and Sharpey-Schafer (1963), only one had postural hypotension. Low et al. (1975b) found no postural hypotension in 12 patients with clinical and electrophysiological evidence of peripheral nerve disease. In their patients baroreceptor function was only mildly impaired, and the curves relating mean arterial pressure to heart period retained their sigmoid shape and differed only slightly from those of controls in that their slope was mildly reduced (Fig. 13–10). Hypertension is associated with high alcoholic consumption (Klatsky et al., 1977) and this may have contributed to the mild abnormalities of baroreflex function, since the gain of the baroreceptor reflex is reduced by hypertension (Gribbin et al., 1971; Korner et al., 1974). The patients studied pathologically by Novak and Victor (1974) had very severe degrees of peripheral neuropathy associated with hoarseness and weakness of the voice, dysphagia, and autonomic disturbances.

Impairment of sweating occurs in alcoholic peripheral neuropathy, presumably due to the involvement of the postganglionic sympathetic efferent fibers in the peripheral nerves (Low et al., 1975b).

457

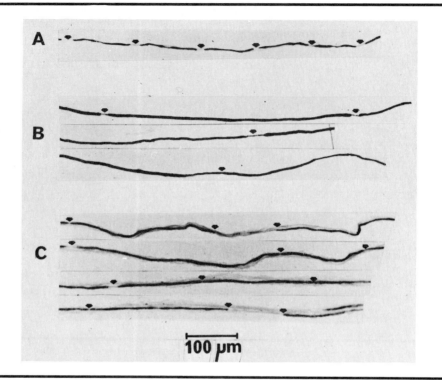

Figure 13–13 Teased single fibers from the greater splanchnic nerve of a subject with diabetes showing paranodal demyelination (*A, B*) and segmental demyelination (*C*). Arrows indicate nodes.

Only a few pathologic studies of the autonomic nervous system have been reported in alcoholic peripheral neuropathy. Degenerating giant neurons were found in the sympathetic ganglia of patients with alcoholic polyneuropathy, similar to those seen in diabetic neuropathy (Appenzeller and Richardson, 1966). Appenzeller and Ogin (1974) found increased numbers of myelinated fibers and short internodes in the white rami of alcoholic patients. Low et al. (1975*b*) found that the histological structure of the splanchnic nerve in patients with alcoholic neuropathy did not differ from that of controls, and contrasted with the marked degenerative changes in the splanchnic nerves of diabetic patients. These workers considered that the absence of postural hypotension and the relatively normal baroreceptor function was consistent with the absence of pathology in the splanchnic nerves, since postural hypotension is more likely to occur if the splanchnic outflow is involved. Novak and Victor (1974) found active myelin degeneration in the paravertebral sympathetic chain as well as degenerative changes in the vagus nerves of one very severely affected patient with hepatic encephalopathy, Wernicke's disease, and polyneuropathy. The impairment of sweating in alcoholic patients without postural hypotension is further evidence that involvement of postganglionic sympathetic efferent fibers of the limbs is not alone sufficient to cause postural hypotension and disturbance of baroreceptor function (Low et al., 1975b). The late involvement of the sympathetic and parasympathetic nervous systems in alcoholic neuropathy is consistent with the dying-back pathology of the disease.

Acute Idiopathic Polyneuritis (Landry-Guillain-Barré Syndrome)

Hypertension, hypotension, and tachycardia are well recognized complications of the Landry-Guillain-Barré syndrome (Haymaker and Kernohan, 1949; Marshall, 1963; Davies and Dingle, 1972). The response to the Valsalva maneuver may be blocked (Watson, 1962; Barraclough and Sharpey-Schafer, 1963), and postural hypotension may occur (Birchfield and Shaw, 1964). There is impairment of the heart rate response to changes in blood pressure (Fig. 13–14). Sweating may be normal or im-

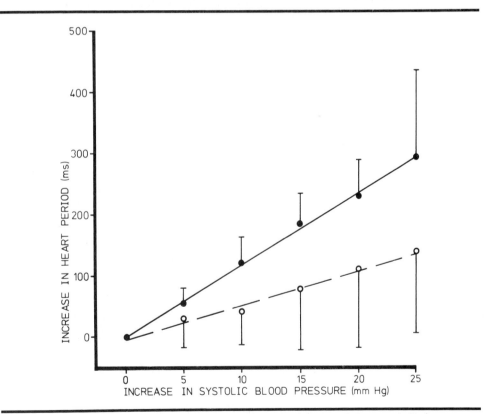

Figure 13–14 Relationship of increase in heart period to increase in systolic blood pressure in control subjects (closed circles) and in patients with the Landry-Guillian-Barré syndrome (open circles). Vertical bars represent one S.D. There is a significant impairment in the baroreceptor reflex in patients with Landry-Guillain-Barré syndrome.

paired (Johnson and Spalding, 1974) and vasomotor responses in the hand may be abnormal (Appenzeller and Marshall, 1963).

The dysautonomia in the Landry-Guillain-Barré syndrome is not found in all patients and is variable in its manifestations. The inconsistencies of the autonomic disturbances probably relate to the patchy nature of the pathology in the peripheral (Haymaker and Kernohan, 1949; Asbury et al., 1969) and autonomic nervous systems (Birchfield and Shaw, 1964; Matsuyama and Haymaker, 1967).

An experimental analogy to the Guillain-Barré syndrome is experimental allergic neuritis (EAN), in which the myelinated sympathetic and parasympathetic fibers may be affected by demyelinating lesions and are associated with changes in conduction (Tuck, 1978).

Acute Autonomic Neuropathy   Cases of acute autonomic neuropathy involving sympathetic and parasympathetic systems, most of which have recovered, have been described by several authors (Tomashefsky et al., 1972; Appenzeller and Kornfeld, 1973; Yahr and Frontera, 1975; Okada et al., 1975; Young et al., 1975). In one case the illness was related to infectious mononucleosis (Yahr and Frontera, 1975). It is probable that the condition is a form of acute polyneuritis restricted to the autonomic nervous system.

Amyloid   Amyloid disease may be associated with postural hypotension (Kyle et al., 1966), abnormalities of sweating, and impaired response to a Valsalva maneuver (Fig. 13–9) (Burns et al., 1971). Abnormal respiratory control, attributed to failure of peripheral chemoreceptor function, has been reported in one patient (Eisele et al., 1971). In the peripheral nerves of patients with primary amyloidosis, there is predominant loss of unmyelinated and small myelinated fibers (Dyck and Lambert, 1969); similar abnormalities in the autonomic efferent fibers would account for the physiological disturbances. Pathological changes have been described in the autonomic nervous system but morphometric studies have not been performed (Kyle et al., 1966; Appenzeller and True, 1967; Burns et al., 1971; Nordborg et al., 1973).

Vincristine   Postural hypotension, constipation, paralytic ileus, and abnormal Valsalva responses may occur in patients with vincristine neuropathy (McLeod and Penny, 1969; Casey et al., 1973; Hancock and Naysmith, 1975). The pathological changes in the peripheral nerves are those of axonal degeneration. Walsh (1971) found no abnormality in the splanchnic nerve of one patient who died with vincristine neuropathy.

Porphyria   Postural hypotension, hypertension, impairment of sweating, and tachycardia may occur in association with the neuropathy of porphyria (Schirger et al., 1962; Ridley et al., 1968).

Malignancy   Impairment of sweating occurs in association with the peripheral neuropathy of remote malignancies. In addition, postural hypotension has been reported in association with carcinoma of the bronchus (Ivy, 1961; Siemsen and Meister, 1963; Park et al., 1972; Ahmed and Carpenter, 1975) and of the pancreas (Thomas and Shields, 1970). Walsh (1971) investigated two patients with lymphoma who had postural hypotension, in one of whom there was a blocked Valsalva response.

Chronic Renal Failure   Autonomic dysfunction, manifested by postural hypertension and impaired response to the Valsalva maneuver and to induced hypotension, has been demonstrated in patients on chronic hemodialysis (Appenzeller and Lueker, 1972; Kersh et al., 1974). There is a reduced sensitivity of the baroreflex mechanisms (Pickering et al., 1972a), and it seems likely that the autonomic disturbances are related to the associated peripheral neuropathy.

Thallium Poisoning   Autonomic dysfunction was reported in three out of five cases of thallium poisoning by Bank et al. (1972). Tachycardia and hypertension were present in association with a peripheral neuropathy. Axonal degeneration appears to be the principal pathological change.

Charcot-Marie-Tooth Disease   Jammes (1972) tested autonomic function in five patients with probable dominantly inherited hypertrophic Charcot-Marie-Tooth disease. Sweating over the extremities was reduced. Reflex and vasomotor responses to body heating and cooling were impaired, and there was evidence of denervation supersensitivity. Abnormalities of pupillary reaction were also noted but there was no postural hypotension. The findings can be explained on the basis of involvement of postganglionic sympathetic efferents, as it is known that the unmyelinated fibers are damaged in this condition (Low et al., 1978).

Riley-Day Syndrome   Familial dysautonomia or Riley-Day syndrome is an autosomal recessive disorder, affecting mainly Jewish children, characterized by the autonomic disturbances of impaired lacrimation, postural hypotension, excessive sweating, and poor temperature control, in addition to reduced corneal and deep tendon reflexes and indifference to pain. The response to the Valsalva maneuver may be blocked and histamine skin reactions abnormal

461

(Aguayo et al., 1971). There may be a pupillary denervation supersensitivity response to methacholine 2.5 per cent and to phenylephrine, indicating involvement of both the sympathetic and parasympathetic fibers (Aguayo et al., 1971; Shinebourne et al., 1967). There is a marked reduction of small myelinated and unmyelinated fibers in the sural nerve (Aguayo et al., 1971; Pearson et al., 1975) and a reduction in neurons in the dorsal root ganglia and sympathetic ganglia (Pearson et al., 1971).

Tetanus

Sympathetic hyperactivity is well documented in tetanus and is manifested by hypertension, tachycardia, sweating, pyrexia, and sometimes hypotension (Kerr et al., 1968). There is no functional or structural peripheral nerve abnormality in the condition.

EXPERIMENTAL AUTONOMIC NEUROPATHY

Apart from surgical sympathectomy, the main techniques which have been employed for damaging the autonomic nervous system have been immunosympathectomy, specific sympathetic tissue antigens, 6-hydroxydopamine sympathectomy, toxic agents, and experimental allergic neuritis (EAN).

Immuno-sympathectomy

Nerve growth factor (NGF) is a protein which was originally isolated from mouse sarcoma, and later from snake venom and mouse submaxillary salivary glands. It is necessary for the growth and maintenance of sympathetic and certain sensory neurons (Levi-Montalcini and Angeletti, 1968; Mobley et al., 1977). Injection of NGF antiserum into newborn mice and other animals causes permanent destruction of about 90 to 95 per cent of sympathetic neurons in the paravertebral ganglia, a technique known as immunosympathectomy (Cohen, 1960; Levi-Montalcini and Booker, 1960; Levi-Montalcini and Angeletti, 1966, 1968). Administration of NGF antiserum to rats causes almost complete destruction of paravertebral ganglia and severe atrophy of the celiac ganglion, but has little effect on the mesenteric ganglion (Zaimis et al., 1965). Electrical activity is reduced in the sympathetic nerves following immunosympathectomy, and there is also a loss of the normal vasoconstrictor response when the nerves are stimulated electrically (Brody, 1963, 1964). After immunosympathectomy, regenerative sprouting of unmyelinated fibers does not occur unless the nerves are subsequently crushed (Aguayo et al., 1972; Bray et al., 1973).

The relationship of immunosympathectomy to human diseases remains uncertain. There has been a report of an increase in serum antigen levels of β-NGF in patients with familial dysautonomia (Riley-Day syndrome) (Siggers et al., 1976), but the significance of these observations has been questioned (Levi-Montalcini, 1976). It has also been suggested that NGF levels in patients with idiopathic orthostatic hypotension should be investigated (Levi-Montalcini, 1976; Kontos, 1977), but in one case no abnormalities were detected (Goedert and Buhler, 1977).

Specific Sympathetic Tissue Antigen

Appenzeller et al. (1965) described an experimental autonomic neuropathy in rabbits induced by a sympathetic tissue antigen. Rabbits were injected with an antigen extracted from human sympathetic nerves and ganglia. In the majority of treated animals, reflex vasodilatation in the ear in response to heating the back was abolished 6 to 14 days after immunization. A circulating antibody which appeared to be specific to sympathetic tissue was absorbed out of the immune sera by sympathetic but not by sciatic nerve, Gasserian ganglion, or liver extracts and, on electrophoresis, it migrated as a beta protein. Vascular reflexes were not affected in animals immunized with sciatic nerve and Gasserian ganglion tissue antigen, although they had clinical evidence of allergic neuritis. Mild pathological lesions of delayed hypersensitivity type were found in the sympathetic chain of some animals but were not considered to be responsible for the disorder. It was suggested that the experimental disease was an immunological disorder, probably affecting efferent sympathetic cholinergic fibers and associated with the presence of a specific circulating antibody. It differed immunologically, pathologically, and functionally from experimental allergic neuritis. The authors suggested that the experimental autonomic neuropathy may resemble the human dysautonomias manifested by orthostatic hypotension and disturbances of sweating, lacrimation, and salivation without morphological change in sympathetic ganglia.

6-Hydroxydopamine Sympathectomy

6-hydroxydopamine (6-OHDA) administered systemically produces a long-standing depletion of noradrenaline from peripheral sympathetic innervated organs (Laverty et al., 1965). In adult animals there is selective destruction of peripheral adrenergic nerve terminals, the cell body remaining morphologically unaffected, and regeneration occurs after cessation of the drug (Tranzer and Thoenen, 1968; Bennett et al., 1970; Eranko and Eranko, 1972). In newborn animals sympathetic ganglion cells are destroyed and regeneration does not occur (Angeletti and Levi-Montalcini, 1970; Angeletti, 1971). There is a failure to generate or conduct nerve impulses in response to electrical stimulation of the sympathetic nerves within 1 hour after 6-OHDA injections but, on recovery, a normal response to sympathetic nerve stimulation is obtained before the noradrenaline tissue stores are replenished (Haeusler, 1971).

463

AUTONOMIC NERVOUS SYSTEM

The effects of 6-OHDA on mesenteric vascular control have been studied in cats (Post and McLeod, 1973; Post, 1976). The animals were given two intraperitoneal injections of 6-OHDA (100 mg per kg) at an interval of 24 hours and the two injections were repeated 7 and 14 days later. On the fifteenth and sixteenth days after the commencement of poisoning, electrophysiological studies were performed. There was no alteration in the motor conduction velocity in the posterior tibial nerve or of the amplitude of the compund muscle action potential recorded from the foot. However, studies of mesenteric blood flow demonstrated that the neural control of the mesenteric vascular bed was abnormal. There was denervation supersensitivity to noradrenaline and phenylephrine, there was no response to intravenous tyramine which releases endogenous noradrenaline from the vesicles in the adrenergic terminals, and there was a markedly impaired vasoconstrictor response to electrical stimulation of the splanchnic nerve (Fig. 13–15). No morphological changes were demonstrated in the posterior tibial or splanchnic nerves.

6-OHDA therefore produces a chemical sympathectomy in animals that results in impairment of vasomotor control. However, there appears to be no precise clinical counterpart in man of the sympathetic failure of animals poisoned with 6-OHDA. In idiopathic orthostatic hypotension and in the Shy-Drager syndrome, in which sympathetic failure occurs, the postganglionic cholinergic fibers are involved as well as the adrenergic fibers.

Acrylamide Neuropathy

Acrylamide is known to damage peripheral myelinated nerve fibers and to cause a dying-back type of degeneration (Fullerton and Barnes, 1966; Prineas, 1969; Hopkins, 1970; Hopkins and Gilliatt, 1971; Schaumburg et al., 1974). Some workers have made brief mention of clinical abnormalities suggestive of involvement of the autonomic nervous system, such as distended bladder in rats (Fullerton and Barnes, 1966) and excessive sweating in man (Auld and Bedwell, 1967). Alteration in the voice, implying involvement of the vagus nerve, has also been noted (Leswing and Ribelin, 1969; Bradley and Asbury, 1970; Hopkins, 1970). Hopkins (1970) found histopathological changes of loss of myelinated fibers in the recurrent laryngeal nerve of one baboon with aphonia.

Systematic studies of the neurophysiological, pathological, and vasomotor changes in cats poisoned with acrylamide have been made (Post and McLeod, 1973, 1977a, b; Post, 1976). The animals were poisoned with 15 mg/kg of acrylamide for periods of up to 16 weeks. They were described as mildly poisoned when they displayed weakness of the hind limbs only, moderately poisoned when forelimbs as well as hind limbs were affected, and severely poisoned when they were unable to walk because of

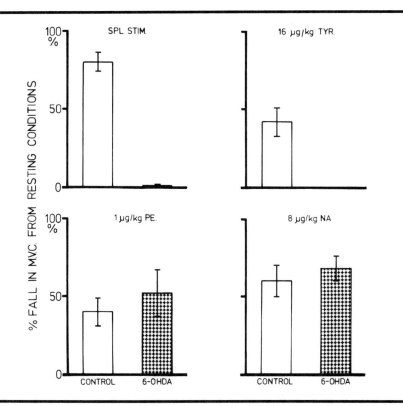

Figure 13–15 Changes in mesenteric vascular conductance (MVC) in control and 6-OHDA-poisoned cats following splanchnic nerve stimulation (SPL. STIM.) and intravenous injection of phenylephrine (PE), tyramine (TYR), and noradrenaline (NA). There is denervation supersensitivity to noradrenaline and phenylephrine, a markedly impaired vasoconstrictor response to splanchnic nerve stimulation, and no response to tyramine in 6-OHDA-poisoned cats. Vertical bars represent ± 1 S.D.

severe paralysis of both forelimbs and hind limbs. The duration of poisoning was 4 to 6 weeks in mildly poisoned animals, 6 to 12 weeks in moderately poisoned animals, and 12 to 16 weeks in the severely poisoned cats. Motor conduction velocities in the posterior tibial nerve and amplitude of the muscle action potential in the small muscles of the foot were reduced in the affected animals. The compound action potential was recorded from the greater splanchnic nerve. Its main components were an Aβ wave, representing conduction in the large myelinated fibers (8 to 16 μm), and a B wave which represented conduction in the small myelinated preganglionic sympathetic efferent fibers (2 to 6 μm) (McLeod, 1958). There was progressive slowing of both the Aβ and B waves as the duration and severity of the poisoning increased. Similar changes were noted in the amplitude and time integral of the waves (Figs. 13–4 and 13–16).

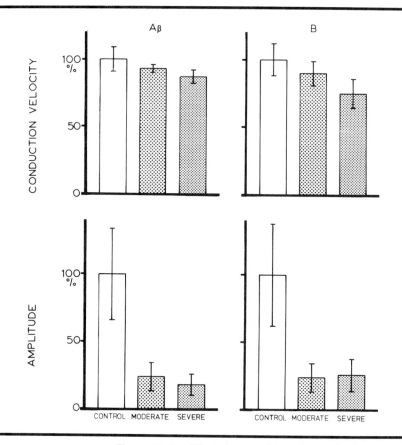

Figure 13–16 Effect of acrylamide on the conduction velocity and amplitude of the Aβ and B waves in the compound action potential of the splanchnic nerve of the cat. The values are expressed as a percentage of mean control values. Vertical bars represent ± 1 S.D.

These neurophysiological findings, which indicate damage to both large and small myelinated fibers in the sympathetic nervous system, were confirmed by histological studies on the splanchnic nerve. Similar histological changes were also noted in the vagus nerve. In order to compare the effect of acrylamide on the somatic, sympathetic, and parasympathetic nervous systems, the density of myelinated fibers that remained in the nerve to medial head of gastrocnemius (NMG), splanchnic, and vagus nerves from each group of poisoned animals was expressed as a percentage of the mean control value. It is clear that, as the duration of the period of intoxication increased, there was a corresponding decrease in the percentage of myelinated fibers remaining in each nerve and also that NMG was damaged the most severely and the splanchnic nerve the least (Fig. 13–17). The findings

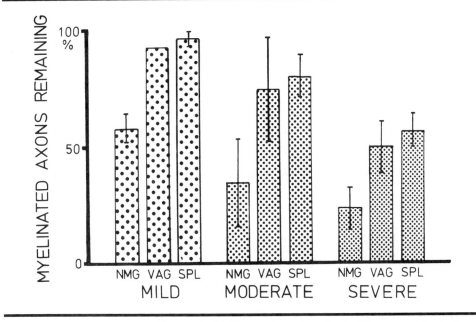

Figure 13–17 The numbers of myelinated fibers remaining in the acrylamide-poisoned nerve to the medial head of gastrocnemius muscle (NMG) and the vagus (VAG) and splanchnic (SPL) nerves expressed as a percentage of the mean total myelinated fiber density of the controls. Vertical bars represent ± 1 S.D. Only two vagus nerves were counted in the mildly poisoned group, and hence no S.D. was calculated.

suggest that acrylamide affects the longest nerve fibers first and most severely, and that the autonomic fibers are not greatly affected until the animals have a severe peripheral neuropathy.

Studies of the vasomotor control of the mesenteric vascular bed were performed on the poisoned animals. There was impairment of the vasoconstrictor response to splanchnic nerve stimulation and a decreased response to tyramine, which releases endogenous noradrenaline from the vesicles in the adrenergic terminals. Denervation supersensitivity was found with phenylephrine and noradrenaline. Abnormalities of vasomotor control were demonstrated in mildly and severely poisoned animals, although these were more pronounced in the latter (Fig. 13–18). There was also histological and pharmacological evidence of damage to the postganglionic sympathetic unmyelinated fibers (Post, 1978), although in a previous study Hopkins and Lambert (1972) had found no electrophysiological changes in the unmyelinated postganglionic sympathetic efferent fibers in the cervical sympathetic chain of the rat following acrylamide intoxication.

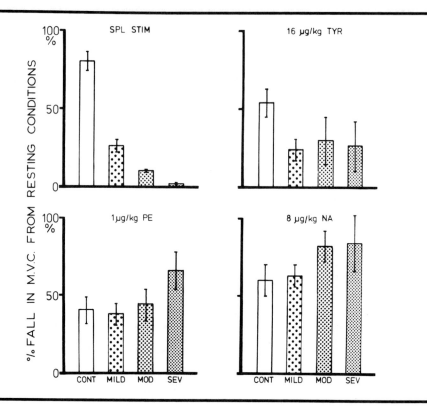

Figure 13–18 Changes in mesenteric vascular conductance (MVC) in control cats and mildly, moderately, and severely acrylamide-poisoned cats following splanchnic nerve stimulation (SPL. STIM) and intravenous injection of phenylephrine (PE), tyramine (TYR), and noradrenaline (NA). There is an impaired vasoconstrictor response to splanchnic nerve stimulation and a decreased response to tyramine. There is an increased vasoconstrictor response (denervation supersensitivity) to phenylephrine and noradrenaline. Abnormalities are most pronounced in severely poisoned animals.

Baroreceptor reflex function has been studied in another series of severely acrylamide-poisoned cats (Post and McLeod, 1977c). The heart rate response to a 60-degree tilt from the horizontal posture, to arterial blood loss of 40 ml, and to 20 μg of phenylephrine was significantly reduced in severely poisoned cats when compared with controls. These findings indicate that autonomic control of the heart is affected in severely poisoned animals (Fig. 13–19).

It may be concluded from these studies that in acrylamide neuropathy, which is a model of dying-back neuropathies in man, the myelinated fibers in the vagus nerve and preganglionic division of the sympathetic nervous system are affected. Postganglionic unmyelinated sympathetic efferent fibers are also involved to some

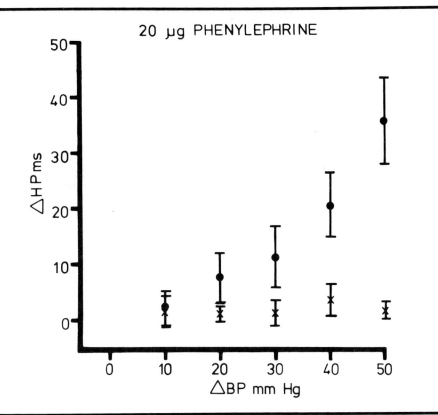

Figure 13–19 Effect of acrylamide on baroreceptor reflex. Change in heart period (△HP) is plotted against rise in systemic blood pressure (△BP) induced by 20 μg phenylephrine. Filled circles represent values in control animals; crosses represent values in acrylamide-poisoned animals. Mean ± 1 S.D.

extent. Autonomic involvement is most pronounced in animals with a severe peripheral neuropathy, since the shorter fibers are not affected until the later stages of the toxic process. There are resulting disturbances in the vasomotor control of the mesenteric vascular bed which plays an important role in the regulation of blood pressure following change in posture. Innervation of the heart is also affected by acrylamide, and this results in impairment of the heart rate response to changes in blood pressure in severely poisoned animals.

Experimental Allergic Neuritis

Tuck (1978) has recently succeeded in producing demyelinated lesions in the splanchnic and vagus nerves of guinea pigs with EAN. In Tuck's experiments, slowing of conduction and dispersion of the compound action potential of the myelinated fibers have been demonstrated. These studies are the first to show experimental demyelination in the autonomic nervous system and are of particular relevance to the clinical disorder of the Landry-Guillain-Barré syndrome, in which autonomic dysfunction may occur.

SUMMARY AND CONCLUSIONS

The autonomic nervous system consists of the sympathetic (thoracolumbar) and parasympathetic (craniosacral) divisions.

In the sympathetic nervous system the preganglionic efferent fibers are myelinated and in man range in diameter from about 1 to 5 μm. The postganglionic efferent fibers are unmyelinated. In the vagus nerve, the motor fibers to the heart are unmyelinated or are small diameter myelinated fibers. Most of the afferent fibers in the carotid sinus and aortic depressor nerves are myelinated and are in the 2 to 6-μm range. Thus, on both afferent and efferent sides of the autonomic nervous system, the fibers concerned with cardiovascular control are predominantly small diameter myelinated or unmyelinated fibers.

In peripheral neuropathies impairment of sweating is common, presumably due to the involvement of the unmyelinated sympathetic fibers in the peripheral nerve. However, disturbances of blood pressure and heart rate control and postural hypotension are less common and occur predominantly in disorders which affect primarily small diameter myelinated and unmyelinated fibers, such as amyloid disease, familial dysautonomia (Riley-Day syndrome), and diabetes. Postural hypotension is most likely to occur when the splanchnic nerve and innervation of the mesenteric vascular bed are affected pathologically, and this has been demonstrated to be the case in diabetes. In acute idiopathic polyneuritis (Landry-Guillain-Barré syndrome) autonomic dysfunction is variable because of the patchy demyelination which occurs throughout the autonomic and peripheral nervous systems, and it is most likely to be present when there is demyelination of the preganglionic sympathetic efferent fibers and of the myelinated fibers in the vagus nerve.

In alcoholic and other dying-back neuropathies, postural hypotension and other major disturbances of autonomic function occur only in severe cases in which the unmyelinated fibers and small myelinated fibers in the autonomic nervous system become involved, and the innervation of the splanchnic bed is affected. The autonomic nerves are shorter than the peripheral nerves and are likely to be affected significantly only late in the course of a dying-back neuropathy.

In acrylamide autonomic neuropathy, myelinated and some unmyelinated fibers in the splanchnic nerve and sympathetic trunk and in the vagus nerve degenerate,

470

particularly in severely poisoned animals. There is slowing of conduction of large and small myelinated fibers in the splanchnic nerve. Disturbances of autonomic function are more pronounced in severely poisoned animals. In experimental allergic neuritis (EAN) the vagus and splanchnic nerves may be demyelinated, and there is slowing of conduction and dispersion of the action potentials. The autonomic neuropathy in EAN may be relevant to the disturbances of autonomic function which occur in the Landry-Guillain-Barré syndrome.

References

Adrian, E. D., Bronk, D. W., and Phillips, G.: Discharge in mammalian sympathetic nerves. J. Physiol. (Lond.), *74*:115, 1932.

Agostoni, E., Chinnock, J. E., Daly, M. de B., and Murray, J. G.: Functional and histological studies of the vagus nerve and its branches to the heart, lungs and abdominal viscera of the cat. J. Physiol. (Lond.), *135*:182, 1957.

Aguayo, A. J., Martin, J. B., and Bray, G. M.: Effects of nerve growth factor antiserum on peripheral unmyelinated fibers. Acta Neuropathol. (Berl.), *20*:288, 1972.

Aguayo, A. J., Nair, C. P. V., and Bray, G. M.: Peripheral nerve abnormalities in the Riley-Day syndrome. Findings in a sural nerve biopsy. Arch. Neurol., *24*:106, 1971.

Ahmed, M. N., and Carpenter, S.: Autonomic neuropathy and carcinoma of the lung. Can. Med. Assoc. J., *113*:410, 1975.

Amassian, V. E.: Fiber groups and spinal pathways of cortically represented visceral afferents. J. Neurophysiol., *14*:445, 1951.

Angell-James, J. E., and Daly, M. de B.: Comparison of the reflex vasomotor responses to separate and combined stimulation of the carotid sinus and aortic arch baroreceptors by pulsatile and non-pulsatile pressures in the dog. J. Physiol., *209*:257, 1970.

Angeletti, P. U.: Chemical sympathectomy in newborn animals. Neuropharmacology, *10*:55, 1971.

Angeletti, P. U., and Levi-Montalcini, R.: Sympathetic nerve cell destruction in newborn mammals by 6-hydroxydopamine. Proc. Natl. Acad. Sci. U.S.A., *65*:114, 1970.

Appenzeller, O.: The Autonomic Nervous System. An Introduction to Basic and Clinical Concepts, 2nd ed. Amsterdam, North Holland, 1976.

Appenzeller, O., Arnason, B. G., and Adams, R. D.: Experimental autonomic neuropathy: An immunologically induced disorder of reflex vasomotor function. J. Neurol. Neurosurg. Psychiatry, *28*:510, 1965.

Appenzeller, O., and Descarries, L.: Circulatory reflexes in patients with cerebrovascular disease. N. Engl. J. Med., *271*:820, 1964.

Appenzeller, O., and Kornfeld, M.: Acute pandysautonomia. Clinical and morphologic study. Arch. Neurol., *29*:334, 1973.

Appenzeller, O., and Lueker, R.: Autonomic dysfunction in patients on chronic hemodialysis. Neurology(Minneap.), *22*:395, 1972.

AUTONOMIC NERVOUS SYSTEM

Appenzeller, O., and Marshall, J.: Vasomotor disturbance in Landry-Guillain-Barré syndrome. Arch. Neurol., 9:368, 1963.

Appenzeller, O., and Ogin, G.: Myelinated fibers in the human paravertebral sympathetic chain: Quantitative studies on white rami communicantes. J. Neurol. Neurosurg. Psychiatry, 36:777, 1973.

Appenzeller, O., and Ogin, G.: Myelinated fibers in human paravertebral sympathetic chain: White rami communicantes in alcoholic and diabetic patients. J. Neurol. Neurosurg. Psychiatry, 37:1155, 1974.

Appenzeller, O., and Richardson, E. P.: The sympathetic chain in patients with diabetic and alcoholic neuropathy. Neurology (Minneap.), 16:1205, 1966.

Appenzeller, O., and Schnieden, H.: Neurogenic pathways concerned in reflex vasodilatation in the head with especial reference to stimuli affecting the afferent pathway. Clin. Sci., 25:413, 1963.

Appenzeller, O., and True, C. W.: Amyloidosis confined to the central and peripheral nervous system. J. Neuropathol. Exp. Neurol., 26:174, 1967.

Asbury, A. K., Arnason, B. G., and Adams, R. D.: The inflammatory lesion in idiopathic polyneuritis — its role in pathogenesis. Medicine (Baltimore), 48:173, 1969.

Auld, R. B., and Bedwell, S. F.: Peripheral neuropathy with sympathetic overactivity from industrial contact with acrylamide. Can. Med. Assoc. J., 96:652, 1967.

Bank, W. J., Pleasure, D. E., Suzuki, K., Nigro, M., and Katz, R.: Thallium poisoning. Arch. Neurol., 26:456, 1972.

Bannister, R., Ardill, L., and Fentem, P.: Defective autonomic control of blood vessels in idiopathic orthostatic hypotension. Brain, 9:725, 1967.

Bannister, R., and Oppenheimer, D. R.: Degenerative diseases of the nervous system associated with autonomic failure. Brain, 95:457, 1972.

Bannister, R., Sever, P., and Gross, M.: Cardiovascular reflexes and biochemical responses in progressive autonomic failure. Brain, 100:327, 1977.

Barany, F. R., and Cooper, E. H.: Pilomotor and sudomotor innervation in diabetes. Clin. Sci., 15:533, 1956.

Barraclough, M. A., and Sharpey-Schafer, E. P.: Hypotension from absent circulatory reflexes. Effects of alcohol, barbiturates, psychotherapeutic drugs and other mechanisms. Lancet, 1:1121, 1963.

Bennett, T., Burnstock, G., Cobb, J. L. S., and Malmfors, T.: An ultrastructural and histochemical study of the short-term effects of 6-hydroxydopamine on adrenergic nerves in the domestic fowl. Br. J. Pharmacol., 38:802, 1970.

Bennett, T., Hosking, D. J., and Hampton, J. R.: Baroreflex sensitivity and responses to the Valsalva manoeuvre in subjects with diabetes mellitus. J. Neurol. Neurosurg. Psychiatry, 39:178, 1976.

Berner, J. H., Jr.: Orthostatic hypotension in diabetes mellitus. Acta Med. Scand., 143:336, 1952.

Birchfield, R. I.: Postural hypotension in Wernicke's disease. Am. J. Med., 36:404, 1964.

AUTONOMIC NERVOUS SYSTEM

Birchfield, R. I., and Shaw, C. M.: Postural hypotension in the Guillain-Barré syndrome. Arch. Neurol., *10*:149, 1964.

Bonica, J. J.: Autonomic innervation of the viscera in relation to nerve block. Anesthesiology, *29*:793, 1968.

Bradley, W. G., and Asbury, A. K.: Radioautographic studies of Schwann cell behavior. Part I. Acrylamide neuropathy in the mouse. J. Neuropathol. Exp. Neurol., *29*:500, 1970.

Bray, G. M., Aguayo, A. J., and Martin, J. B.: Immunosympathectomy: Late effects on the composition of rat cervical sympathetic trunks and influence on axonal regeneration after crush. Acta. Neuropathol. (Berl.), *26*:345, 1973.

Brigden, W., Howarth, S., and Sharpey-Schafer, E. P.: Postural changes in the peripheral blood flow of normal subjects with observations on vasovagal fainting reactions as a result of tilting, the lordotic posture, pregnancy and spinal anaesthesia. Clin. Sci., *9*:79, 1950.

Brody, M. J.: Electrical activity in sympathetic nerves of immunologically sympathectomized rats. Proc. Soc. Exp. Biol. Med., *114*:565, 1963.

Brody, M. J.: Cardiovascular responses following immunological sympathectomy. Circ. Res., *15*:161, 1964.

Brown, E., Goei, J. S., Greenfield, A. D. M., and Plassaras, G.: Circulatory responses to a large but brief increase in venous return in man. J. Physiol., (Lond.), *170*:21P, 1964.

Brown, M. J., Martin, J. R., and Asbury, A. K.: Painful diabetic neuropathy. A morphometric study. Arch. Neurol., *33*:164, 1976.

Buck, A. C., McRae, C. U., Reed, P. I., and Chisholm, G. D.: The diabetic bladder. Proc. R. Soc. Med., *67*:81, 1974.

Bulbring, E., and Burn, J. H.: The sympathetic dilator fibers in the muscles of the cat and dog. J. Physiol. (Lond.), *83*:483, 1935.

Burke, D., Sundlof, G., and Wallin, B. G.: Postural effects on muscle nerve sympathetic activity in man. J. Physiol. (Lond.), *272*:399, 1977.

Burns, R. J., Downey, J. A., Grewin, D. B., and Whelan, R. F.: Autonomic dysfunction with orthostatic hypotension. Aust. N.Z. J. Med., *1*:15, 1971.

Casey, E. B., Jellife, A. M., LeQuesne, P. M., and Millett, Y. L.: Vincristine neuropathy — clinical and electrophysiological observations. Brain, *96*:69, 1973.

Cohen, S.: Purification of a nerve-growth promoting protein from the mouse salivary gland and its neuro-cytotoxic antiserum. Proc. Natl. Acad. Sci. U.S.A., *46*:302, 1960.

Cooper, K. E., and Kerslake, D. M.: Some aspects of the reflex control of the cutaneous circulation. *In* CIBA Foundation Symposium on Peripheral Circulation in Man. London, Churchill, 1954, pp. 143–149.

Cowley, A. W., Jr., and Guyton, A. C.: Quantification of intermediate steps in the renin-angiotensin-vasoconstrictor feedback loop in the dog. Circ. Res., *30*:557, 1972.

Culbertson, J. W., Wilkins, R. W., Ingelfinger, F. J., and Bradley, S. E.: The effect of the upright posture upon hepatic blood flow in normotensive and hypertensive subjects. J. Clin. Invest., *30*:305, 1951.

473

Currens, J. H.: A comparison of the blood pressure in the lying and standing positions: A study of five hundred men and five hundred women. Am. Heart J., *35*:646, 1948.

Davies, A. G., and Dingle, H. R.: Observations on cardiovascular and neuro-endocrine disturbance in the Guillain-Barré syndrome. J. Neurol. Neurosurg. Psychiatry, *35*:176, 1972.

De la Lande, I. S., Parks, V. J., Sandison, A. G., Skinner, S. L., and Whelan, R. F.: The peripheral vasodilator action of reserpine in man. Aust. J. Exp. Biol. Med. Sci., *38*:313, 1960.

Delius, W., Hagbarth, K. E., Hongell, A., and Wallin, B. G.: General characteristics of sympathetic activity in human muscle nerves. Acta Physiol. Scand., *84*:65, 1972*a*.

Delius, W. , Hagbarth, K. E., Hongell, A., and Wallin, B. G.: Manoeuvres affecting sympathetic outflow in human muscles nerves. Acta Physiol. Scand., *84*:82, 1972*b*.

Delius, W., Hagbarth, K. E., Hongell, A., and Wallin, B. G.: Manoeuvres affecting sympathetic outflow in human skin nerves. Acta Physiol. Scand., *84*:177, 1972*c*.

Donald, D. E., and Edis, A. J.: Comparison of aortic and carotid sinus baroreflexes in the dog. J. Physiol. (Lond.), *215*:521, 1971.

Dyck, P. J., and Lambert, E. H.: Dissociated sensation in amyloidosis. Arch. Neurol., *20*:490, 1969.

Eckberg, D. L, Cavanaugh, M. S., Mark, A. L., and Abboud, F. M.: A simplified neck suction device for activation of carotid baroreceptors. J. Lab. Clin. Med., *85*:167, 1975.

Eckberg, D. L., Fletcher, G. F., and Braunwald, E.: Mechanisms of prolongation of the R-R interval with electrical stimulation of the carotid sinus nerves in man. Circ. Res., *30*:131, 1972.

Eisele, J. H., Cross, C. E., Rausch, D. C., Kurpershoek, C. J., and Xelis, R. F.: Abnormal respiratory control in acquired dysautonomia. N. Engl. J. Med., *285*:366, 1971.

Eranko, L., and Eranko, O.: Effect of 6-hydroxydopamine on the ganglion cells and small intensely fluorescent cells in the superior cervical ganglion of the rat. Acta Physiol. Scand., *84*:115, 1972.

Evans, C. L.: Sweating in relation to sympathetic innervation. Br. Med. Bull., *13*:197, 1957.

Evans, D. H. L., and Murray, J. G.: Histological and functional studies on the fiber composition of the vagus nerve in the rabbit. J. Anat., *88*:320, 1954.

Ewing, D. J., Burt, A. A., Williams, I. R., Campbell, I. W., and Clarke, B. F.: Peripheral motor nerve function in diabetic autonomic neuropathy. J. Neurol. Neurosurg. Psychiatry, *39*:453, 1976*a*:

Ewing, D. J., Campbell, I. W., and Clarke, B. F.: Mortality in diabetic autonomic neuropathy. Lancet, *1*:601, 1976*b*.

Ewing, D. J., Irving, J. B., Kerr, F., Wildsmith, J. A. W., and Clarke, B. F.: Cardiovascular responses to sustained handgrip in normal subjects and in patients with diabetes mellitus. A test of autonomic function. Clin. Sci. Mol. Med., *46*:295, 1974.

Ewing, D. J., and Winney, R.: Autonomic function in patients with chronic renal failure on intermittent haemodialysis. Nephron, *15*:424, 1975.

AUTONOMIC NERVOUS SYSTEM

Eyzaguirre, C., and Uchizono, K.: Observations on the fiber content of nerves reaching the carotid body of the cat. J. Physiol. (Lond.), *159*:268, 1961.

Faerman, I., Glocer, L., Fox, D., Jadzinsky, M. N., and Rapaport, M.: Impotence and diabetes. Histological studies of the autonomic nervous fibers of the corpora cavernosa in impotent diabetic males. Diabetes, *23*:971, 1974.

Fekete, T., Rub, D., and Bogdan, E.: Absence of respiratory arrhythmia, a possible symptom of cardiac autonomic neuropathy in diabetes mellitus. Diabetologia, *12*:390, 1976.

Foley, J. O., and Dubois, F. S.: Quantitative studies of the vagus nerve in the cat. I. The ratio of sensory to motor fibers. J. Comp. Neurol., *67*:49, 1937.

Frank, H. J., Frewin, D. B., Robinson, S. M., and Wise, P. H.:Cardiovascular responses in diabetic dysautonomia. Aust. N.Z. J. Med., *2*:1, 1972.

Fraser, D. M., Campbell, I. W., Ewing, D. J., Murray, A., Neilson, J. M. M., and Clarke, B. F.: Peripheral and autonomic nerve function in newly diagnosed diabetes mellitus. Diabetes, *26*:546, 1977.

Fullerton, P. M., and Barnes, J. M.: Peripheral neuropathy in rats produced by acrylamide. Br. J. Ind. Med., *25*:210, 1966.

Gabella, G.: Structure of the Autonomic Nervous System. New York, John Wiley and Sons, 1976.

Gasser, H. S., and Erlanger, J.: The role played by the constituent fibers of a nerve trunk in determining the form of its action potential wave. Am. J. Physiol., *80*:522, 1927.

Gerard, M. W., and Billingsley, P. R.: The innervation of the carotid body. Anat. Res., *25*:391, 1923.

Gilliatt, R. W.: Vasoconstriction in the finger after deep inspiration. J. Physiol. (Lond.), *107*:70, 1948.

Gilliatt, R. W., Guttmann, L., and Whitteridge, D.: Inspiratory vasoconstriction in patients after spinal injuries. J. Physiol. (Lond.), *107*:67, 1948.

Goedert, M., and Buhler, F. R.: Nerve growth factor antibodies in idiopathic orthostatic hypotension. N. Engl. J. Med., *297*:336, 1977.

Gorlin, R., Knowles, J. H., and Storey, C. F.: The Valsalva maneuver as a test of cardiac function. Pathological physiology and clinical significance. Am. J. Med., *22*:197, 1957.

Gravellese, M. A., and Victor, M.: Circulatory studies in Wernicke's encephalopathy. Circ. Res., *15*:836, 1957.

Gribbin, B., Pickering, J. G., Sleight, P., and Peto, R.: Effect of age and high blood pressure on baroreflex sensitivity in man. Circ. Res., *29*:424, 1971.

Gundersen, H. J. G., and Neubauer, B.: A long-term diabetic autonomic nervous abnormality. Reduced variation in resting heart rate measured by a simple and sensitive method. Diabetologia, *13*:137, 1977.

Guttmann, L.: Topographic studies of disturbances of sweat secretion after complete lesion of peripheral nerves. J. Neurol. Psychiatry, *3*:197, 1940.

Guttmann, L.: A demonstration of the study of sweat secretion by the quinizarin method. Proc. R. Soc. Med., *35*:77, 1941.

Guttmann, L., and Whitteridge, D.: Effects of bladder distention on autonomic mechanism after spinal cord injuries. Brain,
70:361, 1947.

Haeusler, G.: Short- and long-term effects of 6-
hydroxydopamine on peripheral organs. In Malmfors, T., and
Thoenen, H. (eds.): 6-Hydroxydopamine and Catecholamine
Neurons. North Holland, Amsterdam, 1971.

Hagbarth, K. E., Hallin, R. G., Hongell, A., Torebjork, H. E., and
Wallin, B. G.: General Characteristics of sympathetic activity in
human skin nerves. Acta Physiol. Scand., 84:164, 1972.

Hagbarth, K. E., and Vallbo, A. B.: Pulse and respiratory
grouping of sympathetic nerve impulses in human muscle
nerves. Acta Physiol. Scand., 74:96, 1968.

Hallin, R. G., and Torebjork, H. E.: Single unit sympathetic
activity in human skin nerves during rest and various manoeuvres. Acta Physiol. Scand., 92:303, 1974.

Hancock, B. W., and Naysmith, A.: Vincristine-induced autonomic neuropathy. Br. Med. J., 3:207, 1975.

Haymaker, W., and Kernohan, J. W.: The Landry-Guillain-Barré
syndrome. Medicine (Baltimore), 28:59, 1949.

Hoffman, H. H., and Schnitzlein, H. N.: The number of nerve
fibers in the vagus nerve of man. Anat. Rec., 139:429, 1961.

Holman, M. E., and McLean, A.: The innervation of sheep
mesenteric veins. J. Physiol. (Lond.), 190:55, 1967.

Hopkins, A. P.: The effects of acrylamide on the peripheral
nervous system of the baboon. J. Neurol. Neurosurg. Psychiatry. 33:805, 1970.

Hopkins, A. P., and Gilliatt, R. W.: Motor and sensory conduction velocity in the baboon. Normal values and changes during acrylamide neuropathy. J. Neurol. Neurosurg. Psychiatry,
34:415, 1971.

Hopkins, A. P., and Lambert, E. H.: Conduction in unmyelinated fibres in experimental neuropathy. J. Neurol. Neurosurg.
Psychiatry, 35:163, 1972.

Ivy, H. K.: Renal sodium loss and bronchogenic carcinoma.
Associated autonomic neuropathy. Arch. Intern. Med., 108:47,
1961.

Jamieson, G. G., Ludbrook, J., and Wilson, A.: The response
of hand blood flow to distant ice application. Aust. J. Exp.
Biol. Med. Sci., 49:145, 1971.

Jammes, J. L.: The autonomic nervous system in peroneal
muscular atrophy. Arch. Neurol., 27:213, 1972.

Johnson, J. M., Rowell, L. B., Niederberg, M., and Eisman, M.
M.: Human splanchnic and forearm vasoconstrictor responses
to reduction of right atrial and aortic pressures. Circ. Res.,
34:515, 1974.

Johnson, R. H., Lee, G. de J., Oppenheimer, D. R., and Spalding, J. M. K.: Autonomic failure with orthostatic hypotension
due to intermediolateral column degeneration. A report of two
cases with autopsies. Q. J. Med., 35:276, 1966.

Johnson, R. H., McLellan, D. L., and Love, D. R.: Orthostatic
hypotension and the Holmes-Adie syndrome: A study of two
patients with afferent baroreceptor block. J. Neurol. Neurosurg. Psychiatry, 34:562, 1971.

Johnson, R. H., Smith, A. C., and Spalding, J. M. K.: Blood pressure response to standing and to Valsalva's manoeuvre: Independence of the two mechanisms in neurological diseases including cervical cord lesions. Clin. Sci., 36:77, 1969.

Johnson, R. H., and Spalding, J. M. K.: Disorders of the Autonomic Nervous System. Oxford, Blackwell, 1974.

Kendrick, E., Oberg, B., and Wennergren, G.: Extent of engagement of various cardiovascular effectors to alterations of carotid sinus pressure. Acta Physiol. Scand., 86:410, 1972a.

Kendrick, E., Oberg, B., and Wennergren, G.: Vasoconstrictor fibre discharge to skeletal muscle, kidney, intestine and skin at varying levels of arterial baroreceptor activity in the cat. Acta Physiol Scand., 85:464, 1972b.

Kerr, J. H., Corbett, J. L., Prys-Roberts, C., Smith, A. C., and Spalding, J. M. K.: Involvement of the sympathetic nervous system in tetanus. Studies on 82 cases. Lancet, 2:236, 1968.

Kersh, E. S., Kornfield, S. J., Unger, A., Popper, R. W., Cantor, S., and Cohn, K.: Autonomic insufficiency in uremia as a cause of hemodialysis-induced hypotension. N. Engl. J. Med., 290:650, 1974.

Kerslake, D. M.: Factors concerned in the regulation of sweat production in man. J. Physiol. (Lond.), 127:280, 1955.

Kerslake, D. M., and Cooper, K. E.: Vasodilatation in the hand in response to heating the skin elsewhere. Clin. Sci., 9:31, 1950.

Kirchheim, H. R.: Systemic arterial baroreceptor reflexes. Physiol. Rev., 56:100, 1976.

Klatsky, A. L., Friedman, G. D., Siegelaub, A. B., and Gerard, M. J.: Alcohol consumption and blood pressure. Kaiser-Permanente multiphasic health examination data. N. Engl. J. Med., 296:1194, 1977.

Kontos, H. A.: Orthostatic hypotension and nerve-growth factor. N. Engl. J. Med., 296:343, 1976.

Korner, P. I.: Integrative neural cardiovascular control. Physiol. Rev., 51:312, 1971.

Korner, P. I., Shaw, J., West, M. J., and Oliver, J. R.: Central nervous system control of baroreceptor reflexes in the rabbit. Circ. Res., 31:637, 1972.

Korner, P. I., West, M. J., Shaw, J., and Uther, J. B.: "Steady-state" properties of the baroreceptor heart rate reflex in essential hypertension in man. Clin. Exp. Pharmacol. Physiol., 1:65, 1974.

Kuntz, A.: The Autonomic Nervous System. Philadelphia, Lea and Febiger, 1953.

Kuru, M.: Nervous control of micturition. Physiol. Rev., 45:425, 1965.

Kyle, R. A., Kottke, B. A., and Schirger, A.: Orthostatic hypotension as a clue to primary systemic amyloidosis. Circulation, 34:883, 1966.

Laverty, R., Sharman, D. F., and Vogt, M.: Action of 2,4,5-trihydroxyphenylethylamine on the storage and release of noradrenaline. Br. J. Pharmacol., 24:549, 1965.

Leswing, R. J., and Ribelin, W. E.: Physiologic and pathologic changes in acrylamide neuropathy. Arch. Environ. Health, 18:22, 1969.

477

Levi-Montalcini, R.: Nerve growth factor in familial dysautonomia. N. Engl. J. Med., *295*:671, 1976.

Levi-Montalcini, R., and Angeletti, P. U.: Immmunosympathectomy. Pharmacol. Rev., *18*:619, 1966.

Levi-Montalcini, R., and Angeletti, P. U.: Nerve growth factor. Physiol. Rev., *48*:534, 1968.

Levi-Montalcini, R., and Booker, B.: Destruction of the sympathetic ganglia in mammals by an antiserum to a nerve-growth protein. Proc. Natl. Acad. Sci. U.S.A., *46*:384, 1960.

Levin, A. B.: A simple test of cardiac function based upon the heart rate changes induced by the Valsalva maneuver. Am. J. Cardiol., *18*:90, 1966.

Li, C. L., Mathews, G., and Bak, A. F.: Action potential of somatic and autonomic nerves. Exp. Neurol., *56*:527, 1977.

List, C. F., and Peet, M. M.: Sweat secretion in man. II. Anatomic distribution of disturbance in sweating associated with lesions of the sympathetic nervous system. Arch. Neurol. Psychiatry, *40*:27–43, 1938.

Lloyd-Mostyn, R. G., and Watkins, P. J.: Defective innervation of heart in diabetic autonomic neuropathy. Br. Med. J., *3*:15, 1975.

Lloyd-Mostyn, R. H., and Watkins, P. J.: Total cardiac denervation in diabetic autonomic neuropathy. Diabetes, *25*:748, 1976.

Loggie, L. M. H., and Van Maanen, E. F.: The autonomic nervous system and some aspects of the use of autonomic drugs in children. J. Pediatr., *81*:205, 1972.

Low, P. A., and Dyck, P. J.: Splanchnic preganglionic neurons in man. II. Morphometry of myelinated fibers of T7 ventral spinal root. Acta Neuropathol. (Berl.), *40*:219, 1977.

Low, P. A., McLeod, J. G., and Prineas, J. W.: Hypertrophic Charcot-Marie-Tooth disease. Light and electron microscope studies of the sural nerve. J. Neurol. Sci., *35*:93, 1978.

Low, P. A., Okazaki, H., and Dyck, P. J.: The splanchnic preganglionic outflow in man. I. Morphometry of preganglionic neurons. Acta. Neuropathol. (Berl.), *40*:55, 1977.

Low, P. A., Walsh, J. C., Huang, C. Y., and McLeod, J. G.: The sympathetic nervous system in diabetic neuropathy. A clinical and pathological study. Brain, *98*:341, 1975*a*.

Low, P. A., Walsh, J. C., Huang, C. Y., and McLeod, J. G.: The sympathetic nervous system in alcoholic neuropathy. A clinical and pathological study. Brain, *98*:357, 1975*b*.

Ludbrook, J., Mancia, G., Ferrari, A., and Zanchetti, A.: The variable pressure neck chamber method for studying the carotid baroreflex in man. Clin. Sci. Mol. Med., *53*:165, 1977.

Ludbrook, J., and Vincent, A. H.: The effects of mental arithmetic on hand blood flow. Aust. J. Exp. Biol. Med. Sci., *52*:679, 1974.

Ludbrook, J., Vincent, A., and Walsh. J. A.: Effects of mental arithmetic on arterial pressure and hand blood flow. Clin. Exp. Pharmacol. Physiol. (Suppl.), *2*:67, 1975.

MacMillan, A. L., and Spalding, J. M. K.: Human sweating response to electrophoresed acetylcholine: A test of postganglionic sympathetic function. J. Neurol. Neurosurg. Psychiatry, *32*:155, 1969.

Malins, J. M., and French, J. J.: Diabetic diarrhoea. Q. J. Med. 26:467, 1957.

Marshall, J.: The Landry-Guillain-Barré syndrome. Brain, 86:55, 1963.

Martin, J. B., Travis, R. H., and Van den Noort, S.: Centrally mediated orthostatic hypotension. Arch. Neurol., 19:163, 1968.

Martin, M. M.: Involvement of autonomic nerve fibres in diabetic neuropathy. Lancet, 1:560, 1953.

Matsuyama, H., and Haymaker, W.: Distribution of lesions in the Landry-Guillain-Barré syndrome, with emphasis on involvement of the sympathetic system. Acta. Neuropathol. (Berl.), 8:230, 1967.

McLeod, J. G.: The representation of the splanchnic afferent pathways in the thalamus of the cat. J. Physiol. (Lond.), 140:462, 1958.

McLeod, J. G.: The physiology of visceral sensation and referred pain. Aust. N.Z. J. Surg., 30:298, 1961.

McLeod, J. G., and Penny, R.: Vincristine neuropathy — an electrophysiological and histological study. J. Neurol. Neurosurg. Psychiatry, 32:297, 1969.

Mitchell, G. A. G.: Anatomy of the Autonomic Nervous System. London, Livingstone, 1953.

Mobley, W. C., Server, A. C., Ishii, D. N., Ropelle, R. J., and Shooter, E. M.: Nerve growth factor. N. Engl. J. Med., 297:1096, 1149, 1977.

Moorhouse, J. A., Carter, S. A., and Doupe, J.: Vascular responses in diabetic peripheral neuropathy. Br. Med. J., 1:883, 1966.

Neubauer, B., and Gundersen, H. J.: Early and progressive loss of autonomic control of the heart in diabetics measured on a standard resting ECG. Diabetologia, 12:412, 1976.

Ninomiya, I., and Irisawa, H.: Non-uniformity of the sympathetic nerve activity in response to baroreceptor inputs. Brain Res., 87:313, 1975.

Ninomiya, I., Nisimaru, N., and Irisawa, H.: Sympathetic nerve activity to the spleen, kidney and heart in response to baroreceptor input. Am. J. Physiol., 221:1346, 1971.

Njå, A., and Purves, D.: Specific innervation of guinea pig superior cervical ganglion cells by preganglionic fibres from different levels of the splanchnic cord. J. Physiol. (Lond.), 264:565, 1977.

Nordborg, G., Kristensson, K., Olsson, Y., and Sourander, P.: Involvement of the autonomic nervous system in primary and secondary amyloidosis. Acta Neurol. Scand., 49:31, 1973.

Novak, D. J., and Victor, M.: The vagus and sympathetic nerves in alcoholic polyneuropathy. Arch. Neurol., 30:273, 1974.

Nyberg-Hansen, R.: Innervation and nervous control of the urinary bladder. Acta Neurol. Scand. [Suppl. 20], 42:7, 1966.

Oberg, B.: Overall cardiovascular regulation. Annu. Rev. Physiol., 38:537, 1976.

Odel, H. M., Roth, G. M., and Keating, F. R., Jr.: Autonomic neuropathy simulating the effects of sympathectomy as a complication of diabetes mellitus. Diabetes, 4:92, 1955.

Okada, F., Yamashita, I., and Suwa, N.: Two cases of acute pandysautonomia. Arch. Neurol., *32*:146, 1975.

Page, E. B., Hickam, J. B., Sieker, H. O., McIntosh, H. D., and Pryor, W. W.: Reflex venomotor activity in normal persons and in patients with postural hypotension. Circulation, *11*:262, 1955.

Paintal, A. S.: Conduction in mammalian nerve fibres. *In* Desmedt, J. E. (ed.): New Developments in Electromyography and Clinical Neurophysiology, Vol. 2. Basel, S. Karger, 1973*a*, p. 19.

Paintal, A. S.: Vagal sensory receptors and their reflex effects. Physiol. Rev., *53*:159, 1973*b*.

Park, D. M., Johnson, R. H., Crean, G. P., and Robinson, J. F.: Orthostatic hypotension in bronchial carcinoma. Br. Med. J., *3*:510, 1972.

Pearson, J., Budzilovich, G., and Finegold, M. J.: Sensory, motor and autonomic dysfunction. The nervous system in familial dysautonomia. Neurology (Minneap.), *21*:486, 1971.

Pearson, J., Dancis, J., Axelrod, F., and Grover, N.: The sural nerve in familial dysautonomia. J. Neuropathol. Exp. Neurol., *34*:413, 1975.

Pick, J.: The Autonomic Nervous System. J. B. Lippincott, Philadelphia, 1970.

Pick, J. O., and Sheehan, D.: Sympathetic rami in man. J. Anat., *80*:12, 1946.

Pickering, G. W.: The vasomotor regulation of heat loss from the skin in relation to external temperature. Heart, *16*:115, 1932.

Pickering, G. W., Sleight, P., and Smyth, H. S.: The reflex regulation of arterial blood pressure during sleep in man. J. Physiol. (Lond.) *194*:46P, 1967.

Pickering, T. G., Gribbin, B., and Oliver, D. O.: Baroreflex sensitivity in patients on long-term haemodialysis. Clin. Sci., *43*:645, 1972*a*.

Pickering, T. G., Gribbin, B., Petersen, E. S., Cunningham, D. J. C., and Sleight, P.: Effects of autonomic blockade on the baroreflex in man at rest and during exercise. Circ. Res., *30*:177, 1972*b*.

Pickering, T. G., Gribbin, B., and Sleight, P.: Comparison of the reflex heart rate response to rising and falling arterial pressure in man. Cardiovasc. Res., *6*:277, 1972*c*.

Plum, F.: Bladder dysfunction. *In* Williams, D. (ed.): Modern Trends in Neurology, Vol. 3. London, Butterworth, 1962, p. 151.

Pool, J. L.: Unilateral thoracic hyperhidrosis caused by osteoma of the tenth dorsal vertebra: Case report. J. Neurosurg., *13*:111, 1956.

Post, E. J.: Experimental autonomic neuropathy. Ph.D. Thesis, University of Sydney, 1976.

Post, E. J.: Unmyelinated nerve fibres in feline acrylamide neuropathy. Acta Neuropathol. (Berl.), *42*:19, 1978.

Post, E. J., and McLeod, J. G.: Experimental autonomic neuropathy. Proc. Aust. Assoc. Neurol., *10*:109, 1973.

Post, E. J., and McLeod, J. G.: Acrylamide autonomic neuropathy in the cat. Part 1. Neurophysiological and histological studies. J. Neurol. Sci., *33*:353, 1977*a*.

Post, E. J., and McLeod, J. G.: Acrylamide autonomic neuropathy in the cat. Part II. Effects on mesenteric vascular control. J. Neurol. Sci., *33*:375, 1977*b*.

Post, E. J., and McLeod, J. G.: The baroreceptor heart rate reflex in acrylamide-poisoned cats. Proc. Aust. Physiol. Pharmacol. Soc., *5*:198, 1977*c*.

Prineas, J. W.: The pathogenesis of dying-back polyneuopathies. Part 2. (An ultrastructural study of experimental acrylamide intoxication.) J. Neuropathol. Exp. Neurol., *28*:598, 1969.

Randall, W. C., Alexander, W. F., Coldwater, K. P., Hertzman, A. B., and Cox, J. W.: Sweating patterns in the lower extremity of man elicited by stimulation of the sympathetic trunk. Fed. Proc., *11*:127, 1952.

Ranson, S. W., and Billingsley, P.: The truncus sympatheticus, rami communicantes, and splanchnic nerves in the cat. J. Comp. Neurol., *29*:405, 1918*a*.

Ranson, S. W., and Billingsley, P. R.: An experimental analysis of the sympathetic trunk and greater splanchnic nerve in the cat. J. Comp. Neurol., *29*:441, 1918*b*.

Ratcliffe, A. H., and Jepson, R. P.: Skin resistance changes in the lower limb after lumbar ganglionectomy. J. Neurosurg., *7*:97, 1950.

Richter, C. P.: Instructions for using the cutaneous resistance recorder or dermometer on peripheral nerve injuries and sympathectomies and paravertebral blocks. J. Neurosurg., *3*:181, 1946.

Richter, C. P., and Otenasek, F. J.: Thoracolumbar sympathectomies examined with the electrical skin resistance method. J. Neurosurg., *3*:120, 1946.

Ridley, A., Hierons, R., and Cavanagh, J. B.: Tachycardia and the neuropathy of porphyria. Lancet, *2*:708, 1968.

Robinson, B. F., Epstein, S. E., Beiser, G. D., and Braunwald, E.: Control of heart rate by the autonomic nervous system. Studies in man on the interrelationship between baroreceptor mechanisms and exercise. Circ. Res., *19*:400, 1966.

Roddie, I. C., Shepherd, J. T., and Whelan, R. F.: The vasomotor nerve supply to the skin and muscle of the human forearm. Clin. Sci., *16*:67, 1957.

Rowell, L. B., Detry, J. M., Blackman, J. R., and Wyss, C.: Importance of the splanchnic vascular bed in human blood pressure regulation. J. Appl. Physiol., *32*:213, 1972.

Rundles, R. W.: Diabetic neuropathy. General review with report of 125 cases. Medicine (Baltimore), *24*:111, 1945.

Samueloff, S. L., Browse, N. L., and Shepherd, J. G.: Response of capacity vessels in human limbs to head-up tilt and suction on lower body. J. Appl. Physiol., *21*:47, 1966.

Sarnoff, S. J., Hardenbergh, E., and Whittenberger, J. L.: Mechanism of the arterial response to the Valsalva test. The basis for its use as an indicator of the intactness of the sympathetic outflow. Am. J. Physiol., *154*:316, 1948.

Schaumburg, H. H., Wisniewski, H., and Spencer, P. S.: Ultrastructural studies of the dying-back process. Part I (peripheral nerve terminal and axon degeneration in systemic acrylamide intoxication). J. Neuropathol. Exp. Neurol., *33*:260, 1974.

Schirger, A., Martin, W. J., Goldstein, N. P., and Huezenga, K. A.: Orthostatic hypotension in association with acute exacerbations of porphyria. Mayo Clin. Proc., 37:7, 1962.

Schnitzlein, H. N., Rowe, L. C., and Hoffman, H. H.: The myelinated component of the vagus nerves in man. Anat. Rec., 131:649, 1958.

Sharpey-Schafer, E. P.: Effects of coughing on intrathoracic pressure. arterial pressure, and peripheral blood flow. J. Physiol. (Lond.), 122:351, 1953.

Sharpey-Schafer, E. P.: Effects of Valsalva's manoeuvre on the normal and failing circulation. Br. Med. J., 1:693, 1955.

Sharpey-Schafer, E. P.: Circulatory reflexes in chronic disease of the afferent nervous system. J. Physiol. (Lond.), 134:1, 1956.

Sharpey-Schafer, E. P., and Taylor, D. J.: Absent circulatory reflexes in diabetic neuritis. Lancet, 1:559, 1960.

Shinebourne, E., Sneddon, J. M., and Turner, P.: Evidence for autonomic denervation in familial dysautonomia, the Riley-Day syndrome. Br. Med. J., 4:91, 1967.

Siemsen, J. K., and Meister, L.: Bronchogenic carcinoma associated with severe orthostatic hypotension. Ann. Intern. Med., 58:669, 1963.

Siggers, D. C., Rogers, J. G., Boyer, S. H., Margolet, L., Dorkin, H., Banerjee, S. P., and Shooter, E. M.: Increased nerve growth factor β-chain cross-reacting material in familial dysautonomia. N. Engl. J. Med., 295:629, 1976.

Sjostrand, R.: The significance of the pulmonary blood volume in the regulation of the blood circulation under normal and pathological conditions. Acta Med. Scand., 145:155, 1953.

Smith, A. A., and Dancis, J.: Exaggerated response to infused norepinephrine in familial dysautonomia. N. Engl. J. Med., 270:704, 1964.

Smith, B.: Neuropathy of the oesophagus in diabetes mellitus. J. Neurol. Neurosurg. Psychiatry, 37:1151, 1974.

Smyth, H. S., Sleight, P., and Pickering, G. W.: The reflex regulation of arterial pressure during sleep in man: A quantitative method of assessing baroreflex sensitivity. Circ. Res., 24:109, 1969.

Stone, D. J., Lyon, A. F., and Tierstein, A. S.: A reappraisal of the circulatory effects of the Valsalva maneuver. Am. J. Med., 34:923, 1965.

Szurszewski, J. H., and Weems, W. A.: A study of peripheral input to and its control by post-ganglionic neurones of the inferior mesenteric ganglion. J. Physiol. (Lond.), 256:541, 1976.

Takahashi, K.: A clinicopathological study of the peripheral nervous system in the aged. Geriatrics, 21:123, 1966.

Telford, E. D.: Cervical rib and hyperhidrosis. Br. Med. J., 2:96, 1942.

Thomas, J. P., and Shields, R.: Associated autonomic dysfunction and carcinoma of the pancreas. Br. Med. J., 4:32, 1970.

Thorén, P., Saum, W. R., and Brown, A. R.: Characteristics of rat aortic baroreceptors with non-medullated afferent nerve fibers. Circ. Res., 40:231, 1977.

AUTONOMIC NERVOUS SYSTEM

Tomashefsky, A. J., Horwitz, S. J., and Feingold, M. H.: Acute autonomic neuropathy. Neurology (Minneap.), *22*:251, 1972.

Tranzer, J. P., and Thoenen, H.: An electron microscopic study of selective, acute degeneration of sympathetic nerve terminals after administration of 6-hydroxydopamine. Experientia, *24*:155, 1968.

Tuck, R. R.: Autonomic neuropathy in experimental allergic neuritis. Clin. Exp. Neurol., *15*:197, 1978.

Varma, S., Johnsen, S. D., Sherman, D. E., and Youmans, W. W.: Mechanisms of inhibition of heart rate by phenylephrine. Circ. Res. *8*:1182, 1960.

Vela, A. R., and Balart, L. A.: Esophageal motor manifestations in diabetes mellitus. Am. J. Surg., *119*:21, 1970.

Victor, M., Adams, R. D., and Collins, G. H.: The Wernicke-Korsakoff Syndrome. Philadelphia, F. A. Davis, 1971.

Wallin, B. G., Sundlof, G., and Delius, W.: The effect of carotid sinus nerve stimulation on muscle and skin nerve sympathetic activity in man. Pfluegers Arch., *358*:101, 1975.

Walsh, J. C.: The peripheral nervous system in lymphoma and multiple myeloma. M.D. Thesis, University of Sydney, 1971.

Walsh, J. C., Low, P. A., and Allsop, J. L.: Localised sympathetic overactivity: An uncommon complication of lung cancer. J. Neurol. Neurosurg. Psychiatry, *39*:93, 1976.

Watkins, P. J.: Facial sweating after food: A new sign of diabetic autonomic neuropathy. Br. Med. J., *1*:583, 1973.

Watson, W. E.: Some circulatory response to Valsalva's manoeuvre in patients with polyneuritis and spinal cord disease. J. Neurol. Neurosurg. Psychiatry, *25*:19, 1962.

Whalen, G. E., Soergel, K. H., and Geenen, J. E.: Diabetic diarrhea. A clinical and pathophysiological study. Gastroenterology, *56*:1021, 1969.

Wheeler, T., and Watkins, P. J.: Cardiac denervation in diabetes. Br. Med. J., *2*:584, 1973.

White, J. C., and Smithwick, R. H.: The Autonomic Nervous System. Anatomy, Physiology and Surgical Application, 2nd ed. London. McMillan, 1944.

Widen, L.: Cerebellar representation of high threshold afferents in the splanchnic nerve. Acta Physiol. Scand [Suppl. 117], *33*:1, 1955.

Wilkins, R. W., Culbertson, J. W., and Ingelfinger, F. J.: The effect of splanchnic sympathectomy in hypertensive patients upon estimated hepatic blood flow in the upright as contrasted with the horizontal posture. J. Clin. Invest., *30*:312, 1951.

Yahr, M., and Frontera, A. T.: Acute autonomic neuropathy. Its occurrence in infectious mononucleosis. Arch. Neurol., *32*:132, 1975.

Young, R. R., Asbury, A. K., Corbett, J. L., and Adams, R. D.: Pure pan-dysautonomia with recovery. Description and discussion of diagnostic criteria. Brain. *98*:613, 1975.

Zaimis, E., Berk, L., and Callingham, B. A.: Biochemical and functional changes in the sympathetic nervous system of rats treated with nerve growth factor antiserum. Nature, *206*:1220, 1965.

483

The Clinical View of Neuromuscular Electrophysiology

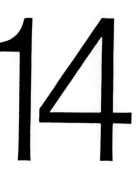

14

Arthur K. Asbury

INTRODUCTION   This volume brings together the experimental observations and investigations by which the pathophysiology of peripheral nervous system disorders may be understood. Put in another way, it describes the conceptual skeleton upon which the flesh of clinical electrodiagnosis is laid. The emphasis here is upon neurophysiological investigation of laboratory animals, both normals and those with experimental analogs of human neuromuscular disorders.

Research strategies employed in investigations described in the preceding chapters are of two quite different types. The first is a basic laboratory approach in which the normal neuromuscular system in animals has been studied by neurophysiological and biophysical techniques. Such studies have been stimulated by, and are extensions of, previous research in normal animals. As information has grown concerning normal electrophysiology in experimental animals, confirmation that similar mechanisms are at play in the human neuromuscular system has been made only secondarily, as chance would permit. An example of the clinical application of this first type of basic neurophysiology is the recent development of microneurography in which single unit responses may be recorded from intact human nerves by percutaneous insertion of tungsten microelectrodes (Hagbarth, and Vallbo, 1969). The second strategy involves investigation of experimental animals in which a disorder mimicking a given human disorder has been induced. In this situation, questions raised by initial observations of human diseases have been studied to better advantage in the appropriate animal model. It then has been possible to extrapolate back to the human condition any new insight or information derived from its experimental counterpart. A classic example of this approach was the electrophysiological investigation in experimental animals of allergic neuritis, diptheria toxin poisoning, thallium intoxication, and Wallerian degeneration carried out by Kaeser and Lambert (1962)

484

Although these two research approaches differ, they complement one another in a highly effective fashion. The outcome has been to enlarge extraordinarily our knowledge of the phenomena encountered in human neuropathies, and to provide a substantial infrastructure upon which clinical electrodiagnosis rests.

DEVELOPMENT OF CLINICAL ELECTRO-DIAGNOSIS

In recent years the key to evaluating nerve and muscle disorders is the patient history and neurological assessment coupled with its extension to the clinical laboratory, specifically the electrodiagnostic examination. It cannot be emphasized too strongly that electrodiagnostic evaluation is a physician-directed extension of the physical examination, and not merely a laboratory test. Neurological physicians have become heavily dependent upon the information extractable from skilled and well directed diagnostic electromyography. The term electromyography, as used here, is meant in the broadest sense to include the evaluation of motor and sensory nerve function, neuromuscular junction, and sensory endings (by inference), as well as voluntary muscle. This remarkable dependence upon clinical electrodiagnosis has not always existed; rather, the shift toward reliance on EMG has evolved rapidly over the past 15 or 20 years.

Many factors have converged to bring diagnostic electromyography to its present state of development and role of importance. First, in the postwar era, the early observations of Gasser and Erlanger were rapidly expanded upon by a host of pioneer investigators, including Buchthal, Lambert, Gilliatt, McDonald, Sears, and many others, and were brought to bear upon clinical problems. Second, new and associated areas of neurobiological interest appeared, including axoplasmic transport and the biophysical study of excitable membranes. Third, striking technical innovations occurred in quick succession in the equipment available to carry out diagnostic electromyography. Fourth, a concurrent surge of interest in neuromuscular disorders using other approaches took place, primarily the use of morphological methods to study peripheral nerve diseases and the use of both morphological and biochemical methods to study muscle diseases. In addition, investigation of peripheral neuropathies has been marked in recent years by many efforts to correlate morphological appearances with their associated electrophysiological features, a point which will be dealt with below in greater detail.

One effect of all these converging factors has been the emergence of an evergrowing cadre of seasoned clinical electrodiagnosticians, knowledgeable in the tenets of basic neurophysiology, familiar with the anatomy of the peripheral nervous system, versed in the clinical features of neuromuscular diseases, and experienced in the pitfalls and artifacts of diagnostic electromyography. All

485

these qualities are requisite for an electromyographer to be worthy of the name, although it is to be admitted that there are many who practice this technique who are less than so qualified. Perhaps it is to the electromyographer, and those who aspire to become one, that the preceding chapters will be of most use, although many others should also find them of interest.

USES OF CLINICAL ELECTRO-DIAGNOSIS

As has been alluded to previously, the purpose here is to illuminate the physiological basis for neuromuscular disorders, and not to produce yet another how-to-do-it primer on the technique of electromyography. Nevertheless, it is worth reviewing the current uses of clinical electromyography in order to provide a context for the preceding chapters. What kinds of clinical questions may be satisfactorily answered electrodiagnostically? How specific is the information derived, particularly in terms of establishing discrete diagnosis?

The following listing of the uses of clinical electrodiagnosis is probably incomplete, but indicates many of the important types of information adducible by the technique.

1. The distinction between disorders primary either to nerve or to muscle.
2. The distinction between upper and lower motor neuron weakness.
3. The distinction between root involvement and more distal nerve trunk involvement.
4. The distinction between generalized polyneuropathic processes and widespread multifocal nerve trunk affection.
5. The distinction, given a generalized polyneuropathic process, between a primary demyelinative neuropathy and axonal degeneration.
6. The assessment, in both primary and demyelinative neuropathies, of many factors bearing on the nature, activity, and likely prognosis of the neuropathy.
7. The assessment, in mononeuropathies, of the site of the lesion and its major effect on nerve fibers, especially the distinction between conduction block (neuropraxia) and Wallerian degeneration (axonotmesis).
8. The characterization of disorders of the neuromuscular junction.
9. The identification, often in muscle of normal bulk and strength, of chronic partial denervation, fasciculations, and myotonia.
10. The analysis of cramp, and its distinction from physiological contracture.

It may be noted from the above list that the electromyographer can usually identify processes and generic groups of disorders, and not specific diseases. For instance, in a given case of polyneuropathy, it may be learned through electrodiagnosis that the disorder is an axonal degeneration, that denervative activity is ongoing, and that a certain amount of reinnervation has occurred. Helpful as these observations might be, they say nothing of the likely basis for the neuropathy. Primary axonal polyneuropathies are usually dysmetabolic or toxic in origin, and the specific neurotoxins and metabolic states are legion. Electrodiagnosis can rarely lead us to the correct one. In other neuromuscular disorders, the combined clinical and electrophysiological features add up to specific diagnoses, particularly in neuromuscular junction diseases such as myasthenia gravis, botulism, and Eaton-Lambert syndrome. The same is true of the myotonias and a number of the demyelinative neuropathies. In addition to these general observations, more can be said of each of the ten items in this list.

NERVE VERSUS MUSCLE DISORDERS Although there are both theoretical and practical problems in making the distinction between neuropathic and myopathic disorders, it is a useful clinical separation, and it is possible to make a satisfactory one in more than 90 per cent of cases. This overall statement is corroborated by the careful quantitative EMG and biopsy histochemical study of Black et al. (1974). When difficulty is encountered in distinguishing myopathy from a neurogenic disorder, it usually occurs in very chronically evolving motor neuron disorders or myopathies where the late EMG and histochemical studies of biopsied muscle may be confusing. In addition, the subjective and interpretational reporting of needle EMG observations has on occasion led to unnecessary errors, and also has given rise to considerable terminological controversy (Engel, 1973, 1975; Daube, 1978). If quantitative description of motor unit potentials and their behavior is given by the electromyographer prior to any attempt at interpretation, as has been strongly suggested by Daube (1978), it is likely that both the controversy and the errors will be effectively reduced.

UPPER VERSUS LOWER MOTOR NEURON WEAKNESS In the presence of pure upper motor neuron weakness, the only important electromyographic observation is reduction of interference pattern on voluntary contraction of muscle, while reflexly or electrically induced activity may be normal. Ordinarily the recognition of upper motor neuron-type weakness rests upon the correlation of the clinical examination and electrodiagnostic considerations. However, the presence of lower motor neuron findings which may not be evident by clinical examination, in conjunction with upper motor neuron findings in the same limb, raises other diagnostic considerations, particularly motor neuron disease. In addition, in the known coexistence of both

487

upper and lower motor findings in the same limb, the electromyographer often can make a useful assessment of the relative proportions to which each process is contributing to the overall degree of weakness. As an aside, psychogenic weakness may be distinguished from lower motor neuron weakness with certainty.

ROOT VERSUS NERVE TRUNK INVOLVEMENT

Nerve root lesions are usually partial. Therefore, considerable difficulty may be encountered using clinical features alone in determining whether one is dealing with one or more partial root lesions or one or more partial nerve trunk lesions placed more distally. In this situation, the distribution of denervative changes in key muscles, amplitude of sensory nerve action potentials, and presence or absence of paraspinous muscle denervative changes are all very helpful electrodiagnostic criteria by which this particular distinction can be made. In addition, lesions proximal to the dorsal root ganglion, such as in tabes dorsalis, are attended by normal peripheral sensory nerve action potentials, whereas lesions distal will manifest reduced or absent potentials.

POLYNEUROPATHY VERSUS MULTIFOCAL PROC-ESSES

Widespread multifocal involvement of peripheral nerve trunks may produce a clinical stocking glove pattern which resembles a polyneuropathy by neurological examination. The distinction may be made by nerve conduction studies if the patchy and variable pattern produced by multifocal processes is recognized. We have encountered two groups of subacute and chronic neuropathies which are marked by electrical multifocality: (1) those with evidence of multifocal demyelinative lesions, often with sites of persistent conduction block placed away from the usual loci of entrapment; and (2) those with evidence mainly of Wallerian degeneration in a multifocal pattern. These latter are usually ischemic in origin, as in cases of systemic vasculitis affecting vasa nervorum.

DEMYELINATION VERSUS AXONAL DEGENERA-TION

There are frequently only subtle clues on clinical examination which will allow the clinician to distinguish between a primary demyelinative versus a primary axonal polyneuropathy. The electrodiagnostic distinctions are much more clearcut. In axonal degenerations, only slight decreases in conduction velocities are found in those nerve trunks whose muscles of innervation are still excitable. More striking are the graded decreases in amplitude of nerve and muscle action potentials. In demyelinative polyneuropathies slowing of motor and sensory nerve conduction velocities is the hallmark, but there are many other helpful features in making this distinction. The presence and degree of conduction block, dispersion of both muscle and nerve action potentials, disproportionate prolongation of distal latencies, and slowing of F wave potentials are all features consistent with a demyelinative neuropathy. Correlation between electrodiagnostic findings and morphological assessment of sural nerve biopsies in the same patients is generally quite satisfying (McLeod et al., 1973). In polyneuropathies in which demyelination is admixed with degenerating fibers, the electrodiagnostic features of both processes will be evident. This finding, when present, is also of use to the clinician.

OTHER FACTORS IN POLYNEUROPATHY The electromyographer is not restricted simply to making a distinction between primary demyelinative and primary axonal neuropathies. Other types of observations may be made as well which bear upon the activity and outlook for the disorder. For instance, in a given axonal degeneration-type polyneuropathy, the electromyographer may make an estimate of the number of functional fibers remaining in a given nerve trunk, can often give some indication of the activity of the process, and may also be able to describe electrophysiological evidence of reinnervative phenomena. Likewise, in demyelinative neuropathies, prognosis can at times be guessed at, particularly several weeks into the illness, on the basis of the degree of coexisting Wallerian degeneration. This is particularly true in acute idiopathic polyneuritis (Guillain-Barré syndrome) as shown by Eisen and Humphreys (1974).

MONONEUROPATHIES Electrophysiological assessment of mononeuropathies is of the greatest use to the clinician in determining the site and severity of the lesion. Mononeuropathies are almost always due to local causes, usually compression or entrapment. Their basic nature is neuropractic but, if severe enough, extensive Wallerian degeneration may also take place secondarily. Such factors are obviously of importance in making management decisions.

NEUROMUSCULAR JUNCTION In cases of neuromuscular weakness in which neuromuscular junction disorders are suspected, electrodiagnostic study may illuminate the clinical problem in a highly satisfactory fashion. Characteristic patterns seen with repetitive nerve stimulation can be expected in myasthenia gravis, botulism, Eaton-Lambert syndrome, and aminoglycoside antibiotic intoxication. In fact, electrophysiological features are as central to the diagnosis and classification of disorders of neuromuscular transmission as are electroencephalographic patterns in the definition of the epilepsies. If a disorder of neuromuscular transmission is suspected clinically, it is impera-

489

tive that the clinician convey this suspicion to the electromyographer in order that the proper array and sequence of repetitive stimulation can be performed.

"NORMAL" MUSCLE Muscles which by clinical examination appear to be of normal bulk and strength may nevertheless betray the features of neuromuscular disorder upon electrophysiological examination. Such features include chronic partial denervation and other denervative phenomena, such as fasciculations. Myotonia may also be detected by electrical means, even when it is not elicitable by percussion techniques clincally, but this is in general the only myopathic process which is discoverable in normally strong muscle. Other myopathic affections are almost always associated with weakness of a given muscle.

CRAMP AND PHYSIOLOGICAL CONTRACTURE Although a discussion of the clinical syndromes manifesting cramp of striated muscle is beyond the scope of this review, it is worth pointing out that ordinary cramp exhibits a full interference pattern electrophysiologically, whereas physiological contracture, such as that associated with McArdle's syndrome, is attended by electrical silence. The latter observation indicates that muscular contraction coupling is taking place without excitation of muscle membrane.

SUMMARY This overview of the clinical uses of neuromuscular electrophysiology addresses itself purely to the service and diagnostic issues, and omits any mention of the numerous clinical investigative ways in which this technology may be employed. In the past, EMG has been used in a highly successful fashion to help define the basic mechanisms in asterixis, action myoclonus, postural mechanisms during sleep, and many other normal and abnormal neurophysiological phenomena.

References Black, J. T., Bhatt, G. P., DeJesus, P. V., Schotland, D. L., and Rowland, L. P.: Diagnostic accuracy of clinical data, quantitative electromyography and histochemistry in neuromuscular disease. A study of 105 cases. J. Neurol. Sci., 21:59, 1974.

Daube, J. R.: The description of motor unit potentials in electromyography. Neurology, 28:623, 1978.

Eisen, A., and Humphreys, P.: The Guillain-Barré syndrome. A clinical and electrodiagnostic study of 25 cases. Arch. Neurol., 30:438, 1974.

Engel, W. K.: "Myopathic EMG"; none-such animal. New Engl. J. Med., 289:485, 1973.

Engel, W. K.: Brief small abundant motor unit potentials: A further critique of electromyographic interpretation. Neurology, 25:173, 1975.

Hagbarth, K. E., and Vallbo, A. B.: Single unit recordings from muscle nerves in human subjects. Acta Physiol. Scand., 76:321, 1969.

Kaeser, H. E., and Lambert, E. H.: Nerve function studies in experimental polyneuritis. Electroencephalogr. Clin. Neurophysiol. (Suppl.) 22:29, 1962.

McLeod, J. G., Prineas, J. W., and Walsh, J. C.: The relationship of conduction velocity to pathology in peripheral nerves. A study of the sural nerve in 90 patients. In Desmedt, J. E. (ed.): New Developments in Electromyography and Clinical Neurophysiology, Vol. 2, Basel, S. Karger, p. 248. 1973.

INDEX

NOTE: Numbers in *italics* indicate illustrations; those followed by t indicate tables.

496